Canine and Feline Neurology

The What's Your Diagnosis? Series

What's Your Diagnosis? is an exciting new series of short books that combine problem-based learning, case studies, and questions and answers.

The books are entirely case-based, with theory, background, and analysis interwoven into each case. Questions are used to test the reader's knowledge in identifying signs, underlying differential diagnoses, diagnostic plans, and treatment options. Answers are then provided to guide the reader through the rationale for the choices made.

Other What's Your Diagnosis? Series Titles

Small Animal Ophthalmology: What's Your Diagnosis?
By Heidi Featherstone and Elaine Holt
978-1-405-15161-0

Canine Internal Medicine: What's Your Diagnosis?
By Jon Wray
978-1-118-91816-6

Small Animal Dermatology: What's Your Diagnosis?
By Jane Coatesworth
978-1-119-31111-9

Canine and Feline Neurology

What's Your Diagnosis?

Edited by

Simon R. Platt
Department of Veterinary Clinical Sciences, College of Veterinary Medicine, Oklahoma State University, Stillwater, OK, USA

Susan A. Arnold
Department of Veterinary Clinical Sciences, University of Minnesota, St. Paul, MN, USA

WILEY

Published by John Wiley & Sons, Inc., Hoboken, New Jersey.

Library of Congress Cataloging-in-Publication Data applied for:

Paperback ISBN: 9781119803126

Cover Design: Wiley
Cover Images: Dan Leon, Amanda Brenna, Susan A. Arnold

Set in 9.5/12pt STIXTwoText by Straive, Pondicherry, India

Printed in Singapore
M116586050826

I dedicate this book to all the teachers, residents, interns, and students I have had the privilege of interacting with and who have taught me more than any book I have read.

—Simon R. Platt

I dedicate this book to my husband, our two daughters, and Farley, my steadfast canine companion.

—Susan A. Arnold

Contents

List of Contributors

Juliet Armstrong
Blue Pearl Pet Hospital
Richmond
VA
USA

Susan A. Arnold
Department of Veterinary Clinical Sciences
University of Minnesota
St. Paul
MN
USA

Katherine Bibi
Blue Pearl Pet Hospital
Kirkland
WA
USA

Amanda Brenna
Puget Sound Veterinary Specialty and Emergency
Gig Harbor
WA
USA

Danielle Daw
MissionVet Specialty and Emergency
San Antonio
TX
USA

Sergio A. Gomes
Dovecote Veterinary Referrals
Derby
UK

Tom Jukier
Department of Clinical Sciences, College of Veterinary Medicine
Auburn University
Auburn
AL
USA

Vivian Lau
Sage Veterinary Centers
Redwood City
CA
USA

Edward MacKillop
BluePearl Pet Hospital
Pittsburgh
PA
USA

Talisha Moore
University of Tennessee
College of Veterinary Medicine
Department of Clinical Science
Knoxville
TN
USA

Jill Niederhuth
BluePearl
Des Moines
IA
USA

Rose K. Peters
Veterinary Clinical Neurology
University of Illinois at Urbana-Champaign
Champaign
IL
USA

Simon R. Platt
Department of Veterinary Clinical Sciences
College of Veterinary Medicine
Oklahoma State University
Stillwater
OK
USA

and

VetOracle Teleradiology, UK
Hallmarq Veterinary Imaging, UK
North American Veterinary Community (NAVC), USA

Koen Santifort
IVC Evidensia Small Animal Hospital Arnhem
Arnhem
The Netherlands

and

IVC Evidensia Small Animal Hospital Hart van Brabant
Waalwijk
The Netherlands

Georgina Stewart
Neurology Department
ARC – Animal Referral Centre
Auckland
New Zealand

Anna Tauro
Access Specialty Animal Hospital
Pasadena
CA
USA

Amanda R. Taylor
Southeast Veterinary Neurology
Miami
FL
USA

Joshua Warren
Head of Neurology and Neurosurgery
Triangle Veterinary Referral Hospital
Durham
NC
USA

Fred Wininger
The Animal Neurology Center
Saint Louis
MO
USA

Preface

Neurology often represents a formidable challenge in general veterinary practice. The perceived complexity of neuroanatomy, the challenge of precise lesion localization, and the rapid evolution of diagnostic and therapeutic options can make this discipline feel daunting for most veterinarians. Yet, neurological patients are a daily reality in our clinics. Our goal in creating this book is to bridge that gap – to transform neurology from a source of anxiety into a structured, approachable, and clinically empowering part of your practice.

This textbook was born from a simple observation: traditional neurology texts, while excellent for foundational knowledge, often do not mirror the dynamic, case-based way we think in the busy clinical setting. Practitioners do not encounter diseases in isolation; they encounter *patients* with specific *presentations* – the acutely paralyzed cat, the dog with a head tilt, the puppy with seizures.

To reflect this reality, we have embraced a fundamentally new format. This book is organized around the most common neurological presentations in dogs and cats. Each chapter dives deep into a single presentation, not just through text and images, but through the power of real-time observation. We have integrated multiple video-based case challenges for every topic. These videos are the heart of the book, allowing you to see the subtle gait abnormalities, the nystagmus, and the proprioceptive deficits – just as you would in your own examination room.

Each case follows a familiar and engaging "What's Your Diagnosis?" structure. After the initial presentation, you will be guided through a series of targeted questions:

1. **What is your lesion localization?** Reinforcing the critical, step-by-step neurological exam.
2. **What are your primary differential diagnoses?** Focusing on a pragmatic, evidence-based list for that specific scenario.
3. **What diagnostic pathway is most logical and feasible?** Balancing ideal-world neurology with real-world constraints of general practice.
4. **What are your initial management and treatment options?** Providing immediate, actionable steps.

This iterative, case-based approach is designed for active learning. We encourage you to engage with each case, formulate your own answers, and then compare them with our detailed discussions. The repetition across multiple cases for each presentation will build a robust, intuitive clinical pattern recognition that you can directly apply the next time a neurological patient walks through your door.

This project is the culmination of the dedication and expertise of a remarkable team of clinician authors who share a passion for teaching and for improving patient care at the primary care level.

We are also indebted to the many contributors who generously shared their clinical videos, making this innovative format possible.

Our hope is that this book will live not on a shelf, but on your desk or tablet – a trusted, practical resource that demystifies veterinary neurology and gives you the confidence to assess, diagnose, and manage these challenging cases with greater skill and clarity. We welcome you to this new way of learning and look forward to hearing how it impacts your practice.

Acknowledgments

Personally, I must offer my particular gratitude to my co-editor, Dr. Susan Arnold, now of the University of Minnesota College of Veterinary Medicine. What began as a mentor-resident relationship has flourished into a truly collaborative partnership. Her dynamic energy, unwavering enthusiasm, and brilliant clinical mind have been the driving force behind this ambitious project's success. Her inspiration is woven into every chapter —*Simon R. Platt*

I gratefully count myself among the many veterinary neurologists that Dr. Simon Platt has inspired. There are few mentors in my life who have had as great of a positive impact on my career as Dr. Platt. I aspire to deserve the praise he bestows upon me and to pass on all the valuable lessons he has instilled in me to the next generation of veterinary neurologists —*Susan A. Arnold*

About the Companion Website

This book includes access to a companion website at

www.wiley.com/go/platt/neurology

To access the website materials, click on the link under Related Resources on the book's page on wiley.com. You can also find this by searching www.wiley.com for the ISBN 9781119803126.

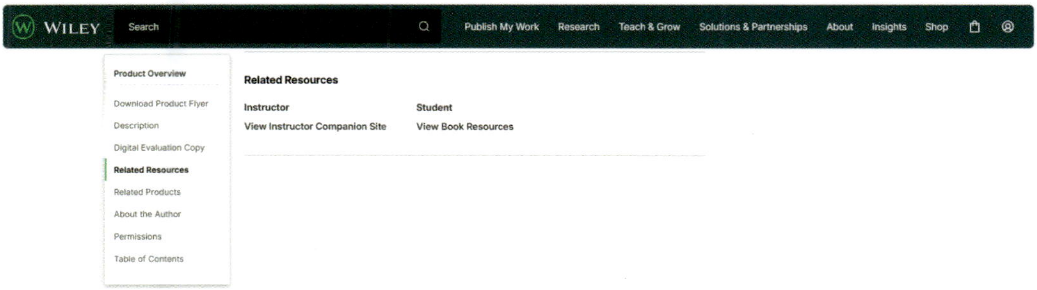

The companion website features video clips showing neurological conditions in motion, demonstrating gait abnormalities, seizures, and vestibular dysfunction.

How to Perform the Neurological Examination

CHAPTER 1

Simon R. Platt[1] and Susan A. Arnold[2]

[1] *Department of Veterinary Clinical Sciences, College of Veterinary Medicine, Oklahoma State University, Stillwater, OK, USA*

[2] *Department of Veterinary Clinical Sciences, University of Minnesota, St. Paul, MN, USA*

The main components of the neurological examination can be divided into an observation portion and a hands-on portion (Table 1.1). The results of the examination can be recorded in a standardized neurological examination form (Table 1.2). This form can be downloaded for use in your clinic or hospital using this QR code.

General observation of mental status and behavior, gait, and posture can be performed while taking the history, but may necessitate changing the clinical environment, waiting for the patient to become comfortable with their new surroundings, or going outside. Based on the presenting complaint, it may be necessary to modify portions of the examination. For example, a patient that is non-ambulatory after being hit by a car is not subjected to postural reaction testing for fear of exacerbating a possible unstable vertebral fracture.

Table 1.1 An overview of the components of the neurological examination.

The observation portion of the examination includes:
(i) Evaluation of mental status and behavior
(ii) Evaluation of gait
(iii) Evaluation of the patient's posture
The hands-on components of the examination include:
(i) Postural reactions
(ii) Cranial nerve evaluation
(iii) Spinal reflex evaluation
(iv) Palpation
(v) Pain perception (reserved for patients demonstrating plegia)

Table 1.2 Neurological examination sheet.

Veterinary Neurological Examination Form

Pet	Owner

Pet Species	Pet Breed

Pet Age (years)	Pet Weight (kg)

Reason for Examination / Presenting Symptoms

Level of Consciousness

- ◯ Alert
- ◯ Dull
- ◯ Stuporous
- ◯ Comatose

Posture

- ☐ Left Head Tilt
- ☐ Right Head Tilt
- ☐ Left Head Turn
- ☐ Right Head Turn
- ☐ Wide-Based Stance
- ☐ Nerve root Signature
- ☐ Kyphosis / Scoliosis
- ☐ Ventroflexed neck
- ☐ Palmigrade / Plantigrade
- ☐ Schiff-Sherrington
- ☐ Decerebellate
- ☐ Decerebrate

Table 1.2 (Continued)

Gait

- [ ] Normal
- [ ] Ataxia
- [ ] Hypermetria
- [ ] Hypometria
- [ ] Ambulatory Paraparesis
- [ ] Ambulatory Tetraparesis
- [ ] Non-Ambulatory Paraparesis
- [ ] Non-Ambulatory Tetraparesis
- [ ] Paraplegia
- [ ] Hemiparesis
- [ ] Hemiplegia

Cranial Nerve Assessment

	Left	Right
Menace Response (II, Cerebrum, VII)		
Dazzle (II, Thalamus, VII)		
Pupillary Light Reflex (II, III)		
Palpebral Reflex (V, VII)		
Corneal Reflex (V, VI)		
Physiological Nystagmus (III, IV, VI, VIII)		
Nasal Stimulation (V, Forebrain)		
Gag Reflex (IX, X)		
Tongue Size and Movement (XII)		
Jaw Tone (V)		
Masticatory Muscle Mass (V)		
Other Observations		

(*Continued*)

Table 1.2 (Continued)

Postural Reactions

	Left Thoracic	Right Thoracic	Left Pelvic	Right Pelvic
Proprioceptive Positioning				
Hopping				
Wheelbarrow / Extensor Postural Thrust				
Visual Placing				
Tactile Placing				

Spinal Reflexes

	Left	Right
Extensor Carpi Radialis		
Thoracic Withdrawal		
Patellar		
Cranial Tibial		
Gastrocnemius		
Pelvic Withdrawal		
Cutaneous Trunci		
Perineal		

Pain Assessment

	Left Thoracic	Right Thoracic	Left Pelvic	Right Pelvic?	Tail Head / Perineal
Nociception					

Lesion Localization

OBSERVATION OF THE PATIENT

MENTAL STATUS AND BEHAVIOR

Before handling the patient, let the patient explore the examination room, if ambulatory, and observe the patient's reaction to the surroundings (Video 1.1). Mental status should be evaluated in terms of both the level of consciousness and the patient's behavior.

VIDEO 1.1 Allowing the patient to roam around the consulting room or a protected space outside can provide insight into the animal's level of consciousness, reaction to stimulation, and behavior. This normal dog demonstrates exploratory behavior as well as a bright and alert demeanor.

Level of Consciousness

- Normal/alert – the patient responds appropriately to environmental stimuli.
- Depressed/obtunded – the animal is drowsy but arousable. Depressed/obtunded dogs and cats are typically inattentive and display little spontaneous activity.
- Stuporous – the patient is unconscious, but arousable with a strong (typically painful) stimulus.
- Comatose – the patient is unconscious and cannot be aroused even with painful stimuli.

Patient Behavior

The patient may have a normal level of consciousness but exhibits abnormal behavior and responds inappropriately to stimuli. Abnormal behavior is identified by comparing the patient's behavior to expected behavior for animals of a similar breed and age (Video 1.2). The owner/caretaker is often able to bring subtle changes in behavior to the veterinarian's attention.

VIDEO 1.2 A 5-year-old Dalmatian dog is seen to exhibit compulsive pacing with a reduced level of consciousness from that expected in a normal dog and confusion as suggested by getting "stuck" in corners.

POSTURE

Posture is the position of the body with respect to gravity. Abnormal postures, such as a head tilt or wide-based stance, are common in dogs and cats with neurologic disease.

Several classic abnormal postures indicative of neurologic dysfunction have been described.

- Abnormal head position is often manifested as a head tilt or a head turn. In a patient with a head tilt, one ear is held lower than the other and the eyes are not parallel to the floor. Unilateral vestibular dysfunction will often cause a head tilt. In a patient with a head turn, the head is held with eyes parallel to the ground , but the nose is turned right or left, indicating intracranial disease, most often prosencephalic.
- Decerebrate rigidity is due to a brainstem lesion causing recumbency and is characterized by extension of all limbs, occasionally with opisthotonus (dorsiflexion of the head and neck) (Figure 1.1). A decreased level of consciousness (often stupor or coma) usually accompanies this posture.
- Decerebellate rigidity is due to an acute cerebellar lesion and is also characterized by recumbency with opisthotonus, thoracic limb extension, and flexion of the hips (Figure 1.2). Consciousness is not impaired due to a lack of brainstem involvement.
- Schiff–Sherrington posture is caused by an acute lesion in the thoracic or lumbar spinal cord segments. Extension of the thoracic limbs with paralysis of the pelvic limbs characterizes Schiff–Sherrington posture (Figure 1.3).

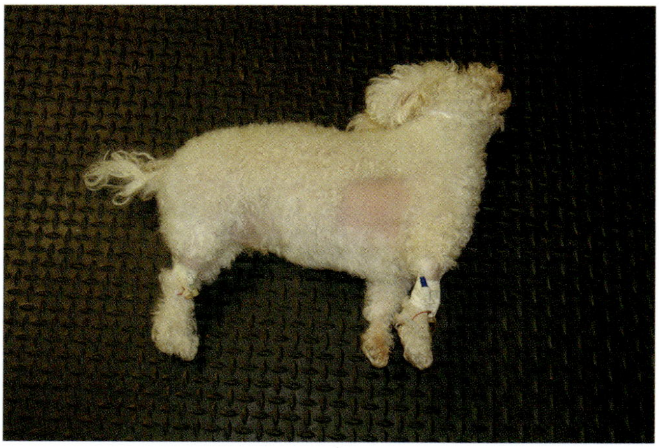

FIGURE 1.1 An 11-year-old miniature poodle exhibits recumbency with rigidity of all four limbs and extension of the neck compatible with decerebrate rigidity and opisthotonus. The dog was in a coma on presentation.

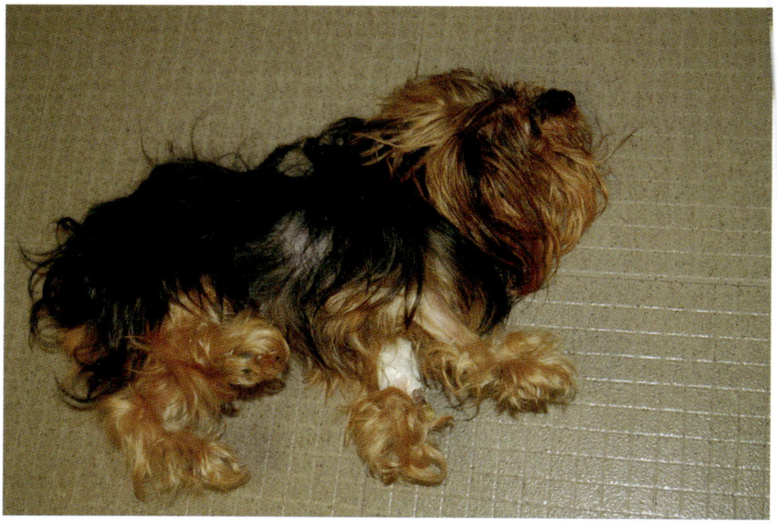

FIGURE 1.2 A 7-year-old Yorkshire terrier with an inflammatory disease predominantly affecting the cerebellum exhibits a spastic flexion of the pelvic limb with increased extensor tone in the thoracic limbs and the cervical musculature, compatible with decerebellate rigidity. This patient had normal mentation.

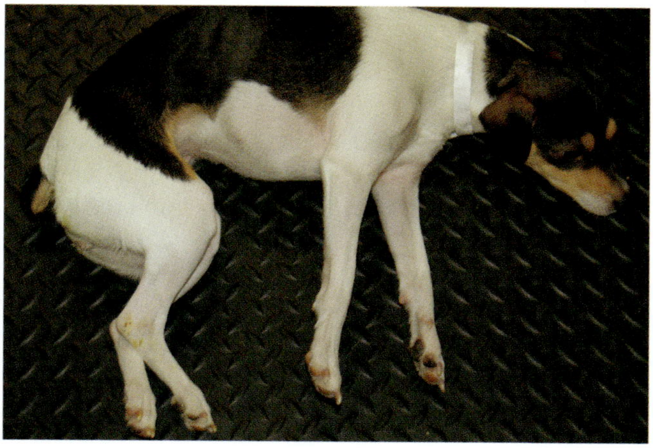

FIGURE 1.3 A 4-year-old terrier mix presented with acute flaccid paralysis and extensor rigidity of the thoracic limbs secondary to an acute thoracolumbar intervertebral disc extrusion. This is compatible with the Schiff–Sherrington posture.

GAIT

Several abnormalities of gait can be observed. These include lameness, ataxia, paresis or paralysis, and involuntary movements.

Lameness

Lameness is decreased leg function, making walking difficult, and is often associated with pain. Such pain can cause limb dysfunction when the patient tries to bear weight on it, resulting in reduced weight bearing and rapid use of the contralateral limb to relieve the pain. As a result, the stride of the painful limb is often shortened. When a single limb is severely painful, it is often carried. This is in contrast to a paretic limb (see next), which is often dragged. Lameness is usually caused by orthopedic, musculoskeletal, or regional vascular disease and by some neurologic lesions, such as inflammation of a nerve root, compression of the nerve root by an intervertebral disc extrusion, or a neoplasia such as a nerve sheath tumor. This neurogenic type of lameness is often referred to as a "root signature."

Patients with bilateral limb pain, such as hip disease or ruptured cruciate ligaments, may not walk at all or have short-strided, stilted gaits. This can mimic weakness due to neurologic disease.

Ataxia

This is the inability to perform normal, coordinated motor activity that is not caused by weakness, musculoskeletal problems, or abnormal movements, such as tremor. There are three types of ataxia.

- **Proprioceptive ataxia**
  This is associated with the loss of the sense of limb and body position due to interruption of ascending proprioceptive pathways (primarily unconscious proprioception). It is caused by a lesion affecting the general proprioceptive pathways in the peripheral nerve, dorsal nerve root, spinal cord, and brainstem.
  It is characterized by clumsiness and incoordination, resulting in a wide-based stance and a swaying gait of the body. The stride of the affected limb(s) is often longer than normal, and the toes may drag or scuff the ground (Video 1.3).

VIDEO 1.3 A 9-year-old dachshund with a thoracolumbar myelopathy exhibits mild proprioceptive ataxia of the pelvic limbs, especially noted when the dog makes a turn.

- **Cerebellar ataxia**
  This is the inability to regulate the rate and range of movement (unconscious proprioception) and is characterized by dysmetria, especially hypermetria, which is an overreaching, high-stepping gait (Video 1.4). Cerebellar ataxia is caused by cerebellar disease or selective dysfunction of spinocerebellar tracts (less common).

VIDEO 1.4 A young American Staffordshire terrier exhibits a hypermetric ataxia affecting all four limbs, compatible with cerebellar dysfunction.

- **Vestibular ataxia**
  Unilateral vestibular lesions cause an ataxia that is accompanied by leaning and falling to one side (Video 1.5). Other signs of vestibular disease, such as head tilt and abnormal nystagmus, may be evident. A severe form of this type of ataxia can result in rolling while recumbent. With bilateral vestibular dysfunction, the patient maintains a crouched position, is reluctant to move, and exhibits side-to-side head movements.

VIDEO 1.5 A young Chihuahua exhibits a left-sided head tilt, a wide-based stance with a leaning and falling ataxia to the left, compatible with vestibular ataxia.

Paresis/Paralysis

Paresis is a partial loss of voluntary movement, while paralysis (plegia) is a complete loss of voluntary movement (Videos 1.6–1.9). Paresis or paralysis indicates a lesion of either the upper motor neuron (UMN) system or the lower motor neuron (LMN) system (see lesion localization chapter). It is not possible to discriminate between UMN and LMN dysfunction based solely on severity, but UMN and LMN dysfunction result in different qualities of gait abnormality. UMN dysfunction leads to spastic, stiff movements, whereas LMN dysfunction leads to weak, short movements. Further, a loss of ability to support weight is a feature of LMN disease, and an inability to generate gait is a feature of UMN disease.

VIDEO 1.6 A mixed-breed dog exhibits non-ambulatory tetraparesis secondary to a C1–C5 myelopathy. There is plegia of the thoracic limbs (no motor function) and paresis of the pelvic limbs (some motor function noted). The increased tone noted in the limbs is compatible with an upper motor neuron lesion.

VIDEO 1.7 A Weimaraner with a C6–T2 myelopathy exhibits ambulatory tetraparesis. There is a short stride in the thoracic limbs and a long stride in the pelvic limbs.

VIDEO 1.8 An 11-year-old dachshund exhibits ambulatory paraparesis and proprioceptive ataxia secondary to a T3–L3 myelopathy.

VIDEO 1.9 A 3-year-old domestic long-haired cat exhibits non-ambulatory tetraparesis secondary to a polyneuropathy. There is carpal flexion and a generalized loss of tone in the limbs.

Abnormal Movements

There are many types of abnormal, involuntary movements. Those that can occur constantly rather than episodically include tremors, myoclonus, and myotonia.

- Tremor – a rhythmical, oscillatory movement localized to one region of the body or generalized to involve the entire body. Tremors can be classified by their distribution and frequency, as well as whether the problem occurs at rest, with posture, on action, or with intention

  Resting tremors: These are observed when the affected body part is supported against gravity and is not voluntarily activated. This form of tremor has not been reported in dogs and cats. The best example of a resting tremor in people would be the tremor associated with Parkinson's disease.

  Action-related tremors: These are diffuse, high-frequency skeletal muscle tremors that worsen with activity and resolve with sleep.

  Postural tremors: These occur during voluntary maintenance of a position against gravity (e.g. a tremor of the limbs when standing that dissipates on activity or lying down). Examples of these include (1) orthostatic tremors, (2) idiopathic head tremor syndrome, and (3) benign, idiopathic, rapid postural tremor (Video 1.10).

VIDEO 1.10 An older beagle dog exhibits high-frequency, low-amplitude pelvic limb tremors. This was only noted when the dog was standing and is compatible with a benign, idiopathic, rapid postural tremor seen in older dogs.

  Kinetic tremors: These occur during any aspect of voluntary movement. They can be present when the movement begins, during the course of movement, and as the target is reached. These are often termed intention tremors most commonly seen as a tremor of the head and neck that occurs when focusing on something such as a food bowl. They are associated with cerebellar disorders and as such, other localizing signs (e.g. hypermetria, disequilibrium) can also be present.

- Myoclonus – this may be physiological (e.g. hiccups or movements on falling asleep referred to as hypnic jerks) or pathological. A common method for classifying pathological myoclonus is by its neuroanatomical localization, subdivided into cortical, subcortical (brainstem and spinal cord), and peripheral types. However, this is not always intuitive, and it has been proposed that myoclonus can also be classified according to its association with epilepsy as an epileptic myoclonus or as a non-epileptic myoclonus. An example of a non-epileptic myoclonus is constant repetitive myoclonus. This is a constant rhythmic jerking, usually of one limb every 1 to several seconds, which persists during activity, rest, and sleep, and may involve several limbs or muscles such as the diaphragm or masticatory muscles.

- Myotonia – this is a delayed relaxation of muscle following voluntary contraction. Myotonia is manifested as muscle stiffness that is relieved by exercise. Attacks of myotonia may culminate in recumbency with rigid extension of the limbs. Some patients with myotonia will display "dimpling" of sustained indentation of affected muscle when percussed.

THE HANDS-ON EXAMINATION

POSTURAL REACTION TESTING

The primary aim of testing postural reactions is to detect any subtle deficits that were not obvious on gait evaluation. Postural reactions test proprioception. Proprioception is the awareness of the precise position and movements of the body and especially the limbs. Proprioceptors are specific receptors sensitive to these movements. They are located in the joint, tendon, and muscles (general proprioception), as well as in the inner ear (special proprioception). The information collected by these receptors is transmitted to the cerebral cortex, where it is consciously perceived (conscious proprioception).

Proprioception involves complex pathways but generally includes an afferent arc and an efferent arc:

The afferent arc: This consists of a proprioceptive receptor, a peripheral sensory nerve, the spinothalamic ascending pathways, and the contralateral somatic sensory area of the cerebral cortex (integration center) (Figure 1.4).

The efferent arc: This consists of the motor cortex contralateral to the tested limb, descending motor pathways within the brainstem and spinal cord (UMN pathways), and the peripheral motor nerve (LMN pathway), as well as the skeletal effector muscles.

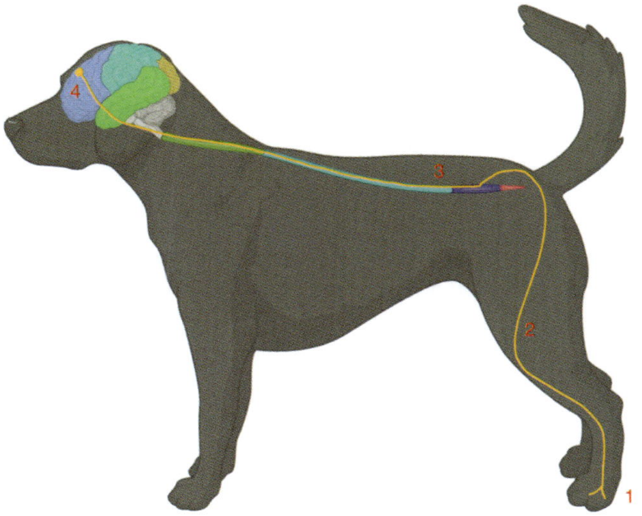

FIGURE 1.4 An illustration of the afferent arc of the conscious proprioceptive pathway. This consists of a (1) proprioceptive receptor, (2) a peripheral sensory nerve, (3) the spinothalamic ascending pathways, and (4) the contralateral somatic sensory area of the cerebral cortex (integration center). Source: Created with www.biorender.com.

Lesions affecting any of the aforementioned anatomical sensory and motor components could result in abnormal postural reactions; therefore, the tests are not very discriminatory for lesion localization purposes. The importance of testing them is in the detection of subtle dysfunction and asymmetries, as well as confirming that a neurological disease is present. In general, postural reactions remain normal in neuromuscular junction and muscular diseases, as long as the animal has the strength to support its weight.

Proprioceptive placing: This is the most commonly performed test in the dog and is designed to evaluate the conscious awareness of the limb position and its movement. It is particularly difficult to perform in cats, which resent having their feet handled during proprioceptive positioning, and so an alternative test is most often performed in this species (see next).

Conscious proprioception is evaluated by placing the paw in an abnormal position (turned over so that the dorsal surface is in contact with the ground) and determining how quickly the animal corrects the paw position (Video 1.11). When performing this test, the animal should be standing squarely on all four limbs, and it is fundamental to support the majority of the animal's weight in order to improve test sensitivity. Failure to do so causes flexion of the limb, which results in the stimulation of many proprioceptors within the different flexed joints. Supporting their weight is also helpful for animals that are reluctant to bear weight because of a painful limb (as seen with some orthopedic diseases). The test should be repeated until the examiner is confident with the result.

VIDEO 1.11 As the patient is supported, the digits can be turned over to test proprioceptive positioning. A normal response is seen in this dog with a rapid replacement of the foot to the standing position.

Hopping: This test is the preferred postural reaction test in cats. It can be particularly difficult to perform in large breeds of dog. The hopping reaction is tested by holding the patient so that the majority of its weight is placed on one limb while the animal is moved laterally (Video 1.12). Normal animals hop on the tested limb to accommodate a new body position as their center of gravity is displaced laterally. An equal response should be seen on both sides, and a normal response consists of hopping the limb before it is located past midline toward the contralateral side of the limb being tested. Subtle ataxia or weakness of one limb may be detected. Animals with severe orthopedic disease will have difficulty performing this test unless their weight is supported adequately.

VIDEO 1.12 Hopping the patient on each of its legs laterally is another test of proprioception. This can be achieved by lifting the animal up completely and letting it bear weight on the tested limb, or in larger patients, simply by picking the contralateral limb up and gently pushing the animal away to initiate the hop. A quick pick up of the paw and a smooth placement of the paw into the weight-bearing position should be seen.

Placing response: Visual placing and tactile placing are, in principle, much more complex postural reaction tests. They are mainly used when proprioceptive positioning or hopping reactions do not confirm a disorder. Visual placing can also be useful in assessing visual function in an animal where the menace response or obstacle course testing is difficult to interpret. Tactile placing is tested with the animal's eyes covered. The animal is lifted, and the distal part of the thoracic limb is brought in contact with the edge of a table. When the dorsal surface of the paw makes contact with the edge of the surface, the animal should immediately place its foot on the surface. Visual placing is tested by allowing the animal to see the table surface. Normal animals will reach for the surface before the paw touches the table.

Hemiwalking, extensor postural thrust, and wheelbarrowing: These are also more complex postural reaction tests.

- *Wheelbarrowing tests the thoracic limbs:* The animal's pelvic limbs are lifted off the ground by supporting the animal under the abdomen and forcing it to walk forwards. This test highlights subtle thoracic limb weakness and ataxia. Subtle vestibular dysfunction can be detected by extending the animal's head and neck while testing.

- *Extensor postural thrust tests the pelvic limbs:* It is elicited by supporting the animal by the chest caudal to the thoracic limbs and lowering the pelvic limbs to the floor, forcing it to walk backwards, thus testing pelvic limb weakness and ataxia.
- Hemiwalking tests the ability of the animal to walk on the thoracic and pelvic limbs on one side while holding the limbs on the other side. The animal should be pushed away from the side on which its limbs are supported and the speed and coordination of the movements assessed. This is best performed on a nonslip surface.

CRANIAL NERVE ASSESSMENT

Tests of cranial nerve (CN) function are summarized in Table 1.3. The following is an overview of each cranial nerve's function, clinical evaluation, and signs of dysfunction. Testing of these nerves

Table 1.3 Cranial nerve function and testing.

Cranial nerve	Nerve Target / Function	Applicable tests
I Olfactory	Smell	Blindfold the animal and monitor behavioral response to food placed near the nose; loss of smell is usually due to nasal disease rather than neurological disease.
II Optic	Vision	i. Menace response ii. Pupillary light reflex iii. Obstacle course iv. Dropping cotton wool balls in front of each eye
III Oculomotor	Extrinsic and intrinsic ocular muscles/upper eyelid muscle	i. Eyeball position ii. Pupil size (mydriatic in disease) iii. Physiological nystagmus iv. Pupillary light reflex
IV Trochlear	Extrinsic ocular muscles	i. Eyeball position
V Trigeminal	Facial sensation/ jaw movement	ii. Palpebral reflex iii. Jaw and masticatory muscle palpation
VI Abducent	Extrinsic ocular muscles	i. Eyeball position ii. Physiological nystagmus
VII Facial	Muscles of facial expression/ parasympathetic supply to lacrimal glands	i. Palpebral response ii. Evaluation of facial symmetry iii. Schirmer tear test
VIII Vestibulocochlear	Hearing and balance	i. Oculocephalic reflexes ii. Assessment for head tilt
IX Glossopharyngeal	Muscles of the pharynx and larynx	Gag reflex
X Vagus	Muscles of the larynx and pharynx	Gag reflex
XI Accessory	Superficial neck muscles	None applicable
XII Hypoglossal	Muscles of the tongue	Tongue grab/inspection

should be done in conjunction with the assessment of proprioception and mentation to determine whether there is brainstem (central) disease or peripheral cranial nerve disease.

OLFACTORY NERVE – CN I

Anatomy and function: CN I is involved in the conscious perception of smell. It is a unique sensory cranial nerve in that its cell bodies lie in the olfactory epithelium on the ethmoturbinate bones rather than in a ganglion. Its axons pass through the cribriform plate to synapse with secondary neurons in the olfactory bulb. These secondary neurons pass successively into the olfactory peduncle and olfactory tracts before they synapse with third-order neurons in the olfactory tubercle. This final neuron projects to the piriform lobe in the olfactory region of the brain.

Clinical evaluation: Evaluation of smell is difficult in animals and remains a subjective assessment. As such, it is rarely performed in clinical cases. This sensory function can be assessed by testing the animal's response (sniffing or licking of the nose, aversion of the head) to aromatic substances while blindfolded. Care should be taken not to use irritating substances that could stimulate the trigeminal nerve (CN V) and cause similar responses.

Clinical signs of dysfunction: Decreased or absent sense of smell is defined as hyposmia or anosmia, respectively. Detecting deficits in smell is difficult and often based on historical findings (e.g. decreased appetite). Non-neurological causes (such as rhinitis and other nasal diseases) are more common causes than central nervous system (CNS) disease.

OPTIC NERVE – CN II

Anatomy and function: The optic nerve is not a "true" nerve but an extension of the brain. It is part of the central visual pathway (involved in sensory visual perception) and the afferent component of the menace response and pupillary light reflex (PLR).

The visual pathway involves three consecutive neurons (see Chapter 6).

- The first neuron represents the bipolar cells of the retina and receives visual information from the neuroepithelial cells of the retina (e.g. rods and cones).
- The second neuron corresponds to the ganglion cell of the retina. Its axon lies in the optic nerve and continues through the optic chiasm and proximal part of the optic tract on the opposite side (55% decussation in humans, 66% in cats, and 75% in dogs).
- The third neuron has its cell body in the lateral geniculate nucleus in the thalamus. Its axon projects to the visual cortex (mostly contralateral occipital cortex) in a band of fibers called the optic radiations.

The menace response is a cortically mediated blink produced by a threatening or unexpected image suddenly appearing in the near visual field. It is present from about 10–12 weeks of age in dogs and cats. The afferent part of this response involves the same structures as the visual pathways. The information generated in the visual cortex is forwarded to the motor cortex to initiate a motor response. The corticobulbar pathways to the facial nerve nucleus (CN VII) then transmit the motor information. This response requires intact facial nerve function and an intact cerebellum (ipsilateral function). The neuronal pathways through the cerebellum are not known.

The afferent part of the PLR shares some common pathways (up to the level of the optic tract) with the visual pathways. While axons involved in vision reach the conscious level after synapse with the lateral geniculate nucleus of the thalamus, the axons involved in the PLR synapse with a third neuron in the pretectal nucleus of the dorsal midbrain. Most of the axons arising from this nucleus decussate again and synapse in the parasympathetic component of the oculomotor nucleus (ipsilateral to the stimulated eye), also in the midbrain. There are also neurons that do not decussate and that project to the oculomotor nucleus on the contralateral side to the stimulated eye. The majority of axons decussate, and this explains why the direct response (constriction in the eye receiving the light stimulus) is greater than the consensual response (constriction in the eye not receiving the light stimulus). The efferent arm of the PLR involves parasympathetic axons in CN III (oculomotor), causing constriction of the pupil.

Clinical evaluation: The optic nerve is the common component of the afferent pathways involved in vision, menace response, visual placing, and the PLR. These tests use different integration centers within the brain and different efferent pathways. The integrity of the optic nerve can be determined by combining the results of these tests.

- Vision in animals is evaluated by observing the animal navigating around the examination room.
- In dogs, the menace response is tested by making a threatening gesture toward the eye via the extreme visual fields (temporal and nasal, which project to different cortical hemispheres), while the other eye is covered; closure of the eyelids should be observed (Video 1.13). In cats, however, it is preferable to stand behind the animal with the contralateral eye uncovered, as up to 40% of cats with vision fail to have a menace response when the contralateral eye is covered. If unilateral visual loss is suspected, each eye can be blindfolded in turn prior to completion of an obstacle course.

VIDEO 1.13 In dogs, the menace response is often performed when standing in front of the patient. One eye is shielded, and the other eye is threatened with an open or closed hand without trying to create a current of air that can be felt by the patient. The normal response is a rapid blinking of the eyelids with a slight avoidant movement of the head.

- At the time of the PLR, the pupils should be examined for symmetry. Resting pupils should be equal in diameter, although slight differences are insignificant. Unequal pupil size is called anisocoria. When performing the PLR examination, a bright light is shined into one eye at a time (Video 1.14). Both pupils should constrict, with a direct response in the tested eye being slightly stronger than a consensual response in the opposite eye. When a bright light is initially flashed into the eye, a blink response may occur. This is referred to as the dazzle reflex and probably does not involve the cerebrum but rather thalamic nuclei. If a poor quality light source is used, the stimulated pupil may dilate slightly with continued stimulation. This is referred to as pupillary escape.

VIDEO 1.14 The pupillary light reflex is performed by shining a bright light into each eye and monitoring the response of the ipsilateral and contralateral pupil for the direct and consensual response, respectively.

Clinical signs of dysfunction: Lesions of the optic nerve can be manifest as partial or complete loss of vision and/or dilated and unresponsive pupils.

OCULOMOTOR NERVE – CN III

Anatomy and function: CN III innervates the ipsilateral dorsal, ventral, and medial recti (extraocular) muscles as well as the ventral oblique muscle (Figure 1.5). The oculomotor nerve also plays an important role in the efferent arm of the PLR and eyelid movement. It is involved in

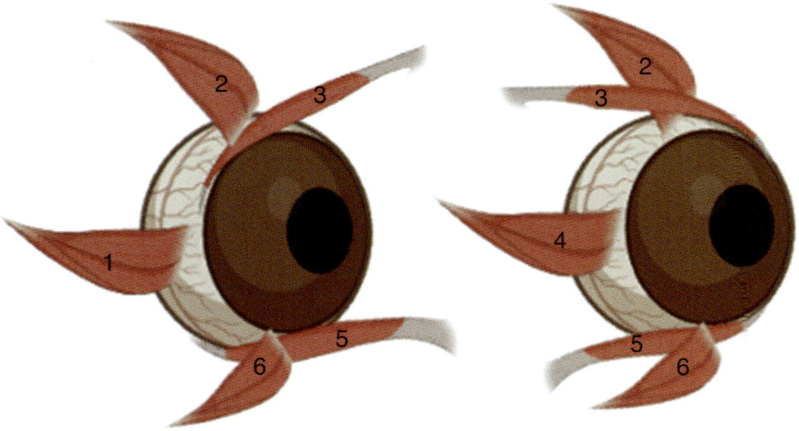

FIGURE 1.5 The extraocular muscles of the eyes are innervated by one of the three cranial nerves (III, IV and VI). (1) Lateral rectus – VI, (2) dorsal rectus – III, (3) dorsal oblique – IV, (4) medial rectus – III, (5) ventral oblique – III, and (6) ventral rectus – III. The retractor bulbi (VI) is not visible in this illustration. *Source:* Created with www.biorender.com.

the elevation of the upper eyelid (levator palpebrae superioris) and controls pupillary constriction via its parasympathetic component. The oculomotor nuclei are located in the rostral midbrain. Their axons exit the brainstem and traverse the middle cranial fossa lateral to the hypophysis before they exit the skull through the orbital fissure.

Clinical evaluation: CN III function can be assessed by observing eye position and movements at rest and by testing for normal physiological nystagmus (vestibuloocular reflex) by moving the head from side to side and up and down (see Vestibulocochlear nerve – CN VIII) (Video 1.15). The parasympathetic function of CN III can be assessed by observing the pupil size and evaluating the PLR.

VIDEO 1.15 Physiological nystagmus is tested by moving the patient's head from one side to the other, as well as up and down. The response of each eye is assessed for a normal response, which is a rapid movement to the side of the head turn and a slow movement back to the center of the gaze.

Clinical signs of dysfunction: Lesions of the oculomotor nerve produce a ventrolateral strabismus and an inability to rotate the eye dorsally, ventrally, or medially during oculovestibular testing (external ophthalmoplegia). This strabismus must be differentiated from a vestibular strabismus that only occurs in certain head positions and is termed positional strabismus. The aforementioned signs can also be associated with a dilated unresponsive pupil (referred to as internal ophthalmoplegia) and/or narrowing of the palpebral fissure (ptosis of the upper eyelid). However, any of these signs can exist on their own.

TROCHLEAR NERVE – CN IV

Anatomy and function: CN IV innervates the contralateral dorsal oblique muscle. This muscle is responsible for the inward rotation of the eyeball. The trochlear nucleus is located in the caudal midbrain. After leaving the brainstem, its axons decussate on the dorsal surface of the brainstem and course rostrally through the middle cranial fossa before they exit the skull via the orbital fissure.

Clinical evaluation: As for CN III, CN IV can be assessed by observing the eye position at rest and by testing for normal physiological nystagmus.

Clinical signs of dysfunction: Lesions of the trochlear nerve produce a dorsolateral strabismus (extorsion) of the contralateral eye. In dogs, this is best evaluated by fundoscopic examination, observing temporal deviation of the dorsal retinal vessels. In cats, it can be seen as an alteration in pupil orientation. This is a very rare isolated finding: lesions of this nerve usually occur in combination with CN III and CN VI lesions, producing complete internal and external ophthalmoplegia.

TRIGEMINAL NERVE – CN V

Anatomy and function: CN V provides sensory innervation to the face (cutaneous elements of the face and the cornea, mucosa of the nasal septum, and mucosa of the oral cavity) and motor innervation of the masticatory muscles (temporalis, masseter, medial and lateral pterygoid, and rostral part of the digastric muscles). The cell body of the sensory part of CN V lies in the trigeminal ganglion. Its sensory nuclei form a large, separate, continuous, and elongated nuclear column extending along the brainstem. Its motor nuclei are located in the pons. CN V consists of three branches: ophthalmic, maxillary, and mandibular. Each branch provides sensation to specific areas of the face:

- Ophthalmic (cornea, medial canthus of the eye, nasal septal mucosa, and skin on the dorsum of the nose)
- Maxillary (lateral canthus of the eye, skin of the cheek, side of the nose, muzzle, palates, mucous membrane of the nasopharynx, teeth, and gingiva of the upper jaw)
- Mandibular (mandibular portion of the face and oral cavity)
  The ophthalmic and maxillary branches are in close proximity to the cavernous sinus before they exit the skull through the orbital fissure and round foramen, respectively. These two branches have only sensory function. The mandibular branch exits the skull through the oval foramen and serves both a motor and sensory function.

Clinical evaluation: The motor function of CN V is assessed by evaluating the size and symmetry of the masticatory muscles and testing the resistance of the jaw to opening the mouth. The sensory function (sensation of the face) can be individually tested by:

- The corneal reflex (ophthalmic branch) – this is performed with a cotton-tipped applicator lightly applied to the surface of the cornea. Sometimes it is necessary to distract the palpebrae with your fingers to ensure that they do not close while you are attempting this reflex. When the stimulation is applied to the cornea, the eyeball is seen to retract, and the eyelids close.
- The palpebral reflex (ophthalmic or maxillary branch when touching the medial or lateral canthus of the eye, respectively) – both the medial and lateral canthus of each eye are touched with the finger, and in response, there should be a rapid and complete closure of the eyelids (Video 1.16).

VIDEO 1.16 The palpebral reflex is tested by touching both the medial and lateral canthi with the response being closure of the eyelids.

- The response to stimulation of the nasal mucosa (ophthalmic and maxillary branches) – as another way to assess head and face sensation and behavioral reaction to cranial stimulation, a blunt instrument or cotton-tipped applicator is gently inserted into each nostril while trying to blindfold the animal with the other hand. A normal response to this stimulation is an immediate retraction of the head from the stimulus (Video 1.17).

VIDEO 1.17 Nasal stimulation tests the ophthalmic branch of the trigeminal nerve (CN V) and cortical response to obnoxious stimuli. It is not a reflex, but a behavioral response, similar to the menace response. A withdrawal of the head away from the stimulus is the expected normal response.

- Pinching the skin of the face with hemostat forceps and observing an ipsilateral blink or facial twitch.

A reflex response is best distinguished from a conscious response by stimulating the nasal mucosa: the normal animal will pull its head away, while the animal with forebrain disease may blink or show a facial twitch, but not show a conscious reaction.

Clinical signs of dysfunction: Unilateral involvement of the motor part of CN V causes ipsilateral masticatory muscle atrophy and decreased jaw tone. Enophthalmia and protrusion of the third eyelid can be observed in the ipsilateral eye (passive retraction of the eyeball due to the loss of the temporalis muscle mass). Bilateral involvement of the motor branches produces a dropped jaw with inability to close the mouth voluntarily, associated with various degrees of masticatory muscle atrophy depending on the duration of signs. Decreased or complete loss of facial sensation is defined as facial hypoesthesia or anesthesia. Involvement of the ophthalmic branch of CN V can also produce decreased tear secretion and neurotropic keratitis secondary to the loss of afferent stimulation to the lacrimal reflex.

ABDUCENT NERVE – CN VI

Anatomy and function: CN VI innervates the ipsilateral lateral rectus and retractor bulbi muscles. The CN VI nucleus is located in the rostral medulla oblongata. Its axons follow the same pathway as the axons of CN III and CN IV. The abducent nerve leaves the cranial cavity through the orbital fissure.

Clinical evaluation: CN VI function can be assessed by observing the eye position and movement at rest, testing for normal physiological nystagmus, and testing for normal eyeball retraction during the corneal reflex.

Clinical signs of dysfunction: Lesions of the abducent nerve result in an ipsilateral convergent strabismus, an inability of the eye to cross the midline when evaluating the horizontal physiological nystagmus, and an inability to retract the eyeball. Isolated lesions are rare, as for CN IV.

FACIAL NERVE – CN VII

Anatomy and function: CN VII provides motor function to the muscles of facial expression and sensory function (providing the sense of taste) to the rostral two-thirds of the tongue and palate. Its parasympathetic component innervates the lacrimal glands and the mandibular and sublingual salivary glands. Neurons innervating the muscles of facial expression are located in the facial nucleus in the rostral medulla oblongata. The axons pass through the internal acoustic meatus of the petrosal bone on the dorsal surface of the vestibulocochlear nerve and leave the skull through the stylomastoid foramen. The facial nerve courses through the middle ear before branches are distributed to the muscles of facial expression (ear, eyelids, nose, cheeks, and lips) as well as the caudal portion of the digastric muscle. The parasympathetic fibers (which produce lacrimal gland secretion) leave the facial nerve as it courses through the middle ear.

Clinical evaluation: The motor function of CN VII is primarily assessed by observing the face for symmetry (position of the ears and lip commissure on each side within the same plane, symmetry of the palpebral fissure), spontaneous blinking, and movement of the nostrils. The facial nerve also provides the motor response (efferent part) of the following tests:

- Palpebral reflex (CN V and VII)
- Corneal reflex (CN V, VI and VII)
- Menace response (CN II and VII)
- Pinching of the face (CN V and VII) – the lip pinch is evaluated by pinching the upper lip at the level of the canine tooth using a hemostat. The afferent sensory impulse travels along the infraorbital nerve (a branch of the maxillary branch of the trigeminal nerve, CN V). The efferent response is mediated by the facial nerve (CN VII).

The Schirmer tear test can evaluate the parasympathetic supply of the lacrimal gland associated with CN VII. Examining the mouth for a moist mucosa can subjectively assess salivation.

Clinical signs of dysfunction: Motor dysfunction of CN VII produces ipsilateral drooping of and inability to move the ear and lip, widened palpebral fissure and absent spontaneous and provoked blinking, absent abduction of the nostril during inspiration, and deviation of the nose toward the normal side due to the unopposed muscle tone on the unaffected side. With chronic denervation, the lips are retracted further than normal and the nostril is deviated to the affected side as a result of muscle fibrosis.

Facial spasm can also be seen, causing retraction of the lips and nostril to the affected side, and narrowing of the palpebral fissure on the affected side. This can be distinguished from chronic denervation by performing the palpebral test: in facial spasm the eye can blink.

Unilateral involvement can be seen in the asymmetry of the ears, eyelids, lips, and nose. Lesions of the individual branches of the facial nerve along their course produce paresis or paralysis of the specific muscles they innervate. Dysfunction of the parasympathetic supply of the lacrimal gland produces keratoconjunctivitis sicca. This is mainly seen with lesions of the facial nerve located between the medulla and the middle ear. Lesions distal to the facial canal in the temporal bone will not affect these parasympathetic neurons.

VESTIBULOCOCHLEAR NERVE – CN VIII

Anatomy and function: The vestibulocochlear nerve is involved in hearing and vestibular function (adaptation of the position of the eye and body with respect to the position and movement of the head).

The vestibular system consists of special proprioceptors within the petrous temporal bone (inner ear) (Figure 1.6A), the vestibular nerve, and four brainstem nuclei located in the rostral medulla oblongata on each side of the fourth ventricle. The receptor organs (saccule, utricle, and semicircular canals) detect the position and movement of the head. The neurons of the vestibular ganglia receive impulses from these receptors and project into the vestibular nuclei via the internal acoustic meatus, where this special proprioceptive information is integrated. The vestibular nuclei connect to the nuclei of the cranial nerves responsible for eye movement (CN III, IV, and VI) via the medial longitudinal fasciculus. They also project to the ipsilateral extensor muscles of the limb via the vestibulospinal tract. Finally, these neurons project to the ipsilateral flocculonodular lobe of the cerebellum via the caudal cerebellar peduncles. Through these pathways, the vestibular system controls the position of the eyes, trunk, and limbs depending on the position and movements of the head.

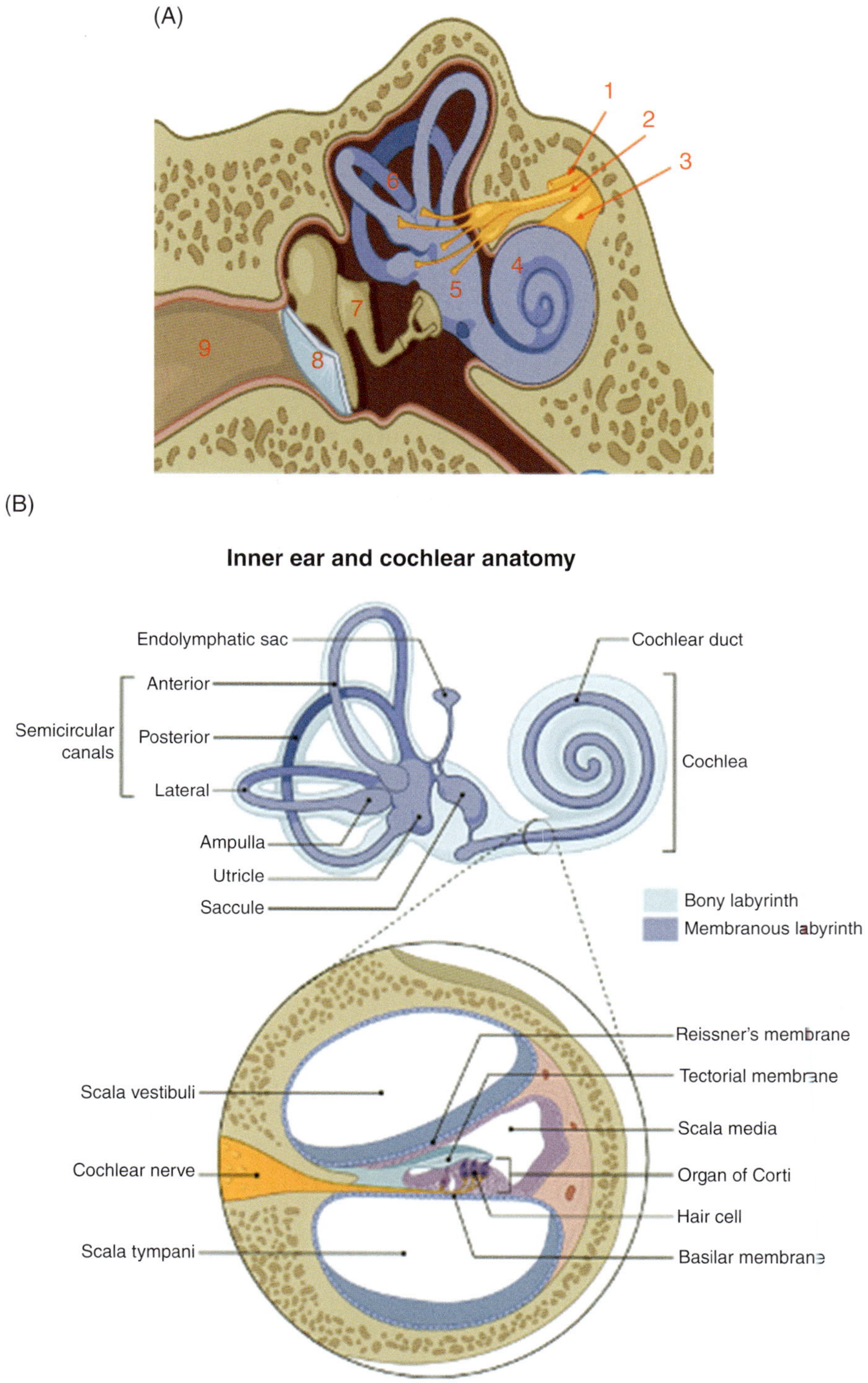

FIGURE 1.6 The peripheral components of the vestibular system originate in the petrous temporal bone and are adjacent to the receptors for auditory function within the inner ear. (A) (1) Facial nerve, (2) vestibular nerve, and (3) cochlear nerve – this nerve joins the vestibular nerve to become the vestibulocochlear nerve (CN VIII) and travels through the internal acoustic meatus with CN VII into the cranial cavity to the brainstem. (4) Cochlea, (5) vestibule housing the saccule and utricle, (6) semicircular canals, (7) ear ossicles, (8) tympanic membrane, and (9) horizontal portion of the external ear canal. (B) Inner ear and cochlear anatomy. *Source:* Created with www.biorender.com.

The hearing system involves the sensory receptor organ (organ of Corti) within the cochlea of the inner ear (Figure 1.6B). The neurons forming the cochlear branch of CN VIII have their cell bodies in the spiral ganglion of CN VIII. They receive impulses from the neuroepithelial hair cells of the organ of Corti and enter the brainstem and synapse with the cochlear nuclei. The auditory information is transmitted through bilateral ascending auditory pathways to the medial geniculate nucleus of the thalamus via the lateral lemniscus. From this nucleus, a third neuron projects via the auditory radiation to the contralateral auditory cortex.

Clinical evaluation: Observation of the animal's body and head posture at rest, and evaluation of its gait, can provide significant information about the vestibular function of CN VIII. This function can also be more specifically assessed by testing the vestibulo-ocular reflex (also known as physiological nystagmus; "Physiological Nystagmus" video 1.15). This type of nystagmus (also called "jerk" nystagmus) is an involuntary rhythmic movement of the eyes, which typically presents with a slow phase in one direction and a quick phase in the other direction. It can occur in normal animals (physiological or vestibular nystagmus) or may be associated with an underlying abnormality (pathological nystagmus). The direction of the nystagmus is classically described by that of the fast-phase movement. A physiological nystagmus can be induced in normal individuals by lateral rotation of the head. With a feline patient, this is best done by holding the animal at arm's length and rotating it from side to side. This physiological nystagmus stabilizes images on the retina during head movement. It is always observed in the plane of head rotation and consists of a slow phase in the direction opposite to head rotation and a fast phase in the same direction. In the absence of any head movement, nystagmus should never be present in a normal animal.

The auditory function of CN VIII is difficult to assess clinically. The startle reaction involves observing the animal's response to a noise stimulus (e.g. a handclap or whistle). Unilateral or partial deafness is virtually impossible to detect using this test. The best assessment is the animal's response to noise when asleep: most owners can report whether they have to touch their animal to wake them. Electrophysiological assessment (such as the brainstem auditory evoked response test) is necessary to confirm and assess the severity of the hearing loss.

Clinical signs of dysfunction: Vestibular dysfunction may result in any or all of the following clinical signs: head tilt, falling, leaning, rolling, circling, abnormal and/or positional nystagmus, positional strabismus, and asymmetrical ataxia. Clinical signs may be a result of lesions involving the receptor organs in the inner ear or the vestibular portion of CN VIII (e.g. peripheral vestibular dysfunction) or lesions involving the brainstem vestibular nuclei (e.g. central vestibular dysfunction). Less frequently, lesions affecting the caudal cerebellar peduncle, the fastigial nucleus, or the flocculonodular lobes of the cerebellum can cause central vestibular dysfunction with a resulting paradoxical head tilt. Bilateral vestibular disease is characterized by head sway from side to side, loss of balance on both sides, and symmetrical ataxia with a wide-based stance. A physiological nystagmus cannot be elicited.

The presence of spontaneous or positional jerk nystagmus indicates vestibular dysfunction but does not further localize the lesion to the peripheral or central vestibular system. Some exceptions are worth mentioning:

- Positional, spontaneous, and physiological nystagmus are usually absent with bilateral lesions.
- Vertical nystagmus and nystagmus that changes direction with different head positions are most commonly seen with central lesions.

GLOSSOPHARYNGEAL AND VAGUS NERVES – CN IX AND CN X

Anatomy and function: The glossopharyngeal and vagus nerves share sensory (nucleus tractus solitarius) and motor (nucleus ambiguus) nuclei. CN IX innervates the musculature of the pharynx and palatine structures. It provides sensory innervation to the caudal third of the tongue and pharyngeal mucosa (taste). Its parasympathetic component innervates the parotid and zygomatic salivary glands. CN X controls motor function of the larynx (recurrent laryngeal branch), pharynx, and esophagus (the cervical esophagus is innervated by the pharyngeal and recurrent laryngeal branches, while the thoracic esophagus is innervated by the vagal branches). It provides sensory function to the larynx, pharynx, and thoracic and abdominal viscera. Its parasympathetic component provides innervation to all thoracic and abdominal viscera, except those of the pelvic region. Both nerves leave the skull through the jugular foramen continuing into the tympano-occipital fissure which lies behind the osseous bulla.

Clinical evaluation: The pharyngeal (swallowing or gag) reflex can assess the function of CN IX and CN X. It is evaluated by applying external pressure to the hyoid bones to stimulate swallowing or by stimulating the pharynx with a finger to elicit a gag reflex. It can also be evaluated by watching the animal eat or drink or by opening its mouth wide; the animal will usually close its mouth, swallow, and lick its nose, allowing simultaneous evaluation of the tongue. The parasympathetic portion of CN X can be evaluated by testing the oculocardiac reflex. This is achieved by applying digital pressure to both eyeballs and observing simultaneously a reflex bradycardia (also mediated by CN V).

Clinical signs of dysfunction: CN IX dysfunction results in dysphagia, absent gag reflex, and reduced pharyngeal tone. Animals frequently cough after drinking and swallow repeatedly because of an accumulation of saliva in their pharynx. CN X dysfunction results in dysphagia, inspiratory dyspnea (due to laryngeal paralysis), voice changes (dysphonia), and regurgitation (due to megaesophagus in the case of a bilateral vagal disorder). The pharyngeal and oculocardiac reflexes are absent.

ACCESSORY NERVE – CN XI

Anatomy and function: CN XI provides motor innervation to the trapezius and part of the sternocephalicus and brachiocephalicus muscles. It leaves the skull with CNs IX and X.

Clinical signs of dysfunction: Lesions of this nerve result in trapezius muscle atrophy. The neck may be deviated toward the affected side in chronic cases. Isolated lesions of the accessory nerve are an extremely rare finding.

HYPOGLOSSAL NERVE – CN XII

Anatomy and function: CN XII provides motor innervation to the muscles of the tongue. The nucleus is in the caudal medulla and can therefore be affected by cervical lesions located cranially. This cranial nerve exits the skull by the hypoglossal canal foramen.

Clinical evaluation: CN XII function can be evaluated by inspecting the tongue for atrophy, asymmetry, or deviation to one side. Manually stretching the tongue and observing a voluntary retraction assesses the tongue's tone. Applying food paste to the nose and observing the animal licking assesses the tongue's movement, as does watching it prehend food or drink water from a clear, colorless bowl.

Clinical signs of dysfunction: Lesions affecting CN XII can result in problems with prehension, mastication, and deglutition. With unilateral and recent lesions, the tongue tends to deviate toward the contralateral side. With unilateral and chronic lesions, the tongue protrudes toward the side of the lesion, and atrophy is observed ipsilaterally. Muscle fasciculations may be obvious on the affected side in the denervated tongue.

SPINAL REFLEXES

Spinal reflexes evaluate reflex arcs and can provide information about the influence of descending UMN pathways. A reflex arc consists of an afferent sensory nerve that synapses directly or indirectly with an efferent motor nerve. The synapse for a given spinal reflex occurs within specific spinal cord segments.

Spinal Cord Reflex Grading

Spinal cord reflexes are graded as absent, weak (present but reduced), normal, exaggerated, and clonic.

Causes of absent and weak reflexes include a lesion affecting any part along the local reflex arc (afferent sensory component, spinal cord segment, efferent motor component). Reflexes can be difficult to assess in patients with severe limb rigidity, range of motion, or muscle extension (either due to loss of UMN inhibition or due to fibrosis of a joint or muscle).

Causes of exaggerated reflexes and clonus include a UMN lesion in the spinal cord cranial to the spinal cord segment involved in the reflex. In testing the patellar reflex, an exaggerated response, called pseudohyperreflexia, can also be seen with lesions in the L6–S1 region of the spinal cord. This region is the source of efferent motor neurons to the stifle flexors that ordinarily dampen stifle extension during the patellar reflex. This patellar pseudohyperreflexia is accompanied by a decreased pelvic limb withdrawal reflex.

Ideally, spinal reflexes should be performed with the patient in lateral recumbency. If this is not possible, the withdrawal reflexes and the patellar reflex can be performed with the patient standing with adequate support provided, but beware that it can be difficult to isolate spinal reflex activity in patients that resist or lose their balance. The perineal reflex can be performed with the patient in any position. The cutaneous trunci reflex is generally performed with the patient standing or sitting.

Thoracic Limb Spinal Reflex Testing

The spinal cord segments for thoracic limb spinal reflexes are C6–T2. Although an exhaustive list of thoracic limb reflex testing is provided subsequently, the authors generally limit their testing to the withdrawal reflex, as it reliably provides sufficient information to assess the nerves and spinal cord segments pertinent to thoracic limb reflex arc evaluation.

Withdrawal (Flexor) Reflex

Anatomy: (Figure 1.7)

- Afferent, sensory nerves: Median nerve, ulnar nerve, and radial nerve
- Spinal cord segments: C6–T2
- Efferent, motor nerves: Median nerve, ulnar nerve, musculocutaneous nerve, and axillary nerve

Clinical evaluation: To perform the withdrawal reflex, use your fingers to pinch the webbing between toes or pinch a digit on the upper limb (do not attempt to perform the withdrawal reflex on the limb touching the ground) (Video 1.18). If you do not observe the reflex with a light pinch, you might need to pinch harder. With an intact reflex, you will observe flexion at every joint (shoulder, elbow, and carpus) in conjunction with the pinching stimulus.

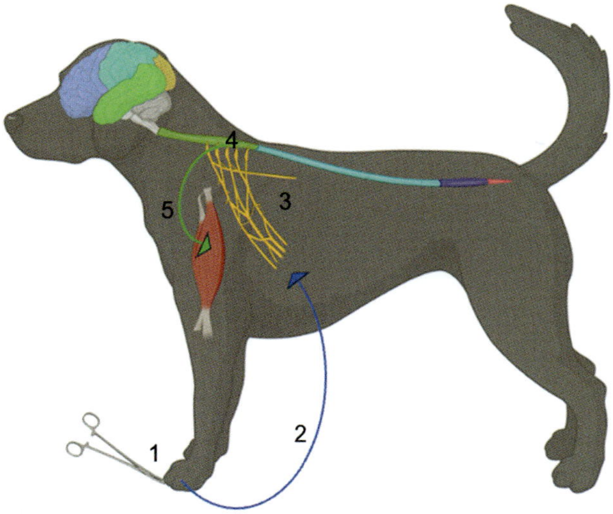

FIGURE 1.7 An illustration of the flexor withdrawal reflex anatomy of the thoracic limb. (1) Nociceptors are stimulated in the digits; (2) sensory input through the median, ulnar, and radial nerves (depending on where the noxious stimulus is applied) and travels through the brachial plexus (3) to the C6–T2 spinal cord segments (4). Motor output is then through the nerve roots of the axillary, musculocutaneous, median, and ulnar nerves (5) to the flexor muscles of the limb. *Source:* Created with www.biorender.com.

VIDEO 1.18 A flexor withdrawal reflex is often performed with the patient in lateral recumbency and initiated with a noxious stimulus to the digits. The entire limb should be withdrawn to the body with good strength, and there should be complete flexion of the carpus and elbow visible.

Biceps Tendon Reflex

Anatomy:

- Afferent, sensory nerve: Musculocutaneous nerve
- Spinal cord segments: C6–C8
- Efferent, motor nerve: Musculocutaneous nerve

Clinical evaluation: To perform the biceps reflex, gently extend the upper limb at the level of the shoulder and the elbow. Place your thumb at the cranial aspect of the elbow joint over the tendon of insertion for the biceps reflex. Using a reflex hammer, gently strike your thumb. In an intact reflex, you will observe a slight contraction of the biceps muscle in conjunction with striking your thumb. However, this reflex is difficult to elicit/not always present in normal dogs and cats, and is challenging to visualize in long-haired animals.

Triceps Tendon Reflex

Anatomy:

- Afferent, sensory nerve: Radial nerve
- Spinal cord segments: C7–T2
- Efferent, motor nerve: Radial nerve

Clinical evaluation: To perform the triceps reflex, hold the upper antebrachium and gently internally rotate it and flex the elbow to expose the tendon of insertion for the triceps reflex on the caudal aspect of the elbow. Using the blunt end of a reflex hammer, gently strike the tendon. In an intact reflex, you will observe a slight contraction of the triceps muscle in conjunction with striking the tendon. However, this reflex is difficult to elicit/not always present, even in normal dogs and cats.

Extensor Carpi Radialis Reflex

Anatomy:

- Afferent, sensory nerve: Radial nerve
- Spinal cord segments: C7–T2
- Efferent, motor nerve: Radial nerve

Clinical evaluation: To perform the extensor carpi radialis reflex, place one hand underneath the upper elbow to provide support. Use the pointed end of a reflex hammer to gently strike the extensor carpi radialis muscle at its origin. In an intact reflex, you will observe carpal extension in conjunction with striking the muscle. This reflex is difficult to elicit/not always present, even in normal dogs and cats. This may not be a true myotatic reflex, though, as it can be elicited in dogs that have had their radial nerves transected.

Pelvic Limb Spinal Reflex Testing

The spinal cord segments for pelvic limb spinal reflexes are the L4–S1 segments of the spinal cord. Although an exhaustive list of pelvic limb reflex testing is provided subsequently, the authors generally limit their pelvic limb reflex testing to the patellar and withdrawal reflexes, as they reliably provide sufficient information for assessing the nerves and spinal cord segments pertinent to pelvic limb reflex arc evaluation.

Patellar Reflex

Anatomy: (Figure 1.8)

- Afferent, sensory nerve: Femoral nerve
- Spinal cord segments: L4–L6
- Efferent, motor nerve: Femoral nerve

Clinical evaluation: To perform the patellar reflex, place one hand underneath the upper limb to provide support. The limb should be held in gentle flexion. Using the blunt end of a reflex hammer, gently strike the patellar tendon. In an intact reflex, you will observe stifle extension in conjunction with striking the tendon (Videos 1.19 and 1.20). Occasionally, the patellar reflex is absent in the limb when it is upright. The patellar reflex is the only reflex that can be performed on the dependent limb and can sometimes be present in this position despite being absent in the upper limb. A subset of normal, geriatric dogs lack patellar reflexes despite having normal femoral nerve and L4–L6 spinal cord segment function.

VIDEO 1.19 The patella reflex is performed by striking the patella tendon when the animal is in lateral recumbency, with the stifle slightly flexed. The response should be a brisk extension of the limb due to a reflex contraction of the quadriceps muscle.

VIDEO 1.20 A dog with acute flaccid paralysis and Schiff–Sherrington exhibits reduced to absent pelvic limb patella and flexor withdrawal reflexes.

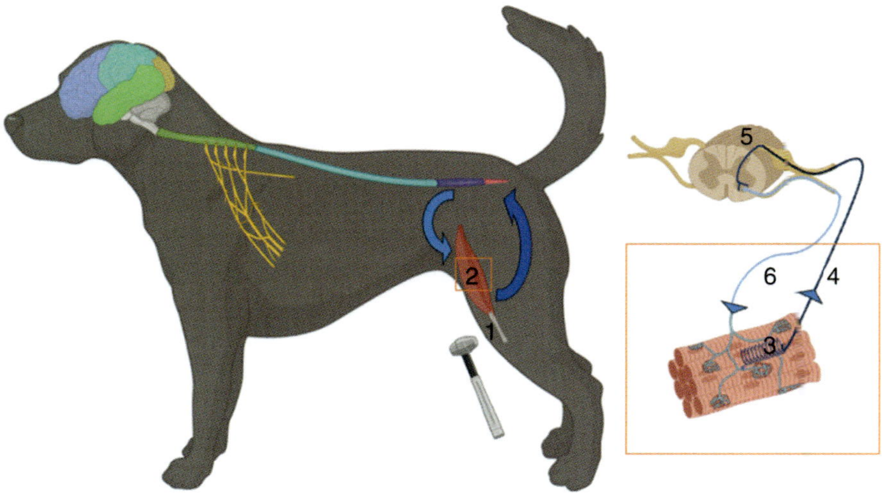

FIGURE 1.8 An illustration of the neuroanatomy responsible for the patella reflex. (1) The patella tendon is struck, which causes contraction of the quadriceps muscle (2) by indirectly stretching the muscle spindles (3), which activate the 1A afferent fibers (4) sending a sensory message to the L4–L6 spinal cord segments (5). The sensory fibers synapse directly onto the motor neurons (6) of the femoral nerve. *Source:* Created with www.biorender.com.

Withdrawal (Flexor) Reflex

Anatomy:

- Afferent, sensory nerve: Sciatic nerve
- Spinal cord segments: L6–S1
- Efferent, motor nerve: Sciatic nerve

Clinical evaluation: To perform the withdrawal reflex, use your fingers to pinch the webbing between digits 4 and 5 or the fifth digit on the upper limb (do not attempt to perform the withdrawal reflex on the limb touching the ground). Afferent information from the dorsal aspect of this digit is carried via the cutaneous branches of the fibular nerve, and information from the plantar aspect is carried via the cutaneous branches of the tibial nerve. If you do not observe the reflex with a light pinch, you might need to pinch harder. In an intact reflex, you will observe flexion at every joint (hip, stifle, tarsus) in conjunction with the pinching stimulus.

The flexion of all joints in the pelvic limb is mediated via the sciatic nerve, with the exception of the hip. The main flexors of the hip are the iliopsoas muscle and the rectus femoris. Both receive efferent innervation from the femoral nerve, which originates from the L4–L6 spinal cord segments. The iliopsoas muscle is also innervated by all of the nerves originating from the lumbar spinal cord segments cranial to L4. The skin of the first digit is innervated by cutaneous branches of the saphenous nerve branch of the femoral nerve. In patients with complete sciatic dysfunction, they will lack the ability to flex the stifle and the hock (and will lack sensation) when the fifth digit is pinched but will flex the hip when the first digit is pinched.

Cranial Tibial Reflex

Anatomy:

- Afferent, sensory nerve: Fibular nerve (branch of the sciatic nerve)

- Spinal cord segments: L6–L7
- Efferent, motor nerve: Fibular nerve

Clinical evaluation: To perform the cranial tibial reflex, gently support the upper pelvic limb. Using the pointed end of a reflex hammer, gently strike the muscles running along the cranial tibia. In an intact reflex, you will observe slight tarsal flexion. However, this reflex is difficult to elicit/not always present, even in normal dogs and cats. Like the extensor carpi radialis reflex, this also might not be a true reflex.

Gastrocnemius Reflex

Anatomy:

- Afferent, sensory nerve: Tibial nerve (branch of the sciatic nerve)
- Spinal cord segments: L7–S1
- Efferent, motor nerve: Tibial nerve

Clinical evaluation: To perform the gastrocnemius reflex, gently grasp the metatarsal region and flex and internally rotate the tarsus to expose the common calcaneal tendon. Using the blunt end of a reflex hammer, strike the tendon. In an intact reflex, you will observe a slight extension of the tarsus, and you may also observe a brief twitch of the caudal thigh muscles. However, this reflex is difficult to elicit/not always present, even in normal dogs and cats.

Other Segmental Spinal Reflexes

Cutaneous Trunci Muscle Reflex

Anatomy:

- Afferent, sensory nerves: segmental spinal nerves of T2–L5
- Spinal cord segments: C8–T1
- Efferent, motor nerve: Lateral thoracic nerve

Clinical evaluation: To perform the cutaneous trunci muscle reflex, use a pair of hemostats to lightly pinch the skin. Start on one side at the level of the wing of the ilium, slightly off midline. In an intact reflex, you will observe the skin over both sides of the thorax twitch (Video 1.21). If you do not observe this reflex at this level, then continue to pinch skin more progressively further cranially until the reflex is observed, or until you reach the cervicothoracic junction. The location at which the cutaneous trunci reflex is observed is called the "cutaneous trunci cutoff" (Video 1.22). Once you determine the cutaneous trunci cutoff on one side, repeat on the other side.

VIDEO 1.21 The cutaneous trunci muscle reflex (formerly the panniculus reflex) is evaluated by pinching the skin on the dorsal trunk between T2 and the sixth lumbar vertebra, observing the contraction of the cutaneous trunci muscles bilaterally, which produces a twitch in the overlying skin as seen in this normal dog.

VIDEO 1.22 An English bulldog exhibits an absent cutaneous trunci muscle (panniculus) reflex bilaterally until the skin is pinched on the left side in the cranial thoracic region. This indicates a lesion is likely immediately cranial to the site.

This reflex involves segmental spinal nerves that carry sensory information into the spinal cord at approximately the level being pinched from its most caudal aspect over the L6 vertebral body. An interneuron travels from the segment cranially on both sides of the spinal cord to synapse with the motor neuron cell bodies, which are located in the ventral horns of the spinal cord in segments C8–T1. These motor neurons comprise the lateral thoracic nerve, which innervates the cutaneous trunci muscle. Because the impulse travels to both sides, pinching the skin on one side will lead to bilateral contraction of the cutaneous trunci muscles. The caudal extent for which the reflex can be elicited varies in dogs. In most normal dogs, the cutaneous trunci reflex begins at the level of the L6 vertebra. This reflex is not always reliably elicited, even in normal dogs, and is difficult to elicit in cats. Gently pulling on a small bunch of fur rather than pinching the skin may be more effective in cats.

Perineal Reflex

Anatomy:

- Afferent, sensory nerve: Pudendal nerve
- Spinal cord segments: S1–S3
- Efferent, motor nerve: Pudendal nerve

Clinical evaluation: To perform the perineal reflex, gently pinch the skin of the perineal region using a hemostat on both sides. In an intact reflex, you will observe immediate tail flexion and contraction of the external anal sphincter.

Head and Spinal Palpation

Palpation of the head is useful in finding masses, muscle atrophy, pain, persistent fontanelles, and abnormal skull conformation. In addition to palpating for masses, gently retropulse each eye to check for discomfort and/or retrobulbar mass effects. Palpate the temporalis muscles to look for either unilateral or bilateral atrophy. Gently open the mouth to assess for any pain associated with the temporomandibular joints, decreased range of motion, or decreased jaw tone. To check for a persistent fontanelle, gently palpate the dorsal-most aspect of the skull. Persistent fontanelles may be accompanied by a domed head that extends laterally past the zygomatic arches in dogs and cats with hydrocephalus. Pressing on the skull slightly dorsal to the zygomatic arches can sometimes lead to a painful response in animals with structural brain disease.

Palpation of the vertebral column is useful for detecting painful regions, masses, epaxial muscle atrophy, swelling, and abnormal vertebral curvature (e.g. kyphosis or scoliosis). Palpation and range of motion assessments are generally performed at the end of the neurological examination, since they are capable of inducing discomfort that may make the animal more difficult to examine further. Generally, if a region is suspected to be painful based on the patient's history and posture, it should be evaluated last. To palpate the thoracolumbar vertebral column, place the dominant hand over the patient's back, and use the nondominant hand to apply light counter support ventral to the thorax/abdomen. Avoid pushing dorsally on the abdomen, as this can reveal abdominal pain that may be confused as back pain. If no pain develops with light palpation, then proceed with stronger palpation. Place one finger or knuckle on either side of the midline, and gently apply pressure ventrally *in between spinous processes*, and travel cranially or caudally. To check for lumbosacral pain, place one hand ventral to the pelvis to extend the lumbosacral joint, raise the pelvis, and use your other hand to apply pressure ventrally over the L7. Performing the tail range of motion can also help in disclosing lumbosacral discomfort. Subtle evidence of thoracolumbar/lumbosacral pain or discomfort may consist of mild abdominal/epaxial muscle tensing. More overt evidence may include vocalizations, the patient trying to bite/escape.

In dogs or cats with obvious signs of neck pain (low head carriage, cervical muscle fasciculations), cervical palpation can be skipped. To palpate the cervical vertebral column, place one hand on either side of the dog's neck and palpate the articular processes. Direct pressure toward midline, working caudally to cranially from the cervicothoracic junction to the craniocervical junction. If no overt evidence of neck pain is observed with palpation, then cervical range of motion can be performed to assess for neck pain. Turn the patient's head toward either side. A normal dog or cat can touch its nose to its lateral thorax. Extending the head upward is also acceptable. The authors advise against flexing the neck ventrally, as this maneuver can lead to exacerbation of neurological dysfunction in patients with abnormal atlantoaxial joints. In cases where patient disposition precludes performing cervical range of motion, a treat can be waved slowly in front of the patient to see if it turns its neck to track it. Subtle evidence of cervical pain may consist of cervical muscle fasciculations or tensing during palpation or reluctance to have the head moved in one or multiple directions. More overt evidence may consist of vocalization/the patient trying to bite/escape or exacerbation of a thoracic limb nerve root signature.

NOCICEPTION TESTING

For pain to be perceived consciously, the sensory component of the peripheral nerves and their spinal cord segments, the spinal cord and brainstem and the related thalamocortex system must all be intact and functional (Figure 1.9). The nociceptive fibers are located deep in the spinal cord white matter and project to both sides of the spinal cord, forming a multisynaptic bilateral network. Therefore, only a severe bilateral spinal cord lesion impairs nociception in cases of

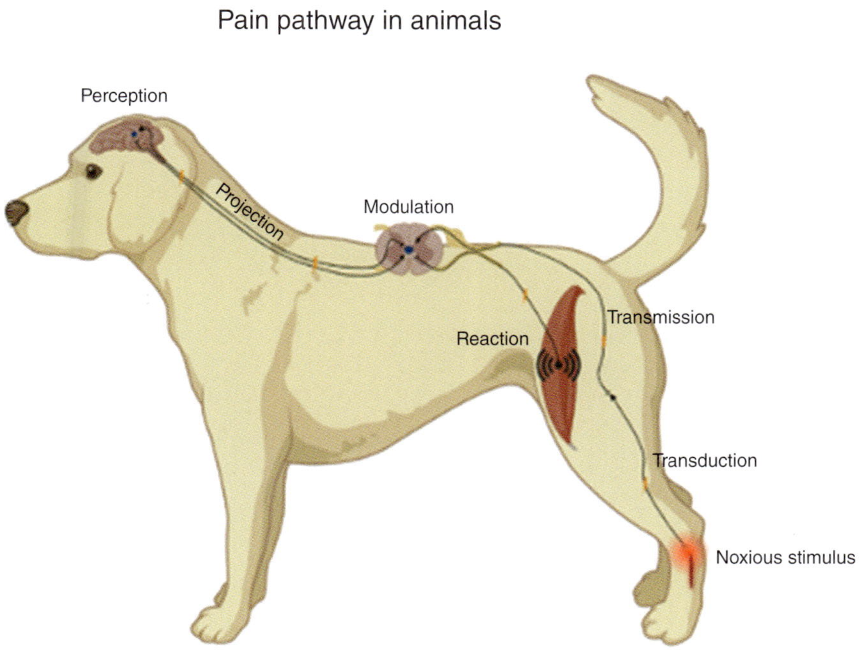

FIGURE 1.9 An illustration of the pain pathways in a dog and the mechanisms of transmission. *Source:* Created with www.biorender.com.

spinal cord dysfunction, or severe damage to a nerve in the periphery for patients displaying monoplegia. For this reason, nociception testing is a useful prognostic indicator in cases of disease. Pain perception must be assessed in any region demonstrating plegia (limb(s), tail, and the perineal region). The expected reaction is a behavioral response such as turning the head, trying to bite, or vocalization. The animal is placed on its side, ideally with a second person talking to it or stroking it to distract its attention. A gentle squeeze is applied initially to the digits to elicit the withdrawal reflex. If the animal does not exhibit a behavioral response to a gentle squeeze, heavy pressure is then applied.

Withdrawal of the limb is only the flexor reflex and should not be taken as evidence of pain sensation. Other areas of cutaneous sensory testing are the tail, perineum, and perianal region, as well as the cutaneous sensory distribution of the thoracic and pelvic limb nerves.

Lesion Localization, Clinical Reasoning, and the Differential Diagnosis

CHAPTER 2

Simon R. Platt[1] and Susan A. Arnold[2]

[1] *Department of Veterinary Clinical Sciences, College of Veterinary Medicine, Oklahoma State University, Stillwater, OK, USA*

[2] *Department of Veterinary Clinical Sciences, University of Minnesota, St. Paul, MN, USA*

This chapter details the functional neuroanatomical components of the nervous system necessary for clinical lesion localization after performing the neurological examination. Additionally, we discuss the principles of clinical reasoning in veterinary neurology, emphasizing how lesion localization, patient signalment, the temporal evolution of clinical signs, the symmetry of clinical signs, and the presence of pain can all contribute to refining a differential diagnosis list. The clinical characteristics of the main mechanisms of neurological disease – vascular, inflammatory, traumatic, toxic, anomalous, metabolic, idiopathic, neoplastic, nutritional, and degenerative – are reviewed.

LESION LOCALIZATION

Lesion localization involves associating the abnormalities found on the neurological exam with specific regions of the nervous system (Figure 2.1). This can help with establishing a differential diagnosis list, in determining the most appropriate diagnostic tests, and in assessing the prognosis.

Each region is associated with specific clinical signs when affected by disease and some non-specific signs. The following sections outline the key localizations and their associated clinical signs:

1. **Forebrain** (Chapter 1)
   The forebrain includes the cerebrum and thalamus. Lesions in this region result in:
   - *Mental status:* Altered behavior and/or a decreased level of consciousness.
   - *Posture:* Head pressing, head turn, and body turn (pleurothotonus) toward the side of dysfunction.
   - *Gait:* Circling or pacing, often toward the side of the lesion without motor deficits or ataxia.
   - *Postural reactions:* Contralateral deficits in proprioceptive placing and hopping tests.
   - *Cranial nerves (CNs):* Contralateral menace response deficit with normal vision and palpebral reflex; facial hypoalgesia on the contralateral side.
   - *Spinal reflexes:* Intact.

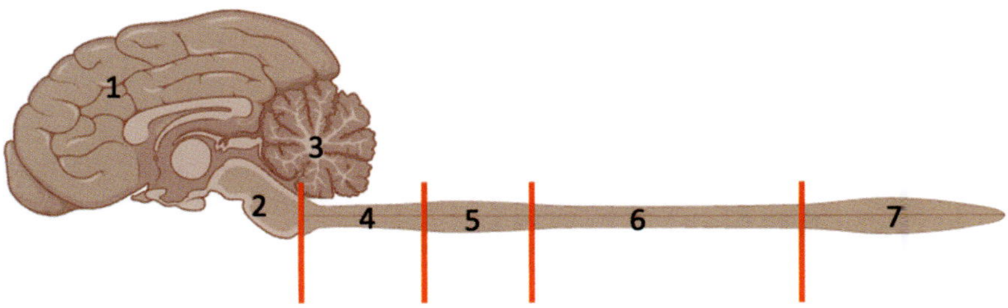

FIGURE 2.1 Localization segments of the central nervous system. (1) Forebrain (cerebrum and thalamus). (2) Brainstem (see Figure 2.2). (3) Cerebellum. (4) C1–C5 spinal cord segments. (5) C6–T2 spinal cord segments. (6) T3–L3 spinal cord segments. (7) L4–S3 spinal cord segments – this is often further divided into L4–L5 and L6–S2, relating to the femoral and sciatic origins, respectively. S1–S3 segments are sometimes dealt with separately as being the origin of the pelvic and pudendal nerves. The caudal segments (previously called coccygeal segments) are caudal to the S1–S3, giving rise to the caudal nerves innervating the tail. *Source:* Created with www.biorender.com.

- *Other findings:* Seizures (focal or generalized), narcolepsy-cataplexy, cervical hyperaesthesia, and movement disorders.

2. Cerebellum

The cerebellum coordinates movement and balance. Lesions in this region result in:

- *Mental status:* May be disoriented due to vestibular dysfunction; otherwise, no effect on the level of consciousness or behavior.
- *Posture:* Wide-based stance, head tilt (contralateral to the side of the cerebellar dysfunction), opisthotonus, decerebrate rigidity (rostral cerebellar dysfunction).
- *Gait:* Cerebellar ataxia: Dysmetria (hypermetria or hypometria) without weakness.
- *Postural reactions:* Delayed initiation and then exaggerated, dysmetric response.
- *CNs:* Vestibular signs – typically absent unless the lesion extends to the flocculonodular lobe and caudal peduncles. A paradoxical vestibular syndrome is possible. Menace response – decreased ipsilateral to the cerebellar dysfunction with normal vision and palpebral reflex. Mydriatic pupil possible with ipsilateral interpositel nucleus lesion.
- *Spinal reflexes:* Intact.

3. **Vestibular System**

The vestibular system maintains balance and spatial orientation. Lesions can be peripheral (inner ear or vestibular nerve; CN VIII) or central (brainstem or cerebellum).

- *Peripheral vestibular signs:* Head tilt, horizontal or rotary nystagmus, falling or rolling toward the side of the lesion.
- *Central vestibular signs (brainstem):* Horizontal, rotary, vertical, or variable nystagmus; ipsilateral proprioceptive deficits; and mentation changes, along with the potential for other ipsilateral CN deficits. With cerebellar lesions, proprioceptive deficits are generally ipsilateral to the cerebellar lesion but contralateral to the direction of the head tilt.

4. **Brainstem (Non-vestibular)** (Figure 2.2)

The brainstem controls cardiovascular and respiratory function and is the location for most of the CN nuclei. Lesions in this region result in:

- *Mental status:* A decreased level of consciousness is possible.
- *Posture:* Decerebrate rigidity (dorsal midbrain dysfunction), opisthotonus, and head tilt possible.

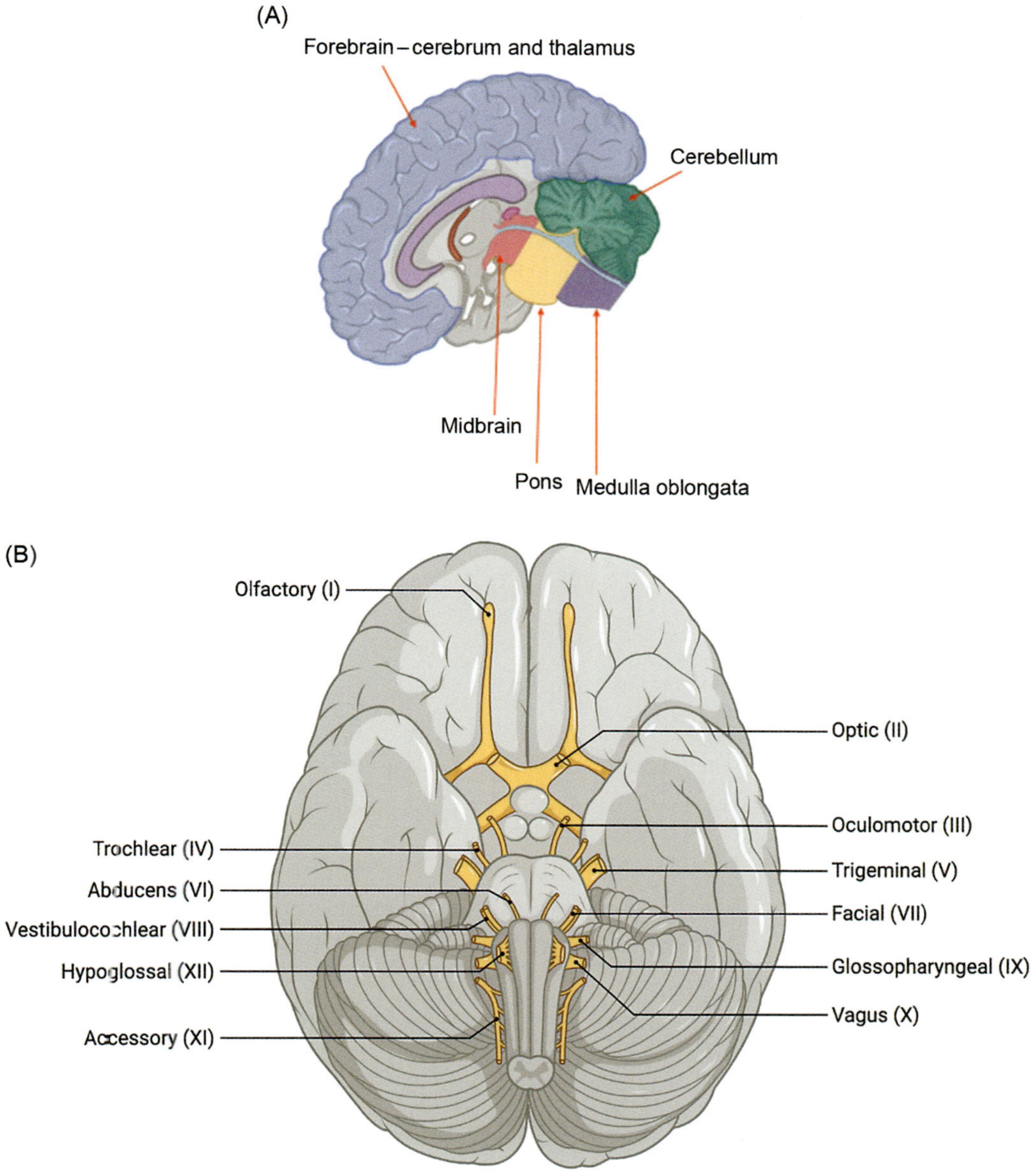

FIGURE 2.2 (A) The intracranial central nervous system anatomy, including the segments of the brainstem. (B) The peripheral portions of the cranial nerves (CNs) and their relation to the forebrain (CNs I and II) and the brainstem (CNs III–XII). *Source:* Created with www.biorender.com.

- *Gait:* Proprioceptive ataxia, vestibular ataxia. Hemiparesis/-plegia or tetraparesis/-plegia.
- *Postural reactions:* Deficits ipsilateral to the side of dysfunction or in all four limbs.
- *CNs:* Multiple ipsilateral CNs from CN III-XII may be affected.
- *Spinal reflexes:* Intact.
- *Other findings:* Respiratory or cardiovascular abnormalities in severe cases. Neck pain may be present.

5. **C1–C5 Spinal Cord Segments**
   Lesions in this region affect the cervical spinal cord and result in:

   - *Mental status:* Normal.
   - *Posture:* Ipsilateral spontaneous knuckling, low head carriage, cervical ventroflexion, torticollis, scoliosis.
   - *Gait:* Proprioceptive ataxia. Hemiparesis/-plegia or tetraparesis/-plegia.
   - *Postural reactions:* Deficits ipsilateral to the side of dysfunction or in all four limbs.
   - *CNs:* Normal.
   - *Spinal reflexes:* Intact; occasionally, the withdrawal reflex may be reduced.
   - *Other findings:* Hypoventilation in tetraplegic patients due to the involvement of the axons that lead to the phrenic and intercostal nerves. Ipsilateral Horner syndrome with severe myelopathies. Phantom scratching associated with a large mid-cervical syringomyelia extending to the superficial dorsal horn ipsilateral to the scratching. Pain may be present at the site of the lesion.

6. **C6–T2 Spinal Cord Segments**
   Lesions in this region affect the cervicothoracic spinal cord and result in:

   - *Mental status:* Normal.
   - *Posture:* Ipsilateral spontaneous knuckling.
   - *Gait:* Proprioceptive ataxia. Hemiparesis/-plegia or tetraparesis/-plegia. Lameness (nerve root signature). Two-engine gait: short, choppy thoracic limb gait; long, lopey pelvic limb gait.
   - *Postural reactions:* Deficits ipsilateral to the side of dysfunction or in all four limbs.
   - *CNs:* Normal.
   - *Spinal reflexes:* Decreased or absent in the thoracic limbs. Normal to increased in the pelvic limbs. Reduced or absent cutaneous trunci reflex ipsilaterally if a lesion affects the C8–T1 segments.
   - *Other findings:* Muscle tone decreased or absent in the thoracic limbs, increased in the pelvic limbs. Muscle atrophy in the thoracic limbs (ipsilateral). Pain may be present at the site of the lesion. Horner syndrome – second-order neuron if the T1–T3 segments are affected. Hypoventilation possible in tetraplegic patients.

7. **T3–L3 Spinal Cord Segments**
   Lesions in this region affect the thoracolumbar spinal cord and result in:

   - *Mental status:* Normal.
   - *Posture:* Ipsilateral spontaneous knuckling, kyphosis, lordosis, scoliosis; Schiff–Sherrington posture with acute and severe myelopathy.
   - *Gait:* Proprioceptive ataxia. Paraparesis/-plegia, monoparesis/-plegia of one pelvic limb.
   - *Postural reactions:* Delayed or absent in pelvic limbs (ipsilateral to the lesion). Thoracic limbs are normal.
   - *CNs:* Normal.
   - *Spinal reflexes:* Normal in the thoracic limbs. Normal to increased in the pelvic limbs. Reduced or absent cutaneous trunci reflex caudal to the spinal cord segment affected. Pinching the skin (dermatome) at the level of two vertebrae caudal to the lesion does not elicit any reflex.

- *Other findings:* Muscle tone is normal to increased in the pelvic limbs. Pain may be present at the site of the lesion. Urinary retention is possible.

8. **L4–L6 Spinal Cord Segments**
   Lesions in this region affect the lumbar spinal cord and result in:
   - *Mental status:* Normal.
   - *Posture:* Non-weight-bearing lameness (Nerve root signature).
   - *Gait:* Paraparesis/-plegia, monoparesis/-plegia of one pelvic limb.
   - *Postural reactions:* Delayed or absent in pelvic limbs (ipsilateral to the lesion). Thoracic limbs normal.
   - *CNs:* Normal.
   - *Spinal reflexes:* Normal in the thoracic limbs. Intact withdrawal reflex with decreased or absent ipsilateral patellar reflex.
   - *Other findings:* Muscle tone is decreased or absent in the quadriceps group with possible atrophy of these muscles. Pain may be present at the site of the lesion. Urinary retention is possible.
9. **L6-Cd Spinal Cord Segments**
   Lesions in this region affect the lumbosacral spinal cord and result in:
   - *Mental status:* Normal.
   - *Posture:* Spontaneous knuckling, low tail carriage, plantigrade stance.
   - *Gait:* Paresis of both pelvic limbs (paraparesis) or one pelvic limb (monoparesis). Difficulty rising, but the ability to walk typically remains intact. Paresis/-plegia of the tail is possible.
   - *Postural reactions:* Delayed or absent in pelvic limbs (ipsilateral to the lesion). Thoracic limbs normal.
   - *CNs:* Normal.
   - *Spinal reflexes:* Normal in thoracic limbs. Decreased or absent withdrawal reflex in the ipsilateral pelvic limb, decreased or absent perineal reflex. Patellar reflex present in both pelvic limbs and can sometimes appear exaggerated (termed “pseudohyperreflexia”) due to a reduction in the antagonistic sciatic-innervated muscles.
   - *Other findings:* Muscle tone is decreased or absent in the sciatic-innervated muscles. Pain may be present at the site of the lesion. Urinary and fecal incontinence is possible.

NEUROMUSCULAR SYSTEM

Lesions in the neuromuscular system affect the peripheral nerves, neuromuscular junction, or muscles and result in:

- *Mental status:* Normal.
- *Posture:* Spontaneous knuckling, palmigrade, and plantigrade stance. May be unable to bear weight.
- *Gait:* Paresis/-plegia (flaccid) in the affected limbs with polyneuropathies, but exercise-induced weakness can be seen with muscle and neuromuscular junction diseases.
- *Postural reactions:* Can be normal with motor peripheral neuropathies, neuromuscular junction

and muscle disease, but delayed with sensory peripheral neuropathies. If there is severe generalized weakness, postural reactions can appear reduced or absent.

- *CNs:* Variable involvement depending on disease; CN VII, VIII, IX, and X might be affected with polyneuropathy.
- *Spinal reflexes:* Decreased or absent in affected limbs with polyneuropathies, but can appear intact with myopathies and with neuromuscular junction diseases unless repeatedly challenged.
- *Other findings:* Muscle atrophy may be present and reduced muscle tone in affected limbs. Self-mutilation may be seen with sensory peripheral neuropathies.

DIFFERENTIAL DIAGNOSIS

The process of distinguishing a particular disease or condition from others that present with similar clinical features underlies the creation of a differential diagnosis list. The mnemonic **VITAMIN D** (Vascular, Inflammatory, Toxic, Traumatic, Anomalous, Metabolic, Idiopathic, Neoplastic, Nutritional, Degenerative) is commonly used to categorize neurological disorders. Each category has distinct clinical characteristics that aid in their consideration for a specific case especially when using the concepts of clinical reasoning (see next).

CLINICAL CHARACTERISTICS OF THE NEUROLOGICAL DIFFERENTIAL DIAGNOSES

1. **Vascular**
   Vascular disorders result from disruptions in blood flow to the nervous system, such as strokes (ischemic or hemorrhagic) or thromboembolism.
   - *Clinical signs:* Peracute or acute onset, nonprogressive or improving, focal, often asymmetric (lateralizing) neurological deficits (e.g. hemiparesis and circling).
2. **Inflammatory**
   Inflammatory disorders include infectious (bacteria, rickettsia, fungi, protozoa, viruses) and noninfectious causes, such as immune-mediated meningoencephalitis.
   - *Clinical signs:* Signs usually progress without medical treatment, although they may wax and wane in some cases early after onset. Neurological deficits can refer to a focal or multifocal lesion, can be asymmetrical or symmetrical, and can be accompanied by fever and pain.
3. **Traumatic**
   Traumatic injuries result from physical damage to the nervous system, such as fractures, contusions, or lacerations.
   - *Clinical signs:* Peracute or acute onset. Signs usually remain static or improve over time with supportive treatment. Neurological deficits can be bilateral or lateralized and often refer to a focal lesion; however, multiple lesions frequently exist. Due to the secondary injury associated with central nervous system (CNS) trauma, clinical signs can progress during the first 24–72 hours, and undetected vertebral column instability can cause delayed deterioration in clinical signs. The injury is usually accompanied by pain.
4. **Toxic**
   Toxic disorders are caused by exposure to neurotoxins, such as lead, organophosphates, or certain medications.

- *Clinical signs:* Acute or subacute onset, bilaterally symmetrical or diffuse, nonpainful and nonprogressive neurological signs, often accompanied by systemic signs (e.g. vomiting and diarrhea).

5. **Anomalous**
Anomalous disorders are congenital or developmental abnormalities of the nervous system. Malformations of the cranium and vertebral column do not always affect the nervous system and are often incidental findings on imaging.

   - *Clinical signs:* Onset in young animals (<2 years old); nonprogressive or slowly progressive, bilateral/diffuse with breed predispositions helpful in their recognition.

6. **Metabolic**

   Metabolic disorders result from systemic diseases that affect the nervous system, such as hepatic encephalopathy or hypoglycemia.

   - *Clinical signs:* Clinical onset of neurological signs is variable but is most often acute, even though accompanying signs of systemic disease are often subacute to chronic. Diffuse nonspecific signs, bilateral (often symmetrical) deficits referable to the forebrain or peripheral neuropathies without clinical signs of pain are the most common. Most of these conditions tend to wax and wane with time, with accompanying systemic signs.

7. **Idiopathic**
Idiopathic disorders have no known cause and are often diagnoses of exclusion. The term should be reserved for specific documented conditions or syndromes of unknown etiology rather than for cases where a diagnosis could not be or has not been confirmed.

   - *Clinical signs:* Variable, often breed-specific or episodic.

8. **Neoplastic**
Neoplastic disorders involve primary or metastatic tumors of the nervous system. Neoplasia is more common in animals >5 years old, but can occur at any age.

   - *Clinical signs:* Chronic progressive neurological deficits, although acute decompensation can occur. Neurological deficits can be asymmetrical or symmetrical, and often suggest a focal lesion.

9. **Nutritional**
Nutritional disorders result from deficiencies or imbalances in essential nutrients.

   - *Clinical signs:* Neurological signs are typically bilateral (often symmetrical), and no pain is noted (except in patients with pathological vertebral fractures due to nutritional secondary hyperparathyroidism). The onset of signs is variable (acute or chronic), and they are often slowly progressive. The distribution of signs can be diffuse or multifocal, as some nutritional diseases can affect selective areas of the CNS. On the other hand, painful pathological vertebral fractures following a relatively minor trauma are unfortunately still seen in puppies and kittens due to secondary nutritional hyperparathyroidism.

10. **Degenerative**
Degenerative disorders involve progressive loss of nervous tissue due to genetic or age-related factors.

    - *Clinical signs:* The clinical signs typically have a chronic onset; they are bilateral (often symmetrical), with slow progression. The age of onset is variable: some diseases may affect young, mainly purebred animals shortly after birth (such as cerebellar cortical degeneration); less frequently, adult animals may be affected (e.g. degenerative myelopathy). Degenerative diseases can also affect structures that surround the nervous system (bones, intervertebral discs, articular joints) and secondarily cause neurological deficits, mainly due to compression of the nervous tissue, as seen with cervical spondylomyelopathy, intervertebral disc protrusion, intervertebral disc extrusion (Hansen type I), synovial cysts, and degenerative lumbosacral stenosis.

CLINICAL REASONING AND THE DIFFERENTIAL DIAGNOSIS

The neurological exam provides the initial data necessary for clinical reasoning. For example, a dog with paraparesis, absent proprioception, and hyperreflexia in the pelvic limbs localizes the lesion to the T3–L3 spinal cord segment. By considering the clinical characteristics of the VITAMIN D categories (see earlier), the clinician can prioritize differential diagnoses. In this case, vascular (ischemic myelopathy), inflammatory (discospondylitis), degenerative (intervertebral disc disease), and neoplastic causes would be considered.

Advanced diagnostic tools, such as MRI, cerebrospinal fluid (CSF) analysis, and bloodwork, are often required to confirm the diagnosis. However, clinical reasoning guides the selection of appropriate tests and ensures a systematic approach to diagnosis.

Clinical reasoning in veterinary neurology is a multifaceted process that integrates a wide range of information to arrive at an accurate diagnosis. Beyond the neurological examination itself, factors such as the patient's breed, age, sex, the symmetry or asymmetry of clinical signs, and the presence of pain during the examination play critical roles in refining the differential diagnosis list. These elements provide additional layers of context that help clinicians prioritize potential causes of neurological dysfunction and tailor their diagnostic approach.

THE ROLE OF SIGNALMENT IN CLINICAL REASONING

1. **Breed Predispositions**
   Certain neurological disorders have a strong breed predisposition, making the patient's breed a valuable clue in clinical reasoning. For example:
   - *Degenerative myelopathy:* Commonly seen in German shepherds, boxers, and Pembroke Welsh Corgis.
   - *Chiari-like malformation and syringomyelia:* Frequently diagnosed in Cavalier King Charles spaniels, Chihuahuas, and French bulldogs.
   - *Idiopathic epilepsy:* Common in breeds such as border collies, Labrador retrievers, and beagles.
   - *Intervertebral disc extrusion:* Predominantly affects chondrodystrophic breeds like dachshunds, Shih Tzus, and French bulldogs.

   Recognizing these breed-specific tendencies allows clinicians to prioritize certain differentials early in the diagnostic process.
2. **Age of the Patient**
   The age of the patient is another critical factor in clinical reasoning, as certain neurological disorders are more likely to occur in specific age groups:
   - *Young animals:* Congenital or anomalous conditions (e.g. hydrocephalus and portosystemic shunts) and infectious diseases (e.g. canine distemper and feline infectious peritonitis) are more common.

- *Adult animals:* Inflammatory, traumatic, and idiopathic conditions (e.g. idiopathic epilepsy and intervertebral disc disease [IVDD]) are frequently seen.
- *Older animals:* Degenerative, neoplastic, and vascular disorders (e.g. degenerative myelopathy, brain tumors, and strokes) are more likely.

For example, a 10-year-old dog with progressive pelvic limb weakness and ataxia would raise suspicion for degenerative myelopathy or a spinal cord tumor, whereas a 6-month-old puppy with similar signs might suggest a congenital anomaly like a spinal malformation.

NEUROLOGICAL SYMMETRY IN CLINICAL REASONING

The symmetry or asymmetry of neurological signs is a key element in localizing lesions and narrowing differential diagnoses. Asymmetrical signs often indicate focal lesions, whereas symmetrical signs may suggest diffuse or systemic disease.

1. **Asymmetrical Signs**
   Asymmetrical deficits, such as circling, hemiparesis, unilateral CN deficits, or unilateral proprioceptive deficits, typically point to a focal lesion in the brain, brainstem, or spinal cord. The most common differentials to consider in this case would be vascular, neoplastic, and inflammatory, unless there has been trauma in the history.
2. **Symmetrical Signs**
   Symmetrical deficits often suggest diffuse or systemic disease. Examples include metabolic disorders (e.g. hepatic encephalopathy), toxicities, nutritional deficiencies, or inflammatory conditions affecting the entire nervous system.

THE PRESENCE OF PAIN AND CLINICAL REASONING

The presence or absence of pain during the neurological examination is a critical diagnostic clue for the location and type of disease. Pain can indicate inflammation, trauma, or compression of neural structures, while the absence of pain may suggest noninflammatory or degenerative conditions or indicate an intramedullary spinal cord localization.

1. **Painful Conditions**
   - *Inflammatory diseases:* Conditions such as meningoencephalitis or discospondylitis often present with significant pain.
   - *Trauma:* Spinal fractures, intervertebral disc herniation, or soft tissue injuries are typically painful.
   - *Neoplasia:* Tumors affecting the vertebrae or peripheral nerves may be painful and cause pain due to compression or invasion of surrounding tissues.
2. **Nonpainful Conditions**
   - *Vascular events:* Strokes or ischemic myelopathies are usually nonpainful unless accompanied by secondary complications.
   - *Anomalous structural lesions*: Syringomyelia, subarachnoid diverticulum, and vertebral anomalies are usually non-painful unless the latter are accompanied by disc herniations.
   - *Nutritional deficiencies:* Commonly nonpainful unless there is a secondary complication such as epidural hemorrhage or fracture.

THE ROLE OF TEMPORAL EVOLUTION OF NEUROLOGICAL DEFICITS IN CLINICAL REASONING

The temporal evolution of clinical signs – how they develop and change over time – is a critical component of clinical reasoning in veterinary neurology. Understanding whether neurological signs are acute or chronic, progressive, improving, static, or waxing and waning provides valuable insights into the underlying disease process. This information, when combined with the aforementioned other factors, such as lesion localization and signalment, helps refine the list of differential diagnoses and guides diagnostic and therapeutic decisions.

1. **Acute Onset**
   Acute neurological signs develop over minutes to hours and are often associated with specific disease processes, which include a vascular, traumatic, or toxic event.

2. **Chronic Onset**
   Chronic neurological signs develop over weeks to months and are often associated with degenerative, neoplastic, or metabolic conditions.

3. **Progressive Signs**
   Progressive neurological signs worsen over time and are characteristic of diseases that continue to damage the nervous system. Progression suggests an ongoing disease process, such as inflammation, neoplasia, or degeneration.

4. **Improving Signs**
   Improving neurological signs indicate a disease process that is resolving or responding to treatment. Improvement suggests a reversible condition, such as a vascular, traumatic, or toxic disorder.

5. **Static Signs**
   Static neurological signs remain unchanged over time and suggest a nonprogressive or stable condition, such as a previous vascular event or congenital anomaly.

6. **Waxing and Waning Signs**
   Waxing and waning neurological signs fluctuate in severity over time and are often associated with metabolic or episodic conditions. Mild compressive lesions (often degenerative) can cause fluctuating clinical signs based on the level of activity of the pet, getting better with rest and reappearing with exercise.

CONCLUSION

Localizing the neurological lesion responsible for the clinical signs depends on the neurological examination. Once this has been achieved, the main aim becomes to develop a list of potential differential diagnoses for which a diagnostic plan can be constructed. Clinical reasoning is an essential skill in veterinary neurology, enabling clinicians to interpret the neurological exam and develop a logical list of differential diagnoses. By understanding the clinical characteristics of the main classifications of neurological disorders (VITAMIN D), veterinarians can systematically approach even the most complex cases. This process not only improves diagnostic accuracy but also enhances patient care by ensuring timely and appropriate treatment.

Circling and Altered Mentation

Case 1—Dog with Progressive Circling and Personality Change

CHAPTER 3.1

Simon R. Platt

Department of Veterinary Clinical Sciences, College of Veterinary Medicine, Oklahoma State University, Stillwater, OK, USA

CASE HISTORY

A 7-year-old spayed female mixed-breed canine was presented for a progressive loss of awareness, a change in behavior, and an acute onset of circling and pacing. The condition was first noted 1 week earlier.

She had otherwise been healthy and was an indoor dog with no exposure to toxins or history of trauma and with no other pets in the house. She had been routinely vaccinated and had received regular prophylactic anti-parasitic medications, with the last dose given 3 weeks earlier. She was being fed a commercial complete canine diet with no supplements and no recent changes.

Her current appetite was considered slightly reduced, but her water intake was assessed as normal. There had been no body-weight changes recently, with a normal urination and defecation history described. There were no respiratory or upper gastrointestinal signs of recent note.

Physical examination was unremarkable.

NEUROLOGICAL EXAMINATION (Video 3.1.1)

VIDEO 3.1.1 Neurological examination of a 7-year-old female spayed mixed breed that presented with circling and behavior change. Aspects of the neurological examination not covered by the video are presumed normal.

The dog was considered mentally dull and confused, getting trapped in between the furniture. She exhibited a mild, intermittent right-sided head and body turn. On gait assessment, she was ambulatory with normal strength and motor function with circles to the right, occasionally becoming aimless with constant pacing.

Postural reactions were reduced on the left side, especially in the pelvic limbs, with a slow initiation to hop on this side and slow, inconsistent recovery of paw placement when the digits were turned over. The right side was not considered normal, but the postural reaction deficits were milder.

Spinal reflexes and the perineal reflex were intact.

There was a reduced or absent left-sided menace response with an intact palpebral reflex. The pupillary light reflex and pupil size were normal bilaterally. Nasal stimulation was normal. There was no cranial muscle atrophy noted, and the jaw tone was appropriate. Tongue movement and the gag reflex were normal. Normal physiologic nystagmus was seen when her head was moved from side to side, and her eyes tracked toward the ceiling when her neck was extended.

There was mild pain on palpation of the neck.

1. **Where is the lesion localization?**
2. **What major disease processes should be considered?**
3. **What tests could you perform to help determine the diagnosis?**

WHERE IS THE LESION LOCALIZATION?

The neurological examination is suggestive of a lesion affecting the forebrain, lateralized to the right (Figure 3.1.1). A multifocal disease cannot be ruled out. The localization is based on a combination of signs exhibited and the neurological examination deficits:

- **Dull and confused mentation**
  These two terms have different connotations. Dullness, sometimes referred to as drowsiness, depression, lethargy, or obtundation, implies a reduced ability to sustain a normal level of consciousness without external stimulation. An improved level of arousal in these cases is usually elicited by speaking to the animal or applying a tactile stimulus. A state of drowsiness does not necessarily imply primary dysfunction of the central nervous system (CNS), but disorders of the brainstem and forebrain are usually responsible. The term confusion implies an inability to think with appropriate speed and clarity. The word "inappropriate" is sometimes used in place of this term. Assessing an animal to be either normally aware or confused relies on an interpretation of an animal's behavior. Behavior suggestive of confusion includes getting trapped in corners or under furniture, unprovoked vocalization, staring at the floor or wall for

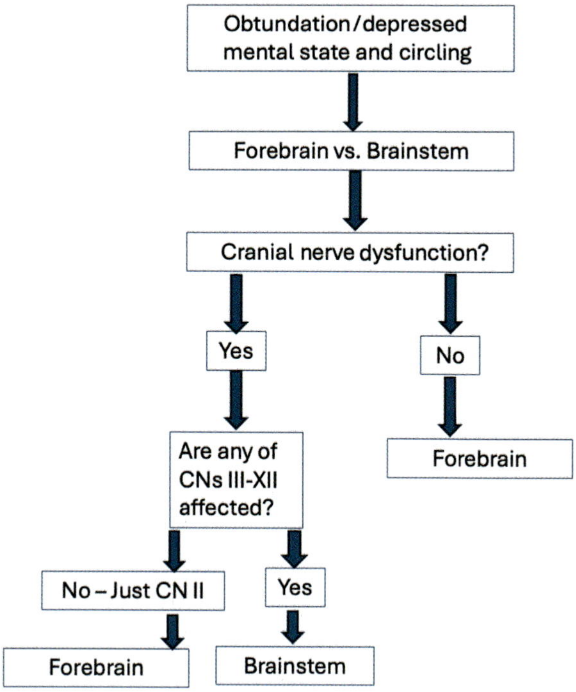

FIGURE 3.1.1 Simplified algorithmic overview of localization for obtundation.

protracted periods of time, and loss of house training. Such activity strongly suggests a forebrain lesion.

- **Circling to the right**
  Circling in relation to a structural neurological disease is related to an intracranial disease. This can be associated with forebrain, brainstem, or cerebellar disease. Most commonly, the latter two locations are associated with vestibular dysfunction when circling is noted. Forebrain lesions (cerebrum and thalamus) that are unilateral or asymmetric may cause the pet to walk in circles or turn predominantly in one direction. The circles with cerebral disease are usually wide and *toward* the side of the lesion, while the circles with thalamic disease are most often tight in nature. It is rare that circles from a forebrain lesion would not be associated with a change in consciousness and/or behavior, and such associated signs can help with the lesion localization (Figure 3.1.2). In this dog's case, the circling can be compatible with a right-sided cerebral lesion. An important distinction between the circling observed with forebrain lesions and that with brainstem or cerebellar lesions is that animals with forebrain lesions do not display overt paresis or ataxia, unlike those with brainstem or cerebellar lesions.

- **Head and body turn to the right**
  The terms head turn and pleurothotonus are often used interchangeably to refer to postural abnormalities. A head turn specifically refers to the deviation of the head and neck in the horizontal plane, whereas pleurothotonus involves a twisting of the head, neck, and trunk to one side. It is important to differentiate a head turn from a head tilt, with the latter being an abnormal head posture characterized by rotation of the median plane of the head along the axis of the body (one ear is held lower than the other). Additional terms that can describe similar deviations in head and neck posture include torticollis, laterocollis, and scoliosis. The presence of a head turn has been attributable to lesions affecting the ipsilateral forebrain, either the cerebrum or rostral thalamus. The understanding of why a head turn manifests itself in cats and dogs remains elusive. Infrequently, a head turn can be associated with vestibular, cerebellar, or cervical spinal cord localization. In dogs with brainstem disease, a head turn is accompanied by either a head tilt only, a body turn only, or both a head tilt and a body turn. Cerebellar disease causes an ipsilateral body turn with a contralateral head tilt and, rarely, a head turn. With cervical spinal cord disease, it is also rare to have a head turn in isolation. This finding could be a result of denervation and atrophy of the ipsilateral paraspinal muscles, causing an imbalance of muscle tone, which could lead to deviation of the head and neck away from the lesion. In this dog's case, the findings are compatible with a right-sided forebrain lesion.

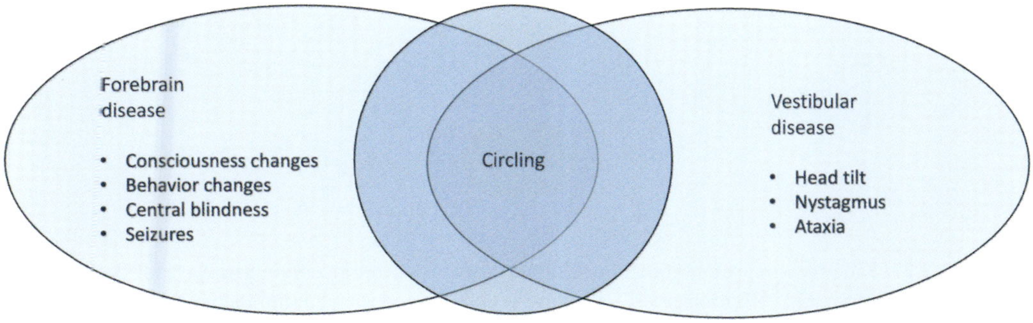

FIGURE 3.1.2 Circling is most often the result of an asymmetrical forebrain lesion or a vestibular lesion. The associated neurological dysfunctions of each localization can help determine the origin of the circling.

- **Postural reaction deficits – worse on the left**

  These tests have complex pathways but generally involve a proprioceptive receptor in the limb being evaluated, a peripheral sensory nerve, the ipsilateral ascending proprioceptive pathways, and the contralateral somatic sensory area of the cerebral cortex (integration center in the forebrain) (Figure 3.1.3). The response to testing involves the contralateral motor cortex in the forebrain, the descending motor pathways within the ipsilateral brainstem and spinal cord (upper motor neuron [UMN]), the peripheral motor nerve, and the limb muscles. Therefore, the entire nervous system is needed to be able to perform postural reactions. Testing them is very important for detecting subtle dysfunction and asymmetry, and for confirming the presence of a neurological disease. Lesions affecting any of the above anatomical sensory and/or motor components could result in abnormal postural reactions. Although abnormalities of these reactions indicate neurological dysfunction, they do not provide specific information for lesion localization, and other neurological deficits need to be considered in order to narrow down the responsible neuroanatomy. In this dog's case, if there is a focal lesion, left-sided postural reaction deficits could be compatible with a right-sided forebrain lesion.

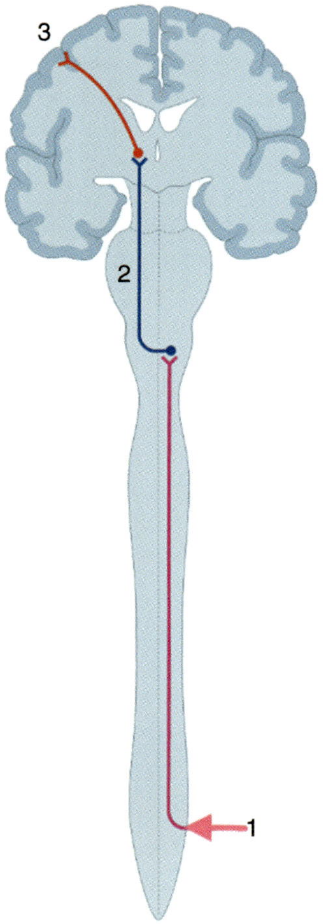

FIGURE 3.1.3 Schematic representation of one of the conscious proprioception pathways for the pelvic limb. (1) Receptors for joint proprioception (mechanoreceptors) send a signal into the dorsal horn of the spinal cord, which then ascends in the dorsal spinal cord columns (gracile fascicle of the dorsal funiculus); (2) the second neuron arises from the gracile nucleus and crosses over in the brainstem, projecting to neuron 3 in the thalamus; (3) the third neuron projects to the primary sensory area of the brain (remaining contralateral to the limb that was tested). *Source:* Created with www.biorender.com.

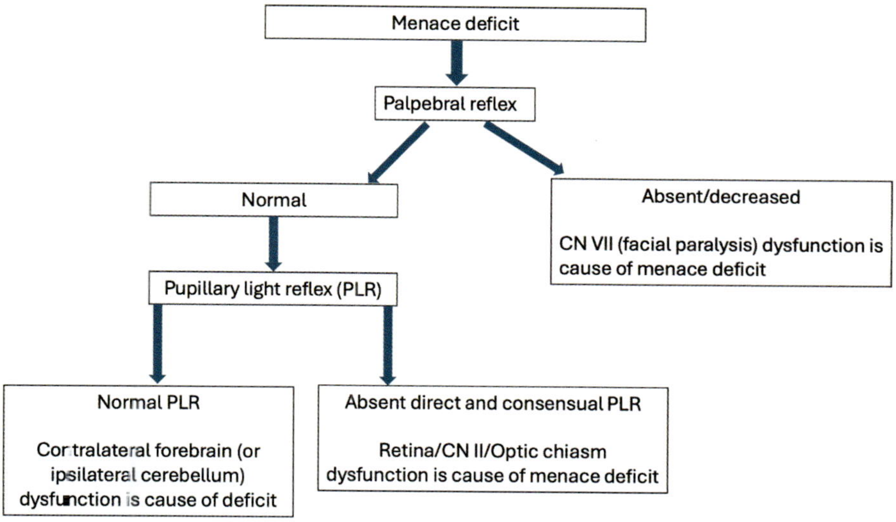

FIGURE 3.1.4 An algorithmic approach to a menace response deficit on neurological examination.

- **Inconsistent or absent menace response on the left**
  The afferent part of this response involves the same structures as the visual pathway. The efferent part of the response is not well understood. The information generated in the visual cortex is forwarded to the motor cortex to initiate a motor response. The corticobulbar pathways then transmit the motor information to the facial nerve (CN VII) nucleus. This response requires intact ipsilateral facial nerve function as well as an intact cerebellum (ipsilateral function) (see Chapter 6, Case 2, Figure 4). An abnormal menace response could indicate a lesion in any component of this neuroanatomy. In this dog's case, with normal palpebral and pupillary light reflex assessments, the finding is compatible with a right forebrain lesion (Figure 3.1.4).

- **Neck pain**
  The detection of neck pain, in addition to signs consistent with brain disease, can suggest a multifocal disease, most commonly due to inflammation. However, there are three other considerations in this instance:

  i. A chronic unrelated disease affecting the structures of the neck, such as intervertebral disc disease, may be responsible for the pain.

  ii. Intracranial disease may cause a "referred" type of neck pain in circumstances or diseases that result in elevated intracranial pressure (ICP) as a result of compression or stretching of the brain vasculature and meninges, which are densely innervated with nociceptors.

  iii. Some diseases may alter the cerebrospinal fluid (CSF) dynamics and result in cervical spinal cord syringomyelia and associated pain syndromes, much like those described in association with Chiari-like malformation.

WHAT IS THE DIFFERENTIAL DIAGNOSIS?

The differential diagnosis for a lesion causing a subacute progressive lateralizing forebrain lesion includes (1) inflammatory (infectious or sterile/immune dysfunction) disease and (2) neoplasia. Vascular lesions (strokes) are acute in onset and typically nonprogressive, as is trauma. Toxicity, metabolic disease, and nutritional disease are most often symmetrical. Anomalous disease of the forebrain can be asymmetrical but is usually insidious in onset and progressive. Degenerative brain disease is more often a chronic, progressive, and often symmetrical condition. There are no idiopathic asymmetrical forebrain syndromes that could be responsible.

INFLAMMATORY DISEASE OF THE BRAIN

Meningoencephalitis refers to inflammation of the brain and surrounding meninges. The majority of dogs with meningoencephalitis do not have a definable infectious cause and are often collectively referred to as meningoencephalitis of undetermined origin (MUO). The MUO umbrella includes distinct neuropathological entities, including granulomatous meningoencephalitis (GME), necrotizing meningoencephalitis (NME), necrotizing leukoencephalitis (NLE), and other nonspecific entities.

- GME is most common in middle-aged toy and small-breed dogs, with a possible breed predisposition in poodles and terriers. However, any age or breed of dog and cat can be affected.
- NME presents with seizures and other signs of forebrain dysfunction. It has been reported in the Brussels Griffon, Coton de Tulear, Chihuahua, Japanese Spitz, Maltese, Miniature Pinscher, Papillon, Pekingese, Pug, Shih Tzu, and Yorkshire terrier. Multifocal asymmetrical areas of necrosis or collapse in both the gray and white matter of the cerebral hemispheres are seen on post-mortem examination.
- NLE has been described in French bulldogs and Yorkshire terriers and is characterized by clinical signs referable to both the forebrain and brainstem. Brainstem involvement frequently manifests as a central vestibular syndrome. Histopathology demonstrates inflammation and necrosis confined to the white matter of the cerebrum and brainstem.

Infectious causes of CNS inflammation in small animals include viral, protozoal, fungal, parasitic, rickettsial, and bacterial organisms.

As a general rule, inflammatory diseases tend to be acute in onset and progressive, with a multifocal or diffuse, often asymmetrical, distribution within the CNS. Neurological manifestations are quite variable and reflect the location of the inflammatory foci within the nervous system. Neck pain can also be present as a manifestation of meningeal inflammation. Animals with CNS infections frequently do not have evidence of systemic involvement. Therefore, the absence of fever, anorexia, and lethargy, and the presence of normal hematology, cannot be used to exclude the possibility of an infectious etiology in an animal with neurological signs.

NEOPLASIA OF THE BRAIN

A brain tumor should be considered a differential diagnosis in any middle-aged or older dog with a clinical history consistent with brain dysfunction, especially when clinical signs are progressive. Primary brain tumors (PBTs) arise from the tissues of the brain, such as neurons, glia, and the meninges. The majority of PBTs in dogs are either meningiomas, gliomas (including astrocytomas, oligodendrogliomas, and undefined gliomas), or choroid plexus tumors. Secondary brain tumors (SBT) include those that metastasize to the brain from a distant primary site or those that have a direct extension from adjacent tissue (skull, nose, ear). Numerous tumors in older animals metastasize to the brain, including hemangiosarcomas, lymphomas, mammary gland adenocarcinomas, and other carcinomas.

Brain tumors primarily affect middle-aged to older dogs. Retrospective studies indicate 95% of dogs affected by brain tumors will be >5 years of age, with a median age of 9 years at diagnosis.

Approximately 75% of canine PBTs are found in the forebrain. Brain tumors cause clinical signs either via compression or invasion of brain tissue or because of a multitude of secondary pathophysiological events such as inflammation, edema, and hemorrhage, ultimately causing intracranial hypertension. In dogs, seizures are the most common clinical manifestation of intracranial neoplasia, being observed in approximately 50% of dogs with forebrain tumors. Central vestibular dysfunction is the most common clinical sign associated with brain tumors originating in the caudal brainstem. Brain tumors may also cause nonspecific clinical signs, such as lethargy, inappetence, and weight loss. Tumors in the fronto-olfactory region or piriform lobe are often associated with only historical evidence of brain disease, such as seizures or behavioral changes, and a normal interictal neurological examination. As the majority of canine PBTs are solitary mass lesions, many cases will also have neurological examination abnormalities related to the area of the brain containing the tumor.

- **Meningiomas**
  Meningiomas are the most common brain tumors in dogs, with Golden Retrievers, Boxer dogs, Miniature Schnauzers, and rat terriers overrepresented. These tumors arise from the arachnoid layer of the meninges, originating at the periphery of the brain parenchyma and expanding inward. Meningiomas can exhibit a wide array of histological subtypes, and any potential differences in the biological behaviors of these subtypes remain to be elucidated.
- **Gliomas**
  Gliomas arise from the supporting cells of the brain parenchyma, which include astrocytes and oligodendrocytes, forming astrocytomas and oligodendrogliomas, respectively. Gliomas commonly affect middle-aged (median 8 years) and brachycephalic breeds of dogs, such as Boxers and Boston terriers. Based on histopathology, gliomas are graded as high or low grade and subtyped as astrocytomas, oligodendrogliomas, and undefined tumors.
- **Choroid plexus tumors (CPTs)**
  CPTs tend to be diagnosed in young to middle-aged dogs (median age 5.5 years), and golden retrievers may be predisposed. CPTs originate in or around the ventricular system, in areas where the choroid plexus is concentrated (the lateral, third, and fourth ventricles). Due to their association with the ventricular system, obstructive hydrocephalus is commonly seen with choroid plexus tumors. These tumors are divided into papilloma, atypical papilloma, and carcinoma.
- **Pituitary gland tumors**
  Pituitary tumors (PT) may be functional or nonfunctional. Nonfunctional tumors usually present with signs primarily related to CNS dysfunction, mainly in the form of progressive obtundation that can also acutely decline. Functional and nonfunctional PTs may enlarge dorsally from the sella and compress the overlying thalamus. Neurological clinical signs of PTs in dogs include abnormal mentation and behavior, cranial nerve abnormalities, postural abnormalities, pain and/or hyperesthesia, gait abnormalities, and abnormal postural reactions. These signs can acutely worsen in cases of pituitary apoplexy, which is a hemorrhage of the PT. Cranial nerve deficits are rare but can be associated with compression of the optic chiasm, optic nerves, post-chiasmal tracts, or oculomotor nerves, leading to decreased or absent pupillary light reflexes and loss of menace response, with associated blindness, and anisocoria may occur.

WHAT DIAGNOSTIC TESTS ARE APPROPRIATE?

The diagnostic tests recommended based on this lesion localization and the potential differentials include a minimum database of hematology, serum chemistry, urinalysis, and infectious disease titers/polymerase chain reaction (PCR), in addition to thoracic and abdominal radiographs.

Abdominal ultrasonography may also be useful in evaluating for a systemic focus of infection or neoplasia. Survey radiographs of the skull are rarely warranted or helpful unless a traumatic incident has occurred.

INFLAMMATORY DISEASE OF THE BRAIN

Investigate for Infectious Disease

Serology and/or PCR should be performed when infectious agents are suspected to be the cause of CNS inflammation, and the infectious agents to be considered should be based on (1) vaccination status; (2) systemic health abnormalities detected; (3) regional prevalence of specific infections; and sometimes (4) CSF results and magnetic resonance imaging (MRI) characteristics of CNS lesions.

IgM and IgG antibodies reflect acute and chronic infections, respectively, and can be evaluated in the serum and/or CSF. Although positive antibody titers reflect direct exposure to an organism, a positive titer does not confirm active infection. Serum and CSF serology and PCR may be pursued for *Toxoplasma gondii*, *Neospora caninum*, *Ehrlichia* spp., and *Rickettsia rickettsii*. *Cryptococcus, Aspergillus, Blastomyces, Coccidioides*, and *Histoplasma* spp. also have specific tests available.

Imaging

There can be considerable variability in computed tomography (CT) or MRI findings among dogs and cats with infectious meningoencephalitis and MUO. There are no definitive findings, with there being much overlap in the descriptions of all the underlying etiologies. However, multiple, single, or diffuse intraparenchymal hyperintense lesions on T2-weighted (T2-W) or fluid attenuated inversion recovery (FLAIR) images are identified most frequently on MRI, with variable contrast enhancement (Figure 3.1.5).

MRI lesions are often distributed throughout both gray and white matter. Vasogenic edema in the white matter is commonly appreciable on T2-W and T1-weighted (T1-W) images as hyper- and hypointense to cerebral parenchyma, respectively.

MUO may be associated with contrast enhancement of the parenchyma and meninges on CT, and mass effect may be observed as displacement of surrounding brain tissue. Some lesions may be associated with hypoattenuating vasogenic (white matter) edema.

MUO, infectious meningoencephalitis, CNS lymphoma, and glial and metastatic neoplasms may present with similar clinical and MRI findings, and discriminating among these differentials may be challenging unless tissue biopsy is obtained.

Diagnosing necrotizing encephalitis, with its subcategories of NLE and NME, based on MRI alone, can be challenging. However, there are breed-specific imaging characteristics in both subcategories that allow the establishment of a clinical diagnosis with a relatively high degree of certainty. Typical breed-specific imaging features, such as lesion distribution, signal intensity, contrast enhancement, and gross changes of brain structure (midline shift, ventriculomegaly, and brain herniation), are documented in the literature for the most commonly affected canine breeds: Yorkshire terrier, French bulldog, Pug, and Chihuahua.

MRI findings have been reported to be normal in approximately 25% of dogs with evidence of inflammation on CSF analysis, demonstrating that normal imaging does not rule out a diagnosis of MUO. However, dogs diagnosed with MUO with no detectable lesions on MRI have reduced disease-related death compared with dogs with abnormal MRI, suggesting the presence or absence of MRI lesions is prognostically relevant.

For MRI descriptions reported with the individual infectious diseases, readers are referred to the further reading section below.

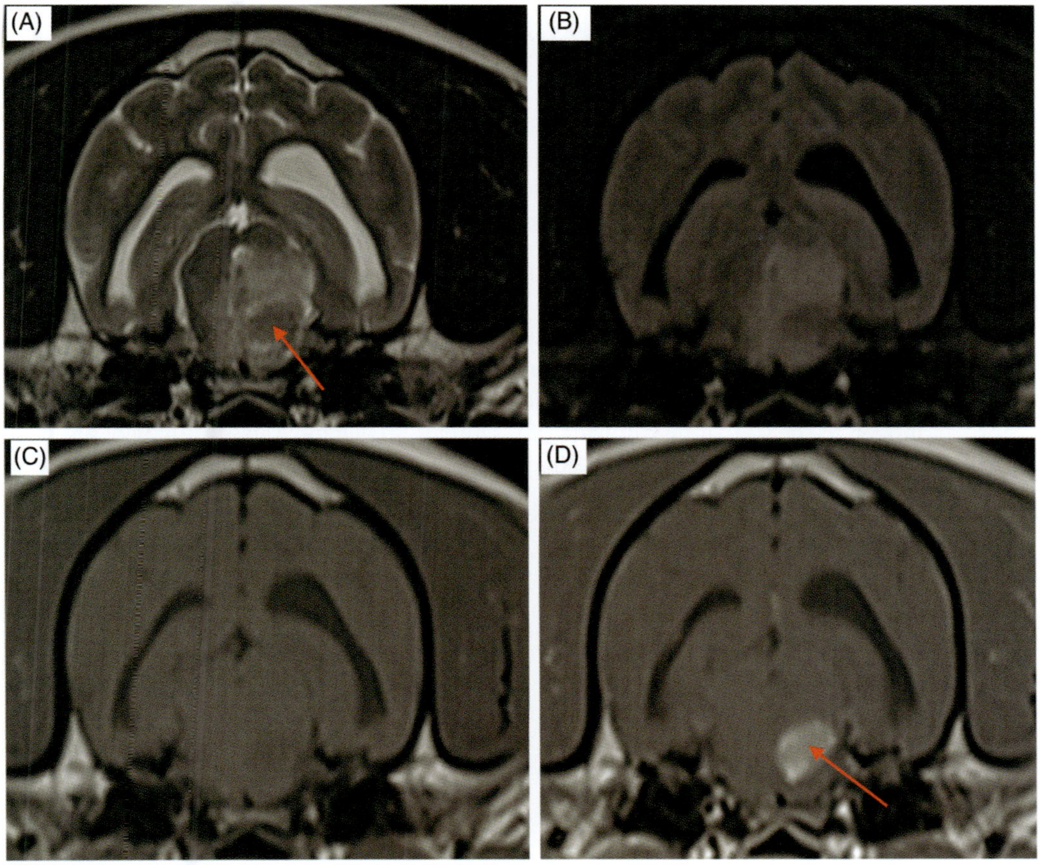

FIGURE 3.1.5 (A) T2-W, (B) FLAIR, (C) T1-W pre-contrast, and (D) T1-W post-contrast transverse brain MR images at the level of the rostral brainstem of a 4-year-old West Highland white terrier. There is a focal left-sided intraparenchymal lesion (arrow), which is iso- to hyperintense on T2-W and FLAIR sequences, T1-W hypointense, and strongly enhanced post-contrast. There is a moderate amount of peri-lesional edema seen on T2-W and FLAIR. Histopathology confirmed GME.

Cerebrospinal Fluid (CSF) Analysis

MUO

CSF analysis typically reveals moderately elevated total protein levels and a mononuclear, lymphocytic, or mixed pleocytosis. However, neutrophilic or eosinophilic pleocytosis and even normal CSF analysis can be seen. Although classic patterns have been associated with the variants of MUO, there is much overlap in the characteristics between the diseases.

Infectious disease testing can be performed on CSF as well as blood.

Protozoal meningoencephalitis

CSF analysis typically demonstrates pleocytosis with a mixed population of neutrophils and the presence of small and large mononuclear cells. Eosinophils can also be seen. With CNS toxoplasmosis, a presumptive diagnosis is based on positive antibody titers in the CSF. However, a positive titer can be seen in animals previously exposed to the organism following nonspecific immune stimulation and, therefore, is not definitive evidence of active disease. A positive serum IgM titer or an increasing IgG titer (fourfold) can confirm a recent infection. Serum and CSF anti-*Neospora* antibody titers are more reliable than serum titers alone. However, as is the case for toxoplasmosis, evidence of a rising titer should be obtained. PCR assays performed on CSF samples can aid in the antemortem diagnosis of these protozoal infections.

Viral meningoencephalitis

Canine Distemper Virus (CDV) – Results of CSF analysis are variable. During the acute stage of the disease, an inflammatory response is lacking, and thus, the cell count and protein levels can be normal. In the chronic stage of the disease, lymphocytic pleocytosis is more frequently identified. An elevated CSF titer of antibodies against CDV relative to the serum titer is supportive of a diagnosis.

Fungal meningoencephalitis

CSF analysis can be normal or show mixed, neutrophilic, eosinophilic, or mononuclear pleocytosis. The encapsulated *Cryptococcus* organism might be identified in the CSF. In cases in which the organism is not observed on cytology, diagnosis can be made either by detecting the cryptococcal capsular antigen in the CSF or by culturing CSF samples. In general, the sensitivity of antibody testing for fungal infections is considered poor.

Bacterial and rickettsial meningoencephalitis

Typically, there is a marked elevation in the protein level and total nucleated cell count, and the majority of cells are degenerate neutrophils. Bacteria may be visible in the spinal fluid. However, CSF analysis can be unremarkable or show more nonspecific inflammatory changes. CSF should be cultured if it contains degenerate neutrophils, although it is common for the cultures to be negative.

NEOPLASIA OF THE BRAIN

Imaging

Cross-sectional diagnostic imaging techniques, such as CT and MRI, have revolutionized the clinical diagnosis and management of brain tumors in veterinary medicine, although MRI is the preferred modality for the assessment of animals with intracranial disease. Accurate presumptive diagnoses of the general tumor type can be extrapolated from MRI features in many dogs.

- *Meningiomas:* Meningiomas most often appear as solitary, broad-based, well-marginated, extra-parenchymal contrast-enhancing masses on CT and MRI (Figure 3.1.6). These tumors may contain intratumoral fluid/cysts, mineralization, hemorrhage, or be predominantly cystic. Meningiomas may also be associated with adjacent calvarial hyperostosis or a dural tail sign. On pre-contrast CT images, hemorrhage and calcification have a hyperattenuating (white) appearance. Histiocytic sarcomas and granular cell tumors share many overlapping imaging features significant with those of meningiomas.

- *Gliomas*: As gliomas may infiltrate or displace the neuroparenchyma, they may appear as poorly or well-marginated lesions and may or may not demonstrate contrast enhancement. Oligodendrogliomas tend to be strongly T2-W hyperintense to surrounding brain tissue as a result of a high mucin content. Among contrast-enhancing gliomas, the patterns and degree of enhancement can be highly variable. A "ring-enhancing" pattern, in which a circular ring of contrast enhancement surrounds nonenhancing abnormal tissue, is often associated with gliomas. However, ring enhancement is a nonspecific finding that has been associated with several neoplastic, vascular, and inflammatory brain diseases. The different histologic subtypes of gliomas cannot be reliably differentiated using conventional MRI sequences, although high-grade gliomas are more likely to demonstrate contrast enhancement (Figure 3.1.7). Gliomas can be difficult to identify using CT; thus, MRI is the preferred imaging modality for their evaluation.

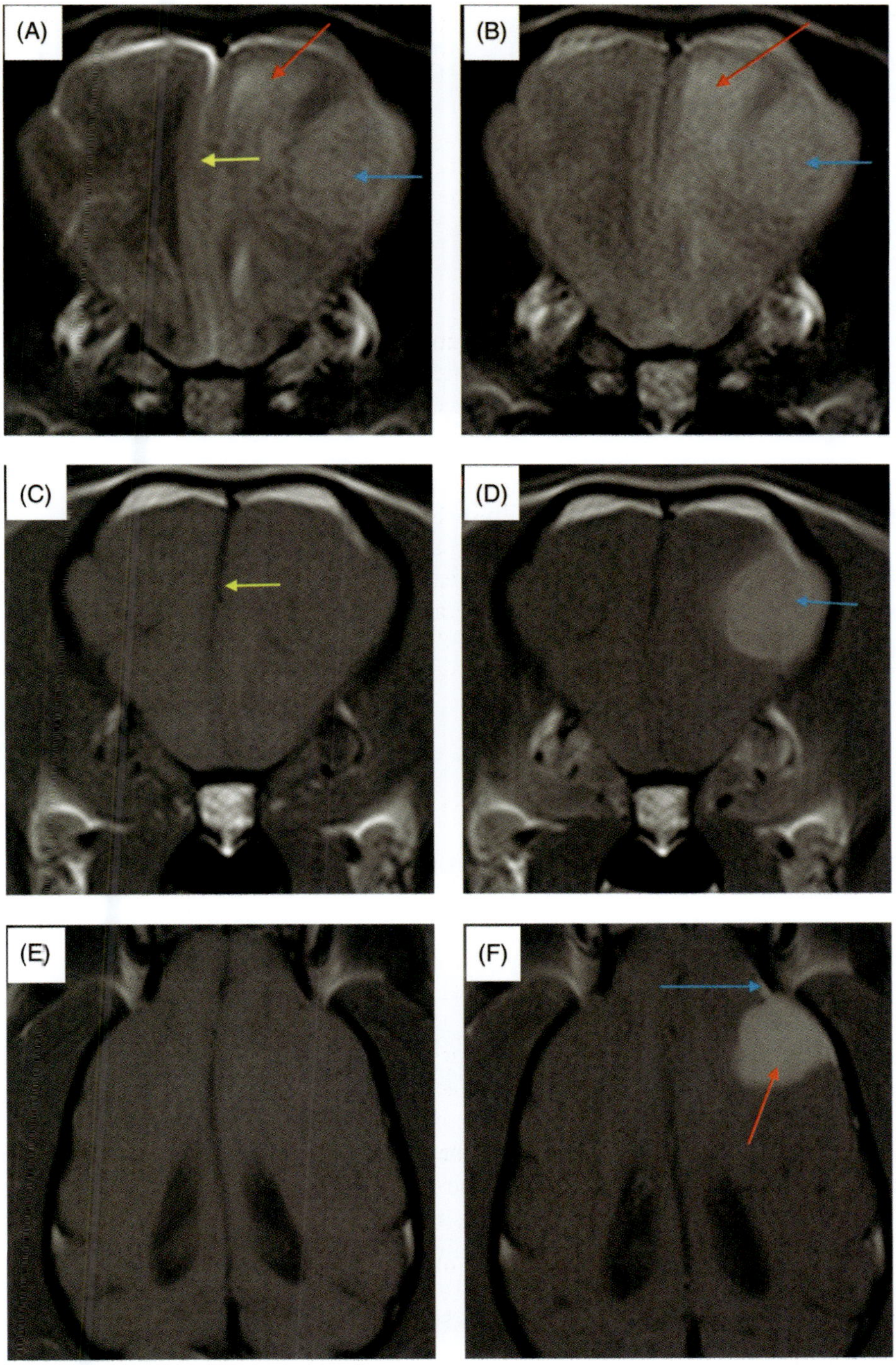

FIGURE 3.1.6 (A) Transverse T2-W, (B) Transverse FLAIR, (C) Transverse T1-W pre-contrast, and (D) Transverse T1-W post-contrast images of the brain at the level of the frontal lobe. Red arrow – perilesional edema, blue arrow – mass lesion, and yellow arrow – midline shift. Dorsal T1-W images of the brain (E) pre-contrast and (F) post-contrast. Blue arrow – dural tail, red arrow – mass lesion. There is an extra-parenchymal and broad-based space-occupying lesion confirmed to be a meningioma, centered on the left frontal lobe. This lesion is well-defined, and it shows a rounded to oval shape. It is homogeneous, hyperintense in T2-W when compared to gray matter, hyperintense in FLAIR, and isointense in T1-W. After contrast, there is moderate to severe and homogeneous contrast enhancement. Caudally and rostrally, a short dural tail sign is seen, suggesting attachment to the meninges. This lesion causes moderate perilesional edema, which tracks along the white matter to reach the rostral occipital lobe and causes mild mass effect, with mild midline shift.

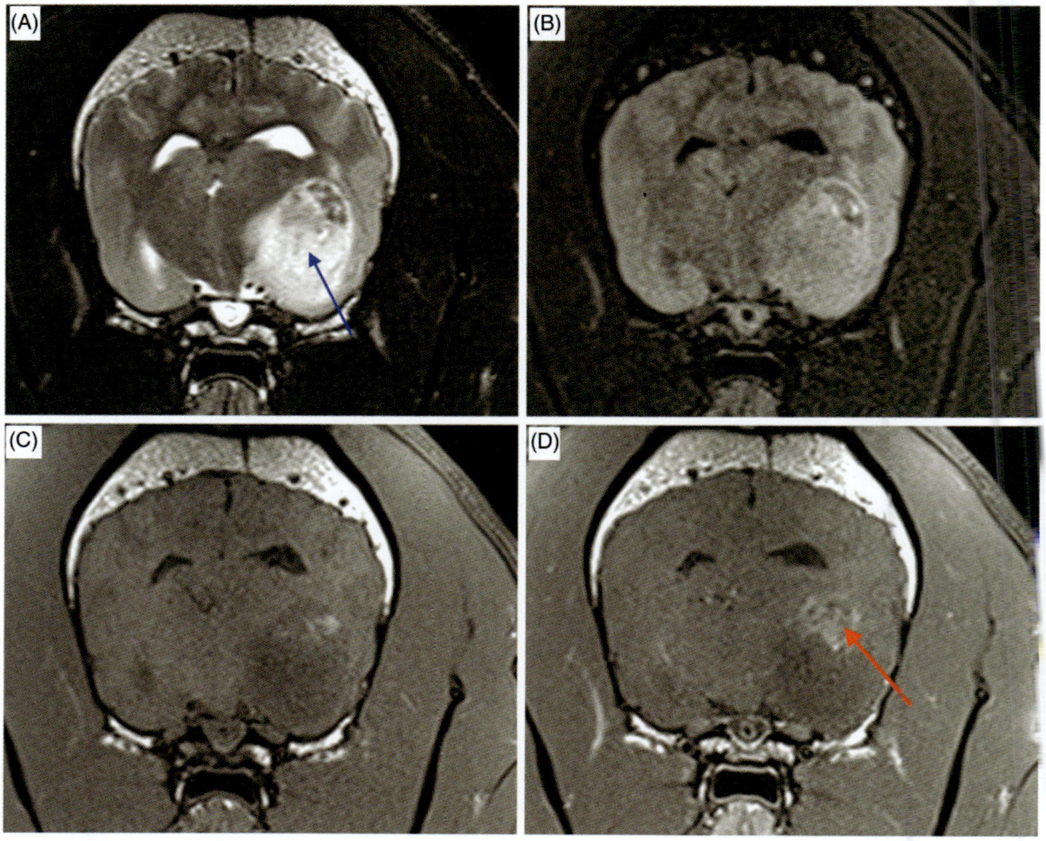

FIGURE 3.1.7 There is a large, relatively well-defined, irregular intraparenchymal lesion centered on the left piriform lobe. The lesion is markedly heterogeneous, being predominantly (A) T2-W hyperintense to gray matter (blue arrow), (B) FLAIR hyperintense, and (C) T1-W hypointense with ill-defined, irregular patchy contrast enhancement (red arrow) (D). The lesion was confirmed to be a high-grade glioma.

- *Choroid plexus tumors*: Choroid plexus tumors are the most common tumors found in an intraventricular location and often demonstrate marked contrast enhancement (Figure 3.1.8).
- *Pituitary gland tumors*: These tumors may be identified within the sella or extend into the parasellar or suprasellar locations. Magnetic resonance (MR) imaging features of pituitary adenomas include isointensity to hyperintensity on T2-W images, isointensity to hypointensity on T1-W images, and avid homogeneous contrast enhancement on T1-W postcontrast images (Figure 3.1.9). MR may detect pituitary tumors as small as 3 mm. With conventional CT, 40% of dogs with microadenomas have a normal-appearing pituitary gland.

CSF Analysis

CSF is frequently abnormal in patients with brain tumors. However, white blood cell (WBC) counts, WBC differentials, and total protein concentrations are highly variable and are often nonspecific for the presence of intracranial neoplasia. Exfoliated neoplastic cells may be observed in the CSF cytology of animals with any type of brain tumor, but choroid plexus tumors, lymphoma, and histiocytic sarcoma are the most commonly reported to be detected with CSF analysis.

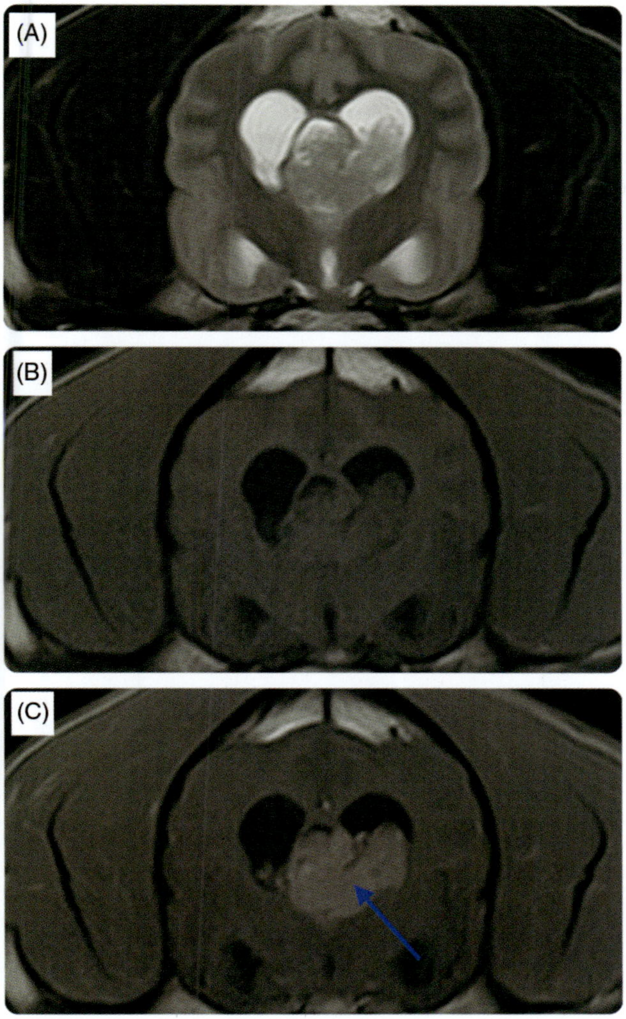

FIGURE 3.1.8 There is a large, well-defined, reasonably homogeneous extra-parenchymal mass in the dorsal part of the third ventricle. This mass (arrow) is T2-W (A) and FLAIR hyperintense compared to gray matter, T1-W (B) isointense to hyperintense markedly/homogeneously contrast-enhancing (C). The lesion is midline, extending caudally from the level of the optic chiasm toward the mesencephalic aqueduct and laterally into the left lateral ventricle. The mass was confirmed to be a choroid plexus tumor.

OUTCOME

In our case, MRI confirmed a large, ill-defined, ring-enhancing, and space-occupying intraparenchymal mass centered on the right-sided piriform lobe, compatible with a high-grade glioma. The owners chose to attempt therapy with radiation, which improved the dog's quality of life for another 8 months, after which time they elected euthanasia.

A recent study evaluated 38 dogs with suspected symptomatic primary solitary intracranial glioma, treated with a complete uniform fractionated megavoltage radiation protocol of 15×3Gy over 5 weeks. The disease-specific median survival time was 698 days, and survival at 1 and 2 years was, respectively, 74.2% ± 7.4% and 49.0% ± 9.8%. Radiation therapy is deemed a safe and effective treatment for canine intracranial gliomas, allowing long-term tumor control, improvement in patient quality of life, and management of associated clinical signs. Treatment for seizure activity in these cases should also be considered, although radiotherapy can help improve this clinical sign, and palliative therapy with anti-inflammatory corticosteroids should be considered for all similar patients.

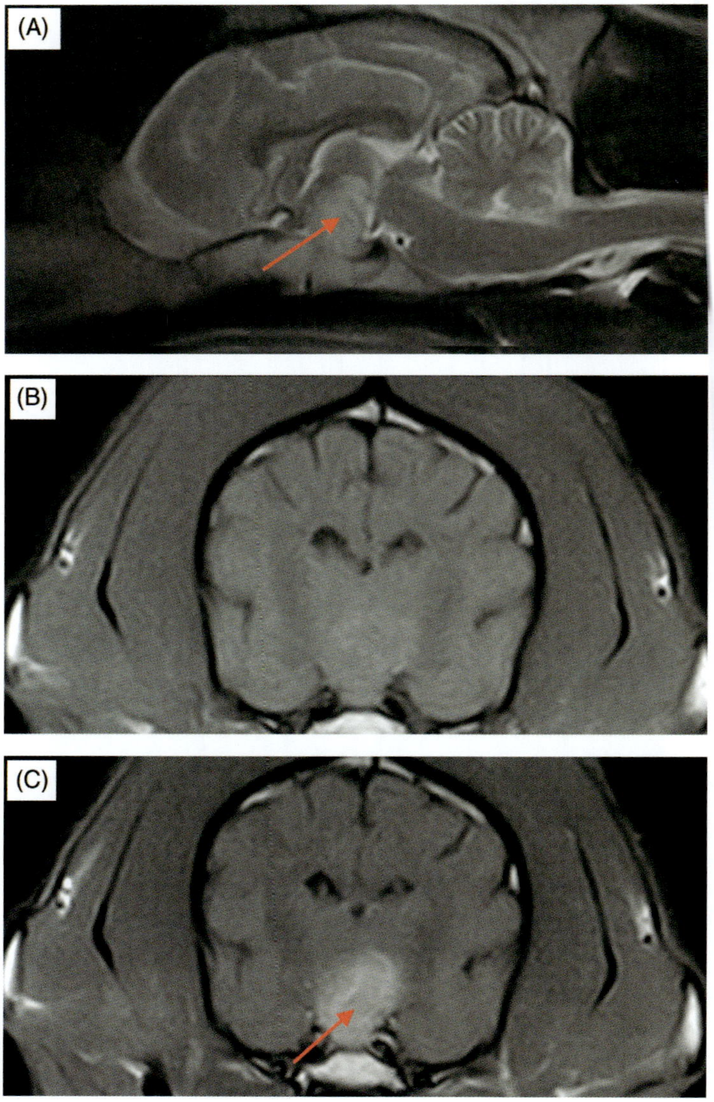

FIGURE 3.1.9 (A) Sagittal T2-W, (B) transverse T1-W pre-contrast, and (C) transverse T1-W post-contrast images of a 7-year-old Lurcher with a chronic, progressive dull mentation. There is a relatively well-defined, ovoid pituitary-based mass lesion that is fairly homogenous, being T2-W hyperintense to gray matter, T1-W iso- to hyperintense with strong contrast enhancement. The lesion is compatible with a pituitary macroadenoma.

SUGGESTED READING

Andersen-Ranberg, E., Berendt, M., and Gredal, H. (2021). Biomarkers of non-infectious inflammatory CNS diseases in dogs - where are we now? Part I: meningoencephalitis of unknown origin. *Vet. J.* 273: 105678.

Beckmann, O., Golini, S., and Kircher, C. (2014). MRI findings in a case of canine tick born meningo-encephalomyelitis. *Schweiz. Arch. Tierheilkd.* 156 (8): 395–399.

Butterfield, S., Whittaker, D., Tabanez, J. et al. (2023). Bacterial meningitis secondary to otogenic infection in 10 French bulldogs: a retrospective case series. *Vet. Rec. Open* 10 (1): e263.

Cardy, T.J.A. and Cornelis, I. (2018). Clinical presentation and magnetic resonance imaging findings in 11 dogs with eosinophilic meningoencephalitis of unknown aetiology. *J. Small Anim. Pract.* 59 (7): 422–431:https://doi.org/10.1111/jsap.12837.

Cornelis, I., Van Ham, L., Gielen, I. et al. (2019). Clinical presentation, diagnostic findings, prognostic factors, treatment and outcome in dogs with meningoencephalomyelitis of unknown origin: a review. *Vet. J.* 244: 37–44.

deLahunta, A., Glass, E., and Kent, M. (2021). *Veterinary Neuroanatomy and Clinical Neurology*, 5e. Philadelphia: Elsevier.

Debreuque, M., De Fornel, P., David, I. et al. (2020). Definitive-intent uniform megavoltage fractioned radiotherapy protocol for presumed canine intracranial gliomas retrospective analysis of survival and prognostic factors in 38 cases (2013–2019). *BMC Vet. Res.* 16 (1): 412.

Flegel, T. (2017). Breed-specific magnetic resonance imaging characteristics of necrotizing encephalitis in dogs. *Front. Vet. Sci.* 4: 203.

Galer, J., Forward, A.K., Hughes, J. et al. (2024). Clinical features, treatment, and outcome of juvenile dogs with meningoencephalitis of unknown etiology. *J. Vet. Intern. Med.* 38 (4): 2214–2220.

Gonçalves, R., De Decker, S., Walmsley, G., and Maddox, T.W. (2024). Magnetic resonance imaging prognostic factors for survival and relapse in dogs with meningoencephalitis of unknown origin. *Front. Vet. Sci.* 11: 1370882.

Gonçalves, R., De Decker, S., Walmsley, G. et al. (2022). Inflammatory disease affecting the central nervous system in dogs: a retrospective study in England (2010-2019). *Front. Vet. Sci.* 8: 819945.

Gonzalo-Nadal, V., Kohl, A., Rocchi, M. et al. (2024). Suspected tick-borne flavivirus meningoencephalomyelitis in dogs from the UK: six cases (2021). *J. Small Anim. Pract.* 65 (2): 132–143.

Hecht, S. and Adams, W.H. (2010). MRI of brain disease in veterinary patients part 2: acquired brain disorders. *Vet. Clin. N. Am. Small Anim. Pract.* 40 (1): 39–63.

Kelley, A.J., Stainback, L.B., Knowles, K.E. et al. (2021). Clinical characteristics, magnetic resonance imaging features treatment, and outcome for presumed intracranial coccidioidomycosis in 45 dogs (2009–2019). *J. Vet. Intern. Med.* 35 (5): 2222–2231.

Menchetti, M., De Risio, L., Galli, G. et al. (2019). Neurological abnormalities in 97 dogs with detectable pituitary masses. *Vet. Q.* 39 (1): 57–64.

Miller, A.D., Miller, C.R., and Rossmeisl, J.H. (2019). Canine primary intracranial cancer: a clinicopathologic and comparative review of glioma, meningioma, and choroid plexus tumors. *Front. Oncol.* 9: 1151.

Nagendran, A., José López, R., Suñol, A. et al. (2024). The value of a head turn in neurolocalization. *J. Vet. Intern. Med.* 38 (1): 268–276.

Ostrager, A., Bentley, R.T., Lewis, M.J., and Moore, G.E. (2024). Survival in dogs with meningoencephalomyelitis of unknown etiology with and without lesions detected by magnetic resonance imaging. *J. Vet. Intern. Med.* 38 (4): 2204–2213.

Schwartz, M., Lamb, C.R., Brodbelt, D.C., and Volk, H.A. (2011). Canine intracranial neoplasia: clinical risk factors for development of epileptic seizures. *J. Small Anim. Pract.* 52 (12): 632–637.

Snyder, J.M., Lipitz, L., Skorupski, K.A. et al. (2008). Secondary intracranial neoplasia in the dog: 177 cases (1986–2003). *J. Vet. Intern. Med.* 22 (1): 172–177.

Song, R.B., Vite, C.H., Bradley, C.W., and Cross, J.R. (2013). Postmortem evaluation of 435 cases of intracranial neoplasia in dogs and relationship of neoplasm with breed, age, and body weight. *J. Vet. Intern. Med.* 27 (5): 1143–1152.

Sturges, B.K., Dickinson, P.J., Bollen, A.W. et al. (2008). Magnetic resonance imaging and histological classification of intracranial meningiomas in 112 dogs. *J. Vet. Intern. Med.* 22 (3): 586–595.

Toyoda, I., Vernau, W., Sturges, B.K. et al. (2020). Clinicopathological characteristics of histiocytic sarcoma affecting the central nervous system in dogs. *J. Vet. Intern. Med.* 34: 828–837.

Westworth, D.R., Dickinson, P.J., Vernau, W. et al. (2008). Choroid plexus tumours in 56 dogs (1985–2007). *J. Vet. Intern. Med.* 22 (5): 1157–1165.

Young, B.D., Levine, J.M., Fosgate, G.T. et al. (2009). Magnetic resonance imaging characteristics of necrotizing meningoencephalitis in Pug dogs. *J. Vet. Intern. Med.* 23 (3): 527–535.

Young, B.D., Fosgate, G.T., Holmes, S.P. et al. (2014). Evaluation of standard magnetic resonance characteristics used to differentiate neoplastic, inflammatory, and vascular brain lesions in dogs. *Vet. Radiol. Ultrasound* 55 (4): 399–406.

CHAPTER 3.2

Circling and Altered Mentation

Case 2—A Cat with Acute Circling

Simon R. Platt

Department of Veterinary Clinical Sciences, College of Veterinary Medicine, Oklahoma State University, Stillwater, OK, USA

CASE HISTORY

A 12-year-old neutered male domestic short-haired cat was presented for an acute onset of pacing, circling to the left, and dull mentation. This happened one week earlier, and there had been no perceptible change, according to the owner's opinion.

The cat had otherwise been healthy, was allowed to roam outside every day, and lived with three other cats in the house; the three other cats were currently considered healthy. He had been routinely vaccinated but did not receive regular prophylactic anti-parasitic medications. He ate a commercial complete diet with no supplements or recent changes and was allowed to eat ad lib.

The owner was not aware of the cat's current appetite or water intake, with all four cats eating and drinking from the same source. There may have been a mild weight loss in the owner's opinion. Urination and defecation history were unknown based on the cat's outdoor lifestyle. There were no respiratory or upper gastrointestinal signs of recent note.

A general physical examination revealed a slightly thin cat (body condition score 4/9), with palpable thyroid glands and moderate periodontal disease.

NEUROLOGICAL EXAMINATION

The cat was considered mentally dull, in the owner's opinion, which was appreciated on initial observation. He had a normal posture, and on gait assessment, he was ambulatory with normal strength and motor function. When he became comfortable with the examination room environment, he intermittently circled to the left with constant pacing, which occasionally was aimless. Postural reactions were reduced on the cat's right side based on the hopping examination (Video 3.2.1).

VIDEO 3.2.1 Neurological examination of a 12-year-old male neutered domestic shorthaired cat that presented with acute circling to the left and pacing. Postural reactions are notably decreased on the cat's right side. Aspects of the neurological examination not covered by the video are presumed normal.

Spinal reflexes were performed while the cat was standing by stimulating the digits, and these were considered intact. Muscle mass and tone were appropriate.

There was an inconsistent right-sided menace response with an intact palpebral reflex. The pupillary light reflex and pupil size were normal bilaterally. Nasal stimulation was not performed. There was no cranial muscle atrophy noted, and the jaw tone was appropriate. Tongue movement and the gag reflex were normal. There was normal physiologic nystagmus seen when his head was moved from side to side.

There was no cervical pain on palpation of the neck.

When the cat was observed eating in his cage, food was only taken out of the left side of the bowl, compatible with a hemineglect syndrome (Video 3.2.2).

VIDEO 3.2.2 A 9-year-old domestic longhaired cat with dull mentation demonstrates hemi-neglect syndrome; the cat only eats out of the left side of the food bowl, compatible with a left-sided forebrain lesion.

1. **Where is the lesion localization?**
2. **What major disease processes should be considered?**
3. **What tests could you perform to help determine the diagnosis?**

WHERE IS THE LESION LOCALIZATION?

The neurological examination is suggestive of a lesion affecting the forebrain, lateralized to the left (Figure 3.2.1). A multifocal disease cannot be ruled out. This localization is based on the following considerations:

- **Dull mentation**
  Mental status encompasses the way an animal responds to environmental stimuli and its level of arousal or consciousness. The two anatomical structures involved in maintaining an adequate level of arousal are the ascending reticular activating system (ARAS), located in the brainstem, and the forebrain. The ARAS receives input from all sensory modalities (except muscle and joint proprioception) at both the levels of the spinal cord and brainstem. It then projects

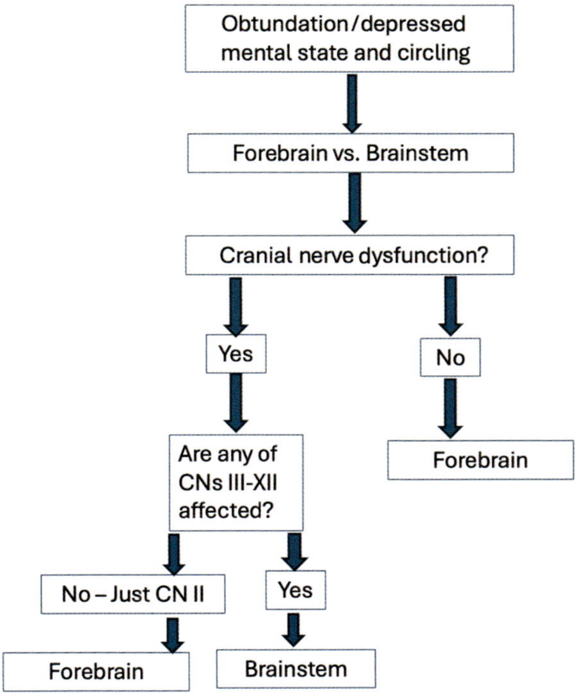

FIGURE 3.2.1 Simplified algorithmic overview of localization for obtundation.

stimulatory input diffusely to all areas of the cerebral cortex via the thalamus to maintain a state of consciousness. The region of the forebrain commonly associated with behavior is the limbic system, which consists of portions of the cerebrum and thalamus. Based heavily on the owner's opinion of her own cat's normal mental status, and in part on our examination, a forebrain or brainstem lesion was suspected.

- **Pacing**
  Pacing or compulsive walking is considered a change in behavior even in the absence of obvious signs of confusion. This is a stereotypical behavior that can arise from various neuroanatomical abnormalities. The primary neuroanatomical structures believed to be implicated in compulsive behaviors, including pacing, are the basal nuclei of the forebrain, the frontal cortex of the forebrain, the limbic system (amygdala, hippocampus), and the thalamus.

- **Circling to the left**
  Circling can be caused by lesions in the vestibular system (central or peripheral) or by an asymmetrical/focal lesion in the forebrain. Tight circles are usually, but not exclusively, associated with a vestibular syndrome, whilst wide circles are often associated with a forebrain lesion. Other signs of vestibular dysfunction (head tilt, nystagmus) should also be present (see Chapter 3, Case 1, Figure 2). However, thalamic lesions can also result in tight circles and, therefore, in the absence of other vestibular signs, tight circles might represent an ipsilateral thalamic dysfunction. Wide circles reflect a forebrain lesion caused by an aversion against the area that the patient cannot consciously perceive. The cat being discussed is circling toward the left side. This means that the patient has an aversion syndrome against the right side, which is controlled by the right forebrain. Therefore, the patient circles toward the area that can be perceived. Conventionally, this is summarized as a patient "circling toward the lesion." The leftward circling in this patient's case is compatible with a left-sided cerebral lesion.

- **Postural reaction deficits on the right**
  As discussed in this chapter's Case 1, postural reactions evaluate proprioceptive pathways. Multiple components of the peripheral and central nervous system (CNS) that affect limb function are tested with postural reactions (see Chapter 3, Case 1, Figure 3). In this cat's case, the significant deficits noted on its right side in both thoracic and pelvic limbs can be compatible with a right-sided cervical cord lesion, a right-sided brainstem lesion, or a left-sided forebrain lesion. In the presence of the other clinical signs, a left-sided forebrain disease is most likely if this is a focal disease process.

- **Inconsistent or absent menace on the right**
  In cats, it is preferable to stand behind the animal with the contralateral eye uncovered when performing this test, as up to 40% of cats with vision fail to have a menace response when the contralateral eye is covered. The neuroanatomy, which is tested by the menace response, is covered in Case 1 in this chapter, and the reader is also referred to see Chapter 6, Case 2, Figure 4. An abnormal menace response could indicate a lesion in any component of this neuroanatomy. In this cat's case, with normal palpebral and pupillary light reflex assessments, the finding is compatible with a left forebrain lesion (Figure 3.2.2).

- **Hemineglect/hemi-inattention**
  Hemineglect syndrome, also known as hemi-inattention syndrome, refers to an abnormal behavior in which animals with structural forebrain disease ignore sensory input from the contralateral part of their environment (e.g. eating from one half of the bowl, turning in the wrong direction in response to sound). This syndrome indicates a forebrain lesion contralateral to the side apparently "ignored" by the animal. In this cat's case, the consumption of food only from the left side of the bowl is again compatible with a left forebrain lesion.

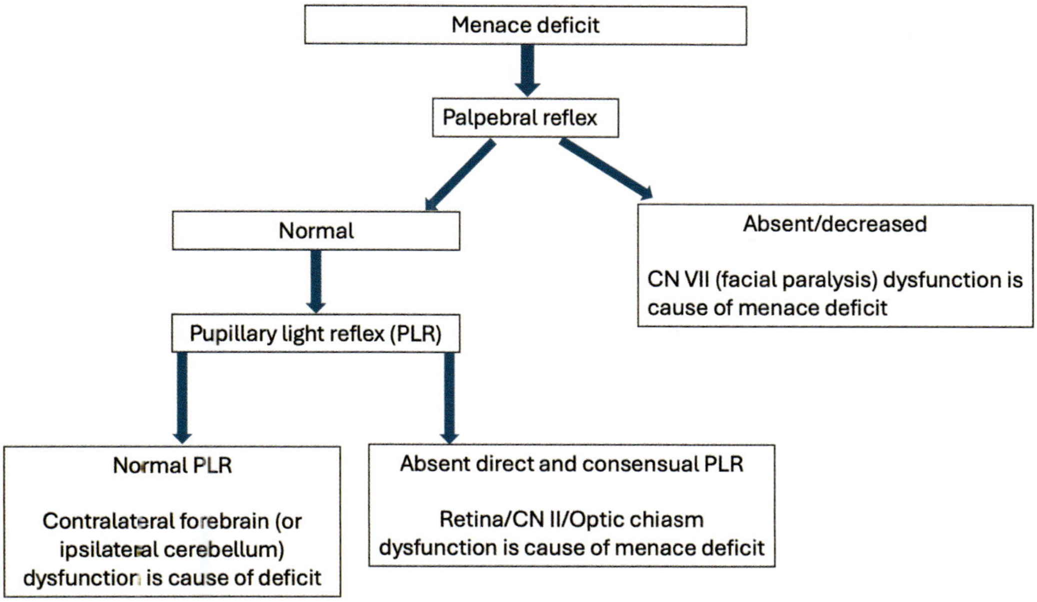

FIGURE 3.2.2 An algorithmic approach to a menace response deficit on neurological examination.

WHAT IS THE DIFFERENTIAL DIAGNOSIS?

The differential diagnosis for a lesion causing an acute forebrain lesion includes (1) trauma and (2) vascular lesions (strokes and hypertensive encephalopathy). Hypertensive encephalopathy can be asymmetric and can wax and wane. Inflammatory diseases are usually more subacute in onset, but cannot be ruled out in this case based on the intermittent observation by the owners that occurs with outdoor-living cats. Although neoplasia causing an asymmetric forebrain disease could be suspected in older cats, the acute onset again makes this less likely (see Case 4 in this chapter for more information on feline brain tumors).

Metabolic diseases such as hepatic encephalopathy are usually relatively symmetric, so they are not considered likely in this cat. Intoxication should always be considered for an acute onset forebrain disease, especially if this cannot be ruled out historically; most toxicities are, however, relatively symmetric. Anomalous disease of the forebrain can be asymmetric but is usually insidious in onset and progressive, and is unlikely to manifest after the first 2 years of life. Degenerative disease of the brain is more of a chronic, progressive, and most often symmetrical presentation. There are no idiopathic asymmetrical forebrain syndromes that could be responsible.

1. **Vascular disease of the brain**

   Cerebrovascular accidents (CVA) or strokes, both ischemic and hemorrhagic, are being increasingly recognized as a cause of brain dysfunction in cats. Strokes are rapidly developing clinical signs of focal (or global) disturbance of brain function, lasting more than 24 hours or leading to death, with no apparent cause other than that of vascular origin. A vascular disorder in cats termed feline ischemic encephalopathy has historically been described as an infarction frequently localized in the area of the brain supplied by the middle cerebral artery. It is likely that this is not a specific condition and may just represent a topographic variant of CVAs in cats.

   Ischemic strokes are most common and result from vascular obstruction from emboli originating in other vascular beds, from the heart, or local thrombus formation within a blood vessel.

Clinical signs are acute in onset and asymmetric. They may be initially progressive but are often static after the first 24 hours. If the degree of ischemia and the associated pathophysiological sequelae are more severe, clinical signs may be rapidly progressive and often fatal. The clinical signs typically reflect a focal abnormality referable to the area of the CNS affected. CVAs have been documented to affect all neuroanatomic regions of the brain. The median age of cats affected with presumed ischemic CVAs is 12 years.
Ischemic brain CVAs in cats may be associated with:

- Hypertrophic cardiomyopathy, neoplasia, and hyperthyroidism.
- Hypercoagulable states (such as protein-losing nephropathy or enteropathy, hyperadrenocorticism, immune-mediated hemolytic anemia, and polycythemia vera), which may result in intramural emboli and subsequent thrombosis of cerebral blood vessels.
- Bacteremia (e.g. sepsis and endocarditis), which may predispose to septic embolization of intracranial blood vessels.
- Neoplastic infiltration of blood vessels, including intravascular lymphoma
- Vasculitis due to systemic disease (e.g. Leishmania) or local CNS inflammation
- Migrating parasites (*Cuterebra larva*)
- The use of mouth gags.

In cats with hemorrhagic brain infarcts, significant liver pathology and nephritis have been identified in 100% and 25% of cases, respectively. Hypertension (associated with a variety of conditions such as renal disease, hyperthyroidism, primary hyperaldosteronism, and pheochromocytoma) can result in an increase in cerebrovascular hydrostatic forces leading to intracranial hemorrhage and edema. Disorders of coagulation (e.g. disseminated intravascular coagulation (DIC) and thrombocytopenia) can also result in brain hemorrhage.

Systemic hypertension is increasingly recognized in small animals. The pathological effect of systemic hypertension on tissues is referred to as target organ damage. Target organ damage can result when the systolic blood pressure reaches 150–160 mmHg. A variety of tissues can be affected, including the kidneys, eyes, cardiovascular system, and the CNS. The clinical signs of hypertensive encephalopathy are often reversible, with resolution of the neurological signs occurring within hours to the first few days following initiation of therapy. Hypertensive encephalopathy in cats is associated with either an acute (>30 mmHg from resting rate) or a sustained (>160 mmHg) elevation in systolic arterial blood pressure. The clinical signs reflect involvement of the forebrain and include seizures, altered mental status, decreased level of consciousness, and blindness.

2. **Traumatic brain injury (TBI)**
Severe head trauma causing TBI is associated with high mortality rates in animals. Common causes of head injuries in cats and dogs include road traffic accidents, falls from height, kicks, gunshot or pellet wounds, and bites from larger animals. Traumatic injuries to the brain may result from blunt or penetrating insults; most feline head trauma is associated with crush injury. For more specific information on TBI, the reader is referred to Chapter 15.

3. **Inflammatory disease of the brain**
Encephalitis and meningitis often coexist (meningoencephalitis) and have infectious and immune-mediated causes. Feline meningoencephalitis of unknown origin (MUO) has also been described, although it is rarer than MUO in dogs. The incidence of infectious agents causing meningoencephalitis varies with geographic location. Infectious agents that most

commonly cause meningoencephalitis in cats include viruses (e.g. rabies and feline infectious peritonitis virus [FIP]), bacteria, protozoa (*Toxoplasma gondii*), and fungal organisms (e.g. cryptococcosis).

- FIP typically affects animals less than 3 years of age from multi-cat environments. However, cats as old as 15 years have been diagnosed with the disease. The causative agent, the FIP virus, is a mutant of the ubiquitous feline enteric coronavirus. The disease often has an insidious onset with progressive clinical signs. Neurological signs most commonly include altered mental status, visual deficits, vestibular syndrome, seizures, ataxia, and paresis. Three distinct clinical neurological syndromes affecting cats with FIP have been identified: multifocal CNS disease, central vestibular syndrome, and T3–L3 myelopathy. Affected cats may have concurrent systemic signs, including lethargy, anorexia, weight loss, and fluctuating pyrexia. Ocular lesions have also been identified, including anterior uveitis, iritis, keratic precipitates, and retinitis.

  Two forms of the disease are recognized: the effusive or "wet" form (associated with serous exudates into the abdominal cavity) and the noneffusive or "dry" form (associated with granulomatous parenchymal lesions). Neurological involvement is more common with the noneffusive form of the disease; more than one-third of the cases with the noneffusive form and less than 5% of cases with the effusive form of FIP present with involvement of the CNS. Neurological FIP induces a pyogranulomatous and immune complex-mediated vasculitis involving the leptomeninges, ependymal lining, periventricular brain parenchyma, spinal cord, and choroid plexus of the CNS. Pathological abnormalities are most commonly detected in the caudal cranial fossa, particularly affecting the caudoventral brainstem.

- Bacterial disease – Bacterial infections of the brain are usually a consequence of direct extension of infection from the inner/middle ear or sinuses or a penetrating injury to the skull (surgical or traumatic, such as a bite). Hematogenous spread can occur less commonly. Both aerobic and anaerobic bacteria have been isolated, with culture results typically yielding polymicrobial growth. Abscesses, granulomas, and intracranial empyema can result from bacterial diseases affecting the CNS.

  - A brain abscess is a collection of immune cells, pus, and other materials in the brain, usually from a bacterial, fungal, or protozoan infection.

  - Granulomas are a focal, compact collection of inflammatory cells in which mononuclear cells predominate. Granulomas usually form due to the persistence of a nondegradable substance or a hypersensitivity response. An overlap of the two mechanisms occurs in most infectious diseases since microorganisms can serve both as foreign bodies and as antigens for immunologic responses.

  - Empyema is a collection of pus that does not have a confining capsule. Most commonly, intracranial empyema is subdural in location. Subdural empyema represents a loculated infection between the outermost layer of the meninges, the dura, and the arachnoid.

- Fungal disease – The type of fungal infections affecting the CNS in cats depends on geographical location, but they tend to be uncommon. The major pathogens causing fungal meningoencephalitis include *Cryptococcus* spp., *Blastomyces dermatidis*, *Cladophialophora bantiana*, *Coccidoides*, and *Aspergillus* spp.

  Cryptococcus neoformans is a saprophytic yeast with a worldwide distribution and is the most common fungal disease of cats. The onset is usually chronic, with progressive neurological deficits that will depend on the localization of the lesion. Nonspecific signs include anorexia, weight loss, lethargy, lymphadenopathy, and pyrexia. Respiratory signs, skin lesions, and ocular disease can be seen in association with neurological signs. Neurological signs often reflect a focal or multifocal meningoencephalitis.

- Protozoal – *Toxoplasma gondii* is an intracellular protozoan parasite that can cause encephalitis in infected cats. Signs of disease are most frequently seen in young or immunocompromised animals and may occur concurrently with FIP. Neurological signs include seizures, behavioral changes, cranial nerve deficits, cerebellar signs, and multifocal or diffuse neuromuscular disease.

4. **Intoxication**

Toxins that cause neurological signs include plant or environmental toxins, envenomation, pesticides, herbicides, medications, or food. The suspected toxin may be based on known exposure, but in many situations, cats will exhibit clinical signs that cause suspicion of toxicity. Prompt recognition and management of the toxicity case are necessary to avoid serious morbidity and mortality. A thorough history is essential in the investigation of possible toxin exposure, which is most often considered with an acute onset of relatively symmetric intracranial disease unless there is associated hemorrhage.

In addition to clinical signs associated with nervous system dysfunction (see below), patients exposed to toxins may also exhibit gastrointestinal signs such as vomiting and diarrhea; cardiovascular signs such as arrhythmias, poor perfusion, discolored mucous membranes, and poor pulse quality. Such multisystem involvement emphasizes the need for a thorough physical examination.

Neurological clinical signs associated with toxicities can be directly due to the toxin itself or secondary to the effects of the toxin on other systems, such as respiratory compromise, causing hypoxic states, and coagulopathies, causing intracranial hemorrhage. Neurotoxins can be broadly categorized into neuro-excitatory and neuro-inhibitory according to the predominant neurological signs present. Neuro-excitatory toxins affect the CNS, causing hyper-excitability and seizures, and/or affect the peripheral nervous system (PNS), causing muscle tremors and fasciculations. Ataxia may also occur. Possible systemic complications associated with neuro-excitatory toxins can also include heat stroke (and subsequent complications such as disseminated intravascular coagulopathy [DIC]), rhabdomyolysis, aspiration pneumonia, and secondary neurologic injury. Neuro-inhibitory toxins either affect the CNS, causing obtundation, stupor, and coma, and/or affect the PNS, causing weakness or flaccid paralysis, which, at its most severe, includes respiratory paralysis.

For further information on toxicities, see Chapter 8.

WHAT DIAGNOSTIC TESTS ARE APPROPRIATE?

The diagnostic tests recommended based on this lesion localization and the potential differentials include a minimum database of hematology, serum chemistry, urinalysis, and infectious disease titers/PCR, in addition to thoracic and abdominal radiographs. A fundic examination in cats with suspected inflammatory or hypertensive encephalopathy is a sensitive test to support the diagnosis. Abdominal ultrasonography may also be of value in investigating a systemic focus of infection. Coagulation screening tests and blood pressure evaluations should be considered in all patients, but especially in those with vascular disease and intoxication, as likely possibilities. Blood and urine cultures could be considered if an inflammatory disease is suspected, particularly if there are systemic signs. Acute phase protein levels may be valuable in these cases as well.

The choice of specific neurodiagnostic techniques depends on the most likely underlying cause and location of the lesion. Although some diagnostic techniques, such as CT or MRI, may be indicated to investigate potential encephalopathy, the overall medical condition of the patient must be assessed and the risks and benefits calculated, particularly when general anesthesia is required (e.g. trauma patients). Skull radiographs are not sensitive or specific for diagnosing intracranial disease in cats or dogs. They may provide some useful corroborating information for animals with skull fractures, cranial bone tumors, otitis-media interna, and nasal disease.

1. **Vascular diseases**

   CSF analysis: Cerebrospinal fluid is often nonspecific and may be normal in the presence of vascular disease, although this helps to rule out inflammation as a cause. Mild increases in protein content, reflecting disruption of the blood–brain barrier, or increases in neutrophilic and mononuclear populations, may be seen.

   Imaging studies: As stroke alters the structural integrity of the brain, advanced imaging studies (such as CT and MRI) are often required. The imaging characteristics of a stroke may vary depending upon the degree of disease (e.g. ischemia versus overt hemorrhage) and the time between the onset of clinical signs and the imaging studies being performed. The appearance of cerebrovascular disease can vary from a focal lesion to diffuse or multifocal changes.

   CT images are frequently normal during the acute phase of ischemia; therefore, the diagnosis of ischemic stroke relies upon the exclusion of other diseases. Conventional MRI can be used to visualize ischemic stroke within hours of the onset of clinical signs and can also distinguish hemorrhagic lesions from infarction (Figure 3.2.3). However, the overall sensitivity and specificity of conventional MRI protocols for ischemic strokes in the first 24–48 hours are poor with focal inflammatory brain disease and some neoplastic lesions having a similar appearance on MR images. More detailed information on the imaging of stroke lesions can be found in the review by Arnold et al.

   Hypertensive encephalopathy has been associated with cerebral vasogenic edema, which typically results in an increased signal intensity within the white matter on T2-weighted (T2-W) MR images. It is most often bilaterally symmetrical and located in the subcortical cerebral white matter. In addition, lesions related to vasogenic edema are hyperintense on both DWI and ADC mapping, which suggests a T2 shine-through phenomenon related to restricted diffusion of protons.

2. **Traumatic brain injury**

   As with all types of trauma, the "ABC" (airway, breathing, circulation) of emergency care is extremely important. The initial physical assessment of the severely brain-injured patient focuses on imminently life-threatening abnormalities. It is important not to focus first on the neurological status of the patient, as many animals will be in a state of hypotensive shock following TBI, which can exacerbate obtunded mentation. Hypotension and hypoxemia need to be recognized and addressed immediately and should be routinely investigated in any animals suspected of experiencing a TBI. Once normotension, normovolemia, and appropriate oxygenation and ventilation are established, and the patient has been thoroughly assessed for traumatic injuries, a neurological examination, head imaging, and intracranial pressure measurement can be considered. Further information on TBI can be found in Chapter 15.

3. **Inflammatory disease of the brain**

   Once infectious etiologies have been investigated and systemic health assessed, specific CNS imaging and CSF analysis are important next diagnostic steps in cats suspected to have an inflammatory disease.

   CSF analysis: If there is evidence or even a suspicion of increased intracranial pressure (anisocoria, lack of pupil response to light, reduced or absent physiological nystagmus, decreased or absent response to noxious stimulation), diagnostic imaging should be performed prior to cisterna magna or lumbar puncture, which may risk promoting further herniation. In these cases, reducing the ICP using mannitol (0.25–1 g/kg IV) should be considered.

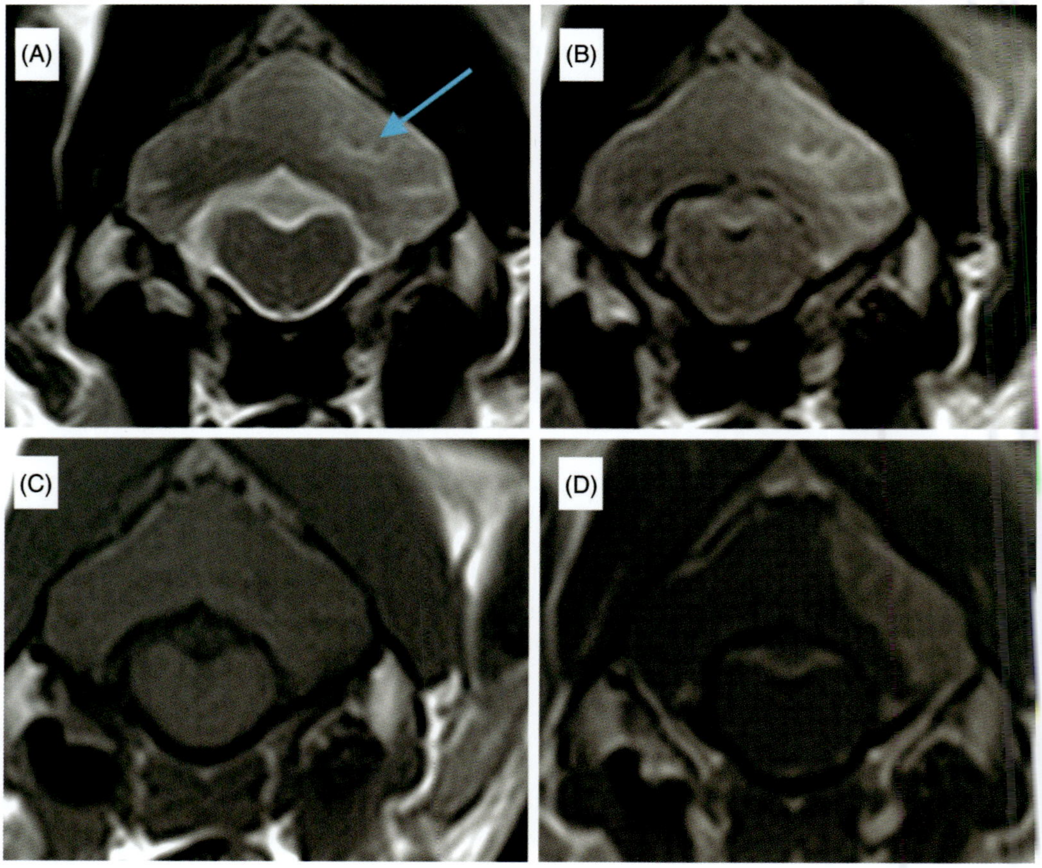

FIGURE 3.2.3 Transverse MR images of the caudal fossa of an 18-year-old European shorthaired cat that presented with an acute onset, 4 days earlier, of generalized ataxia with hypermetria of the left limbs and falling to the right side. There is a fairly well-defined intra-parenchymal lesion affecting the left cerebellar hemisphere and predominantly affecting the gray matter. This lesion is homogeneous, hyperintense in T2-W (A) and FLAIR (B), mildly hypointense in T1-W (C), and with strong parenchymal contrast enhancement (D). The lesion is compatible with an ischemic stroke.

Although CSF analysis is rarely specific, when it is assessed in conjunction with the patient's signalment, history, neurological signs, and the results of other diagnostic tests (such as serological assays), it can help to better define the underlying etiology. While an increased cell count, or pleocytosis, is commonly present in cases of inflammatory CNS disease, cytology rarely provides definitive differentiation among idiopathic, infectious, and neoplastic disorders. On occasion, bacteria, fungi, protozoa, or parasites may be identified on microscopic examination of CSF; however, this is extremely rare. One must be especially cautious not to "overinterpret" the CSF profile. For example, CSF analysis occasionally reveals no abnormalities. Despite its limitations, the CSF WBC differential may help the clinician to narrow down the differential diagnosis, especially when combined with cross-sectional imaging of the CNS.

Eosinophilic pleocytosis: Infectious diseases, such as *Cryptococcus*, *Toxoplasma*, and parasitic migration, can be considered when there is a predominance of eosinophils in the CSF.

Lymphocytic pleocytosis: Viral disease, lymphoma, and immune-mediated diseases should be considered with lymphocytic proliferation in the CSF.

Neutrophilic pleocytosis: Feline infectious peritonitis is an important differential diagnosis in cats when there is a high prevalence of CSF neutrophils. Often, total protein is elevated over 200 mg/dL with over 100 white blood cells/μL, with over 50% being neutrophils. Degenerate neutrophils can be seen with bacterial infections.

Mixed cell and mononuclear pleocytosis: This is a nonspecific finding and may be secondary to any insult to the brain. Immune-mediated diseases (MUO) have been documented with this finding.

Imaging studies: While CT may have diagnostic utility in some cases of inflammatory brain disease, MRI is the gold standard neuroimaging modality.

Encephalitis may cause no detectable abnormalities on MRI or may manifest as multifocal (rather than focal or diffuse) lesions associated with brain parenchyma that typically appear hyperintense on T2-W images, and hypointense on T1-weighted (T1-W) images. Fluid attenuated inversion recovery (FLAIR) has higher sensitivity than conventional spin-echo sequences in detecting subtle brain lesions in dogs with clinical signs of multifocal brain disease, and its use is encouraged in all of these cases. Meningitis may not be detected with MRI or may appear as meningeal enhancement following administration of contrast medium. Most findings are nonspecific for the underlying inflammatory etiology and, in some cases, are not specific for inflammatory disease versus neoplasia or vascular disease.

- In FIP, MRI may show T2 hyperintensity and contrast enhancement of ventricular lining, choroid plexus, and meninges compatible with ependymitis, choroiditis, and meningitis (Figure 3.2.4). Concurrent hydrocephalus is common secondary to obstruction of CSF flow, and herniation of the cerebellum secondary to increased intracranial pressure is possible.

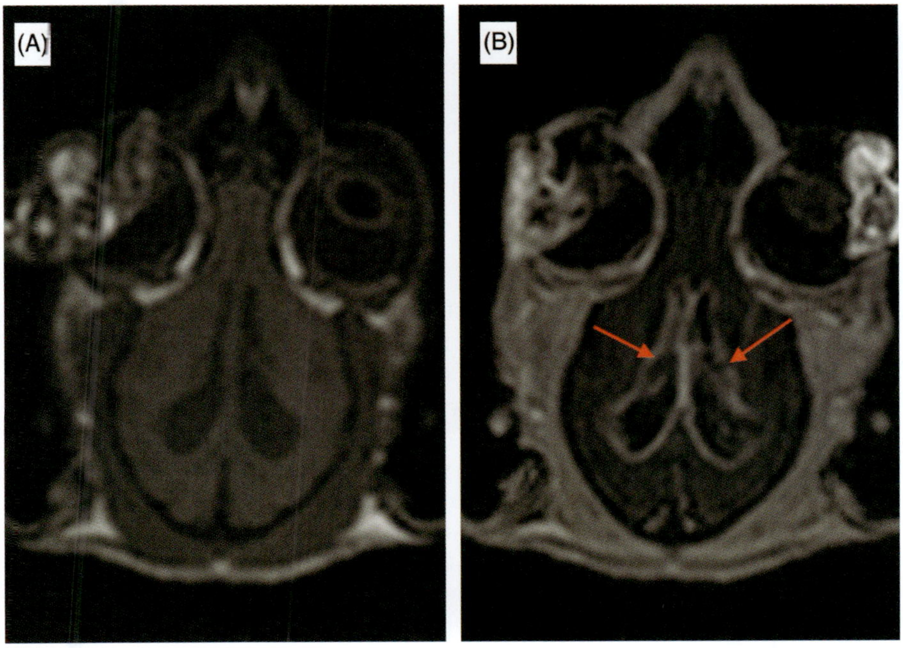

FIGURE 3.2.4 Dorsal T1-W (A) and 3D T1-W post-contrast (B) MR images of an 18-month-old domestic shorthaired cat's brain. The cat presented with a dull and confused mentation. There is a bilateral and relatively symmetrical expansion of the lateral ventricles, which exhibit diffuse ependymal contrast enhancement. FIP was confirmed on post-mortem.

- MRI may help identify a suspected bacterial infection based on concurrent abnormalities of local structures (ears, sinuses, nasal cavity) that are responsible for the origin of the infection. Extension of disease from these structures could give rise to nonspecific signs of meningitis and encephalitis but may also be associated with abscesses and empyema (Figure 3.2.5). Intracranial abscesses are typically hypointense on T1-W and hyperintense on T2-W images, with strong peripheral contrast enhancement and associated brain edema.
- Fungal disease can be associated with focal or multifocal intra-parenchymal mass lesions with dural contact, lesion hypointensity on T2-W images and diffusion-weighted imaging/apparent diffusion coefficient map (DWI/ADC), strong and homogeneous

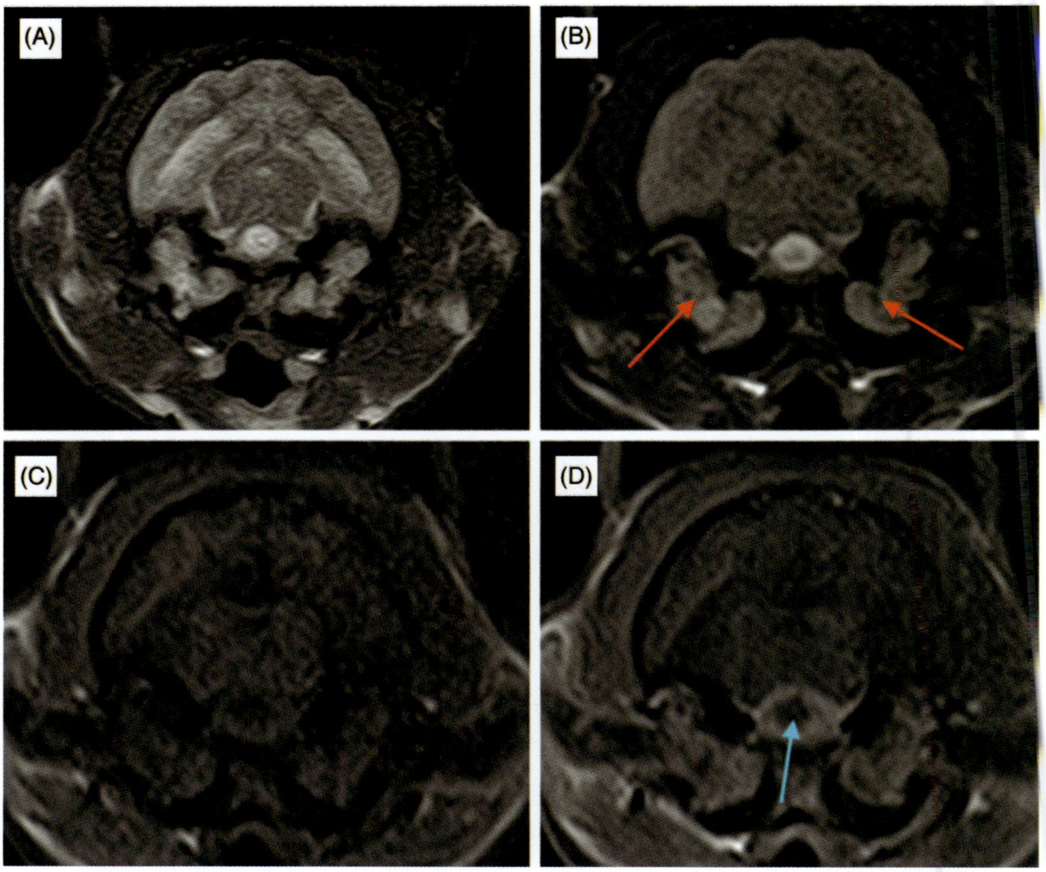

FIGURE 3.2.5 Transverse MR images of the brain at the level of the tympanic cavities and the midbrain of a 3-year-old domestic shorthaired cat, which presented with chronic waxing and waning dull mentation and ataxia. There is a large space-occupying intracranial extra-parenchymal lesion along the ventral aspect of the brainstem (blue arrow). This lesion is mainly T2-W (A), and FLAIR (B) hyperintense, T1 isointense (C), with strong contrast enhancement (D). There is a well-defined strongly T2-W hyperintense, T1-W hypointense, noncontrast-enhancing area in the center of the lesion. There is meningeal thickening and contrast-enhancement in continuity with the lesion along the ventral and lateral aspects of the brainstem. There is a mass effect with marked left ventral compression and dorsal deviation of the brainstem. The tympanic cavities are filled with heterogeneous material (red arrows) with a contrast-enhancing lining along their inner surface. The images are compatible with bilateral otitis media and interna with intracranial extension to caudal fossa empyema and meningitis.

contrast enhancement of the lesion(s), concurrent meningeal enhancement, marked perilesional edema and mass-effect, and ocular abnormalities. Imaging findings in cats with CNS cryptococcosis include solitary or multifocal mass lesions that are typically hyperintense on T2-W images and show variable degrees of contrast enhancement. Diffuse and patchy meningeal, ependymal, and choroid plexus enhancements are also possible.

- Protozoal meningoencephalitis in cats has been documented to cause multifocal, indistinct, contrast-enhancing parenchymal lesions that were iso- to hypointense on T1-W images, hyperintense on T2-W images, and are associated with edema.
- Parasitic meningoencephalitis in cats can appear on MRI as focal or multifocal parenchymal lesions of variable signal intensity and peripheral parenchymal or meningeal contrast enhancement. Intraparenchymal hemorrhage is a common feature in parasite migration, and T2*-W images are useful in establishing a presumptive diagnosis.
- Magnetic resonance imaging shows intraparenchymal infiltrative ill-defined lesions in cats with MUO.

4. **Intoxication**
   In many patients, especially when the exposure to a toxin is uncertain, the diagnostic approach to the patient must proceed in tandem with supportive care, symptomatic treatment, and decontamination procedures.

- A complete minimum database is essential in any animal suspected of having neurotoxicity. At a minimum, a urine dipstick should be performed in addition to electrolyte, glucose, and calcium assessments.
- A bilirubin serum level or bile acid tolerance test may be performed to rule out endogenous toxicity due to liver disease or to investigate the secondary effects of the toxin on the liver itself.
- Ongoing measurement of urine production could be vital to predicting a potential oliguric or anuric state.
- Blood gas, anion gap, and osmolality measurement (where possible) should also be considered. If blood gas is not possible, oxygenation status can be monitored with a pulse oximeter, although certain toxins can demonstrate a normal pulse oximeter reading despite severe poisoning, as is the case with carbon monoxide poisoning.
- Coagulation testing is recommended for rodenticide exposure and envenomation.
- Thoracic and abdominal imaging, inclusive of ultrasonography, may be essential to detect secondary consequences such as aspiration pneumonia and cavity effusions.
- The use of urine testing kits for illegal drug intoxication in cats and dogs should be considered. An on-site urine toxicity screen can accurately detect the presence of amphetamines, barbiturates, benzodiazepines, and opioids, although it may be less accurate for the detection of the more common marijuana toxicity.
- CSF analysis and advanced nervous system imaging may be required to rule out other causes of similar clinical signs, especially inflammatory disease and vascular disease, which can both be acute in onset. It should be recognized that these tests require anesthesia, and this could compromise the patient, who may already have a severe mentally obtunded state, respiratory complications, and/or aberrations of blood pressure.

- Contacting a poison control center – Regional and national animal poison control services should be contacted in all cases where there has been a certain exposure to a known toxin. Such services can provide information on all known pharmacokinetics of the toxin, its metabolism and excretion, expected clinical signs, and recommended therapies. In addition, where the toxin is a manufactured product, the manufacturer can be contacted for specific information.

OUTCOME

In our case, the minimum database was considered normal, but there was an elevated serum T4 concentration, and systolic blood pressure was consistently above 160 mmHg. CSF acquired from the atlanto-occipital cistern was considered normal.

MRI confirmed an ill-defined and irregular intraparenchymal lesion centered on the right paramedian thalamus (Figure 3.2.6). The lesion was homogenously T2-W hyperintense, FLAIR heterogeneously iso- to hyperintense, and T1-W

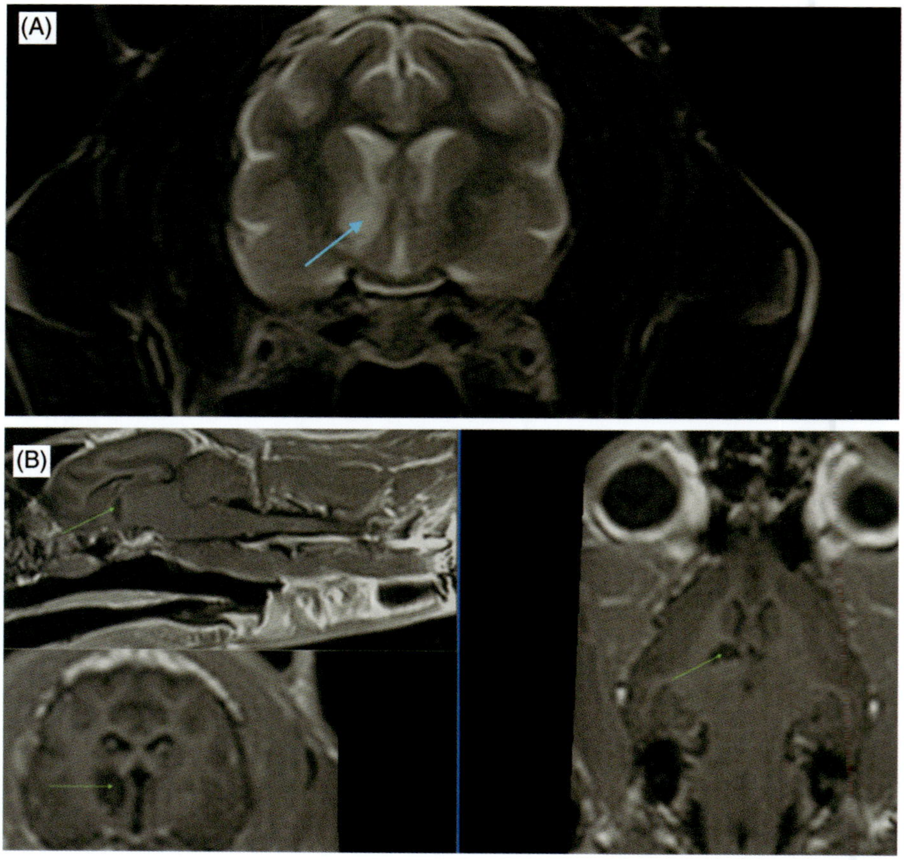

FIGURE 3.2.6 Transverse T2-W (A) and 3D reconstructed T1-W MPRAGE post-contrast (B) MR images of the cat detailed in this case study. There is an ill-defined and irregular, moderately sized intraparenchymal lesion centered on the right paramedian thalamus. The lesion is immediately caudal and ventral to the right caudate nucleus. The lesion is homogenously T2-W hyperintense (blue arrow), T1-W hypointense with no contrast enhancement (green arrows). There is no evident mass effect. The right brain is on the left side of the images in this figure.

hypointense with no contrast enhancement. There was no evident mass effect or SWI signal void. Although not definitive, the diagnostic findings were compatible with an ischemic stroke of several days' duration. The cat was reported to show slow and continuous improvement over the next month without specific treatment apart from that directed at hyperthyroidism and high blood pressure, also compatible with an ischemic event. The short-term prognosis for cats and dogs with ischemic strokes, if they are neither severely affected nor impacted by critical concurrent disease, is good. The long-term prognosis in cats with CVAs is currently unknown, but in dogs, it is considered good if no underlying disease is found. In a single study with a total of 22 dogs with presumed CVAs, 23% died within 30 days; however, those that survived this period had a median survival time of 505 days.

SUGGESTED READING

Acierno, M.J., Brown, S., Coleman, A.E. et al. (2018). ACVIM consensus statement: guidelines for the identification, evaluation, and management of systemic hypertension in dogs and cats. *J. Vet. Intern. Med.* 32 (6): 1803–1822.

Altay, U.M., Skerritt, G.C., Hilbe, M. et al. (2011). Feline cerebrovascular disease: clinical and histopathologic findings in 16 cats. *J. Am. Anim. Hosp. Assoc.* 47 (2): 89–97.

Arnold, S.A., Platt, S.R., Gendron, K.P., and West, F.D. (2020). Imaging ischemic and hemorrhagic disease of the brain in dogs. *Front. Vet. Sci.* 7: 279.

Bentley, R.T., Taylor, A.R., and Thomovsky, S.A. (2018). Fungal infections of the central nervous system in small animals: clinical features, diagnosis, and management. *Vet. Clin. North Am. Small Anim. Pract.* 48 (1): 63–83.

Boudreau, C.E. (2018). An update on cerebrovascular disease in dogs and cats. *Vet. Clin. North Am. Small Anim. Pract.* 48 (1): 45–62.

Church, M.E., Turek, B.J., and Durham, A.C. (2019). Neuropathology of spontaneous hypertensive encephalopathy in cats. *Vet. Pathol.* 56 (5): 778–782.

Crawford, A.H., Stoll, A.L., Sanchez-Masian, D. et al. (2017). Clinicopathologic features and magnetic resonance imaging findings in 24 cats with histopathologically confirmed neurologic feline infectious peritonitis. *J. Vet. Intern. Med.* 31 (5): 1477–1486.

deLahunta, A., Glass, E., and Kent, M. (2021). *Veterinary Neuroanatomy and Clinical Neurology*, 5e. Philadelphia: Elsevier.

Felten, S. and Hartmann, K. (2019). Diagnosis of feline infectious peritonitis: a review of the current literature. *Viruses* 11 (11): 1068.

Garosi, L.S. (2010). Cerebrovascular disease in dogs and cats. *Vet. Clin. North Am. Small Anim. Pract.* 40 (1): 65–79.

Gunn-Moore, D.A. and Reed, N. (2011). CNS disease in the cat: current knowledge of infectious causes. *J. Feline Med. Surg.* 13 (11): 824–836.

Gruendl, S., Matiasek, K., Matiasek, L. et al. (2017). Diagnostic utility of cerebrospinal fluid immunocytochemistry for diagnosis of feline infectious peritonitis manifesting in the central nervous system. *J. Feline Med. Surg.* 19 (6): 576–585.

Hecht, S. and Adams, W.H. (2010). MRI of brain disease in veterinary patients part 2: acquired brain disorders. *Vet. Clin. North Am. Small Anim. Pract.* 40 (1): 39–63.

Hecht, S., Michaels, J.R., and Simon, H. (2022). Case report: MRI findings with CNS blastomycosis in three domestic cats. *Front. Vet. Sci.* 9: 966853.

Kuo, K.W., Bacek, L.M., and Taylor, A.R. (2018). Head trauma. *Vet. Clin. North Am. Small Anim. Pract.* 48 (1): 111–128.

Markert, C., Heilmann, R.M., Kiwitz, D., and Dörfelt, R. (2023). A retrospective evaluation of confirmed and suspected poisonings in 166 cats between 2016 and 2020. *Vet. World* 16 (9): 1940–1951.

Moretto, L., Beckmann, K., Günther, C. et al. (2023). Manifestations of hypertensive encephalopathy in cats. *J. Feline Med. Surg.* 25 (2): 1098612X231153357.

Negrin, A., Spencer, S., and Cherubini, G.B. (2017). Feline meningoencephalomyelitis of unknown origin: a retrospective analysis of 16 cases. *Can. Vet. J.* 58 (10): 1073–1080.

Nessler, J., Wohlsein, P., Junginger, J. et al. (2020). Meningoencephalomyelitis of unknown origin in cats: a case series describing clinical and pathological findings. *Front. Vet. Sci.* 7: 291.

O'Neill, J., Kent, M., Glass, E.N., and Platt, S.R. (2013). Clinicopathologic and MRI characteristics of presumptive hypertensive encephalopathy in two cats and two dogs. *J. Am. Anim. Hosp. Assoc.* 49: 412–420.

Quitt, P.R., Reese, S., Fischer, A. et al. (2019). Assessment of menace response in neurologically and ophthalmologically healthy cats. *J. Feline Med. Surg.* 21 (6): 537–543.

Smolek, T., Vince-Kazmerova, Z., Hanes, J. et al. (2024). On the utility of cerebrospinal fluid biomarkers in canine neurological disorders. *Sci. Rep.* 14 (1): 24129.

Stiles, J., Weil, A.B., Packer, R.A., and Lantz, G.C. (2012). Post-anesthetic cortical blindness in cats: twenty cases. *Vet. J.* 193 (2): 367–373.

Whittaker, D.E., Drees, R., and Beltran, E. (2018). MRI and clinical characteristics of suspected cerebrovascular accident in nine cats. *J. Feline Med. Surg.* 20 (8): 674–684.

Wismer, T. and Means, C. (2018). Toxicology of newer insecticides in small animals. *Vet. Clin. North Am. Small Anim. Pract.* 48 (6): 1013–1026.

Circling and Altered Mentation

Case 3—Dog with Marked Reduction of Consciousness

CHAPTER 3.3

Susan A. Arnold

Department of Veterinary Clinical Sciences, University of Minnesota, St. Paul, MN, USA

CASE HISTORY

A 5-month-old intact female Yorkshire Terrier was presented for lethargy that had been progressing over a period of 4 weeks. The dog was acquired from a breeder at 12 weeks of age. The dog had already received three rounds of distemper–hepatitis–parainfluenza–parvovirus vaccines and received a 1-year rabies vaccine at 16 weeks of age. The dog had no known health concerns, was not receiving any medications other than heartworm and flea/tick preventatives, and ate a commercial puppy kibble for small-breed dogs. The dog had no known access to toxins.

NEUROLOGICAL EXAMINATION

The puppy was severely obtunded to the point that it was nearly stuporous. When stimulated enough to prompt limb movement, she was non-ambulatory and was voluntarily paddling all four limbs while laterally recumbent. Limb tone was considered normal. Postural reactions were abnormal based on delayed hopping observed in all four limbs. Spinal reflexes were normal. All cranial nerve (CN) testing was normal, other than an absent menace bilaterally and a subjectively reduced gag reflex. There was no evidence of pain or discomfort on vertebral column palpation or when testing cervical vertebral range of motion.

1. **Where is the likely lesion localization?**
2. **What major disease processes should be considered?**
3. **What tests could you perform to help determine the diagnosis?**

LESION LOCALIZATION

This dog's severely altered mental state immediately indicates that the lesion affects either the forebrain (cerebrum and thalamus; prosencephalon) or the functional components of the brainstem (midbrain, pons, and medulla oblongata). In this dog's case, severe obtundation could be equally attributable to either the forebrain or the brainstem.

Gait dysfunction can be used to distinguish between the forebrain and the brainstem in milder cases in which the patient is not laterally recumbent; patients with a forebrain lesion will have a normal gait, whereas patients with a brainstem lesion can display hemiparesis or tetraparesis with general proprioceptive ataxia, and sometimes vestibular ataxia. In this case, the patient was too obtunded to be motivated to ambulate, eliminating this component as helpful for delineation between the two lesion localizations.

A key distinction helpful for localization occurs in the form of muscle tone: patients with lesions in the brainstem can exhibit increased extensor tone in their limbs and cervical musculature, whereas these features are not present in patients with lesions in the forebrain.

The delayed postural reactions do not help to distinguish between localizations, as both forebrain and brainstem lesions can cause postural reaction deficits.

The most helpful portion of the exam for this dog is the CN exam. Patients with brainstem lesions often have CN deficits referable to the nerves associated with the midbrain (CN III and IV), pons (CN V), and medulla oblongata (CN VI–XII). The only CN deficit observed in this dog was a menace deficit. Given the normal pupillary light reflex and palpebral reflex, the menace deficit observed in this dog is attributable to the cerebral cortex. Overall, given that the only CN deficit is referable to the cerebrum, this patient's lesion localization can be confirmed to be the forebrain.

DIFFERENTIAL DIAGNOSIS

Metabolic Disease – Hepatic Encephalopathy

This is an extremely likely differential diagnosis for this patient based on her signalment, the lesion localization, and the history.

In young animals, hepatic encephalopathy most often results from the presence of a portosystemic shunt. This is a congenital malformation in which blood carried from the small intestine is diverted away from its normal course to the liver due to the presence of an aberrant vessel. Blood coursing from the intestines contains abundant quantities of ammonia, which is normally processed by the liver before entering the systemic circulation. In animals with portosystemic shunts, excessive ammonia in the circulation readily crosses the blood–brain barrier (BBB). How ammonia in the brain causes hepatic encephalopathy is not completely understood. The prevailing hypothesis is that ammonia leads to astrocyte swelling, which interferes with astrocyte function. In response to ammonia, astrocytes can also release the excitatory neurotransmitter glutamate, which may be responsible for the agitation and seizures seen in some patients with hepatic encephalopathy. Other factors, including increased production of neurosteroids, oxidative stress, manganese accumulation, and amino acid imbalance, may also contribute to the development of hepatic encephalopathy.

A grading scheme for clinical signs has been developed: Grade 0: no clinical signs; Grade 1 mildly decreased mobility, apathy, or both; Grade 2: severe apathy, mild ataxia, or both; Grade 3: hypersalivation, severe ataxia, head pressing, blindness, circling, or some combination of these signs; and Grade 4: seizures, stupor, or coma (1,2).

Metabolic Disease – Hypoglycemia

Hypoglycemia is a common cause of abnormal mental status in young, toy-breed dogs, especially in puppies less than 4 months old. Hypoglycemia can be the result of insufficient carbohydrate intake and depletion of the small glycogen reserves.

Other causes of hypoglycemia that would be unlikely in this puppy but are important to consider include hepatic dysfunction, resulting in impaired glycogenolysis and gluconeogenesis, excessive insulin administration in animals being treated for diabetes mellitus, the production of insulin-like substances from neoplasms such as beta islet cell tumors and leiomyosarcomas, xylitol toxicity, and extreme exercise.

The brain relies primarily on glucose as its sole energy source. Thus, when hypoglycemia develops, patients exhibit the same signs as observed in dogs with hepatic encephalopathy. Seizures generally do not occur until blood glucose levels dip below 40 mg/dL (3).

Anomalous Disease – Hydrocephalus

Hydrocephalus is the most common structural anomalous disorder and is defined as the excessive accumulation of cerebrospinal fluid within the ventricular system of the brain, which results in clinical signs. It can occur as a congenital malformation or secondary to a lesion either within the ventricular system or adjacent to it. These acquired causes of hydrocephalus include tumors, infections in the brain, such as the ventriculitis that develops in cats with feline coronavirus encephalitis, and immune-mediated meningoencephalitis.

Congenital hydrocephalus most commonly occurs due to stenosis of the mesencephalic aqueduct, a narrow tube that connects the third ventricle to the fourth ventricle. As a result of stenosis, cerebrospinal fluid accumulates within the third and lateral ventricles. The fluid accumulation leads to compression of neuroparenchyma and subsequent neurological dysfunction.

Clinical signs can range from mild cognitive dysfunction to incoordination, blindness, and seizures.

Traumatic Disease – Head Trauma

Head trauma, resulting from motor vehicle accidents, falls, and blows to the head, can result in variable degrees of encephalopathy. Neurological signs of head trauma are often apparent immediately after the injury and may worsen over the course of 48–72 hours. The primary injury initiates a cascade of physiologic responses that are collectively referred to as the secondary injury, which includes excessive excitatory neurotransmitter release, the formation of reactive oxygen species, cellular energy depletion, and cellular swelling.

The severity of a traumatic brain injury (TBI) due to head trauma can be assessed using the Modified Glasgow Coma scale, which provides a numerical output correlated with prognosis (4).

See Chapter 15 for a more thorough summary of head trauma.

Toxicity

There are many substances that can lead to acute changes of mental status and other neurologic deficits, such as seizure activity, visual deficits, and tremors. Examples include bromethalin, xylitol (by way of causing hypoglycemia), ivermectin, marijuana, illicit drugs, lead, and neuropsychiatric drugs. Signs of neurotoxicity generally appear within hours of ingestion and may be accompanied by other systemic signs, depending on the ingested toxin.

Vascular Disease – Cerebrovascular Accident or Stroke

Ischemic and hemorrhagic strokes in dogs lead to peracute nonprogressive neurologic dysfunction. Hemorrhagic stroke can also lead to progressive neurological deterioration over the next 24–72 hours.

After the rostral cerebellar artery, the middle cerebral artery is the second most common canine brain artery affected by ischemic stroke (5). The middle cerebral artery supplies a large portion of the ipsilateral cerebral hemisphere. A stroke secondary to middle cerebral artery disease could therefore result in severe abnormality of mental status in addition to other neurological deficits referable to the region of the brain affected.

PATIENT INVESTIGATION

Hepatic Encephalopathy

Episodic signs of cerebral dysfunction, often observed to worsen postprandially, are suggestive of a portosystemic shunt and hepatic encephalopathy. Dogs with portosystemic shunts may have microcytic, normochromic, nonregenerative anemia, hypoalbuminemia, hypocholesterolemia, hypoglycemia, and low blood urea nitrogen (BUN). Liver enzymes are often increased. Coagulation times can also be prolonged. Urinalysis can reveal decreased urine specific gravity and ammonium biurate crystalluria (Figure 3.3.1). Fasting venous ammonia is often elevated in dogs

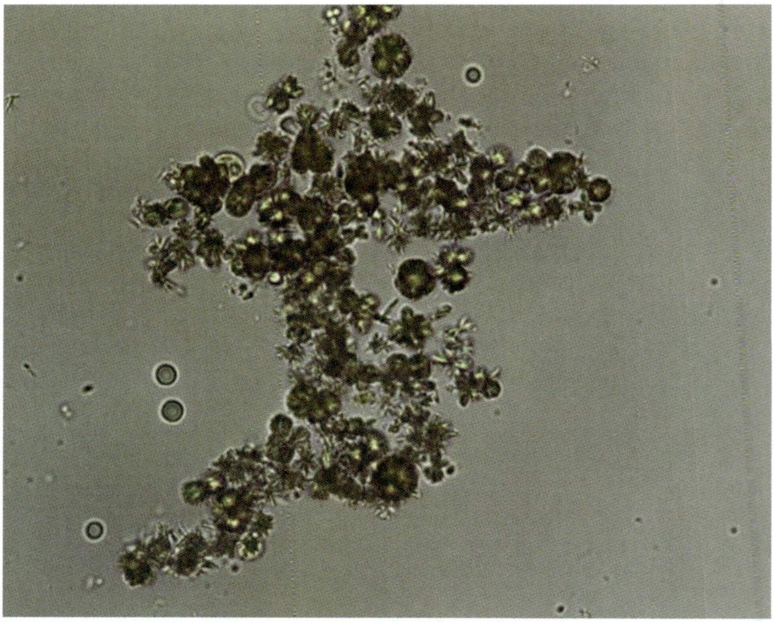

FIGURE 3.3.1 Ammonium biurate crystals in the urine of a dog with a portosystemic shunt.

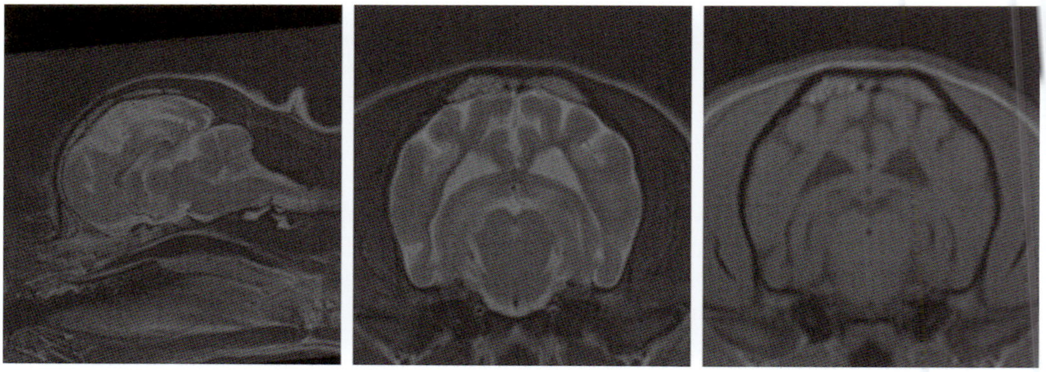

FIGURE 3.3.2 Magnetic resonance images of the brain of a dog with hepatic encephalopathy. Note the widened sulci visible on the T2-weighted transverse image (middle image) and T1-weighted transverse image (right image).

with hepatic encephalopathy, although venous ammonia measurement is less reliable than measuring pre- and postprandial bile acids. In dogs with portosystemic shunts, post-prandial bile acids are elevated. Ultrasonography can be used to evaluate liver size and can often identify the aberrant shunting vessel, but it is overall a less sensitive diagnostic test than computed tomography (CT), which has nearly 100% sensitivity and specificity for the identification of a portosystemic shunt. Magnetic resonance imaging (MRI) of the brain may show widened sulci, as well as T1-weighted hyperintensity in the lentiform nuclei, which is proposed to occur due to manganese deposition (Figure 3.3.2).

Hypoglycemia

Signs that worsen following a period of fasting in a young dog, or are episodic in dogs of any age, are suggestive of hypoglycemia.

Confirmation of hypoglycemia is readily performed by assessing serum blood glucose levels. A minimum database can help in assessing various causes of hypoglycemia, especially hepatic insufficiency associated with a portosystemic shunt, neoplasia, or cirrhosis impeding the normal function of the liver.

Xylitol is a sucrose alternative that is found in many sugar-free products, including some candies, chewing gums, and peanut butter, and can be ruled in or out as the cause of hypoglycemia through thorough historical questioning. Once xylitol toxicity and hepatic dysfunction have been ruled out, a presumptive diagnosis of juvenile fasting hypoglycemia can be made in young, small-breed dogs.

Hypoglycemia of extreme exercise is presumed if a low blood glucose reading is obtained after extreme exercise, but is not repeatable during times of rest.

In older dogs in which a neoplastic cause of hypoglycemia is suspected, a paired insulin-blood glucose measurement is obtained during a period of hypoglycemia. Normal to increased insulin in the face of hypoglycemia is suggestive of an insulin-like substance-producing tumor.

Although ultrasound can be used to evaluate the liver, pancreas, and small intestine for such types of tumors, ultrasound has poor sensitivity for the most common tumor to cause hypoglycemia (beta islet cell tumor). CT is therefore the preferred diagnostic modality for this investigation.

Hydrocephalus

Some dogs with hydrocephalus have external conformational abnormalities, including a fixed, bilateral ventrolateral strabismus and a domed head that extends laterally beyond the zygomatic arches. They may also have a persistently open fontanelle on the top of the head. However, many dogs with hydrocephalus do not have any overt conformational abnormalities.

Radiographs are rarely performed, given the availability of more sensitive imaging techniques. If a persistent fontanelle is present, an ultrasound can be directed through the opening to evaluate the neuroparenchyma. If excessive anechoic fluid is observed (occupying approximately 60% or more of the cranial cavity), a diagnosis of hydrocephalus can be suspected if other diseases are ruled out. CT can also be used to evaluate for hydrocephalus, but MRI is the most sensitive and specific imaging modality for confirming hydrocephalus and ruling out other brain lesions.

Head Trauma

Head trauma is generally confirmed when the traumatic event is witnessed or highly suspected, given environmental contexts.

Gentle palpation may reveal skull fractures. An otoscopic examination should be performed, as hemorrhage within the ear canal can be suggestive of skull fractures. Skull radiographs can be used to confirm skull fractures, but are technically difficult to perform effectively in a traumatized animal. CT and MRI are the imaging modalities of choice for evaluating head trauma. CT has a slight superiority for identifying bone fractures, whereas MRI gives a more comprehensive view of the neuroparenchyma, including identification of edema, tissue laceration, and hemorrhage.

Toxicities

Historical questioning is imperative in ascertaining the possibility of toxin ingestion. Consultation with a veterinary toxicologist, often available through pet poison hotlines, can help to determine if an ingested substance could be the cause of observed neurological dysfunction. Some toxins will cause alterations that can be observed on a minimum database.

Vascular Disease (Stroke)

Stroke itself is not associated with abnormalities that can be detected on a minimum database, but the underlying causes of some strokes, including hyperadrenocorticism and renal disease, can be suspected based on abnormalities on complete blood count, blood chemistry panels, and urinalysis. As systemic hypertension is also a cause of strokes, patients should have their systemic blood pressure measured. Confirming a stroke in dogs and cats requires a brain MRI.

TREATMENT AND PROGNOSIS

Hepatic Encephalopathy

Treatment depends on the cause of hepatic encephalopathy. When it occurs secondary to congenital portosystemic shunts, treatment consists of medical interventions and, in some cases, surgical intervention. Medical treatment for hepatic encephalopathy secondary to a portosystemic shunt consists of feeding a low-protein diet to reduce nitrogenous byproducts, lactulose to trap nitrogenous molecules within the gastrointestinal tract and to speed gastrointestinal transit time, and antimicrobials to reduce the gastrointestinal flora responsible for generating nitrogenous byproducts. In severe cases of hepatic encephalopathy, lactulose retention enemas can also aid in rapidly reducing clinical signs. Surgical treatment for portosystemic shunts consists of shunt attenuation, which can be achieved through several techniques. The reader is directed to surgical textbooks for more information regarding the details of these surgical procedures. An important factor to consider is that following shunt ligation, animals can rarely develop a constellation of signs collectively referred to as post-attenuation neurologic signs (PANS). While prophylactic levetiracetam administration does not necessarily prevent post-attenuation seizures, which are one of the components of PANS, it can prevent death from these often severe seizures. Thus perioperative treatment with levetiracetam is recommended.

Hypoglycemia

Immediate treatment of hypoglycemia consists of glucose replacement, typically either through intravenous dextrose administration or, when unavailable, the application of corn syrup to the oral mucous membranes. Long-term treatment of persistent hypoglycemia is directed at the underlying cause. The reader is referred to internal medicine textbooks and resources for more thorough descriptions of these treatments.

Head Trauma

Please refer to Chapter 15, Case 1, for a comprehensive review of head trauma management.

Toxicities

Treatment is highly variable depending on the toxic substance. Some toxins have antidotes, while the treatment of others consists exclusively of supportive care. Treatment should be guided by a veterinary toxicologist.

Vascular Disease (Stroke)

There is no direct therapy for canine strokes. Most dogs that have experienced ischemic strokes show improvement over several weeks with adequate supportive care. For more details, please see Chapter 5, Case 3.

OUTCOME

The puppy's minimum database was suggestive of portosystemic shunting: a microcytic anemia was observed, along with low serum albumin, glucose, BUN, and cholesterol, and ammonium biurate crystalluria. The dog was treated with a lactulose retention enema, which improved its mentation. Subsequently, the dog received oral metronidazole and lactulose and was fed a low-protein diet. These therapies reduced the patient's clinical signs. Bile acid testing later showed markedly elevated pre- and post-prandial levels. A portosystemic shunt was subsequently confirmed via abdominal ultrasound. Three months after diagnosis, the puppy was referred to a surgical practice for shunt attenuation. Three days prior to surgery, levetiracetam therapy was initiated, and the dog remained on this medication until 2 weeks after surgery. Shunt attenuation was achieved with cellophane banding. Recovery was uneventful, and the observed mentation abnormalities resolved.

SUGGESTED READING

Garosi, L.S. (2010). Cerebrovascular disease in dogs and cats. *Vet. Clin. North Am. Small Anim. Pract.* 40 (1): 65–79.

Idowu, O. and Heading, K. (2018). Hypoglycemia in dogs: causes, management, and diagnosis. *Can. Vet. J.* 59 (6): 642.

Konstantinidis, A.O., Patsikas, M.N., Papazoglou, L.G., and Adamama-Moraitou, K.K. (2023). Congenital portosystemic shunts in dogs and cats: classification, pathophysiology, clinical presentation and diagnosis. *Vet. Sci.* 10 (2): 160.

Lidbury, J.A., Cook, A.K., and Steiner, J.M. (2016). Hepatic encephalopathy in dogs and cats. *J. Vet. Emerg. Crit. Care* 26 (4): 471–487.

Platt, S.R., Radaelli, S.T., and McDonnell, J.J. (2001). The prognostic value of the modified Glasgow coma scale in head trauma in dogs. *J. Vet. Intern. Med.* 15 (6): 581–584.

CHAPTER 3.4

Circling and Altered Mentation

Case 4—Cat with Chronic Reduced Consciousness

Susan A. Arnold

Department of Veterinary Clinical Sciences, University of Minnesota, St. Paul, MN, USA

CASE HISTORY

A 14-year-old neutered male domestic short-haired cat was presented for several months of progressive behavioral changes. Initially, the cat displayed less interest in playing with his toys. Over the course of 3 weeks, he stopped playing with his toys entirely. Additionally, he started wandering around the house, seemingly aimlessly, and vocalizing at random (Video 3.4.1).

VIDEO 3.4.1 Cat displaying obtundation, leftward propulsive circling, and dementia. Source: Video credit: David Dumond.

He was evaluated by his primary veterinarian, and no overt abnormalities were observed on general physical examination. Complete blood count, blood chemistry panel, and urinalysis were normal. Anxiety and cognitive dysfunction were considered potential causes, and the owners were offered anxiolytic medication trial for their pet, which they declined in favor of continued monitoring.

The behavior worsened over 6–7 weeks to the point where the cat routinely interrupted his owners' sleep with his pacing and vocalizations. Although the pacing continued, about 3 months into the cat's change in behavior, he became less energetic and appeared to wake only at feeding time.

Throughout this process, his appetite remained robust, his water intake stayed consistent, and he urinated and defecated normally in his litterbox. Historically, the cat spent time both indoors and outdoors, but had been an indoor-only cat for the last 5 years. He was up to date on all core feline vaccinations, had received a feline leukemia vaccine as a kitten, and consumed a commercial canned cat food.

A general physical examination revealed a body condition score of 6/9 with generalized, severe periodontal disease and an unkempt hair coat.

NEUROLOGICAL EXAMINATION

Upon examination, the cat was moderately obtunded, indicating that he was significantly less responsive to stimuli than expected. Normally, this cat was active in exploring new environments and often required restraint to prevent him from swatting and biting; however, he currently sat on the exam room floor without showing interest in his surroundings. He vocalized intermittently.

When he was encouraged to walk, he hissed lightly. In the limited time he walked around the room, no overt paresis, ataxia, or lameness was appreciated. When asked to describe his gait patterns at home, his owners commented that he tended to walk in broad, leftward (counterclockwise) circles. His head position was normal. Paw placement was not performed, given his historical reluctance to have his feet touched. Other postural reaction tests were subjectively considered normal in all four limbs. His muscle mass and tone were normal in all four limbs, as were spinal reflexes. His cutaneous trunci reflex could not be elicited. His perineal reflex was normal.

On cranial nerve examination, his pupillary light and palpebral reflexes were normal bilaterally. He had an absent menace response bilaterally. All other cranial nerve tests were normal. The cat hissed throughout vertebral column palpation. Normal cervical range of motion was observed.

1. **Where is the likely lesion localization?**
2. **What major disease processes should be considered?**
3. **What tests could you perform to help determine the diagnosis?**

LESION LOCALIZATION

The cat's obtunded mentation immediately suggests that a problem is affecting the forebrain, potentially lateralized to the left. The localization is based on the following considerations:

- *Obtundation:* This decreased level of consciousness can occur due to lesions of the forebrain or the brainstem. Other examination findings are necessary to distinguish between these two possible localizations. The cat is not displaying any gait abnormalities in the form of paresis or ataxia. These could occur in a patient with a brainstem lesion, although they may not be present with minor lesions.
- *Pacing:* A key finding for this patient is that although he lacks gait abnormalities, he is reported to consistently walk in broad circles to the left. This is a common feature in animals with forebrain disease.
- *Menace response:* The menace response in cats is less reliable than in dogs. Thus, for this patient, the lack of menace response bilaterally is difficult to interpret.

Overall, the obtunded mentation and propulsive pacing point to a lesion in the forebrain. The tendency to circle to the left may indicate a unilateral forebrain lesion affecting the left side (see Case 1 in this chapter for further details).

MAJOR DISEASE PROCESSES TO CONSIDER

This cat's main clinical sign is a progressive, chronically reduced consciousness. Because the cat tends to walk in leftward circles, structural diseases affecting one side of the forebrain could be prioritized. However, diffuse and multifocal forebrain conditions in which one side is more affected than the other side could also lead to unidirectional pacing and should also be considered. Given the cat's age and slow progression of signs, a strong consideration is a neoplasm affecting the left forebrain. A variety of infectious diseases can also cause the signs observed in this cat. Congenital or hereditary conditions include brain malformations and inherited neurodegenerative diseases and can cause chronic altered mentation. Several metabolic or systemic diseases can lead to chronic altered mentation in cats: Neurodegenerative diseases and heritable inborn errors of metabolism can also lead to chronically altered mentation in cats. Finally, historical trauma can cause abnormal mentation in patients but generally does not lead to progressive signs, as observed in this cat.

Neoplasia

- The most common primary brain tumor in cats is meningioma. This is a slow-growing, typically "benign" tumor that arises from arachnoid cap cells of the meninges. The average age of cats affected by meningiomas is 12 years. Meningiomas cause compression, rather than invasion, of the surrounding brain tissue. This process typically leads to a gradual onset of clinical signs as observed in this cat, with progressive mentation decline often being the only clinical sign of feline meningioma for months before other deficits may develop.

- Other primary brain neoplasms, including pituitary neoplasms and tumors of the ventricular system (ependymomas and choroid plexus tumors), are also possible but are less common in cats than meningiomas. Tumors of the ventricular system can lead to obstructive hydrocephalus, which can contribute to both progressive and acute neurological deterioration in cats with such tumors. Gliomas, another primary brain tumor, are uncommon in cats.

Inflammation – Infectious diseases

- Feline coronavirus is a widespread virus of cats, with roughly 50% of cats in the United States and Europe possessing antibodies against the virus. Although it typically only causes mild gastrointestinal signs in cats, in a subset of cats, the virus mutates into a virulent form associated with a condition known as feline infectious peritonitis (FIP). Neurological signs occur in approximately 30% of affected cats, typically as a constellation of multifocal neurological signs that can include seizures, altered mental status, gait disturbances, and central vestibular disease. The infection causes a robust immune response, leading to abundant deposition of antigen-antibody complexes. These can obstruct ventricular cerebrospinal fluid outflow, resulting in severe, obstructive hydrocephalus that contributes to neurological signs. Although the disease typically affects young cats, with more than 50% of affected cats being less than 1 year old, it can also affect older cats.

- *Cryptococcus* species are the most common fungal organisms associated with feline encephalopathy and should also be considered in this cat. *C. neoformans* can remain viable for years in bird excreta and lead to infection via inhalation of the basidiospore phase of the fungus life cycle. Once within the respiratory tract, the basidiospores convert to a yeast form that gets disseminated hematogenously within macrophages and can spread to the brain via direct extension through the cribriform plate. As with feline coronavirus, a variety of neurological signs can occur in affected cats, including altered mentation, seizures, vestibular dysfunction, cranial nerve dysfunction, and gait disturbances.

- Bacterial pathogens, typically associated with abscess or granuloma formation secondary to cranial trauma (such as bite wounds), can occasionally cause the signs observed in this cat, but are uncommon. Further information on feline CNS inflammatory diseases can be found in Case 2 of this chapter.

Anomalous – Congenital and hereditary diseases

- Hydrocephalus is the most common brain malformation of small animals, resulting from stenosis of the mesencephalic aqueduct. Congenital hydrocephalus can sometimes cause physical abnormalities in the form of a domed head, fixed ventrolateral strabismus, and persistently open fontanelles; however, it can also occur without any of these overt physical signs. Signs of hydrocephalus become evident early in life as animals begin to walk and include altered mentation, gait disturbances, vision loss, seizures, and sometimes vestibular dysfunction. Given this cat's advanced age, hydrocephalus is considered unlikely but should be considered for young cats with chronic, either static or slowly progressive forebrain dysfunction.

- Other brain malformations, including porencephaly, can also lead to chronic altered mentation but are uncommon.

Metabolic and systemic diseases

- Hepatic encephalopathy is a condition that occurs due to hepatic insufficiency. The most common cause of hepatic encephalopathy is a portosystemic shunt, which is most often congenital, but acquired intrahepatic shunts can also develop. Severe hepatic dysfunction and cirrhosis can also result in hepatic encephalopathy. As a result of hepatic insufficiency, a hyperammonemic state arises, which alters the balance between excitatory and inhibitory neurotransmitters in the brain. Cats with hepatic encephalopathy can display a variety of neurological signs, most often including obtundation and dementia or confusion, seizures, and ataxia.

- Renal encephalopathy is less common than hepatic encephalopathy but can occur in cats with severe acute kidney injury or chronic kidney disease. Similar to hepatic encephalopathy, renal encephalopathy results from excessive nitrogen-containing compounds, principally urea. Neurological signs of renal encephalopathy mirror those of hepatic encephalopathy.
- Systemic hypertension, in which the systolic blood pressure is at least 160 mmHg, can lead to chronically altered mentation in cats. In most cases, systemic hypertension arises secondary to other diseases, most often renal disease and hyperthyroidism in cats. However, an estimated 20% of cats have primary, or idiopathic, hypertension. The nervous system is among those at risk for target organ damage from hypertension. Systemic hypertension is thought to cause vasogenic edema in the white matter of the brain. Vascular changes are also common and predispose to microhemorrhage formation in the brain and elsewhere. In addition to altered mentation, systemic hypertension can also cause seizures, vestibular dysfunction, and generalized ataxia.
- Glucose derangements can lead to chronic altered mentation in cats. Cats with untreated diabetes mellitus can develop marked hyperglycemia and ketoacidosis (diabetic ketoacidosis; DKA). Lethargy is a common clinical sign observed in cats with DKA. In severe cases, other neurological signs may be present, including difficulty walking and weakness, and seizures. Alternatively, diabetic cats receiving insulin supplementation can experience hypoglycemia, either as an acute event in the face of a single accidental overdose or when the cat has entered clinical remission from diabetes. With chronic insulin over-supplementation, hypoglycemia leads to chronic reduced mentation.
- Electrolyte abnormalities can cause chronically reduced mentation in cats. Hypocalcemia, hypokalemia, and both hyper- and hyponatremia can cause disorientation.
- Feline primary erythrocytosis, also called polycythemia, is a rare myeloproliferative disorder that leads to increased red blood cell volume. Mean packed cell volume in these cats often exceeds 70%. Neurological signs are a common presenting complaint with this condition. Although the most common neurological sequela is an acute development of seizures, acute to chronic altered mentation can also occur.

Neurodegenerative diseases

- Cognitive dysfunction is becoming increasingly recognized in cats. Most cats are at least 15 years old at the onset of signs, although signs can develop in cats as young as 10 years old. The major signs of cognitive dysfunction in cats include disorientation, altered interactions with people or other pets, sleep-wake cycle disturbances, house soiling, altered activity, increased anxiety, and impaired learning and memory. Excessive vocalization is the most common sign observed in cats with cognitive dysfunction. This differential diagnosis is a strong consideration for this patient, given his age and the behaviors observed. The consistent leftward circling may suggest that cognitive dysfunction is an unlikely cause of this cat's signs. However, many cats with cognitive dysfunction do have a tendency to propulsively pace unidirectionally.
- Storage disorders are heritable inborn errors of metabolism in which an enzyme, typically involved in carbohydrate metabolism, is lacking due to a homozygous recessive inheritance pattern. In the absence of the given enzyme, its substrate accumulates intracellularly. There are dozens of recognized storage disorders. Mucopolysaccharidosis is perhaps the most common storage disorder observed in cats. It typically affects cats less than 2 years old and causes not

only progressive neurologic dysfunction but can also lead to musculoskeletal malformations, particularly craniofacial malformations and other systemic abnormalities. Storage disorders are unlikely in a cat of advanced age.

DIAGNOSTIC TESTS

All cats with chronic, progressive behavioral changes should undergo thorough physical examinations to investigate non-neurological causes as well as to screen for systemic diseases with secondary neurological signs. Palpation for a 'thyroid slip' (enlargement) should be performed to screen for hyperthyroidism. Fundoscopic examination should be performed to screen for systemic hypertension. A complete blood count, blood chemistry panel, urinalysis, and T4 level should be evaluated to screen for systemic diseases. Intracranial infections are rarely associated with systemic clinical signs or abnormalities in minimum database parameters, and therefore, normal values do not rule out intracranial infections. Mean arterial blood pressure measurements should be obtained to screen for systemic hypertension.

If all systemic diseases are ruled out, then magnetic resonance imaging (MRI) of the brain should be performed. Brain MRI is highly sensitive and specific for evaluating the various potential causes of chronic behavioral changes. Unless contraindicated, such as in the presence of signs of intracranial hypertension or brain herniation, cerebrospinal fluid (CSF) analysis on CSF collected from the atlanto-occipital cistern should also be obtained and assessed for the presence of infectious organisms, inflammatory patterns consistent with infection, and for neoplastic cells. Cerebrospinal fluid can also be cultured for bacterial and fungal pathogens. Infectious disease titers using either serum samples or CSF can also be performed for *Toxoplasma* and *Cryptococcus* spp.

In this patient, the complete blood count, blood chemistry panel, T4, fundoscopic examination, and mean arterial blood pressure were all considered normal.

Brain MRI showed a large, well-defined T2-weighted hyperintense lesion arising from over the left parietal lobe (Figure 3.4.1). This lesion was considered to be extra-parenchymal, meaning that it was arising from outside the brain parenchyma and causing substantial compression and

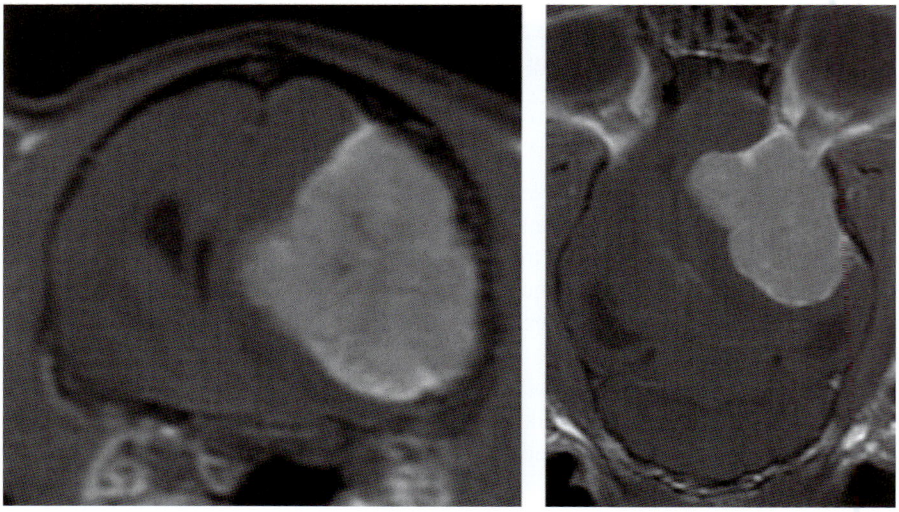

FIGURE 3.4.1 Post-contrast T1-weighted transverse (left) and dorsal (right) magnetic resonance images from a cat. The strongly contrast-enhancing mass, later confirmed to be a meningioma, is well-delineated and is leading to a substantial shifting of the adjacent neuroparenchyma. Note that contrast extends along the meninges from the mass (dural tail sign).

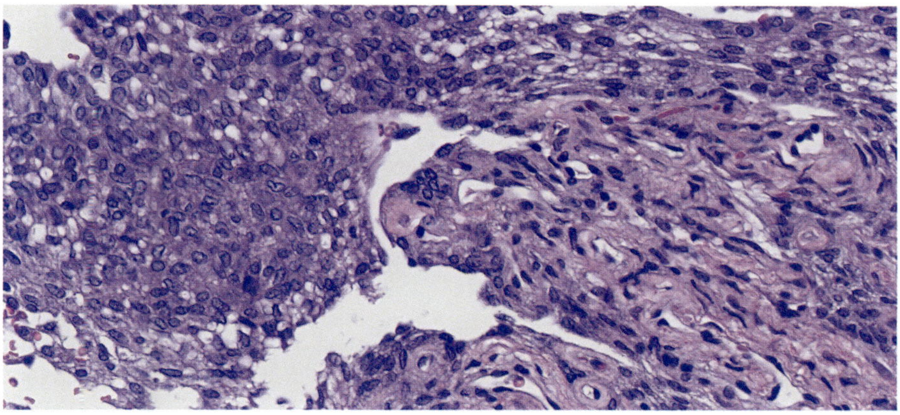

FIGURE 3.4.2 Histopathology from a low-grade feline meningioma. *Source:* Photo credit: Ariel de Aguiar.

deviation of the adjacent neuroparenchyma. The mass was homogeneously and strongly contrast-enhancing. There was a "dural tail" associated with the mass. The collection of these imaging findings was consistent with a meningioma.

Meningiomas are slow-growing tumors in cats and are most often benign when graded (Figure 3.4.2). Surgical resection is the recommended treatment for feline intracranial meningiomas. In most cases, surgical resection is considered "curative," given that the tumors can often be grossly removed, and regrowth occurs very slowly. The average recurrence-free survival time in one study was 826 days and 1,345 days in another study. In cats with tumors that are not amenable to surgical resection, radiation therapy can also yield good results, with one study reporting a median survival time of 339 days following stereotactic radiation therapy. Palliative therapy is an alternative to these definitive therapy options, consisting primarily of glucocorticoids to reduce tumor-associated edema and potentially slow growth. Survival times for cats treated with palliative care are not well documented.

OUTCOME

The cat underwent a left rostrotentorial craniectomy to remove the suspected meningioma. Surgery was uneventful, and all grossly visible tumor tissue was removed. The cat was mildly obtunded the day following surgery and was discharged for continued care at home. Three months after surgery, he had returned to playing with his toys at home (Video 3.4.2). He lived for another 4 years following surgery and was euthanized for an unrelated progression of chronic renal failure.

VIDEO 3.4.2 Cat playing with toys, 3 months following surgical resection of meningioma. *Source:* Photo credit: David Dumond.

SUGGESTED READING

Coady, M., Fletcher, D.J., and Goggs, R. (2019). Severity of ionized hypercalcemia and hypocalcemia is associated with etiology in dogs and cats. *Front Vet Sci.* 6. https://doi.org/10.3389/fvets.2019.00276.

Darcy, H., Simpson, K., Gajanayake, I. et al. (2018). Feline primary erythrocytosis: a multicentre case series of 18 cats. *J. Feline Med. Surg.* 20 (12): 1192–1198. https://doi.org/10.1177/1098612X17750333.

Elliott, J., Barber, P.J., Syme, H.M. et al. (2001). Feline hypertension: clinical findings and response to antihypertensive treatment in 30 cases. *J. Small Anim. Pract.* 42 (3): 122–129. https://doi.org/10.1111/j.1748-5,827.2001.tb02008.x.

Hartmann, K. (2005). Feline infectious peritonitis. *Vet. Clin. North Am. Small Anim. Pract.* 35 (1): 39–79. vi. https://doi.org/10.1016/j.cvsm.2004.10.011.

Kent, M. (2009). The cat with neurological manifestations of systemic disease. *J. Feline Med. Surg.* 11 (5): 395–407. https://doi.org/10.1016/j.jfms.2009.03.007.

Landsberg, G.M., Denenberg, S., and Araujo, J.A. (2010). Cognitive dysfunction in cats: a syndrome we used to dismiss as "old age." *J. Feline Med. Surg.* 12 (11): 837–848. https://doi.org/10.1016/j.jfms.2010.09.004.

Rudloff, E. (2017). Diabetic ketoacidosis in the cat: recognition and essential treatment. *J. Feline Med. Surg.* 19 (11): 1167–1174. https://doi.org/10.1177/1098612X17735762.

Sordo, L. and Gunn-Moore, D.A. (2021). Cognitive dysfunction in cats: update on neuropathological and behavioural changes plus clinical management. *Vet. Rec.* 188 (1): e3. https://doi.org/10.1002/vetr.3.

Tichenor, M., Hearon, K., and Selmic, L.E. (2024). Characteristics and outcomes for 61 cats that underwent either surgery or stereotactic radiotherapy as treatment for intracranial meningioma (2005–2017). *J. Am. Vet. Med. Assoc.* 262 (1): 1–8. https://doi.org/10.2460/javma.23.02.0083.

Trivedi, S.R., Malik, R., Meyer, W., and Sykes, J.E. (2011). Feline cryptococcosis. *J. Feline Med. Surg.* 13 (3): 163–172. https://doi.org/10.1016/j.jfms.2011.01.009.

Seizures

Case 1—Cluster Seizures in a Dog

CHAPTER 4.1

Talisha Moore[1] and Simon R. Platt[2]

[1] *University of Tennessee, College of Veterinary Medicine, Department of Clinical Science, Knoxville, TN, USA*

[2] *Department of Veterinary Clinical Sciences, College of Veterinary Medicine, Oklahoma State University, Stillwater, OK, USA*

A 1-year-old neutered male Belgian shepherd dog exhibited a generalized tonic-clonic seizure yesterday and today has experienced four further events, returning to normal in the owner's opinion each time. The patient has otherwise been healthy and has never experienced similar events, according to the owner. The dog has been cared for by the owner for 6 months and is up to date on vaccinations. It is currently on flea, tick, and heartworm preventatives, none of which are isoxazolines, and is considered an indoor pet. There are no known toxin exposures and no history of trauma. The physical and neurological examination, performed 3 hours after the last event, is considered normal apart from mild depression.

> CAUTION: This neurologic examination is being performed during the postictal phase; therefore, neurologic abnormalities should be interpreted with caution. It is recommended that a neurologic examination be repeated when the patient is not in a postictal state. The interictal (i.e. time between seizures) examination will be more reliable.

1. **What is a seizure?**
2. **What are cluster seizures?**
3. **What differentials should be considered?**
4. **What treatment options are available for cluster seizures?**

WHAT IS A SEIZURE?

A seizure is a nonspecific, sudden event involving involuntary body activity. An epileptic seizure is a temporary episode characterized by signs resulting from abnormal, excessive neuronal activity in the brain. The clinical features of epileptic seizures can be separated into four components:

i. The prodrome is the period preceding the onset of seizure activity. During this time, increased anxiety-related behavior (i.e. attention-seeking, whining), reluctance to perform normal activity patterns, and increased hiding can be noted.

ii. An aura can occur as the initial manifestation of a seizure. During this period, which may last from minutes to hours, animals may display stereotypical sensory or motor behaviors, such as pacing and licking, as well as autonomic patterns like salivating, urinating, and vomiting. They may also exhibit unusual psychiatric events, including excessive barking or altered attention-seeking behaviors.

iii. The ictal period refers to the actual seizure event, marked by involuntary muscle tone or movement, abnormal sensations, or behavior, and usually lasts from seconds to minutes.

iv. The postictal period follows the actual seizure and can last from minutes to days. During this period, an animal may show unusual or atypical behaviors, such as aggression, disorientation, inappropriate bowel or bladder activity, excessive or reduced thirst and appetite or neurological deficits like weakness, blindness, and sensory or motor issues.

Seizures are divided into either focal or generalized

- Focal seizures can be (1) motor, commonly seen as facial muscle twitching or the involvement of an individual limb (Video 4.1.1); (2) sensory, manifested by abnormal behavioral disorders, or (3) autonomic, with the most common manifestations being mydriasis and salivation.
- Generalized seizures are subdivided into motor or non-motor types. The terms convulsive (*grand mal*) and nonconvulsive (*petit mal*) seizures are no longer in use.
  - Generalized motor seizures are classified into different types, including tonic, tonic–clonic, clonic, myoclonic, and atonic, (Video 4.1.2). Automatisms refer to repeated, mostly coordinated movements with impaired cognition, typically involving oro-alimentary behaviors such as lip-smacking or licking, or pedal movements like running-like actions.
  - Non-motor generalized seizures can be characterized by a loss of sensory processing and environmental responsiveness. These may occur during the aura phase before motor symptoms appear in dogs.

VIDEO 4.1.1 A 3-year-old English bulldog exhibits focal motor (involuntary movements of the facial and masticatory muscles) and autonomic (salivation) seizure activity.

VIDEO 4.1.2 A 6-year-old shepherd-cross dog exhibits a generalized tonic-clonic seizure event with involuntary rigidity and motor movements of the limbs and jaws noted and presumed decreased consciousness.

Reflex seizures can be focal or generalized and occur in response to a trigger. Recognized triggers have been reported in dogs, which include photosensitivity, fear and anxiety and eating. Myoclonic seizures in wire-haired dachshunds with Lafora disease can be triggered by auditory and visual stimuli. Feline Audiogenic Reflex Seizures (FARS) is an epilepsy syndrome in older cats triggered by specific high-pitched or sharp sounds, such as crinkling foil, metal spoons hitting ceramic, or tapping.

WHAT ARE CLUSTER SEIZURES?

Terms like "acute repetitive seizures," "cluster seizures" (CS), "serial seizures," and "flurry seizures" describe a pattern with multiple generalized tonic, clonic, or tonic–clonic seizures, or even several focal seizures, occurring within 24 hours. There is no single clinical definition for a seizure cluster. Studies on seizure clustering use different criteria, such as two to four seizures in less than 48 hours; three seizures in 24 hours; or two generalized tonic–clonic seizures or three complex focal seizures within 4 hours. In between the events, the patient regains consciousness.

Limited data exist documenting the prevalence of cluster seizures in veterinary medicine. Studies have suggested that anywhere between 38% and 77% of dogs with epilepsy can experience CS at some point. Some canine breeds appear predisposed to CS. Up to 94% of border collies and nearly 50% of Australian shepherd dogs diagnosed with idiopathic epilepsy have been reported to experience CS. German shepherds, Rottweilers, and boxer dogs have also been noted with a higher prevalence of CS compared to other breeds with idiopathic epilepsy. Sex, neuter status, and body size are unlikely to be associated with CS occurrence. Dogs experiencing CS are less likely to achieve long-term seizure remission, while experiencing a decreased survival time and an increased likelihood of euthanasia compared to dogs with single epileptic seizure episodes.

Limited research has been conducted to evaluate the prevalence of seizure clustering in cats. One study evaluating 125 cats with primary and secondary causes of seizure activity documented CS in 53% and 59% of cases, respectively.

WHAT DIFFERENTIALS SHOULD BE CONSIDERED?

The main etiological categories responsible for seizure activity are idiopathic, structural, and metabolic.

- **Idiopathic epilepsy**
  A diagnosis of idiopathic epilepsy is most common in purebred dogs with the first onset of seizures between 1 and 5 years old and a normal interictal neurological examination, especially if there is a lengthy initial interictal period (>4 weeks). Additionally, a normal minimum database (complete blood count [CBC], chemistry panel, and liver function testing), a normal magnetic resonance imaging (MRI) scan, and normal cerebrospinal fluid (CSF) analysis are expected.
  A genetic basis has been reported in numerous dog breeds, including Belgian shepherd dogs, poodles, beagles, springer spaniels, vizslas, Irish wolfhounds, Lagotto Romagnolos, Rhodesian ridgebacks, and Labrador retrievers.
- **Structural epilepsy**
  These types of epileptic seizures are the direct result of structural brain pathology such as stroke, inflammation, neoplasia, trauma, or hydrocephalus. Dogs of any age can develop structural epileptic seizures. Younger animals are more prone to developmental anomalies and encephalitic diseases (inflammatory diseases of the brain), whilst older animals (>7 years of age) are more likely to develop intracranial neoplasia and experience strokes. See this chapter, cases 3 and 4, and chapter 3 for more details.

> CAUTION: Many dogs with structural epilepsy will have interictal neurologic deficits. However, if the lesion is located within a "clinically silent" brain region (olfactory bulb, pyriform, and frontal lobes), the neurologic examination may be normal, and seizures may be the only clinical manifestation of the disease. A retrospective clinical comparison of idiopathic versus structural (symptomatic) epilepsy revealed that 64% of dogs with a new onset of seizures and diagnosed with structural brain disease had a normal neurologic examination.

- **Metabolic epileptic seizures**
  Metabolic (formerly reactive) seizures are a reaction of the normal brain to transient systemic insult, toxic reaction, or physiological stress. Animals of any age may be affected. Small-breed dogs are more predisposed to develop seizures secondary to portosystemic shunts at a younger age. Typically, a higher seizure frequency occurs initially until the underlying metabolic or toxic insult is corrected. Evidence of systemic illness is often present concurrently.

Multiple other types of paroxysmal episodes involving changes in behavior, movements, or neurological status can mimic epileptic seizures. It is equally important to differentiate these episodes from true epileptic seizures, as misdiagnosis might cause missed detection of other serious health issues, unnecessary medication for the patient, or excessive emotional and financial stress for the owner.

Some common causes of non-seizure paroxysms include syncope of cardiac origin, metabolic-related weakness (e.g. transient hypoglycemia, endocrine diseases), and acute toxicities. One helpful distinguishing feature is the lack of a postictal period following these "episodes." With syncope, a rapid return to consciousness or the ability to walk within seconds to a minute is typical, although some animals will urinate during or immediately after the event. Neurological episodes that are not epileptic seizures may include acute vestibular attacks (sometimes called vestibular epilepsy and characterized by vestibular ataxia, falling, rolling, etc.), cataplectic/narcoleptic events (sudden loss of consciousness precipitated by excitement), and a variety of canine paroxysmal dyskinesias (see Chapter 8, Case 2).

The conditions that can lead to CS are the same as those underlying isolated epileptic seizures. Studies evaluating cluster seizures in dogs admitted to the hospital have not revealed a specific cause for the seizures in 25–28% of cases and may be called cryptogenic. Approximately 28–37.5% of cases are diagnosed with primary (genetic or idiopathic) epilepsy.

WHAT TREATMENT OPTIONS ARE AVAILABLE FOR CLUSTER SEIZURES?

The management of CS involves both short-term and long-term strategies. Long-term therapy aims to prevent CS through optimal antiseizure management of epilepsy – regular monitoring, dose adjustments, and optimization of maintenance anti-seizure medications such as phenobarbital, potassium bromide, zonisamide, and levetiracetam (see Case 2 in this chapter). However, when CS occur, a short-term treatment plan should be initiated during or immediately after the first seizure (if the animal typically presents with CS) or, more commonly, after the second seizure. The goal is to terminate ongoing seizures and prevent further seizures from occurring. Specifically, the short-term management includes the combined use of short-acting (e.g. midazolam, diazepam) and longer-acting (e.g. levetiracetam) interventions. Different options exist for those patients who present with CS during hospitalization and those who are at home with the owner (Figure 4.1.1).

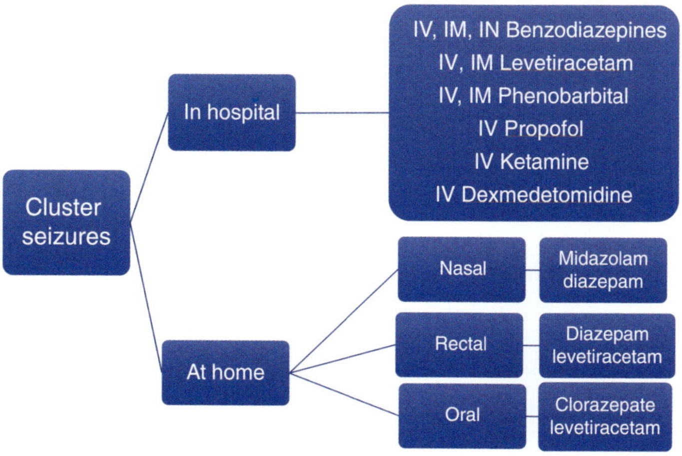

FIGURE 4.1.1 Treatment options for the management of cluster seizures in the hospital or at-home environment.

SHORT-ACTING TREATMENT AT THE TIME OF A CLUSTER EVENT

- **Benzodiazepines**

  Benzodiazepines (diazepam, midazolam) are potent, fast-acting anticonvulsants and are therefore often the preferred initial therapy for emergency seizures. When skilled technicians, veterinary nurses, or veterinarians are present, intravenous (IV) administration is preferred. However, if IV access is not available, the recommendation for emergency seizures in a dog or cat is to consider intramuscular (IM) or intranasal midazolam immediately. Benzodiazepines can also be administered via rectal or buccal routes when parenteral therapy is not feasible, such as in the at-home environment.

  Diazepam can be administered into the rectum using plastic administrators such as teat infusion cannulas or tom-cat catheters with a water-soluble lubricant. The efficacy of rectally delivered diazepam depends on several factors, not least the time that it takes for the drug to reach the therapeutic concentration. Rectal diazepam (0.5–2.0 mg/kg) has been evaluated for the treatment of cluster seizures in dogs, proving a significant decrease in the number of CS in 24 hours as well as a significant decrease in the total cost of emergency care. The intranasal route has been extensively investigated and found to be not only more convenient and socially acceptable than rectal diazepam, but also to yield equal or better results regarding antiepileptic activity and onset of action. Diazepam and midazolam, administered intranasally (IN) to dogs, have both been shown to reach high concentrations rapidly. Gel formulations can be compounded for this purpose, or the liquid formulation can be used with an atomizer attached to a syringe.

  Continuous benzodiazepine infusion may be a necessary and effective mode of in-hospital therapy for frequent CS. The dose should be calculated hourly (diazepam 0.1–0.5 mg/kg of body weight, q1h) and is usually diluted in 0.9% saline or in 5% dextrose in water (D5W), with the volume used being equal to the maintenance fluid requirement over the hour. The dose can be delivered with an infusion pump. The dosage rate should be reduced by 50% every 6 hours for at least two reductions before discontinuing the drug.

- **Levetiracetam**

  Levetiracetam (LEV) (20–60 mg/kg IV, IM, or rectal) is a rapidly acting and safe anticonvulsant that can be used parenterally when benzodiazepines are considered ineffective. It can be effective for 8 hours, at which time it can be repeated. It causes minimal sedation and is not metabolized in the liver, making it a suitable option for older dogs and cats. In addition to its seizure-suppressing activity, previous experiments in chronic epilepsy models in rodents suggested that LEV might also possess anti-epileptogenic or disease-modifying activity.

- **Phenobarbital (PB)**

  The distribution of PB to the central nervous system may take up to 30 minutes because of weaker lipophilicity in comparison with diazepam. If the patient is refractory to benzodiazepines and levetiracetam, a loading dose of PB may be required if the patient is not already being maintained on this drug. The recommended loading dose is 12–24 mg/kg IV, if immediate therapeutic concentrations are desired, but this can induce a profound stupor with concurrent suppression of the cardiovascular and respiratory systems. Alternatively, the dose can initially be 2–6 mg/kg IV, with the dose repeated every 20–30 minutes to effect, and a maximum total 24-hour dose of 24 mg/kg. The parenteral form can also be given IM, which is recommended if diazepam has already been administered. This will avoid the potentiation of profound respiratory and cardiovascular depression.

  Cluster seizures that do not respond to a benzodiazepine, levetiracetam, or PB may be considered refractory and require more aggressive treatment. Short-acting anesthetic drugs are the most commonly used agents for treating resistant SE, as they have a rapid onset of action, short half-lives, and cause reductions in cerebral metabolic rates. These drugs should be used only in an intensive care setting because of the need for continuous blood pressure monitoring and, ideally, central venous pressure monitoring. Propofol, ketamine, and dexmedetomidine have all been suggested as being effective for animals with refractory emergency seizures when used IV at standard doses.

AT-HOME TREATMENT AT THE TIME OF A CLUSTER EVENT

The following options should be considered as home therapies for animals known to exhibit cluster seizures. The treatments are not intended as a method to avoid veterinary care and counseling, but offer an "on the spot" therapy that may prevent cluster seizures from occurring or at least reduce the amount of seizures exhibited within a 24-hour period. As such, the owners can be advised to attempt one of the following options at the time of the first seizure.

- **Benzodiazepines** – Intranasal versus rectal delivery (see above discussion)
- **Oral clorazepate**
  Clorazepate (clorazepate dipotassium) is a benzodiazepine prodrug that acts by enhancing gamma-aminobutyric acid (GABA) activity in the brain. Oral doses between 0.5 and 2 mg/kg every 8 hours can result in sedation and ataxia, but such signs may resolve 3–4 days after treatment. In essence, this drug is a short-term anticonvulsant that can be effective when administered orally. Anecdotally, this drug can be given as a pulsed therapy adjunctively to the animal's maintenance medication. It is recommended to start at the lower end of the dose range to balance cluster seizure management versus the side effects of clorazepate. The success of this approach may depend on the owner's tolerance to the ensuing sedation and the ability to predict a cluster based on the first seizure event. The duration of treatment can be short (1–3 days)
- **Oral or rectal levetiracetam**
  The pharmacokinetics of standard-release levetiracetam appear favorable for oral administration during CS. The bioavailability of oral administration is nearly 100%. The use of an interval or pulsed oral dosing regimen of levetiracetam can be used in the treatment of at-home cluster seizures. If the animal is already on phenobarbital, a higher dose of levetiracetam is advised (more than 20 mg/kg). Similar to the use of clorazepate, the success of this approach in this situation may depend on predicting cluster activity. However, in this drug's case, there will be limited sedation, and liver metabolism is not a concern. A documented protocol involves administering an initial dose of approximately 60 mg/kg after a seizure has occurred or preictal signs are recognized by the owner, followed by approximately 20 mg/kg every 8 hours until seizures do not happen for 48 hours. If the dog is already being prescribed this drug for maintenance seizure control, then a lower dose can be used, which should be tailored to the drug's sedative effects; approximately 40% of dogs receiving 60 mg/kg orally will be ataxic and/or sedated.

  Owners can easily employ the oral route at home. However, the postictal phase in epileptic patients can impair swallowing ability, preventing the use of this route because of aspiration risk, thus delaying the initiation of treatment. For this reason, rectal delivery of this drug has been investigated and has been demonstrated to be successful for CS in dogs when used at 40 mg/kg. In the majority of cases, target plasma concentrations are reached after rapid absorption within 30 minutes after administration of the drug.

OUTCOME

The dog in this case had a systemic health investigation, including a dynamic bile acids study, which was all considered normal. The owners elected not to pursue more advanced diagnostics at this time, based on the normal physical and neurological examinations and their limited financial resources. The dog was immediately initiated on phenobarbital (3 mg/kg per os [PO] q12h), and the owners were provided with an at-home "rescue" protocol, which consisted of intranasal midazolam (0.3 mg/kg as needed with a maximum of three administrations; compounded at a local pharmacy) and a levetiracetam standard-release oral protocol (see above for dosing details). The dog continued to have a high seizure frequency with intermittent CS and was started on potassium bromide as a second maintenance anti-seizure therapy. The seizure frequency improved with only occasional need for an at-home CS rescue protocol, to which the dog responded invariably well by not progressing into high-frequency CS events.

SUGGESTED READING

Al Kafaji, T., Tocco, F., Okonji, S., and Gallucci, A. (2024). Clinical features and outcome of 10 dogs with suspected idiopathic vestibular epilepsy. *J. Vet. Intern. Med* 38 (3): 1591–1597.

Berendt, M., Farquhar, R.G., Mandigers, P.J. et al. (2015). International veterinary epilepsy task force consensus report on epilepsy definition, classification and terminology in companion animals. *BMC Vet. Res.* 11: 182.

Cagnotti, G., Odore, R., Bertone, I. et al. (2019). Open-label clinical trial of rectally administered levetiracetam as supplemental treatment in dogs with cluster seizures. *J. Vet. Intern. Med.* 33: 1714–1718.

Cagnotti, G., Odore, R., Gardini, G. et al. (2018). Pharmacokinetics of rectal levetiracetam as add-on treatment in dogs affected by cluster seizures or status epilepticus. *BMC Vet. Res.* 14: 189.

Charalambous, M., Bhatti, S.F.M., Van Ham, L. et al. (2017). Intranasal midazolam versus rectal diazepam for the management of canine status epilepticus: a multicenter randomized parallel-group clinical trial. *J. Vet. Intern. Med.* 31 (4): 1149–1158.

Charalambous, M., Muñana, K., Patterson, E.E. et al. (2024). ACVIM Consensus Statement on the management of status epilepticus and cluster seizures in dogs and cats. *J. Vet. Intern. Med.* 38 (1): 19–40.

Charalambous, M., Volk, H.A., Tipold, A. et al. (2019). Comparison of intranasal versus intravenous midazolam for management of status epilepticus in dogs: a multi-center randomized parallel group clinical study. *J. Vet. Intern. Med.* 33 (6): 2709–2717.

De Risio, L., Bhatti, S., Muñana, K. et al. (2015). International veterinary epilepsy task force consensus proposal: diagnostic approach to epilepsy in dogs. *BMC Vet. Res.* 11: 148.

Hardy, B.T., Patterson, E.E., Cloyd, J.M. et al. (2012). Double-masked, placebo-controlled study of intravenous levetiracetam for the treatment of status epilepticus and acute repetitive seizures in dogs. *J. Vet. Intern. Med.* 26 (2): 334–340.

Hülsmeyer, V., Zimmermann, R., Brauer, C. et al. (2010). Epilepsy in border collies: clinical manifestation, outcome, and mode of inheritance. *J. Vet. Intern. Med.* 24: 171–178.

Jankauskas, M., Gradeckienė, A., Čižinauskas, S. et al. (2025). Extended analysis of status epilepticus and cluster seizures in dogs in the context of overall epilepsy incidence: 254 cases. *Animals (Basel)* 15 (19): 2807.

Kwiatkowska, M., Tipold, A., Huenerfauth, E., and Pomianowski, A. (2018). Clinical risk factors for early seizure recurrence in dogs hospitalized for seizure evaluation. *J. Vet. Intern. Med.* 32: 757–763.

Monteiro, R., Adams, V., Keys, D., and Platt, S. (2012). Canine idiopathic epilepsy: prevalence, risk factors and outcome associated with cluster seizures and status epilepticus. *J. Small Anim. Pract.* 53: 526–530.

Munguia, G.G., Brooks, A.C., Thomovsky, S.A. et al. (2024). Emergency approach to acute seizures in dogs and cats. *Vet. Sci.* 11 (6): 277.

Packer, R., Shihab, N., Torres, B., and Volk, H. (2014). Clinical risk factors associated with anti-epileptic drug responsiveness in canine epilepsy. *PLoS One* 9: e106026.

Packer, R., Nye, G., Porter, S., and Volk, H. (2015). Assessment into the usage of levetiracetam in a canine epilepsy clinic. *BMC Vet. Res.* 11: 25.

Packer, R., Shihab, N., Torres, B., and Volk, H. (2016). Risk factors for cluster seizures in canine idiopathic epilepsy. *Res. Vet. Sci.* 105: 136–138.

Pákozdy, A., Leschnik, M., Sarchahi, A.A. et al. (2010). Clinical comparison of primary versus secondary epilepsy in 125 cats. *J. Feline Med. Surg.* 12 (12): 910–916.

Patry, F. (1931). The relation of time of day, sleep, and other factors to the incidence of epileptic seizures. *Am. J. Psychiatry* 87: 789–813.

Patterson, E. (2014). Status epilepticus and cluster seizures. *Vet. Clin. North Am. Small Anim. Pract.* 44: 1103–1112.

Peters, R., Schubert, T., Clemmons, R., and Vickroy, T. (2014). Levetiracetam rectal administration in healthy dogs. *J. Vet. Intern. Med.* 28: 504–509.

Platt, S.R. (2014). Pathophysiology and management of cluster seizures. In: *Canine and Feline Epilepsy: Diagnosis and Management* (ed. L. De Risio and S. Platt), 503–518. Cabi Publishing.

Podell, M. (1995). The use of diazepam per rectum at home for the acute management of cluster seizures in dogs. *J. Vet. Intern. Med.* 9: 68–74.

Podell, M., Smeak, D., and Lord, L.K. (1998). Diazepam used to control cluster seizures in dogs. *J. Vet. Intern. Med.* 12: 120–121.

Probst, C., Thomas, W., Moyers, T. et al. (2013). Evaluation of plasma diazepam and nordiazepam concentrations following administration of diazepam intravenously or via suppository per rectum in dogs. *Am. J. Vet. Res.* 74: 611–615.

Seizures

Case 2—Refractory Seizures in a Dog

CHAPTER 4.2

Simon R. Platt[1] and Talisha Moore[2]

[1] *Department of Veterinary Clinical Sciences, College of Veterinary Medicine, Oklahoma State University, Stillwater, OK, USA*

[2] *University of Tennessee, College of Veterinary Medicine, Department of Clinical Science, Knoxville, TN, USA*

CASE HISTORY

A 3-year-old spayed female border collie was presented for high-frequency generalized tonic-clonic seizure activity over the past 9 months. The owners report the episodes last approximately 2 minutes, with a 5–10-minute period of post-ictal confusion. Between episodes, the dog is considered normal in terms of its level of awareness and behavior. At the initial presentation, the dog underwent a brain magnetic resonance imaging (MRI) exam and cerebrospinal fluid (CSF) analysis, which were considered normal, as were the dog's complete blood count (CBC), serum chemistry, and urinalysis. A presumptive diagnosis of idiopathic epilepsy was based on this investigation.

The patient has had 2–3 episodes a week over the last 2 months. This has improved since the time of onset, when the frequency was 4–5 seizures per week. This has been associated with the initiation of oral phenobarbital (3 mg/kg by mouth every 12 hours). There have been 4 days on which the dog has exhibited more than two seizures over these 9 months. Blood work (CBC and serum chemistry), as well as pre- and post-prandial bile acids, were normal 5 months ago. At that time, the serum phenobarbital concentration was 22 µg/mL (reference range 15–35 µg/mL).

The dog's neurological and physical examinations at the time of presentation are considered normal.

1. **What are the indications for initiating anti-seizure medication in a dog?**
2. **What anti-seizure medications can be considered in dogs, and what are the associated dosing regimens, adverse effects, and monitoring guidelines?**
3. **What approach should be considered for this dog?**
4. **What adjunctive treatment options could be considered in a dog refractory to anti-convulsant medication?**

WHAT ARE THE INDICATIONS FOR INITIATING ANTI-SEIZURE MEDICATION IN A DOG?

Administering anti-seizure medication is essential for managing dogs with epilepsy. The main aim is to decrease how often, how long, and how severe the seizures are, while also avoiding significant adverse effects. Dogs with untreated epilepsy or inadequate treatment may face increasing seizure frequency, longer episodes, or more severe signs over time.

While various owner and patient factors might influence the situation, lifelong anti-seizure therapy should be contemplated if a dog shows any of the following:

- Two or more seizures within 3 months
- Status epilepticus (unless associated with intoxication or metabolic disease)
- Cluster seizures (unless associated with intoxication or metabolic disease)
- A severe or lengthy postictal period
- A structural intracranial disease

The author extends the seizure frequency window from 3 to 6 months to establish a clearer pattern of seizure activity, which aids in assessing the impact of anti-seizure medication. Nonetheless, this must be balanced with the understanding that earlier treatment often increases the likelihood of success. Therefore, each dog is managed individually (Figure 4.2.1).

WHAT ANTI-SEIZURE MEDICATIONS CAN BE CONSIDERED IN DOGS, AND WHAT ARE THE ASSOCIATED DOSING REGIMENS, ADVERSE EFFECTS, AND MONITORING GUIDELINES?

Currently, there are limited evidence-based guidelines for selecting anti-seizure medications in dogs. Table 4.2.1 outlines factors to consider when making this choice.

The following medications are commonly used in the treatment of epileptic seizures in dogs (Table 4.2.2). Their mechanisms of action are often based on their site of neuronal action (Figure 4.2.2) and are covered comprehensively in the suggested reading at the end of this case.

PHENOBARBITAL (PB)

Key Pharmacologic Facts

The half-life of phenobarbital in dogs is about 2–3 days, allowing for twice-daily dosing. Steady-state levels are reached in 10–15 days. Notably, phenobarbital can trigger autoinduction, speeding up its own metabolism. This results in a shorter half-life and greater fluctuations in serum levels during the dosing period, potentially reducing seizure control. To counteract this, dosing can be adjusted to every 8 hours. Since PB undergoes hepatic metabolism, impaired liver function may result in increased serum concentrations.

Administration and Monitoring

Phenobarbital is typically started at 2–4 mg/kg per os (PO) every 12 hours in dogs. Dose adjustments depend on therapeutic response, intolerable side effects, or if serum levels exceed 35 μg/mL due to an increased risk of hepatotoxicity. PB can be effective even at serum concentrations below the reference range of 15–45 μg/mL, so doses do not necessarily need to be increased in patients with subtherapeutic PB serum concentration if their seizures are well-controlled on their current dose.

Therapeutic monitoring should be done at steady state, usually 10–15 days after starting treatment. Because of its long half-life, a single blood sample collected at any time during the dosing interval usually suffices. If therapy fails, it may help to measure both a peak (1–2 hours post-dose) and a trough (just before dosing) to calculate half-life. This could lead to increased dosing frequency to reduce fluctuations in serum levels during the dosing interval. Routine serum concentration assessments should be undertaken every 6 months, along with tests for functional bile acids, serum biochemistry, and hematology.

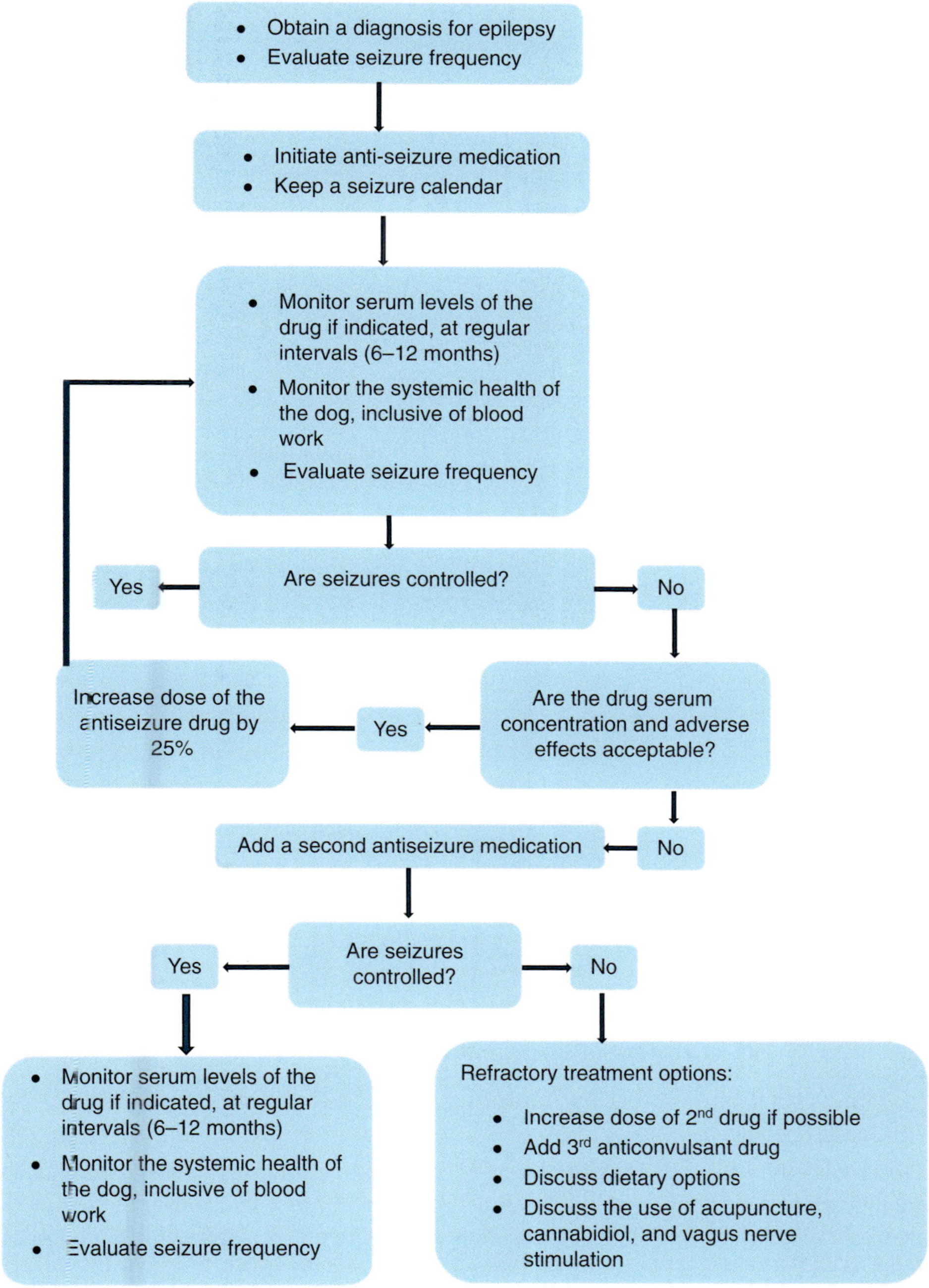

FIGURE 4.2.1 An algorithmic approach to the individualized therapy of dogs presenting with seizure activity.

Table 4.2.1 Factors to consider when choosing an anti-seizure medication.

Drug factors	Patient factors
Safety	Concurrent systemic health (i.e. renal or liver disease
Ease of administration	Owner's ability to dose once versus multiple times a day
Adverse effects	Seizure frequency
Time to maximum efficacy (related to half-life)	
Cost	
Interactions with other medications	

Table 4.2.2 Anti-seizure medications for dogs, their dosing recommendations, and documented efficacy.

Drug	Dosing	Approximate efficacy (% of dogs expected with a seizure reduction)
Phenobarbital	2–4 mg/kg q12h–q8h	90 as monotherapy
Potassium bromide	20–40 mg/kg/day	50–60 as monotherapy
Levetiracetam (standard release)	20–30 mg/kg q8h–q6h	60 as adjunctive medication
Levetiracetam (extended release)	30 mg/kg q12h	Unknown
Zonisamide	5–10 mg/kg q12h	60–76 as monotherapy
Gabapentin	10–20 mg/kg q8h	50 as adjunctive medication
Pregabalin	4–5 mg/kg q12h–q8h	50 as adjunctive medication
Imepitoin	10–30 mg/kg q12h	50–60 as monotherapy
Topiramate	2–10 mg/kg q12h–q8h	50 as adjunctive medication
Felbamate	5–20 mg/kg q12h–q8h	60–75 as adjunctive medication

Adverse Effects

Expected adverse effects that are usually transient include sedation, proprioceptive ataxia, polydipsia, and polyphagia. These can improve with time but may be permanent.

Life-threatening adverse effects of PB include:

1. Hepatotoxicity – A serum phenobarbital concentration > 35 μg/mL is associated with a higher risk of development of liver dysfunction. Dynamic bile acid and/or ammonia concentrations should be analyzed to evaluate liver function if alanine transaminase (ALT) levels suddenly increase or serum albumin levels start to decrease.
2. Neutropenia, thrombocytopenia, and anemia – typically a blood dyscrasia that can reverse upon discontinuation of phenobarbital, occurs within the first 6 months of dosing.

Phenobarbital may also be a risk factor for the development of dyskinesia or superficial necrolytic dermatitis in dogs.

Serum total and free thyroxine (T4) concentrations may be low in dogs treated with phenobarbital (and, in a few dogs, the serum thyroid-stimulating hormone concentration may be elevated), leading to a mistaken diagnosis of hypothyroidism.

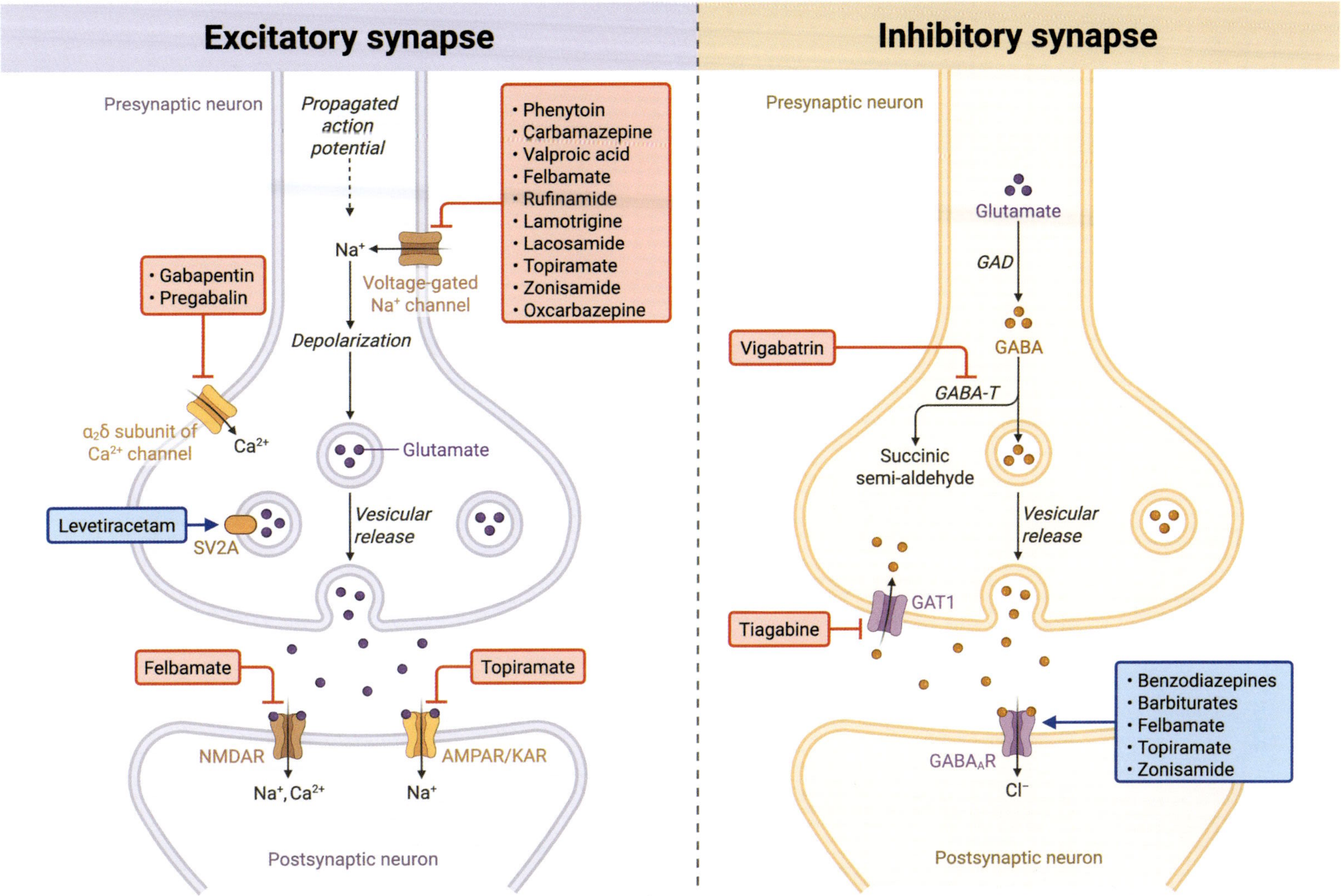

FIGURE 4.2.2 Sites of action of many of the anti-seizure medications available. Those not mentioned in more detail in this chapter are typically human medications that are not currently used for veterinary patients. *Source:* Created with www.biorender.com.

POTASSIUM BROMIDE (KBr)

Key Pharmacologic Facts

Bromide is not metabolized in the body and is excreted unchanged in urine, making it suitable for patients with liver disease. Changes in dietary salt or water intake can affect serum bromide levels – specifically, increasing the chloride content in the diet while keeping the KBr dose constant may lead to increased bromide excretion, resulting in decreased serum bromide concentration. Bromide has a long half-life (median 15.2 days); steady state is typically reached after about 3 months.

Administration and Monitoring

A maintenance dose of 20–40 mg/kg once daily is recommended. Potassium bromide may cause gastric irritation; splitting the daily dose into two doses can improve tolerability.

Serum samples for bromide levels should be taken when the drug reaches a steady state, approximately after 3 months. For patients requiring quicker effectiveness, a loading dose of 400–600 mg/kg can be administered over 4–6 days, followed by standard maintenance doses. Serum KBr levels that control epileptic seizures typically range from 0.8 to 3.4 mg/mL when used alone, but lower levels (0.8–2.5 mg/mL) may suffice when combined with phenobarbital. Higher bromide concentrations are not linked to organ toxicity, unlike with PB.

Adverse Effects

KBr treatment can cause sedation, ataxia, increased thirst, and increased appetite. Bromide intoxication, known as bromism, can present with various neurological deficits, including intracranial signs, myelopathies, or diffuse lower motor neuron disease. Rarely, KBr administration has been linked to pancreatitis and megaesophagus.

LEVETIRACETAM

Key Pharmacologic Facts

Levetiracetam binds to the presynaptic vesicular protein, SV2A, which decreases glutamate neurotransmitter release. In dogs, the drug is well absorbed, is rapidly metabolized with an estimated elimination half-life of 3–4 hours, and is predominantly excreted renally (>80%). An extended-release formulation of levetiracetam has been shown to have a half-life exceeding 7 hours in dogs following oral administration, suggesting the potential for once- or twice-daily administration.

Administration and Monitoring

Oral levetiracetam comes in both standard and extended-release (ER) forms. Typically, it is initiated at 60 mg/kg/day, administered either every 8 hours for the standard version or every 12 hours for the ER version. When the standard dose is administered three times daily, the peak drug level from one dose can drop by 50–90% before the next dose, which may result in poor seizure control. More frequent dosing can reduce these fluctuations, but this may not be practical for clients. The oral dose should be increased when dogs are receiving phenobarbital concurrently, as lower serum levels can potentially be related to the induction of serum hydrolases.

Currently, there is no established reference range for levetiracetam serum concentrations in dogs. The human reference range of 5–45 μg/mL is often used for guidance, but therapeutic drug monitoring is rare. Instead, dose adjustments are typically based on clinical response and tolerability of side effects, which are generally mild.

Adverse Effects

Sedation, ataxia, gastrointestinal-related signs, and behavioral-related changes have been reported following administration.

ZONISAMIDE

Key Pharmacologic Facts

Zonisamide's mechanism of action is believed to be related to the modulation of calcium ion channels and slow sodium channel inactivation. The bioavailability of zonisamide following oral administration is approximately 70%, and the reported elimination half-life is approximately 16 hours. Zonisamide is metabolized hepatically and thus influenced by concurrent administration of other similarly metabolized drugs.

Administration and Monitoring

The initial starting dose of zonisamide should be approximately 5–10 mg/kg q12h. A reference interval for zonisamide has not yet been established, and the human therapeutic range of 10–40 µg/mL is often cited; as with levetiracetam, serum drug monitoring is infrequently performed in veterinary medicine. Stable plasma concentrations are achieved within 3–4 days following oral administration in dogs. Phenobarbital dosages should be reduced by 25% at the time of starting zonisamide due to phenobarbital's enhanced hepatic enzyme induction and associated increased clearance of zonisamide; alternatively, the starting dose of zonisamide when used as an adjunct to phenobarbital should be 10 mg/kg q12h to address phenobarbital-induced metabolism of zonisamide.

Adverse Effects

Zonisamide appears to be well-tolerated in dogs. Sedation, ataxia, dry eye, vomiting, soft stools or constipation, and inappetence are the most common issues. Patients with a history of sulfa drug hypersensitivity should not be prescribed zonisamide. More rare and serious side effects reported include renal tubular acidosis, blood dyscrasias, immune-mediated polyarthritis, uveitis, and hepatotoxicity. Therefore, serum biochemistry, hematology, and liver function evaluations should be considered every 6 months, as for PB.

GABAPENTIN AND PREGABALIN

Key Pharmacologic Facts

Gabapentin and pregabalin are used as pain-relieving medications, sedatives/anxiolytics, and anticonvulsants. Pregabalin is structurally similar to gabapentin, with both drugs being structural analogs of gamma aminobutyric acid (GABA), with the mechanism of action being voltage-gated calcium channel modulation, which decreases depolarization-induced calcium influx at the nerve terminals and ultimately reduces excitatory neurotransmitter release. The mean elimination half-life of gabapentin is 3–4 hours, and that of pregabalin is estimated at 7 hours in dogs.

A major benefit of these drugs is that both the parent compound and its metabolites are excreted renally; thus, there are no drug–drug interactions with other antiseizure medications that undergo hepatic metabolism (e.g. phenobarbital).

Administration and Monitoring

A recommended initial gabapentin dose is 10–20 mg/kg three times daily. The recommended oral dose of pregabalin for dogs is 2–5 mg/kg, 2–3 times daily, starting at the low end of the dosing range and increasing 1 mg/kg/week until the final dose is reached. In patients with renal disease, lower doses are recommended. Serum monitoring is not recommended, as the drug has a very high therapeutic index and little drug–drug interaction.

Adverse Effects

Gabapentin and pregabalin are generally well tolerated in dogs, and the most commonly reported side effects are sedation/lethargy and pelvic limb ataxia.

IMEPITOIN

Key Pharmacologic Facts

Imepitoin was approved for use in dogs with epilepsy in Europe in 2013. In 2018, it was approved by the U.S. Food and Drug Administration for the treatment of noise aversion in dogs. Imepitoin is a low-affinity partial agonist of the $GABA_A$ receptor. The elimination half-life is approximately 1.5–2 hours after a 30 mg/kg dose, but can extend up to 6 hours after chronic twice-daily treatment. Maximal plasma levels occur 2–3 hours after absorption, which may be prolonged. Imepitoin is mainly metabolized by the liver before being excreted in the feces. Kidney or liver dysfunction should not significantly impact the pharmacokinetics of imepitoin. The affinity of phenobarbital or diazepam for the $GABA_A$ receptor is much higher than that of imepitoin. Therefore, switching from phenobarbital to imepitoin should be avoided, while switching from imepitoin to phenobarbital is considered safe.

Administration and Monitoring

The recommended starting dose is 10–20 mg/kg q12h. The dose can be increased up to a maximum of 30 mg/kg q12h. A CBC and serum biochemistry profile are recommended before starting imepitoin treatment and every 6–12 months thereafter. The drug has a wide therapeutic index. Serum drug monitoring is therefore not needed.

Adverse Effects

These commonly include polyphagia and, less commonly, gastrointestinal signs, hyperactivity, ataxia, and a prolapsed third eyelid. No idiosyncratic reactions have yet been demonstrated. Liver enzyme activity does not appear to be induced by imepitoin. Discontinuation of imepitoin does not result in withdrawal seizures.

TOPIRAMATE

Key Pharmacologic Facts

This is a sulfamate-substituted monosaccharide that blocks the spread of seizures by rapidly potentiating GABA activity in the brain. Topiramate is well absorbed and primarily excreted renally as an unchanged drug.

Administration and Monitoring

A suggested starting dose is 2 mg/kg PO q12h. This dose may be slowly increased to 5–10 mg/kg 2–3 times per day, depending on the patient's response.

Adverse Effects

Topiramate is generally well tolerated, with adverse effects including ataxia, sedation, inappetence, and weight loss.

FELBAMATE

Key Pharmacologic Facts

Felbamate's mechanisms of action appear diverse: it inhibits excitatory N-methyl-D-aspartate (NMDA) receptor activity and potentiates inhibitory GABA receptor activity. Felbamate also has neuroprotective effects against neuronal hypoxia in animal models. Felbamate is both excreted unchanged and as metabolites in the urine. The half-life in adult dogs averages around 4–6 hours. Because the drug can induce liver enzyme induction, half-lives may decrease with time, and dosages may need adjustment.

Administration and Monitoring

A suggested starting dose is 5–10 mg/kg PO every 12 hours with titration to every 8 hours up to 20 mg/kg. Upper limits of 60–70 mg/kg PO every 8 hours have been noted.

CBC, chemistry panel, and bile acid tests should be performed at baseline and regularly during treatment. Therapeutic drug levels for felbamate in dogs are not known but appear to be in the 25–100 μg/mL range. The usefulness of monitoring serum levels is uncertain.

Adverse Effects

Ataxia, tremors, vomiting, dry eye, and hypersalivation have been noted, without sedation, but with concerns about liver toxicity and bone marrow suppression, keeping this medication off the main list of traditionally used first-line anti-seizure drugs.

WHAT APPROACH SHOULD BE CONSIDERED FOR THIS DOG?

The dog described in this case has an unacceptable monthly frequency of seizures despite the use of phenobarbital. The serum level of phenobarbital suggests appropriate dosing but needs to be repeated now, and if there is no significant change, it would support an increase in the drug dose. This can be an arbitrary 25% increment, with the serum concentration repeated 2–3 weeks later. The signalment and the current frequency of the events also support the use of a second drug at this time, which could be levetiracetam, zonisamide, or potassium bromide. A higher-end dose of levetiracetam and zonisamide would be required when combined with phenobarbital. The carer should be advised that sedation and ataxia may be prominent with these combinations. However, if seizure frequency can be improved, phenobarbital reduction could be attempted to limit these adverse effects.

An at-home cluster seizure treatment protocol should also be provided to the pet carer (see Case 1), in addition to counseling regarding refractory epilepsy, emergency potentials, as well as the pet and carer's quality of life.

WHAT NONPHARMACOLOGIC TREATMENT OPTIONS COULD BE CONSIDERED IN A DOG REFRACTORY TO ANTI-CONVULSANT MEDICATION?

Although an exact definition has not been established in veterinary medicine, it is generally agreed that a dog that continues to have frequent or severe seizures or intolerable side effects despite appropriate antiseizure drug therapy is considered refractory to treatment.

The term drug-resistant epilepsy has been defined in human medicine as a failure of adequate trials of two tolerated and appropriately chosen and used anti-seizure drugs (whether as monotherapies or in combination) to achieve sustained seizure freedom.

Most of the dogs with epilepsy are successfully treated with the conventional antiseizure medications such as phenobarbital and potassium bromide. However, it has been estimated that up to 30% of dogs have refractory epilepsy and do not attain satisfactory seizure control with conventional therapy. This is an important factor to explain to owners at the start of seizure therapy for their pet, so their expectations can be managed.

Alternative adjunctive therapies have been investigated for refractory patients, with some of these treatment options currently used in veterinary medicine to offer additional ways to manage epilepsy in dogs and cats.

CANNABIDIOL

In recent years, there has been an increasing interest in using cannabidiol for epilepsy management in dogs. Cannabidiol is extracted from *Cannabis sativa* and is one of the cannabinoids (CB) with nonpsychotropic action.

CB1 receptors are widely distributed in the brain and are associated with cannabinoid effects on cognition, appetite, emotions, memory, perception, and control of movement. The mechanism of action of cannabidiol is not clear, but a decrease in glutamate release, activation of 5-hydroxytryptophan 1A receptors, and inhibition of adenosine reuptake are suspected.

Clinical studies have shown some potential effect of cannabidiol in dogs with drug-resistant epilepsy. Seizure frequency was significantly reduced in these studies when cannabidiol was given at 2.0–4.5 mg/kg orally twice daily, with limited adverse effects.

DIETARY MANAGEMENT

Dietary approaches for human epilepsy are well established. The most studied is the ketogenic diet, which in its traditional form is high in fats and low in proteins and carbohydrates. This diet mimics fasting, providing an alternative energy source for the brain, enhancing mitochondrial function, and inhibiting glutamatergic pathways and synaptic activity. In veterinary medicine, a trial with this classic ketogenic diet did not reduce seizure frequency and posed a high risk of pancreatitis. Recently, medium-chain triglyceride (MCT)-enriched diets, similar to the ketogenic diet, have been developed for adult epilepsy because they are more palatable and easier to adhere to. Initially created for canine cognitive dysfunction, these diets have been tested in multiple studies involving drug-resistant canine epilepsy, showing over a 50% reduction in seizure frequency in up to half of the cases. Additionally, comorbidities such as fear, anxiety, impulsivity, and cognitive issues also improved with MCT-enriched diets.

NEUROSTIMULATION

An electrical or magnetic pulse delivered directly to the nervous tissue, either directly (intracranially) or transcranially, has been shown to provide a palliative effect in human patients with epilepsy. This is achieved with vagus nerve stimulation, deep-brain stimulation, and transcranial magnetic stimulation.

Vagus nerve stimulation (VNS) – Over 80% of vagal fibers carry sensory information from the viscera toward the brain (afferent fibers), while only around 20% of fibers are responsible for motor signaling (efferent fibers). An implantable device placed around the cervical part of the vagus nerve can deliver intermittent electrical stimulation, which modulates brain activity detectable on electroencephalography (EEG). Its effect is associated with modulations in serotonin, GABA, dopamine, and noradrenaline, as well as changes in regional cerebral blood flow.

Ten dogs with refractory epilepsy treated with VNS demonstrated a decrease in mean seizure frequency by 34.4% in the last 4 weeks of a 13-week-long therapy. Four of nine dogs showed a reduction of seizure frequency by ≥50%.

ACUPUNCTURE

There are both anecdotal reports and animal studies that suggest acupuncture may inhibit seizures. Antagonism of gamma-aminobutyric acid type A (GABA-A) receptors was found to attenuate the antiepileptic effect of electroacupuncture, whilst electroacupuncture has been shown to act synergistically with the antagonists of non-NMDA receptors. Acupuncture may theoretically affect epilepsy by increasing the release of inhibitory neurotransmitters such as serotonin, GABA, or opioid peptides. Beneficial effects on human epilepsy have been reported in uncontrolled studies. There are no controlled studies in veterinary medicine, but there are several promising case series and reports of an adjunctive benefit of acupuncture for epilepsy.

OUTCOME

The serum phenobarbital concentration was 26 μg/mL (reference range 15–35 μg/mL), supporting an increase of the phenobarbital dosing. This was actually done on a three-times-daily basis rather than twice daily. At the same time, the dog was started on potassium bromide at 30 mg/kg/day. Five months later, the dog had exhibited three cluster seizure days, but the overall frequency of seizure activity was one per month. The relatively young age of this dog, in addition to the breed, suggested that further work needed to be done to improve this seizure frequency; KBr was increased to 35 mg/kg/day, and levetiracetam was added at 30 mg/kg three times daily. A further 3 months later, the dog had only had two seizures.

SUGGESTED READING

Aylón Val, J. and Hernando-Requejo, V. (2025). Drug-resistant epilepsy: which drugs are substrates of P-glycoprotein and which are not? *Curr. Neuropharmacol.* 23.

Baya, P., Press, S., Istvan, S., and Rizzo, K. (2024). Immune-mediated polyarthritis and anterior uveitis secondary to zonisamide administration in a dog with refractory epilepsy. *Vet. Med. Sci.* 10 (2): e1374.

Booth, S., Meller, S., Packer, R.M. et al. (2021). Owner compliance in canine epilepsy. *Vet. Rec.* 188 (4): e16.

Charalambous, M., Brodbelt, D., and Volk, H.A. (2014). Treatment in canine epilepsy--a systematic review. *BMC Vet. Res.* 10: 257.

Charalambous, M., Shivapour, S.K., Brodbelt, D.C., and Volk, H.A. (2016). Antiepileptic drugs' tolerability and safety–a systematic review and meta-analysis of adverse effects in dogs. *BMC Vet. Res.* 12: 79.

Charalambous, M., Hünting, D., Meyerhoff, N. et al. (2025). Application of a novel three-day repetitive transcranial magnetic stimulation protocol for the treatment of drug-resistant epilepsy in dogs: single-blinded randomised sham-controlled clinical trial. *Front. Vet. Sci.* 12: 1598311.

Dewey, C.W., Rishniw, M., and Sakovitch, K. (2022). Felbamate as an oral add-on therapy in six dogs with presumptive idiopathic epilepsy and generalized seizures resistant to drug therapy. *Open Vet. J.* 12 (4): 445–450.

Di Cesare, F., Negro, V., Ravasio, G. et al. (2023). Gabapentin: clinical use and pharmacokinetics in dogs, cats, and horses. *Animals (Basel)* 13 (12): 2045.

Erath, J.R., Nessler, J.N., Riese, F. et al. (2020). Behavioral changes under levetiracetam treatment in dogs. *Front. Vet. Sci.* 7: 169.

Forsgård, J.A., Metsähonkala, L., Kiviranta, A.M. et al. (2019). Seizure-precipitating factors in dogs with idiopathic epilepsy. *J. Vet. Intern. Med.* 33 (2): 701–707.

Fredsø, N., Sabers, A., Toft, N. et al. (2016). A single-blinded phenobarbital-controlled trial of levetiracetam as mono-therapy in dogs with newly diagnosed epilepsy. *Vet. J.* 208: 44–49.

Gouveia, D., Mandigers, P., and Cherubini, G.B. (2024). Bromide: the good, the bad, and the ugly of the oldest antiseizure medication. *Front. Vet. Sci.* 11: 1433191.

Han, F.Y., Conboy-Schmidt, L., Rybachuk, G. et al. (2021). Dietary medium chain triglycerides for management of epilepsy: new data from human, dog, and rodent studies. *Epilepsia* 62 (8): 1790–1806.

Kriechbaumer, S.R.P., Jurina, K., Wielaender, F. et al. (2022). Pregabalin add-on vs. dose increase in levetiracetam add-on treatment: a real-life trial in dogs with drug-resistant epilepsy. *Front. Vet. Sci.* 9: 910038.

Lichtenauer, E.A., Evers, B., van den Broek, J., and Mandigers, P.J.J. (2022). Bromide dose in dogs with epilepsy living close to coastal areas and living more inland: a retrospective observational study. *Front. Vet. Sci.* 9: 906288.

Mastrocco A., Prittie J., West C., Clark M. (2024). A review of the pharmacology and clinical applications of levetiracetam in dogs and cats. *J. Vet. Emerg. Crit. Care* (San Antonio) 34 (1): 9–22.

Muñana, K.R., Thomas, W.B., Inzana, K.D. et al. (2012). Evaluation of levetiracetam as adjunctive treatment for refractory canine epilepsy: a randomized, placebo-controlled, crossover trial. *J. Vet. Intern. Med.* 26 (2): 341–348.

Muñana, K.R., Nettifee-Osborne, J.A., and Papich, M.G. (2015). Effect of chronic administration of phenobarbital, or bromide, on pharmacokinetics of levetiracetam in dogs with epilepsy. *J. Vet. Intern. Med.* 29 (2): 614–619.

Muñana K.R., Vitek S.M., Tarver W.B., et al. (2002) Use of vagal nerve stimulation as a treatment for refractory epilepsy in dogs. *J Am Vet Med Assoc.* 221 (7): 977–83.

Neßler, J., Rundfeldt, C., Löscher, W. et al. (2017). Clinical evaluation of a combination therapy of imepitoin with phenobarbital in dogs with refractory idiopathic epilepsy. *BMC Vet. Res.* 13 (1): 33.

Nowakowska, M., Üçal, M., Charalambous, M. et al. (2022). Neurostimulation as a method of treatment and a preventive measure in canine drug-resistant epilepsy: current state and future prospects. *Front. Vet. Sci.* 9: 889561.

Potschka, H., Bhatti, S.F.M., Tipold, A., and McGrath, S. (2022). Cannabidiol in canine epilepsy. *Vet. J.* 290: 105913.

Potschka, H., Fischer, A., Löscher, W., and Volk, H.A. (2023). Pathophysiology of drug-resistant canine epilepsy. *Vet. J.* 296-297: 10599.

Royaux, E., Van Ham, L., Broeckx, B.J. et al. (2017). Phenobarbital or potassium bromide as an add-on antiepileptic drug for the management of canine idiopathic epilepsy refractory to imepitoin. *Vet. J.* 220: 51–54.

Rozental, A.J., Weisbeck, B.G., Corsato Alvarenga, I. et al. (2023). The efficacy and safety of cannabidiol as adjunct treatment for drug-resistant idiopathic epilepsy in 51 dogs: a double-blinded crossover study. *J. Vet. Intern. Med.* 37 (6): 2291–2300.

Saint-Maxent, M., Juette, T., Parent, J. et al. (2024). Factors influencing serum concentrations of levetiracetam in dogs with epilepsy. *J. Vet. Intern. Med.* 38 (4): 2249–2256.

Saito, M., Nomura, A., Hasegawa, D. et al. (2024). Clinical efficacy and tolerability of zonisamide monotherapy in dogs with newly diagnosed idiopathic epilepsy: prospective open-label uncontrolled multicenter trial. *J. Vet. Intern. Med.* 38 (4): 2228–2236.

Stabile, F., Barnett, C.R., and De Risio, L. (2017) Phenobarbital administration every eight hours: improvement of seizure management in idiopathic epileptic dogs with decreased phenobarbital elimination half-life. *Vet. Rec.* 180 (7): 178.

Stabile, F., van Dijk, J., Barnett, C.R., and De Risio, L. (2019). Epileptic seizure frequency and semiology in dogs with idiopathic epilepsy after initiation of imepitoin or phenobarbital monotherapy. *Vet. J.* 249: 53–57.

Suiter, E.J., Packer, R.M., and Volk, H.A. (2016). Comparing the effects of first-line antiepileptic drugs on the gait of dogs with idiopathic epilepsy. *Vet. Rec.* 178 (26): 652.

Vendramini, T.H.A., Amaral, A.R., Rentas, M.F. et al. (2024). Ketogenic diets: a systematic review of current scientific evidence and possible applicability in dogs and cats. *J. Anim. Physiol. Anim. Nutr. (Berl).* 108 (2): 541–556.

Verdoodt, F., Watanangura, A., Bhatti, S.F.M. et al. (2022). The role of nutrition in canine idiopathic epilepsy management: fact or fiction? *Vet. J.* 290: 105917.

Seizures

Case 3—Status Epilepticus in a Dog

CHAPTER 4.3

Tom Jukier

Department of Clinical Sciences, College of Veterinary Medicine, Auburn University, Auburn, AL, USA

CASE HISTORY

A 5-year-old neutered male Chihuahua was presented to the hospital while experiencing an "episode" that had been ongoing *for the past 2 hours*. The episodes consisted of generalized facial twitches and hypersalivation (See Video 4.3.1). At the beginning of this episode and other similar ones, the client reported that the patient voided urine. However, the two previous episodes were brief, lasting ~30 seconds, before the patient began to move around again. The two previous episodes occurred 6 weeks apart from each other, and 3 weeks prior to this current episode. The owner is unsure about the dog's mental awareness during the episodes, but the patient may have responded to the owner calling its name once. The owner reported that for the past couple of weeks, the dog has appeared to have a slightly different demeanor. He has been hiding more, and he has had a tendency to circle to the left, and sometimes stood with the right thoracic limb in an inappropriate position. The patient has otherwise been healthy and is up-to-date on vaccinations (with the most recent vaccines being administered approximately 6 months ago). The dog is current on flea, tick, and heartworm preventatives, none of which are isoxazolines, and spends most of its time indoors aside from going outside to urinate/defecate and enjoy some sun. There are no known toxin exposures, and no known exposure to other pets or wildlife.

VIDEO 4.3.1 A 5-year-old neutered male Chihuahua exhibits generalized facial twitches and hypersalivation with altered mentation.

NEUROLOGICAL EXAMINATION

Given that the patient is actively experiencing the episode, a neurological examination cannot be performed. However, this episode and the previous ones are compatible with seizure activity. The involuntary facial twitches are known as "automatisms," and the hypersalivation is most likely secondary to the activation of the autonomic nervous system (parasympathetic portion), which may occur during seizures. Seizures are a manifestation of cerebral cortex dysfunction, so the localization should be in the cerebral cortex (also known as the forebrain, prosencephalon, or cerebrum).

1. **What is status epilepticus?**
2. **What treatment options are available for status epilepticus?**
3. **What differentials should be considered?**

WHAT IS STATUS EPILEPTICUS?

Status epilepticus is a seizure that lasts for >5 minutes, or if a patient has a second seizure after the first one within 10 minutes, without fully regaining consciousness in between. Status epilepticus

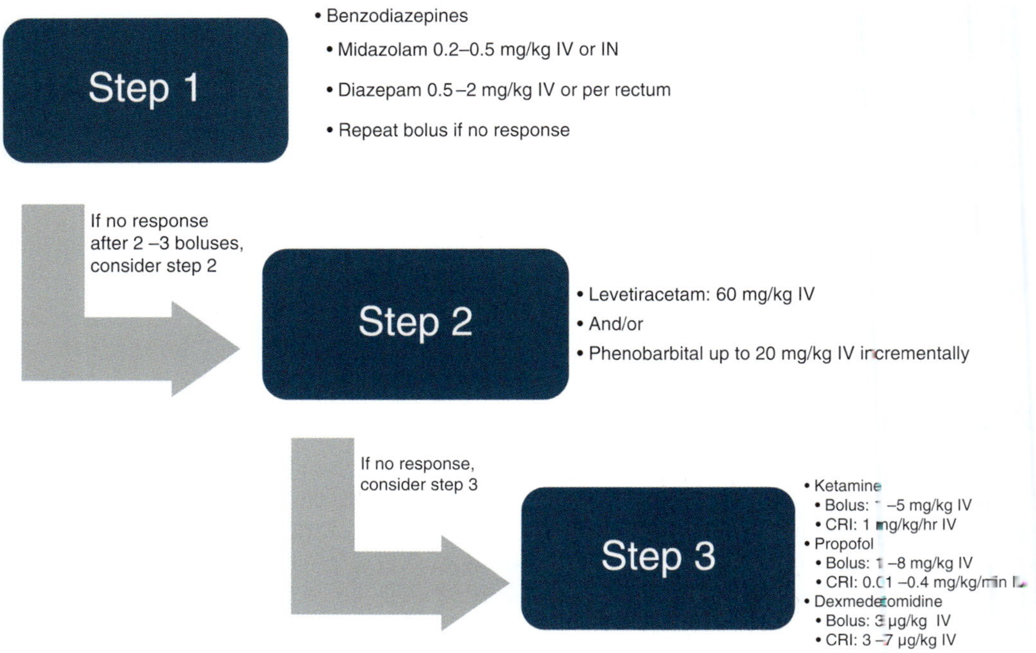

FIGURE 4.3.1 An algorithmic approach to the pharmacological management of emergency seizure activity.

can be caused by a loss of the "natural" mechanisms that result in seizure cessation or by an onset of factors that can lead to prolonged seizures and may have long-term ramifications for the patient. Any disease that can cause seizure activity can cause status epilepticus.

TREATMENT OPTIONS FOR STATUS EPILEPTICUS (Figure 4.3.1)

STEP 1 – When a patient is presented to the hospital experiencing an active seizure, the first-line antiseizure medication (ASM) should be a benzodiazepine. Two main benzodiazepines are commonly used in veterinary medicine: diazepam and midazolam. The antiseizure properties of benzodiazepines are mediated via activation of gamma-aminobutyric acid (GABA) receptors, which then allow chloride ions to enter the neuron, potentiating neuro-inhibition (see Figure 4.2.2 in case 2 of this chapter).

- Diazepam can be administered, intravenously (IV), and rectally using a dose of 0.5–2 mg/kg. The oral route should be avoided in patients who are in an active seizure to prevent the individual administering the medication from being bitten. The intravenous route is the preferred route for diazepam. However, obtaining intravenous access may be challenging in patients who are in an active seizure, particularly if the seizure is a generalized tonic–clonic seizure and if they are smaller in body size.
- Midazolam can be administered via IV, intramuscular, and intranasal (IN) routes using 0.2–0.5 mg/kg. The latter two routes are easier to administer to a patient during an active seizure who does not have an IV catheter. This enables easier intravenous access so that additional medication can be administered as needed.

Based on a recent consensus statement, the IV or IN routes for benzodiazepines are preferable, and redosing should be performed if the seizure has not terminated within 2 minutes. If two benzodiazepine boluses are not effective, a constant rate infusion (CRI) should be initiated, and a third bolus can be attempted. If the patient continues to exhibit seizure activity, a second-line agent should be considered. Tolerance to benzodiazepines can develop within several days of administration. Therefore, if the patient requires continued therapy, a different antiseizure medication should be used.

STEP 2 – Second-line agents include phenobarbital (PB) and levetiracetam (LEV). Similar to benzodiazepines, phenobarbital acts via potentiating GABA receptors, allowing the influx of chloride ions. The administration of up to 20 mg/kg of phenobarbital in increments of 3–6 mg/kg intravenously can be considered at 15-minute intervals. Levetiracetam works via a protein associated with neurotransmitter exocytosis called synaptic vesicle 2A (SV2A) (see Figure 4.2.2 in case 2 of this chapter). The administration of a 60 mg/kg IV dose may lead to shorter hospitalization times for patients with status epilepticus or cluster seizures. This dose can then be followed by the standard starting dose of 20 mg/kg IV (or *per OS* if the patient can swallow) every 8 hours. Both medications are manufactured as IV formulations.

STEP 3 – Third-line treatments should be used if the patient continues to have seizures despite appropriate doses of benzodiazepines, PB, and LEV. Third-line agents include ketamine and/or dexmedetomidine as the first step, followed by propofol. These should be administered as boluses or constant rate infusions. Ketamine has been administered as a 1 mg/kg bolus followed by a 1 mg/kg/hour CRI and a 5 mg/kg IV bolus. For propofol, a bolus of 1–8 mg/kg, or CRI of 0.01–0.4 mg/kg/minute, can be attempted. However, given the possibility of respiratory depression/failure following the administration of propofol, patients receiving this medication should be closely monitored and may require intubation and assisted ventilation if respiratory depression occurs. The administration of dexmedetomidine for seizures has been described by the initial administration of a 3 μg/kg bolus followed by a 3–7 μg/kg/hour CRI. It is important to realize that these medications may stop the physical manifestation of a seizure, but the patient may still be having an electroencephalographic seizure.

Of note, if there is a known toxin exposure that has caused status epilepticus, the patient may benefit from intravenous lipid therapy to help with the removal of the toxin from circulation. However, this may also limit the efficacy of antiseizure medications being administered.

DIFFERENTIALS

When patients are presented with an initial onset of status epilepticus, concern for either a reactive cause for the seizure (e.g. toxin) or a structural cause becomes prominent on the differential list.

Causes of Reactive/Metabolic Seizures

A. Toxins – there are several different toxins that may cause seizures in the dog. These include lead, organophosphates, metaldehyde, and others. In these cases, there is usually some historical aspect that suggests exposure (such as recent local pesticide use).

B. Hypoglycemia – Hypoglycemia can result from several different causes, such as improper use of insulin or excess circulating insulin due to an insulin-secreting tumor, such as pancreatic beta islet cell tumors ("insulinoma") or leiomyosarcoma. Other causes for hypoglycemia include overexertion in working breeds of dogs or younger small breeds of dogs that may have it.

C. Hepatic Encephalopathy – The liver normally clears toxins that are absorbed through the gastrointestinal tract. As such, if the liver is unable to filter blood, these toxins will end up in the capillaries of the brain, and can cross the blood–brain barrier, potentially leading to seizures. A portosystemic shunt (PSS) is a common cause of hepatic encephalopathy. The PSS may be a large vessel (e.g. porto-azygous shunt) or may be microscopic at the level of the sinusoids (e.g. microvascular dysplasia). Lastly, severe and chronic liver disease may lead to cirrhosis and ultimately hepatic encephalopathy.

D. Drug Induced/Idiosyncratic – The administration of any medication can, in theory, lead to seizures if the patient is sensitive to that medication.

Epileptic seizures are the second differential for the seizure itself. Epileptic seizures are the result of inherent neuronal dysfunction that transiently manifests as a seizure. If a patient has two or more epileptic seizures separated by 24 hours, they can be said to have epilepsy. The differentials for epilepsy may include nonstructural (e.g. idiopathic epilepsy), or structural causes such as neoplasia, meningoencephalitis, anomalous (e.g. hydrocephalus), vascular, and traumatic brain injury.

Structural Causes for Epileptic Seizures

A. Meningoencephalitis – Inflammatory conditions of the central nervous system in dogs are common, and a majority of them are immune-mediated in nature. These diseases are more commonly seen in young adults and small breeds of dogs. Females may be overrepresented. These immune-mediated diseases are collectively called meningoencephalitis of unknown origin (MUO). Three distinct forms have been documented, including granulomatous meningoencephalitis (GME), necrotizing meningoencephalitis (NME), and necrotizing leukoencephalitis (NLE). Although magnetic resonance imaging (MRI) may suggest one form over another, definitive diagnosis ultimately requires histopathology. Infectious diseases as a result of fungal, protozoal, rickettsial, viral, and bacterial organisms may also occur in the dog, but are much less common.

B. Neoplasia – Tumors more commonly occur in older dogs but can occur at any age. The most common brain tumor in dogs is meningioma, which is a tumor that arises from the meninges and grows into the brain parenchyma. The second most common brain tumor is glioma. The term "glioma" is a general term used to describe tumors that arise from brain parenchyma. There are several different types of glioma (i.e. oligodendroglioma, astrocytoma, etc.) Gliomas can occur in any breed, but bulldog clade breeds are overrepresented. Other neoplastic disorders that may cause seizures include choroid plexus tumors, ependymomas, lymphoma, granular cell tumors, primitive neuroendocrine tumors, and metastatic tumors. Tumor type can sometimes be judged based on imaging characteristics. For example, meningiomas tend to occur on the surface of the brain, and often display marked contrast enhancement following gadolinium administration. Additionally, a "dural tail" sign may be more common with these types of tumors post-contrast. However, ultimately, histopathology is necessary for definitive diagnosis.

Although any underlying cause for a seizure can cause the clinical manifestation of status epilepticus (SE), when the initial presentation of the seizure is SE, concerns for a reactive seizure or a structural cause for the epileptic seizure should be prioritized.

OUTCOME

The dog was stabilized using a CRI of midazolam and an initial bolus of 60 mg/kg of IV levetiracetam. Eight hours later, the dog was given another bolus of levetiracetam, and the initial weaning of the midazolam CRI commenced. The dog was weaned off the CRI 24 hours after initiation. The dog was initiated on an oral dose of levetiracetam, 8 hours after the second parenteral dose, and this was continued for the next 48 hours. The dog was discharged, having been seizure-free for approximately 3 days. The owners did not want to pursue an MRI or cerebrospinal fluid analysis (CSF) tap at this time. Long-term anticonvulsant medication was discussed with the owner, and the dog was initiated on phenobarbital.

SUGGESTED READING

Blades Golubovic, S. and Rossmeisl, J.H. Jr. (2017). Status epilepticus in dogs and cats, part 2: treatment, monitoring, and prognosis. *J. Vet. Emerg. Crit. Care (San Antonio)* 27: 288–300.

Boothe, D.M. (2012). *Small Animal Clinical Pharmacology and Therapeutics*, 2e. St. Louis Missouri: Elsevier Saunders.

Charalambous, M., Bhatti, S.F.M., Van Ham, L. et al. (2017). Intranasal midazolam versus rectal diazepam for the management of canine status epilepticus: a multicenter randomized parallel-group clinical trial. *J. Vet. Intern. Med.* 31: 1149–1158.

Charalambous, M., Munana, K., Patterson, E.E. et al. (2024) ACVIM consensus statement on the management of status epilepticus and cluster seizures in dogs and cats. *J. Vet. Intern. Med.* 38 (1): 19–40.

Charalambous, M., Volk, H.A., Van Ham, L. et al. (2021). First-line management of canine status epilepticus at home and in hospital: opportunities and limitations of the various administration routes of benzodiazepines. *BMC Vet. Res.* 17: 103.

Gioeni, D., Di Cesare, F., D'Urso, E.S. et al. (2020). Ketamine-dexmedetomidine combination and controlled mild hypothermia for the treatment of long-lasting and super-refractory status epilepticus in 3 dogs suffering from idiopathic epilepsy. *J. Vet. Emerg. Crit. Care (San Antonio)* 30: 455–460.

Hardy, B.T., Patterson, E.E., Cloyd, J.M. et al. (2012). Double-masked, placebo-controlled study of intravenous levetiracetam for the treatment of status epilepticus and acute repetitive seizures in dogs. *J. Vet. Intern. Med.* 26: 334–340.

Heldmann, E., Holt, D.E., Brockman, D.J. et al. (1999). Use of propofol to manage seizure activity after surgical treatment of portosystemic shunts. *J. Small Anim. Pract.* 40: 590–594.

Roynard, P., Bilderback, A., and Dewey, C.W. (2021). Intravenous ketamine bolus(es) for the treatment of status epilepticus, refractory status epilepticus, and cluster seizures: a retrospective study of 15 dogs. *Front. Vet. Sci.* 8: 547279.

Steffen, F. and Grasmueck, S. (2000). Propofol for treatment of refractory seizures in dogs and a cat with intracranial disorders. *J. Small Anim. Pract.* 41: 496–499.

CHAPTER 4.4

Seizures

Case 4—A Cat with Seizures

Tom Jukier

Department of Clinical Sciences, College of Veterinary Medicine, Auburn University, Auburn, AL, USA

CASE HISTORY

A 7-year-old spayed female domestic short-haired cat was presented for recent onset seizures recurring weekly over the past 2 months. The owners report that the episodes last approximately 1 minute, involve the patient freezing in place with the pupils dilated, after which the patient falls to the side, opens its mouth, extends its thoracic limbs, and then begins to "paddle" with its pelvic limbs. During the seizure, the patient appears to hypersalivate and void urine. The patient is a strictly indoor cat and has been otherwise healthy. It is routinely vaccinated and is on flea, tick, and heartworm prevention. The prophylactics have not changed recently, with the last dose being given about 7 months ago. The owners reported that she appeared to be completely normal in between the seizures, but that it takes about 1 day after each event before she is normal again.

NEUROLOGICAL EXAMINATION

The cat was bright, alert, and responsive. She was initially hesitant but began to explore the room after acclimating. She was ambulatory with a normal gait and posture. She jumped on and off the furniture in the room without issue. Postural reactions, spinal reflexes, and cranial nerve examination were all normal. There was no pain on vertebral column or skull palpation, and no evidence of discomfort elicited by cervical range of motion evaluation.

1. **Where do you localize the lesion?**
2. **What are the differentials to consider?**
3. **What diagnostic work-up should be performed?**
4. **What treatment options exist for cats?**

LESION LOCALIZATION

By default, patients experiencing seizures are designated a neurolocalization to the forebrain (cerebrum or thalamus), even if no neurological examination abnormalities are observed. Since no neurological deficits are observed in this patient, the extent of forebrain involvement (and the affected side of the forebrain, if a structural lesion is present) cannot be determined.

DIFFERENTIAL DIAGNOSIS

- **Meningoencephalitis**
  Meningoencephalitis, or inflammation of the meninges and the brain, can be secondary to infectious etiologies or noninfectious, inflammatory etiologies. While in dogs, noninfectious etiologies are far more common than infectious meningoencephalitis, the reverse is true for cats. Although immune-mediated diseases of the brain have been documented in cats, such cases are far less common than those caused by infectious etiologies. Meningoencephalitis in the cat is more likely to be infectious than immune-mediated. In cats, the most common infectious agents to cause meningoencephalitis include feline coronavirus ("feline infectious peritonitis"), *Cryptococcus neoformans*, and *Toxoplasma gondii*. Additionally, bacterial encephalitis can develop as a result of either bite injuries or extension from otitis media/interna. These infectious diseases can affect any portion of the central nervous system, but if the cerebral cortex is affected, it may lead to seizures. Often, cats with infectious meningoencephalitis display interictal abnormalities, such as changes in mentation. They may also display systemic signs of illness, depending on the infectious organism.

- **Unknown cause/idiopathic**
  Idiopathic epilepsy is the most common cause of seizures in dogs and is increasingly recognized as a common cause of seizures in cats. Although seizures in cats are more likely to result from structural abnormalities, including infectious, neoplastic, and traumatic etiologies, idiopathic epilepsy remains a strong differential diagnosis in this cat. Feline idiopathic epilepsy has similar features to canine idiopathic epilepsy: cats are normal interictally and develop epilepsy between late juvenile status and mid-adult status. As opposed to canine epilepsy, which typically causes generalized seizures, feline epilepsy can lead to a broader phenotype in seizures, including focal facial seizures or periods of aggression and disinhibition.

  Feline temporal lobe epilepsy (TLE) and/or feline hippocampal necrosis is an essential subset of epilepsy that accounts for an important and relatively consistent seizure phenotype. TLE arises spontaneously and leads to lip smacking, facial twitching, hypersalivation, and jaw movements, comprising a seizure manifestation called "orofacial automatisms." More recently, this has been termed feline complex partial cluster seizure with orofacial involvement (FEPSO). Interictally, cats with FEPSO and hippocampal necrosis can have substantial unprovoked aggression or periods of rapid, fitful running. FEPSO was first discovered experimentally, as seizures in cats could be induced by creating perturbations in the temporal lobe. Thus, this region of the brain is a known "epileptogenic focus." Over the past 15 years, spontaneous FEPSO and hippocampal necrosis/sclerosis have been increasingly well-described. This condition itself is not a primary entity but rather is secondary to a variety of primary causes, and mimics human autoimmune limbic encephalitis. Although the exact etiology in cats remains unclear, it is associated with specific autoantibodies, notably against the leucine-rich glioma-inactivated 1 (LGI1) protein. In some cats, the condition progresses to generalized seizures, which are typically refractory to conventional treatment. FEPSO and hippocampal necrosis are strong considerations for this cat, given its age and the observed clinical signs.

- **Neoplasia**
  Meningioma is the most common intracranial primary brain tumor in cats. These are slow-growing tumors that occur in older cats. Feline meningiomas differ from canine meningiomas in several ways. First, feline meningiomas are nearly always benign, albeit locally intrusive, whereas canine meningiomas can be more aggressive. Feline meningiomas are typically encapsulated, which adds to their benign nature and facilitates gross total surgical resection more often than encountered in canine meningiomas. Feline meningiomas also rarely cause seizures, unlike canine meningiomas. Finally, feline meningiomas affect

an older patient population than canine meningiomas, which can originate in dogs as young as 5 years old. Most cats with meningiomas are at least 12 years old at the time of diagnosis. Further, since these are slow-growing tumors, they may be found incidentally during necropsy of clinically unaffected cats. Thus, meningioma is an unlikely cause of this cat's seizures.

Contrastingly, lymphoma affects cats at a much younger age than meningiomas, making it an important differential diagnosis for this cat. Lymphoma is the most common neoplasm to metastasize to the feline brain, and can also arise as a primary brain tumor. Other types of tumors (e.g. gliomas) have also been described in the feline brain but are less prevalent.

- **Trauma**
  Post-traumatic epilepsy is a known epileptic syndrome in humans and has been identified in dogs and cats. The prevalence of post-traumatic epilepsy in the dog has been estimated to be ~7%, but the likelihood of post-traumatic epilepsy in the cat appears to be lower.
- **Reactive/metabolic seizures**
  A reactive or metabolic seizure is a seizure caused by extracranial factors, such as toxin exposure, hypoglycemia, or primary organ dysfunction (e.g. liver dysfunction). The appearance of this kind of seizure can be similar to that of an epileptic seizure. Given that the patient has had one seizure a week for 2 months, it is less likely that the seizures are reactive.

DIAGNOSTIC WORKUP

Similar to any patient with new/recent onset seizures, a minimal database including a complete blood count, serum/plasma chemistry, and urinalysis should be performed to assess for possible causes of reactive seizures. Paired fasted and postprandial serum/plasma bile acid concentrations should also be performed, and/or an ammonia concentration to rule out hepatic dysfunction. Liver function tests are also useful to establish baseline liver function before initiation of potentially hepatotoxic drugs (e.g. phenobarbital). Thoracic radiographs and an abdominal ultrasound can be considered prior to more advanced diagnostics based on age, physical examination, and blood work findings.

In order to distinguish a structural cause for the seizures (i.e. neoplasia or meningoencephalitis) from a nonstructural cause (e.g. idiopathic), brain magnetic resonance imaging (MRI) and cerebrospinal fluid (CSF) testing should be performed. Feline hippocampal necrosis leads to distinctive changes on MRI (Figure 4.4.1).

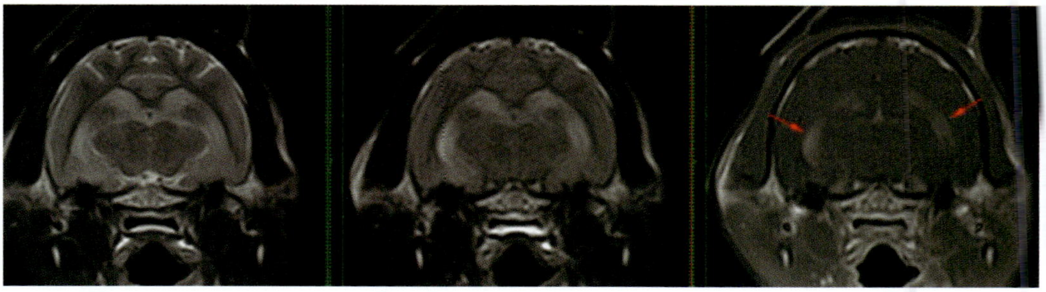

FIGURE 4.4.1 MRI transverse images of a cat's brain with hippocampal necrosis. On T2-weighted imaging (left image) and T2-weighted fluid attenuated inversion recovery (FLAIR) imaging (middle image), the hippocampi are hyperintense. On T1-weighted post-contrast imaging (right image), contrast enhancement is present exclusively in the hippocampi (red arrows).

TREATMENT

Regardless of the underlying cause, the primary clinical signs of an epileptic seizure need to be addressed. This is often done with an antiseizure medication (ASM). Although there are several different medications that can be used, the four most common ASMs are phenobarbital, bromide, levetiracetam, and zonisamide. However, bromide, although effective and safe in the dog, is not safe in the cat and may induce fatal respiratory signs. Therefore, it is best to avoid bromide use in the cat.

- **Phenobarbital**
  Phenobarbital is a barbiturate medication that is commonly used in cats for the treatment of seizures. The mechanism of action is via gamma-aminobutyric acid (GABA) receptor potentiation, allowing an influx of chloride into the neuron (see Figure 4.2.2 in case 2 of this chapter). Based on the evidence in the veterinary literature, phenobarbital may be the most efficacious drug available to the clinician. The exception to this is the epileptic syndrome known as feline audiogenic reflex seizures (FARS), in which case levetiracetam has been demonstrated to be superior in the only study evaluating the treatment of this condition. The half-life of phenobarbital is long enough to justify a 12-hourly dosing interval. A starting dose of 1–2 mg/kg per os (PO) q12h can be used. The cat may be more tolerant of the side effects associated with this medication compared to the dog. However, hepatotoxicity is still possible, and cats on phenobarbital should be routinely monitored for the development of hepatotoxicity. A reference interval (the range of concentrations that are effective and safe in a population of patients) has not been established for cats. However, due to the higher risk of hepatotoxicity at concentrations >35 µg/mL (in dogs), concentrations below this value may be safer in cats as well. Given the half-life of this medication, therapeutic drug monitoring should be performed initially within 10–14 days of therapy initiation, and dose adjustments should be made based on therapeutic outcome, side effects, and plasma drug concentrations.

- **Levetiracetam**
  Levetiracetam is a commonly used ASM in both dogs and cats. Levetiracetam is available as intravenous (IV), immediate-release (IR) oral tablets, and extended-release (ER) oral tablets. The starting dose that is used is often 60 mg/kg/day (20 mg/kg PO q8h for the IR formulation; the ER tablets may physically be too large to administer to many cats). Levetiracetam has been demonstrated to be superior to phenobarbital for the treatment of epileptic seizures as a result of the epileptic syndrome called FARS. Levetiracetam has a short half-life in cats of ~3 hours; therefore, clinicians should be aware that dosing at an interval of every 8 hours will lead to large fluctuations in plasma drug concentrations. A reference interval has not been established in cats (or dogs). Levetiracetam is well-tolerated and has a wide therapeutic window. Therefore, the dose is often increased in response to therapeutic failure.

- **Zonisamide**
  Zonisamide is sometimes used in cats as well. Two reports do suggest some degree of efficacy, and that overall the medication is well tolerated. Zonisamide is only formulated for oral administration; therefore, it cannot be given to patients who cannot swallow (e.g. in the immediate postictal period in some cases). The pharmacokinetics of this drug in the cat support a q12h dosing interval using 5 mg/kg PO. Overall, the medication is well-tolerated in cats. There are rare reports of zonisamide leading to a condition called pseudolymphoma, in which some or all peripheral lymph nodes become enlarged. Microscopic evaluation of the contents obtained by fine needle aspiration in animals with pseudolymphoma will reveal a population of reactive, rather than neoplastic, lymphocytes. Treatment of pseudolymphoma consists of discontinuation of the drug.

OUTCOME

Blood work, inclusive of infectious disease assessments (feline leukemia virus, feline immunodeficiency virus, feline coronavirus, and *Toxoplasma*), was considered normal. An MRI and CSF analysis were performed on the cat, and the results were also considered normal. The cat was thus diagnosed with idiopathic epilepsy. The cat was initiated on phenobarbital 2 mg/kg orally every 12 hours. The seizure frequency over the next 3 months reduced to one event per 6 weeks. The cat tolerated the medication well without significant adverse effects, and so the dose was increased by 25% with a subsequent improvement in seizure control to the point of eradication over the next 3 months.

SUGGESTED READING

Charalambous, M., Pakozdy, A., Bhatti, S.F.M., and Volk, H.A. (2018). Systematic review of antiepileptic drugs' safety and effectiveness in feline epilepsy. *BMC Vet. Res.* 14 (1): 64.

Dayrell-Hart, B., Steinberg, S.A., VanWinkle, T.J., and Farnbach, G.C. (1991). Hepatotoxicity of phenobarbital in dogs: 18 cases (1985-1989). *J. Am. Vet. Med. Assoc.* 199: 1060–1066.

Djani, D.M., Liou, M., Aravamuthan, S. et al. (2024). A retrospective study of the efficacy of zonisamide in controlling seizures in 57 cats. *J. Vet. Intern. Med.* 38: 1092–1100.

Friedenberg, S.G., Butler, A.L., Wei, L. et al. (2012). Seizures following head trauma in dogs: 259 cases (1999-2009). *J. Am. Vet. Med. Assoc.* 241: 1479–1483.

Grohmann, K.S., Schmidt, M.J., Moritz, A., and Kramer, M. (2012). Prevalence of seizures in cats after head trauma. *J. Am. Vet. Med. Assoc.* 241: 1467–1470.

Hasegawa, D., Pakozdy, A., and Volk, H. (2017). Differentiating structural from idiopathic epilepsy in cats. *Vet. Rec.* 180 (25): 608–609. https://doi.org/10.1136/vr.j2896.

Lowrie, M., Thomson, S., Bessant, C. et al. (2017). Levetiracetam in the management of feline audiogenic reflex seizures: a randomised, controlled open-label study. *J. Feline Med. Surg.* 19: 200–206.

Pakozdy, A., Halasz, P., Klang, A. et al. (2023). Temporal lobe epilepsy in cats. *Vet. J.* 291: 105941. https://doi.org/10.1016/j.tvjl.2022.105941. Epub 2022 Dec 19. PMID: 36549606.

Scalia, B., Caine, A., Pittaway, R., and Cherubini, G.B. (2021). Feline temporal lobe epilepsy: seven cases of hippocampal and piriform lobe necrosis in England and literature review. *J. Feline Med. Surg.* 24 (6): 596–608. https://doi.org/10.1177/1098612X211035049.

Thomas, W.B. (2010). Hydrocephalus in dogs and cats. *Vet. Clin. North Am. Small Anim. Pract.* 40: 143–159.

Ukai, M., Hamamoto, Y., Yu, Y. et al. (2018). Efficacy of zonisamide on interictal electroencephalography in familial spontaneous epileptic cats. *J. Feline Med. Surg.* 20: 962–967.

Wahle, A.M., Bruhschwein, A., Matiasek, K. et al. (2014). Clinical characterization of epilepsy of unknown cause in cats. *J. Vet. Intern. Med.* 28 (1): 182–188.

Head Tilt and Imbalance

Case 1—Acute Onset Head Tilt in an Old Dog

CHAPTER 5.1

Susan A. Arnold

Department of Veterinary Clinical Sciences, University of Minnesota, St. Paul, MN, USA

CASE HISTORY

An 11-year-old neutered male German shepherd was presented for an acute onset of inability to walk and a right-sided head tilt of 1-day duration. The dog was reportedly normal the night prior, and when he was let outside on the day of presentation, he was reluctant to get up. Attempting to walk, he rolled over in circles toward the right. A right-sided head tilt was observed (Figure 5.1.1). Prior to the onset of signs, this dog had no known health concerns. He was an indiscriminate eater and had unsupervised outdoor access on a large, rural property. The dog had been routinely vaccinated since 12 weeks of age and was not receiving any medications other than heartworm and flea/tick preventatives.

NEUROLOGICAL AND PHYSICAL EXAMINATION (Video 5.1.1)

VIDEO 5.1.1 A German shepherd dog with a right-sided head tilt.

The dog was bright, alert, and responsive on presentation. He was nonambulatory. When encouraged to stand and walk with support, he consistently fell toward the right and at one point rolled rightward. A moderate right-sided head tilt was observed. His postural reactions, consisting of paw replacement and hopping, were normal in all four limbs. His segmental spinal reflexes were normal. In addition to the right-sided head tilt, his cranial nerve exam also revealed a spontaneous, horizontal nystagmus, fast phase to the left, and a positional ventral strabismus in his right eye. There was no evidence of pain or discomfort on thoracolumbar or cervical palpation or cervical range of motion.

1. **Where is the likely lesion localization?**
2. **What disease processes should be considered?**
3. **What tests could you perform to help determine the diagnosis?**

LESION LOCALIZATION (Figure 5.1.2)

The lesion is likely within the right peripheral vestibular system. The gait abnormality of falling and rolling to one side is consistent with vestibular ataxia. The head tilt, spontaneous nystagmus, and positional ventral strabismus in combination with the vestibular ataxia compose the four

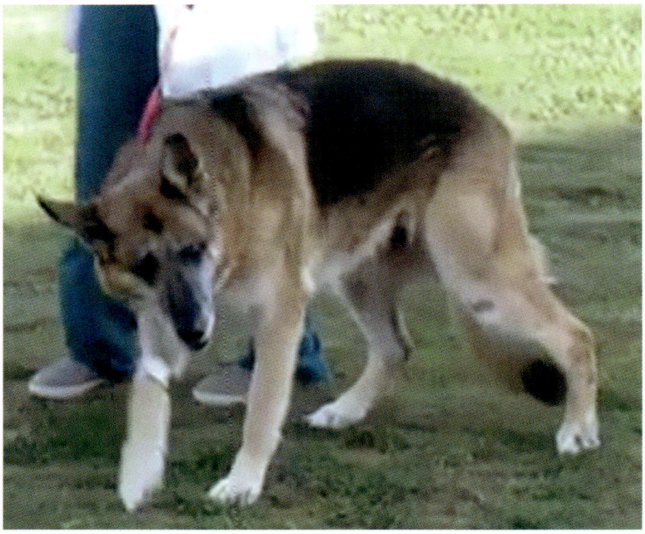

FIGURE 5.1.1 A German shepherd dog with a right-sided head tilt.

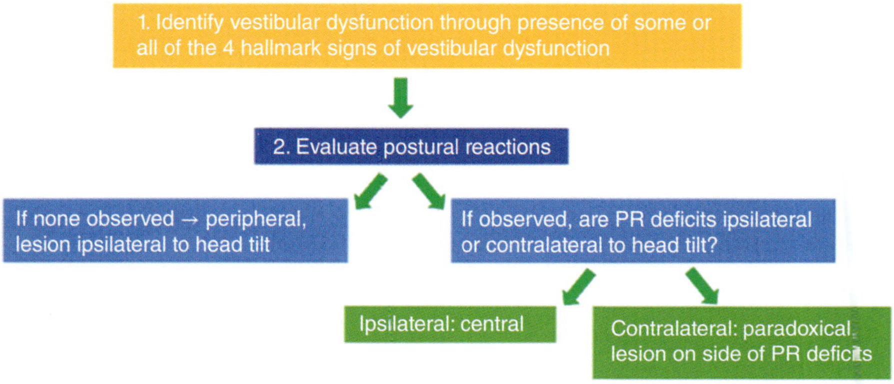

FIGURE 5.1.2 A schematic flowchart for vestibular dysfunction localization. PR = postural reactions.

hallmark signs of vestibular disease. A combination of any or all of these signs will be present in patients with a lesion in any region of the vestibular system. There are several features that make the right peripheral vestibular system (as opposed to a central or paradoxical localization) most likely in this case. Firstly, the dog had normal postural reactions. In central vestibular disease, postural reactions can become affected by lesions interfering with kinesthetic (proprioceptive) pathways traveling through the rostral medulla in the vicinity of the central vestibular system. Secondly, the dog had normal mentation. Lesions interfering with the reticular activating system in the rostral medulla will lead to decreased levels of mentation that are not seen with peripheral localizations. The nuclei for cranial nerves V–XII are also located in the pons (V) and medulla (VI–XII), in the region of the central vestibular system; therefore, clinical signs of dysfunction of these cranial nerves might have also been observed in a case with central vestibular disease.

CAUTION: The absence of signs typically attributed to central vestibular disease does not rule out a lesion affecting the central vestibular system. Up to 25% of dogs demonstrating exclusively signs of peripheral vestibular disease may ultimately be diagnosed with lesions affecting the central vestibular system (1).

The majority of the time, the above considerations will lead to the correct neuroanatomic localization.

In peripheral vestibular disease, the vestibular ataxia will lead to falling/circling toward the affected side. The head tilt is toward the affected side. The positional strabismus develops in the ipsilateral eye. Finally, the horizontal nystagmus fast phase is away from the side of the lesion. In this case, all signs point toward a right peripheral vestibular localization.

The vestibular system is responsible for maintaining balance and equilibrium. It is composed of the peripheral vestibular system, with sensory receptors located bilaterally in the inner ears (utricle, saccule, semicircular ducts) and the vestibulocochlear nerves (CN VIII), and the central vestibular system, composed of four vestibular nuclei located bilaterally in the rostral medulla. Unilateral vestibular system dysfunction will result in a loss of sensory input regarding balance and equilibrium, resulting in the following hallmark signs of vestibular dysfunction:

- *Vestibular ataxia:* The vestibular system is excitatory to ipsilateral limb extensor muscles. Loss of this excitation results in falling/circling toward the side of the lesion.
- *Head tilt:* The vestibular system is excitatory to ipsilateral neck muscles. Loss of excitation on the affected side relative to normal excitation on the contralateral, unaffected side, results in a head tilt toward the side of the lesion.
- *Positional strabismus:* The vestibular system allows for conjugate head and eye movements. Loss of vestibular input on the affected side results in loss of stimulation to conjugate eye movement with head movement. When the head is pointed toward the ceiling, the eye does not reflexively track toward the ceiling, resulting in a positional strabismus.
- *Spontaneous nystagmus:* Normally, physiological nystagmus occurs when the head moves due to the vestibular system providing for conjugate head and eye movements. This means that the fast phase of the physiological nystagmus is in the direction that the head is moving. Loss of vestibular input on the affected side relative to normal input on the unaffected side is interpreted as head movement in the direction of the unaffected side. This results in a spontaneous nystagmus with the fast phase *away from* the affected side.

DIFFERENTIAL DIAGNOSIS

Idiopathic Vestibular Disease

This is an extremely likely differential diagnosis for this patient, based on his age, the speed of onset of clinical signs, and lack of other clinical signs referable to a lesion in the region of the peripheral vestibular system (for example, no facial paresis or Horner syndrome, as may occur in a patient with structural abnormalities in the region of the middle/inner ear). This is a benign, self-limiting condition in dogs and cats. Although sometimes referred to as "old dog vestibular disease," or "geriatric vestibular disease" this can affect dogs of any age, although older dogs are more commonly affected. Cats of any age can be affected and tend to be affected more commonly in the fall/summer months. If evaluated within the first 24 hours of clinical signs, the degree of dysfunction may preclude a complete neurological examination, which should then be repeated 12–24 hours later. Generally, within about 3 days, the spontaneous nystagmus improves/resolves. Within 3 weeks, the ataxia resolves. The head tilt sometimes remains permanently. Although usually animals will have a singular event, repeated episodes are also possible.

Inflammatory – Otitis Media-interna

Infection of the inner ear leads to peripheral vestibular disease. Generally, a peracute onset is less likely with otitis media-interna, but possible. Extension of otitis externa, nasopharyngeal infections via the auditory tube, or hematogenous spread of bacteria can all lead to otitis media-interna. Generally, animals with peripheral vestibular disease secondary to otitis media-interna will also have facial nerve (CN VII) deficits, including decreased lip and ear tone, a palpebral reflex deficit, and Horner syndrome (ptosis, miosis, enophthalmos).

Toxicity – Ototoxicity

Many topical medications and some systemic medications are known ototoxins. Prior to using any potentially ototoxic topical ear medications, an otoscopic examination should be performed to ensure that the tympanic membrane is intact. Chlorhexidine-based ear medications and aminoglycoside-containing ear medications can both lead to ototoxicity, affecting both the vestibular and auditory systems. Systemic administration of aminoglycosides and some chemotherapeutics can also lead to bilateral ototoxicity. In animals that are showing peracute signs of unilateral peripheral vestibular disease, medication history should be obtained to screen for these ototoxins.

Metabolic – Hypothyroidism

Hypothyroidism is an uncommon cause of peripheral vestibular disease in dogs. Most cases have a more chronic onset than what was observed in this case, but it can rarely lead to acute peripheral vestibular disease. Hypothyroidism can lead to ischemic neuropathy of CN VIII, potentially from atherosclerosis or increased blood viscosity in the labyrinthine artery, which supplies CN VIII, but these possibilities remain unconfirmed (2). The presence of severe hypercholesterolemia and other clinical signs of hypothyroidism would support this differential.

Neoplasia

Neoplasms of the ear canal, including squamous cell carcinoma, ceruminous gland adenocarcinoma, carcinomas of undetermined origin, and benign masses can eventually reach the inner ear canal and lead to peripheral vestibular disease. Neoplasms can also originate from primary bone tumors off the tympanic and petrous portions of the temporal bone. Generally, neoplasms lead to a slow onset of clinical signs and CN VIII dysfunction as the sole deficit would be unlikely.

NEXT DIAGNOSTIC STEPS FOR THIS PATIENT

All dogs and cats with peripheral vestibular disease should have an otoscopic examination performed to screen for otitis externa, aural masses, and to evaluate the integrity of the tympanic membrane. A normal otoscopic examination does not rule out otitis media-interna, though. Although most systemic/metabolic diseases are unlikely to lead to peripheral vestibular disease, a minimum database to screen for hypothyroidism should be considered in dogs. Imaging of the head, either as a CT or MRI, is often required to confirm otitis media-interna or neoplasms outside the ear canal (Figures 5.1.3 and 5.1.4). Myringotomy can be performed to aspirate fluid from the middle ear for culture and sensitivity in cases of otitis media-interna. Dogs and cats with idiopathic peripheral vestibular disease will have unremarkable CTs or MRIs. In cases where idiopathic vestibular disease is strongly suspected, monitoring for improvement with exclusively supportive care is a very cost-effective alternative to performing imaging of the head, and other conditions would not resolve spontaneously and would worsen.

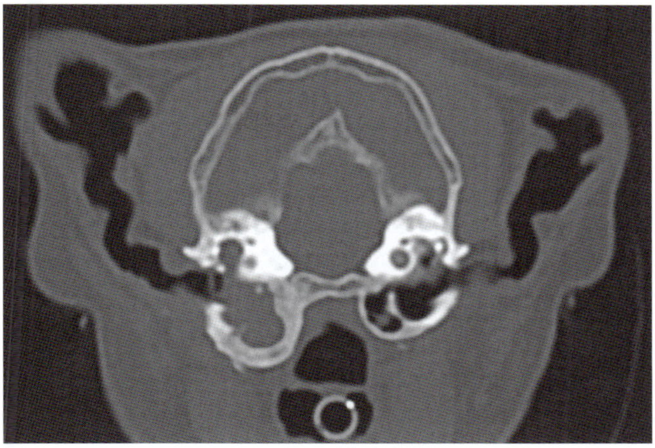

FIGURE 5.1.3 CT (transverse view) of the head of a cat with otitis media/interna in the right ear. Note that compared to the left side, the right tympanic bulla is thickened. The tympanic cavity has soft tissue attenuating material, consistent with effusion in the middle ear.

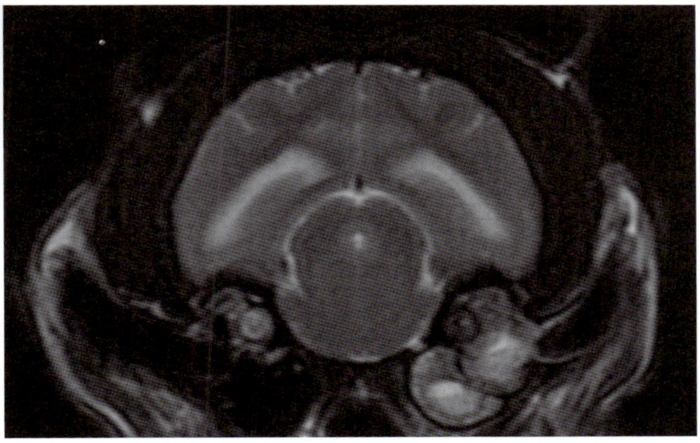

FIGURE 5.1.4 MRI (T2-weighted transverse view) of the head of a cat with otitis media/interna in the left ear. Note that compared to the right side, the left tympanic cavity is filled with hyperintense material, consistent with effusion in the middle ear. The left cochlea is also difficult to visualize and is hypointense compared to the right cochlea. The cochlea contains pure fluid (endolymph and perilymph), which is hyperintense. Hypointensity of the cochlea is consistent with disease of the inner ear.

TREATMENT AND PROGNOSIS

Idiopathic Vestibular Disease

There is no targeted therapy for this benign, self-limiting condition that is associated with an excellent prognosis. Dogs with idiopathic vestibular disease may experience mild to severe nausea and benefit from anti-nausea medication. During the recovery phase, food and water should be placed within reach and dogs should be kept in areas with excellent traction and lighting. Typically, the nystagmus resolves within several days, the ataxia resolves within several weeks, and the head tilt resolves or improves within several months. Clients should be cautioned that even after vestibular ataxia resolves, some dogs with idiopathic vestibular disease retain a head tilt, which most dogs accommodate well. Rarely, idiopathic vestibular disease can recur.

Otitis Media-interna

If myringotomy is performed and reveals a causative bacterial (or rarely, fungal) cause of otitis media-interna, then culture and susceptibility results should guide therapy. Dermatologists with access to video otoscopy can perform deep ear flushes in conjunction with myringotomies, which can remove debris should topical therapy be included in the treatment regimen. Systemic antimicrobials are necessary in the treatment of otitis media-interna. Prioritize antimicrobials with good bone penetration, if possible. Treatment minimally lasts for 4 weeks but is typically 8 weeks or longer. Some dermatologists also recommend a temporary tapering course of systemic corticosteroids to reduce associated inflammation. The starting dose should not exceed an immunosuppressive dose. Treatment success is variable. Some dogs experience complete recovery with medical management but may retain some neurological deficits. Others fail medical management and require surgical intervention with total ear canal ablation and bulla osteotomy (TECA-BO), performed by an experienced general surgeon. Occasionally, untreated or insufficiently treated otitis media-interna can lead to direct extension of the infection through the petrous temporal bone of the skull, resulting in otogenic meningitis or otogenic meningoencephalitis (intracranial abscess or empyema). Patients that experience this sequela may develop clinical signs of central vestibular disease or brainstem disease, but many do not develop signs overtly attributable to a lesion in the brainstem. In the few reports of this complication, its presence does not drastically change the prognosis for patients with otitis media-interna, but some dogs may require surgery to yield a favorable outcome (3–5).

Ototoxicity

There is no direct treatment for ototoxicity. Prompt discontinuation of the causative medication is necessary. The hearing loss that develops from ototoxicity is typically permanent, whereas the vestibular dysfunction tends to improve or resolve.

Hypothyroidism

With levothyroxine supplementation, improvement or resolution of vestibular dysfunction can occur after several weeks of treatment, and generally resolution is maintained with adequate regulation.

Neoplasia

Depending on the tumor type and location, surgical resection or radiation therapy may be investigated as definitive therapy options. Treatment responsiveness is dependent on tumor type, thus, prognosis is variable.

OUTCOME

Due to the acuity and nonprogressive nature of the dog's vestibular dysfunction, supportive care was elected since there was high clinical suspicion of a presumptive diagnosis of idiopathic vestibular disease. Three days after the onset of signs, the dog's nystagmus resolved, and after another 3 weeks, the ataxia had markedly improved. Throughout the course of the disease, the dog displayed a good appetite and did not require extensive support while walking. Six months after the onset of signs, the dog was reportedly normal.

SUGGESTED READING

Bongartz, U., Nessler, J., Maiolini, A. et al. (2020). Vestibular disease in dogs: association between neurological examination, MRI lesion localisation and outcome. *J. Small Anim. Pract.* 61 (1): 57–63.

Butterfield, S., Whittaker, D., Tabanez, J. et al. (2023). Bacterial meningitis secondary to otogenic infection in 10 French bulldogs: a retrospective case series. *Vet. Rec. Open* 10 (1): e263.

Dewey, C.W. and Da Costa, R.C. (2015). *Practical Guide to Canine and Feline Neurology*, 3e. Ames, Iowa: Wiley.

Moral, M., Blanco, C., and Lorenzo, V. (2025). Otogenic meningitis or meningoencephalitis in 30 dogs: association between neurological signs, magnetic resonance imaging findings, and outcome. *Vet. Sci.* 12 (5): 456.

Platt, S.R. and Olby, N.J. (2013). *Manual of Canine and Feline Neurology*, 4e. Quedgeley, Gloucester, UK: British Small Animal Veterinary Association.

Sturges, B.K., Dickinson, P.J., Kortz, G.D. et al. (2006). Clinical signs, magnetic resonance imaging features, and outcome after surgical and medical treatment of otogenic intracranial infection in 11 cats and 4 dogs. *J. Vet. Intern. Med.* 20 (3): 648–656.

Uemura, E.E. (2015). *Fundamentals of Canine Neuroanatomy and Neurophysiology*, 1e. Ames, Iowa: Wiley.

Vitale, C.L. and Olby, N.J. (2007). Neurologic dysfunction in hypothyroid, hyperlipidemic labrador retrievers. *J. Vet. Intern. Med.* 21 (6): 1316–1322.

CHAPTER 5.2

Head Tilt and Imbalance

Case 2—Head Tilt in a Cat

Jill Niederhuth

BluePearl, Des Moines, IA, USA

CASE HISTORY

A 5-year-old spayed female domestic short-haired cat was presented for a 1-week duration of a head tilt (Figure 5.2.1). The cat initially showed a subtle head tilt that had become more significant over the last week. The cat had a history of intermittent upper respiratory infections (URIs) and was evaluated for nasal discharge 5 days before the onset of neurological signs. During that visit, a topical medication was applied to both external ear canals because mild to moderate discharge was observed in both. The cat was reported to be indoors-only since adoption at approximately 12 weeks of age and was up to date on vaccinations but did not receive flea, tick, or heartworm preventatives. There have been no significant health concerns other than the URI history.

NEUROLOGIC AND PHYSICAL EXAMINATION (Video 5.2.1)

VIDEO 5.2.1 Video of a cat with right-sided head tilt. *Source:* Courtesy of Marc Kent.

The cat was bright, alert, and responsive on presentation. The cat had a moderate right-sided head tilt and a mildly wide-based stance with a tendency to stumble toward the right and circle intermittently toward the right. There was mild to moderate ataxia present in all four limbs without any change to the stride length. Postural reactions, including proprioceptive placing and hopping, were normal in all four limbs. Spinal reflexes were not performed, but muscle tone and weight-bearing posture were normal in all four limbs. A cranial nerve exam showed abnormalities, including a moderate positional strabismus in the right eye (OD) and induced nystagmus, when the head and neck were extended. The nystagmus was horizontal with the fast phase to the left. No pain could be elicited on palpation of the cervical or thoracolumbar vertebral column, but palpation of the skull in the region of the right tympanic bulla elicited a moderate reaction.

> ***Exam tip:** A positional strabismus is best identified when the head and neck are extended and the head tilt is corrected, returning the head to its normal orientation.

Key questions to consider

1. Where is the likely lesion localization?
2. What major disease processes should be considered?
3. What tests could you perform to help determine the diagnosis?

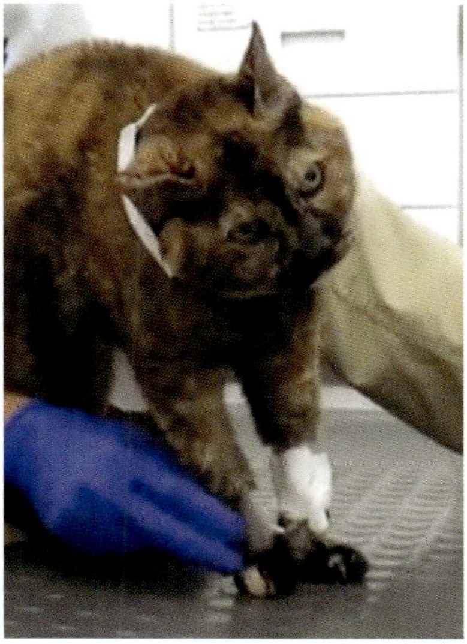

FIGURE 5.2.1 Cat with right-sided head tilt.

LESION LOCALIZATION

This patient is displaying the four hallmark signs of vestibular dysfunction: a head tilt, vestibular ataxia, positional strabismus, and spontaneous nystagmus (in this case, the nystagmus is inducible, which is a form of spontaneous nystagmus). Note that there are two abnormal head positions as they relate to neurological disease: a head tilt and a head turn. A head tilt, where a horizontal line drawn between the eyes is no longer parallel to the floor, is indicative of vestibular dysfunction. The goal of localization once vestibular dysfunction is identified is to determine whether the central vestibular system, primarily located in the brainstem and cerebellum, or the peripheral vestibular system, located within the inner ear, is affected.

Patients with peripheral vestibular disease may also demonstrate Horner syndrome and facial nerve dysfunction due to a lesion affecting the middle/inner ear (Figure 5.2.2). *Note, however, that*

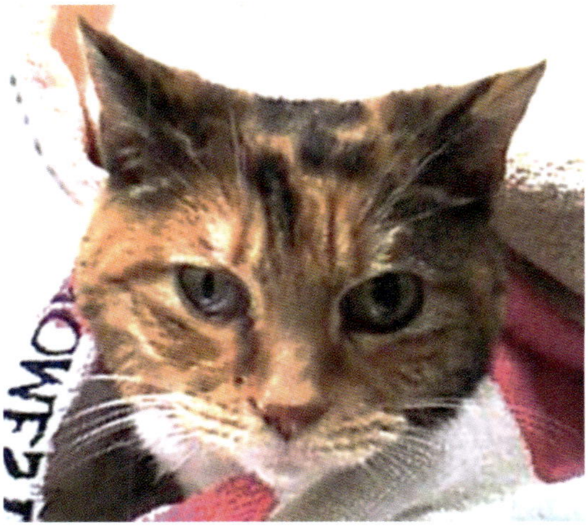

FIGURE 5.2.2 Right-sided Horner syndrome in a cat. Note the ptosis, miosis, and raised third eyelid secondary to enophthalmos. *Source:* Courtesy of Marc Kent.

facial nerve dysfunction (resulting in a decrease or loss of the palpebral reflex and drooping of the lip) can also occur in patients with central vestibular disease of the brainstem. Patients with peripheral vestibular disease have normal mentation and normal postural reactions.

Patients with central vestibular disease of the brainstem may demonstrate a diminished mental status (indicative of brainstem dysfunction in the presence of a head tilt), ipsilateral postural reaction deficits an elongated stride, and their nystagmus can be horizontal, rotary, or vertical.

Patients with central vestibular disease of the cerebellum ("paradoxical vestibular disease") may demonstrate hypermetria of the limbs contralateral to the head tilt, and subtle postural reaction deficits contralateral to the head tilt. More details regarding paradoxical vestibular disease can be found in Chapter 5, Case 3.

More details regarding localizing within the vestibular system are provided in Chapter 5, Case 1.

- Patients with central vestibular disease due to a brainstem lesion may also demonstrate other cranial nerve deficits. However, facial nerve paresis/paralysis, which results in a decrease or loss of the palpebral reflex and drooping of the lip, can also occur in patients with peripheral vestibular disease.
- Patients presenting with vestibular dysfunction, Horner syndrome, and facial nerve dysfunction together have an extremely high likelihood of localizing to the middle/inner ear.
- Sensory deficits to the face, the development of stridor, or evidence of dysphagia in the history would all be consistent with central vestibular disease affecting the caudal brainstem.

Note: Postural reaction deficits suggest a lesion in either the brainstem or the cerebellum. If they are ipsilateral to the head tilt, then the patient's vestibular dysfunction originates from the brainstem. If the postural reaction deficits are contralateral to the head tilt, then the patient's vestibular dysfunction originates from the cerebellum, on the side contralateral to the head tilt ("paradoxical vestibular disease"). The postural reaction deficits that occur with paradoxical vestibular disease are best observed by hopping the patient. Their ability to hop is delayed, then subsequently followed by an overcompensating hop (Chapter 5, Case 3).

This patient shows no clinical signs compatible with central vestibular disease, either in the brainstem or the cerebellum, and is therefore assumed to have peripheral vestibular disease. However, a small proportion of patients that localize to the peripheral vestibular system actually have central lesions confirmed with advanced imaging, so it remains important to consider differentials for central vestibular disease and closely monitor patients for progression to central vestibular signs.

DIFFERENTIAL DIAGNOSES

Inflammatory – Otitis Media/Interna

This is a very likely differential diagnosis in this cat. Otitis media/interna is the most common cause of peripheral vestibular disease in cats, and it is common that affected patients have histories of upper respiratory disease often without histories of otitis externa, which is a more common risk factor in dogs. Additionally, while the disease may present with acute or chronic presentations, it is commonly progressive. The most common organisms that lead to infection are *Pasteurella*, *Staphylococcus* sp., *Pseudomonas*, *Strep* sp., and *Escherichia coli* with multiple-organism infections possible.

Inflammatory – Nasopharyngeal Polyp

This is a reasonable differential diagnosis for a young adult cat with a history of URIs and the development of neurological signs localized to the middle/internal ear. Increased respiratory noise may occur due to the involvement of the nasopharynx depending on the size of the polyp, and it is common that cats have concurrent otitis media/interna. This cat would be at the upper end of the typical age range for presentation.

Toxicity – Ototoxicity

Ototoxicity is an unlikely diagnosis in this cat despite the history of topical medication placed into the ears. Typically, ototoxicity, once it occurs, will be static rather than progressive unless the toxic substance is continued. Ototoxicity could affect one or both ears and besides otitis media/interna is one of the rare causes of bilateral peripheral vestibular disease, which typically presents with wide head excursions and a loss of the physiological nystagmus. Deafness occurs in many patients with ototoxicity, though owners may also perceive that patients with other conditions such as otitis media/interna are acutely deaf. Ototoxicity is most common due to direct toxicity to the inner ear from topically applied medications. Many treatments for otitis externa are not approved for use when the tympanic membrane is perforated, and due to the anatomical challenges of evaluating this structure in dogs and cats with otitis media, accidental toxicity may occur. Single-use concentrated topical treatments may potentially be riskier; the author has treated a cat with bilateral peripheral vestibular disease and bilateral Horner syndrome caused by such a medication administered for otitis externa.

Neoplasia

This differential would be less common in a relatively young cat, but aural neoplasia is a reasonable differential for progressive peripheral vestibular disease in cats and to a lesser extent, dogs. In cats, aural neoplasia is frequently malignant, with adenocarcinoma, squamous cell carcinoma, and lymphoma being the most common forms. Dogs have a malignant disease in fewer cases. Neoplasia more commonly originates from the tissue of the pinna or the external ear canal than the middle/inner ear, but the latter is more likely to lead to neurological deficits.

Presentations of neoplasia can vary, with some patients appearing to have a relatively acute onset and others being more chronically affected. However, clinical signs for greater than 3–6 months are very uncommon with neoplasms that affect the nervous system.

Idiopathic Vestibular Disease

Idiopathic vestibular disease has been reported in cats. Similarly to that seen in dogs, cats have a peracute onset of peripheral vestibular signs that stabilize rapidly and then improve gradually over weeks or months for full improvement. However, this condition appears to happen in cats of any age, including the very young, in contrast to the presentation in dogs and may have a seasonal predilection, with most cases reported in the summer or fall in cats that go outdoors. A regional predisposition has also been reported in the Northeast or mid-Atlantic states, which may account for many practitioners rarely, if ever, encountering the condition.

INVESTIGATION

Otitis Media/Interna

This condition should be highly suspected in a patient with otitis externa, particularly chronically, or in one with a visibly ruptured tympanic membrane or purulent exudate from the ear on the affected side. Pain response when pressure is applied to the affected bulla or on wide opening of the mouth is also common in patients (and can help to differentiate between this and non-painful conditions such as ototoxicity or idiopathic vestibular disease). However, because many cats (and brachycephalic dogs) present without external ear signs, imaging of the bullae is recommended to help confirm disease.

- Skull radiographs and, potentially, ultrasound of the tympanic bullae can be performed by general practitioners, but it is necessary to become adept at acquiring the appropriate images and interpreting them, and the sensitivity may be low. General anesthesia or heavy sedation is needed to take appropriate skull radiographs, and having them evaluated by a radiologist is recommended, as thinning of the cortical bone of the bulla, which may not be apparent to many practitioners, is associated with neoplastic rather than infectious/inflammatory disease.
- Ultrasound can reportedly be performed without sedation or anesthesia in many patients.
- CT is more sensitive for disease of the tympanic bullae than radiographs and MRI provides the additional benefit of identifying the extension of otitis media/interna intracranially more readily than CT or identifying any other condition with reported imaging changes that can cause either peripheral or central vestibular disease in animals (Figure 5.2.3). CT can be performed with heavy sedation in some cases, while general anesthesia is typically required for MRI. Patients with otitis media/interna typically have fluid (or fluid/soft tissue signal on radiographs) visible within their tympanic cavity. Post-contrast imaging on CT or MRI can help distinguish patients with inflammation of the vestibular nerve or associated intracranial meningoencephalitis or abscess formation. It may also help to distinguish non-infectious causes, such as primary secretory otitis media, typically reported in certain small breeds of dog.
- In patients with suspected intracranial extension of otitis media/interna (Figure 5.2.4), CSF evaluation and culture can help to confirm this and may provide an organism diagnosis, which is helpful in treatment.

For patients where otitis media/interna is suspected but owners do not consent to additional testing, treatment with a rationally chosen antibiotic must sometimes be performed to help confirm the disease. Improvement is usually seen within 2 weeks of starting therapy and treatment

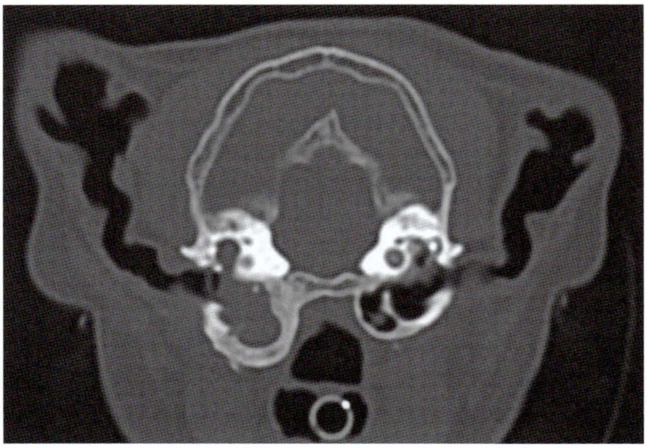

FIGURE 5.2.3 Computed tomography image of right-sided otitis media (and presumably interna) in a cat with right-sided facial paresis, vestibular dysfunction, and Horner syndrome. Note the thickened bone of the tympanic bulla, and soft tissue hyperdensity in the tympanic bulla. In health, this cavity is occupied by air, which is hypodense on CT as is apparent in the unaffected left tympanic bulla in this cat.

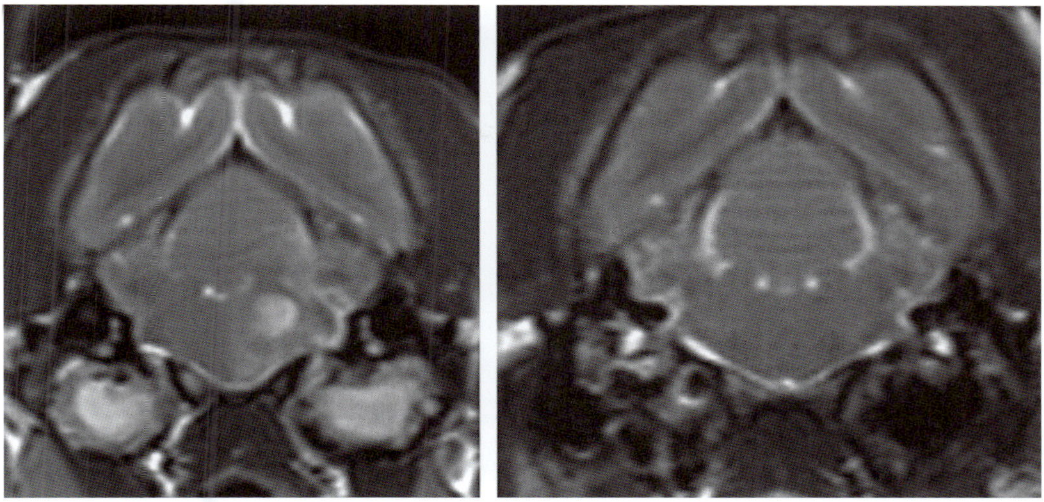

FIGURE 5.2.4 Magnetic resonance images of a cat with bilateral otitis media interna. At the time of diagnosis, T2-weighted hyperintense material was observed in both tympanic cavities, along with direct extension of the presumptive infection through the petrous temporal bone of the left side of the skull. This led to an intracranial abscess at the level of the cerebellum (left image). To treat the cat's bilateral otitis media-interna and otogenic meningoencephalitis, a left ventral bulla osteotomy was performed and the cat was treated with marbofloxacin orally. Six weeks later, a right ventral bulla osteotomy was performed. An MRI was performed 6 weeks after the second surgery, showing complete resolution of otitis media interna in both ears, as well as of the intracranial abscess (right image).

must be continued for 6–8 weeks in many cases to reduce the risk of recurrence. Caution must be used in concurrently starting steroid therapy as this will often benefit any disease with an inflammatory component, including neoplasia.

Nasopharyngeal Polyp

Otoscopic exam may reveal a smooth mass consistent with a polyp. Otherwise, sedated/anesthetized oral exam including a probe exam into the nasopharynx behind the soft palate will often identify a polyp. Occasionally, endoscopy is needed. CT or MRI are both typically able to identify nasopharyngeal polyps, though skull radiographs have also been reported to suggest the diagnosis but require knowledgeable interpretation (Figure 5.2.5). Polyps are not palpable in the soft tissues around the ear/skull and should not extrude from the nasal passages.

Ototoxicity

Ototoxicity can be a challenging diagnosis in some cases, particularly in patients where a potentially toxic cleaner/medication has been applied continually to the ear as clinical signs developed/worsened or in cases where the potential toxin is rarely reported to actually cause ototoxicity (i.e., furosemide). Associated facial nerve dysfunction and Horner syndrome are not likely with ototoxicity, but concurrent deafness is common, which may help to differentiate this condition from otitis media/interna in some cases. If BAER testing (brainstem auditory evoked response) is available, sensorineural deafness can be diagnosed, different from conductive hearing loss associated with severe otitis media. Otherwise, options include discontinuing the potential toxin and monitoring for improvement over several weeks or using diagnostic testing to rule out any other cause of clinical signs that would require a directed therapy.

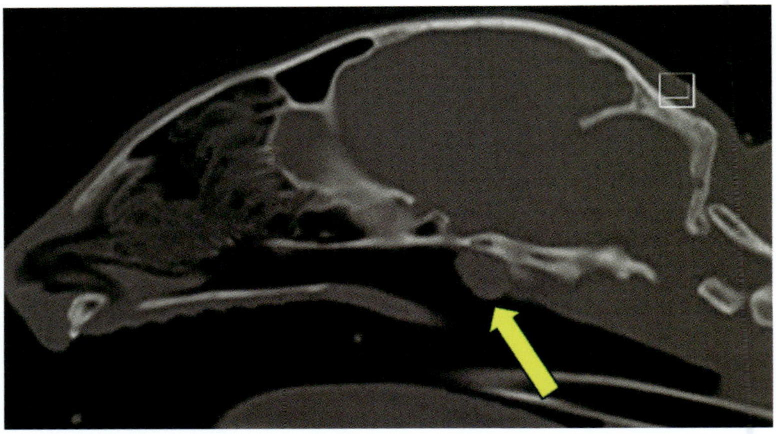

FIGURE 5.2.5 Sagittal CT image of a nasopharyngeal polyp (yellow arrow) in a cat.

Neoplasia

Aural neoplasia can frequently be suspected from otoscopic examination with masses usually appearing papillomatous and irregular. Additionally, if the skull, bulla and submandibular regions are carefully palpated, it is common to feel asymmetry of these structures between the affected and unaffected sides. As with otitis media/interna, skull radiographs, ultrasound, CT, and MRI may all be able to help diagnose aural neoplasia. Frequently, aural neoplasia will extend to an area that is accessible for fine-needle aspirate or biopsy such as the external ear canal or the soft tissues around the bulla. Ultimately, if advanced therapies such as aggressive surgical resection or radiation therapy are being considered, CT and/or MRI will be needed to guide prognosis and recommendations.

Idiopathic Vestibular Disease

This condition is a diagnosis of exclusion but can be suspected in patients that present peracutely and particularly that have already started to improve on their own with only supportive care or that begin to improve shortly after presentation, typically within 1–3 days. Remembering that this condition cannot be diagnosed in patients that show any intracranial signs (such as postural reaction deficits or paresis) is important to differentiate this from stroke in older patients or *Cuterebra* migration in outdoor cats. Additionally, while minimal progression may be possible within the first 24 hours, signs should quickly stabilize and then begin to improve. Imaging findings should be unremarkable; however, neuritis of the vestibulocochlear nerve may be suspected if there is contrast enhancement on MRI or CT, without significant thickening of the nerve.

OUTCOME

A CT of the head confirmed otitis media-interna. No nasopharyngeal polyp was observed. A myringotomy was performed but no bacterial or fungal growth was observed. The cat was started on marbofloxacin and subsequently underwent a right-sided ventral bulla osteotomy. Six weeks after surgery, marbofloxacin was discontinued. The cat made a complete recovery.

SUGGESTED READING

Benigni, L. and Lamb, C. (2006). Diagnostic imaging of ear disease in the dog and cat. *In Pract.* 28 (3): 122–130. https://doi.org/10.1136/inpract.28.3.122.

Bischoff, M.G. and Kneller, S.K. (2004). Diagnostic imaging of the canine and feline ear. *Vet. Clin. North Am. Small Anim. Pract.* 34 (2): 437–458. https://doi.org/10.1016/j cvsm.2003.10.013. PMID: 15062618.

Bongartz, U., Nessler, J., Maiolini, A. et al. (2020). Vestibular disease in dogs: association between neurological examination, MRI lesion localisation and outcome. *J. Small Anim. Pract.* 61: 57–63. https://doi.org/10.1111/jsap.13070.

Classen, J., Bruehschwein, A., Meyer-Lindenberg, A., and Mueller, R.S. (2016). Comparison of ultrasound imaging and video otoscopy with cross-sectional imaging for the diagnosis of canine otitis media. *Vet. J.* 217: 68–71. ISSN 1090-0233, https://doi.org/10.1016/j.tvjl.2016.09.010.

Deleporte S, Briand A, Prelaud P. Clinical outcome of cats with suppurative otitis media and intact tympanum submitted to myringotomy: retrospective findings from 26 cases. *J. Feline Med. Surg.* 2024;26(9), 1098612X241275286. https://doi.org/10.1177/1098612X241275286.

Kirpensteijn, J. (2006). Treatment of aural neoplasia in the dog and cat. *PROC NAVC*, 793–796.

Matz, B.M. and Bellah, J.R. (2023). Aural neoplasia. In: *Small Animal Soft Tissue Surgery* (ed. E. Monnet), 838–845. Wiley https://doi.org/10.1002/9781119693741.ch71.

Milne E, Nuttall T, Marioni-Henry K, et al. Cytological and microbiological characteristics of middle ear effusions in brachycephalic dogs. *J. Vet. Intern. Med.* 2020; 34: 1454–1463. https://doi.org/10.1111/jvim.15792.

Moore, S.A., Bentley, R.T., Carrera-Justiz, S. et al. (2019). Clinical features and short-term outcome of presumptive intracranial complications associated with otitis media/interna: a multi-center retrospective study of 19 cats (2009–2017). *J. Feline Med. Surg.* 21 (2): 148–155. https://doi.org/10.1177/1098612X18764582.

Muilenburg, R.K. et al. (2002). Feline nasopharyngeal polyps. *Vet. Clin. Small Anim. Pract.* 32 (4): 839–849E.

Rossmeisl, J.H. (2010). Vestibular disease in dogs and cats. *Vet. Clin. Small Anim. Pract.* 40 (1): 81–100.

CHAPTER 5.3

Head Tilt and Imbalance

Case 3—Head Tilt and Weakness in a Dog

Jill Niederhuth

BluePearl, Des Moines, IA, USA

CASE HISTORY

A 7-year-old neutered male basset hound was presented for an acute onset of balance dysfunction. The dog was reportedly clinically normal during the day and had just returned from outside when he vomited and began to fall to one side. The dog has a history of mitral valve disease without any history of heart failure. He was on flea/tick/heartworm preventatives and up to date on vaccinations. He had no history of previous neurological concerns. He had a history of antibiotic-responsive diarrhea and had been receiving oral metronidazole 13 mg/kg q12h long-term.

NEUROLOGICAL EXAM (Video 5.3.1)

VIDEO 5.3.1 Video of a 7-year-old basset hound with a head tilt and vestibular ataxia.

The dog appeared to be anxious but otherwise alert and responsive. He had a mild right-sided head tilt and moderate vestibular ataxia with a tendency to stumble and lean towards the right and a moderate base-wide stance. Additionally, there was moderate hypermetria of the left thoracic limb and pelvic limb characterized by a hyperflexion of the limb joints, leading to an exaggerated limb movement. Proprioceptive placement tests were normal in the right limbs, but moderately delayed in the left limbs. Hopping was normal in the right limbs, and delayed and subsequently exaggerated in the left limbs. Spinal reflexes were not performed but there was normal muscle tone and weight-bearing posture of the limbs. Cranial nerve exam showed a slow resting rotary nystagmus with a fast phase to the left. A moderate positional strabismus was present in the right eye (OD). The remainder of the cranial nerve exam was normal. There was no apparent pain on palpation of the vertebral column or range of motion of the cervical vertebral column.

1. **Where is the likely lesion localization?**
2. **What major disease processes should be considered?**
3. **What tests could you perform to help determine the diagnosis?**

LESION LOCALIZATION

This dog presents with right-sided vestibular dysfunction based on the right-sided head tilt. However, the left-sided hypermetria is suggestive of cerebellar dysfunction as are the proprioceptive abnormalities. Because the cerebellum affects the body ipsilaterally, the left-sided hypermetria supports a left-sided cerebellar dysfunction. While a multifocal localization is possible, the combination of signs in this patient can be attributed to a single lesion affecting the cerebellum.

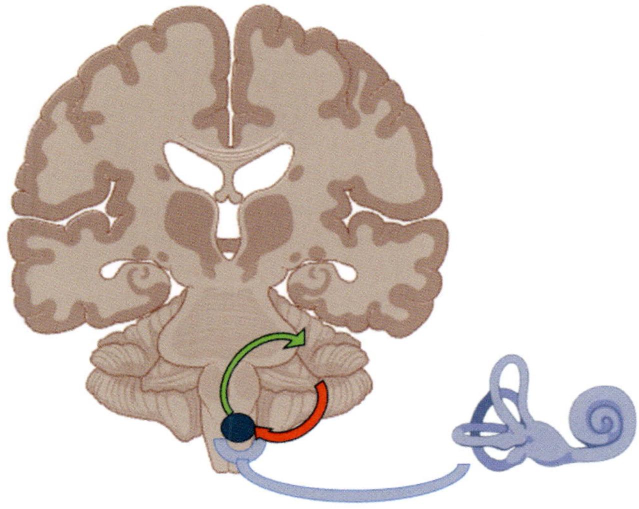

FIGURE 5.3.1 Illustration of the components of the vestibular system. The peripheral vestibular system is comprised of the semicircular ducts and the utricle and saccule, which are the receptors within the inner ear, and the vestibular branch of the vestibulocochlear nerve. This nerve carries special sensory fibers to the vestibular nuclei. The vestibular nuclei (represented by the blue circle in the medulla oblongata) are in constant cross-talk with the ipsilateral cerebellum. Excitatory impulses travel from the vestibular nuclei (green arrow) to the cerebellum, inhibitory impulses travel from the cerebellum (red arrow) to the vestibular nuclei. These inhibitory impulses result in decreased activity of the vestibular nuclei during normal vestibular function. Source: Created with www.biorender.com.

An essential aspect of the vestibular system is that it is a functional system that attempts to maintain balance by altering the amount of excitatory and inhibitory input from each side. While most of the anatomical structures in the peripheral and central vestibular system provide excitatory input, the cerebellum provides inhibitory input (Figure 5.3.1). Ultimately, the side of the vestibular system that has less "function" (i.e., less excitatory input) will be the side that appears dysfunctional. When there is a lesion to the anatomical area of the cerebellum that provides inhibition to the vestibular system, this results in an ipsilateral increase in total excitatory input. This leads to "paradoxical" vestibular signs where the side of the vestibular system *that is normal and without a lesion present* appears dysfunctional. In the case of this patient, it is more likely that this dog is demonstrating signs of right-sided paradoxical vestibular dysfunction from a left-sided cerebellar lesion than a multifocal localization. Note that this is a "central vestibular" localization and warrants significantly different differentials than a peripheral vestibular localization. Additionally, it is important to remember that while a vertical nystagmus is associated with central vestibular disease, it is very common for a pathological nystagmus in patients with central vestibular disease to be horizontal or rotary in direction. Finally, it is the author's experience that there is often a "mismatch" between the severity of the head tilt and the severity of ataxia in patients with central vestibular disease, with the head tilt being milder than it would be in a dog with peripheral vestibular disease displaying a similar level of ataxia. It should be noted, however, that there is no statistically significant difference in the degree of head tilt.

DIFFERENTIAL DIAGNOSIS

Vascular – Cerebrovascular Accident

This is a likely differential diagnosis for this patient given the very sudden onset of signs and the significant asymmetry. These events occur either when a blood clot is formed and then embolizes, causing sudden blockage of a blood vessel (ischemic stroke) or when a blood vessel ruptures and hemorrhage occurs into the brain tissue (hemorrhagic stroke). About 80% of strokes are ischemic, and hemorrhagic stroke has not been reported regularly affecting the cerebellum of dogs or cats. Strokes of the rostral cerebellar artery are particularly common in dogs and affect the region of the cerebellum that result in the development of paradoxical vestibular signs (Figure 5.3.2). Diseases that lead to hypercoagulability or vascular changes are most likely to be diagnosed as suspected predisposing conditions. In dogs, hypertension, hyperadrenocorticism, kidney disease, protein-losing disease (nephropathy, enteropathy), and hypothyroidism are the most diagnosed predisposing conditions. In cats, liver disease, hypertension, kidney disease, cardiomyopathy, pulmonary disease and hyperthyroidism (likely due to cardiomyopathy and hypertension) are documented associated diseases, but paradoxical vestibular disease has not been reported in cats. Ultimately, many patients have no apparent predisposing condition and those in this category appear to be much less likely to have repeated events. While this dog is reported to have heart disease, valvular disease is not known to be a risk factor for stroke, unlike cardiomyopathy.

Neoplasia

Solid brain tumors are common in middle-aged to older dogs and occasionally present relatively acutely. However, a peracute onset of clinical signs is very rare unless hemorrhage associated with the tumor occurs or brain herniation has occurred rapidly and without obvious pre-existing signs of increased intracranial pressure. Neoplasms that occur in this region most commonly include meningiomas, choroid plexus tumors, gliomas, nerve sheath tumors, and medulloblastomas (typically in young patients). Lymphoma, which can form either a mass or have many alternative appearances, can progress very rapidly, but still should not have such a rapid onset of clinical signs.

Trauma

While there is no history of trauma in this patient, damage to the caudal cerebellum is certainly possible with traumatic injury. In smaller breed dogs, this is commonly an "over back" injury where the back of the skull is hit on a hard object, often concrete when the dog flips over backwards during some activity. Traumatic injury has a similar clinical progression to cerebrovascular accident with a peracute onset of signs, rapid stabilization in most cases, and then gradual improvement. With trauma, the secondary injury cascade that develops in the 24-48 hours following the primary injury can lead to progressive or acute deterioration. See Chapter 15, Case 1.

Inflammatory Disease (Infectious)

Infectious encephalitis is uncommon in dogs. Causes include suspected extension of otitis media/interna, recent bite wounds around the head/neck and certain raw diets or eating of dead animals that could predispose to bacterial or protozoal infections. *Neospora caninum*, a protozoal organism that can infect multiple areas of the nervous system in dogs, may have some preference for cerebellar infection, though other reports indicate that the pattern of intracranial infection varies significantly between dogs.

Inflammatory Disease (Noninfectious)

Much more frequently than infectious encephalitis, dogs are diagnosed with inflammatory disease that appears to be immune-mediated. *This disease, often referred to as "meningoencephalitis of unknown etiology" or "MUE," (or unknown origin; MUO), is so common in dogs that it should be on the differential list for virtually all presentations of intracranial disease in adult dogs.* While younger,

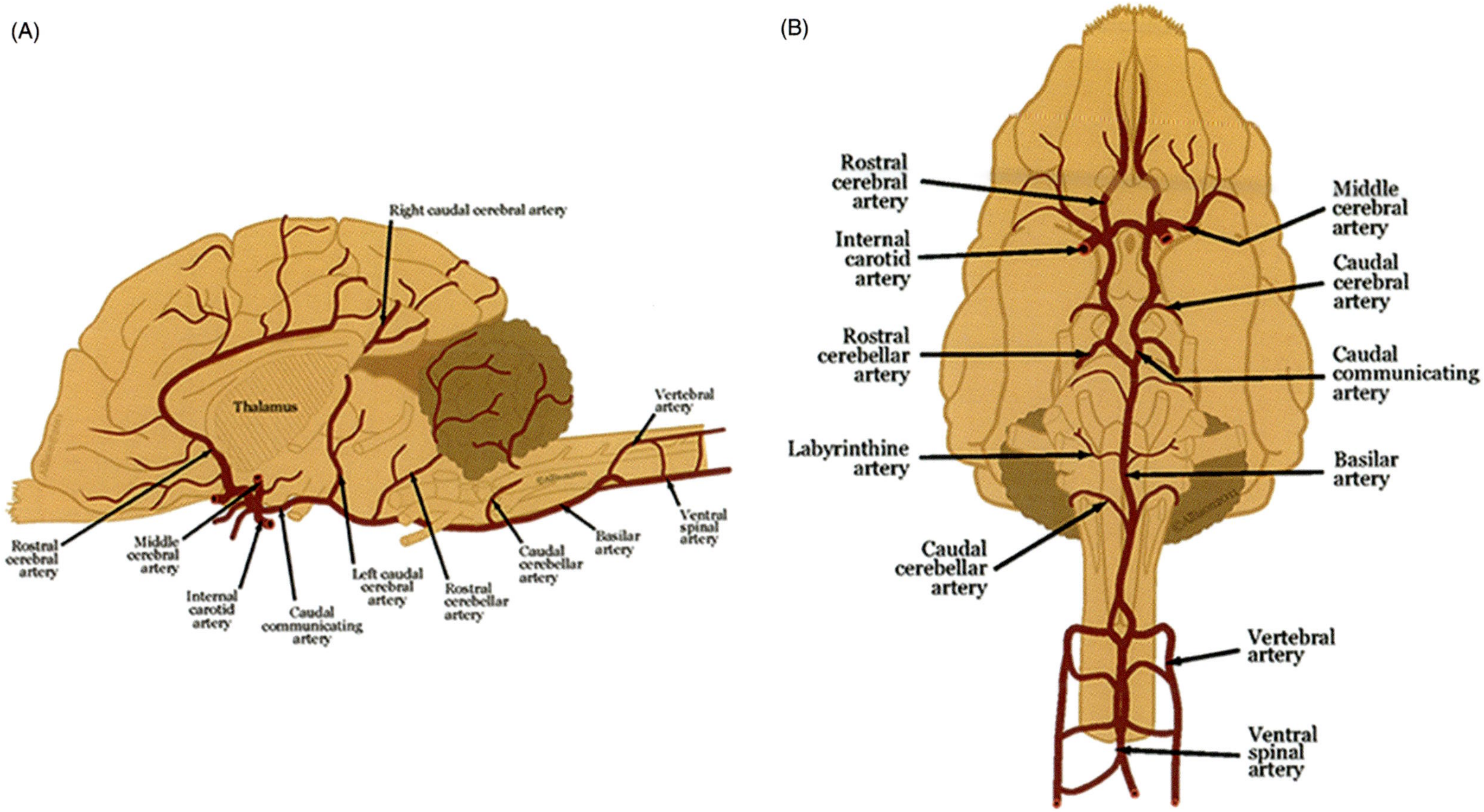

FIGURE 5.3.2 Illustration of the arterial supply of the canine brain (left: lateral view; right: ventral view). The rostral cerebellar artery supplies the region of the cerebellum involved in vestibular system regulation. A stroke affecting this artery is thus responsible for paradoxical vestibular dysfunction. These illustrations were created by Allison L. Wright MS CMI, Athens, Georgia, USA, and are reproduced with permission from the BSAVA Manual of Canine and Feline Neurology fourth edition.

small-breed dogs present more commonly, the author has diagnosed and treated this condition in a wide range of dogs, including very senior and many large breeds. In this dog, this differential should be prioritized lower due to the peracute onset of signs. However, many owners do not recognize that certain other signs seen at home in the days to weeks prior to apparent onset may have indicated a progressive issue, demonstrating the importance of careful assessment of history. Owners will regularly present a patient for an "acute" onset of signs only to indicate when questioned that subtle gait changes, lethargy/mentation changes, or mild balance dysfunction preceded the more severe signs.

Toxicity – Metronidazole

While this patient is receiving metronidazole, this is an unlikely differential given the asymmetry of signs and postural reaction deficits. Metronidazole toxicity does cause mild asymmetry of signs often with a head tilt noted in dogs that present with vestibular or vestibulocerebellar signs. Along with the obvious inconsistencies of the exam with neurotoxicity, it is also more common for dogs or cats to develop signs of metronidazole toxicity when they have received very high doses, often at least 60 mg/kg/day. However, toxicity has been reported as low as 26 mg/kg/day with short courses and even lower doses may lead to toxicity with chronic dosing.

Degenerative – Storage Disease

Cerebellar disease can result due to degenerative changes that occur, often from genetic diseases that lead to a lack of normal metabolism in cells of the body (storage diseases, often lysosomal but sometimes cytoplasmic). While most diseases of this type affect dogs and cats at a very young age, there are conditions affecting the cerebellum that are defined as "late onset," often beginning when dogs are at least several years old. However, the most common of these, neuronal ceroid lipofuscinosis (NCL), affects primarily American Staffordshire terriers or other "bully" mixes and would not be expected in a Basset hound. It would also be extremely uncommon for an owner to report an acute onset of signs, though an owner may notice the onset of mild signs "acutely" before a gradual progression becomes apparent. Lateralization, as observed in this patient, is unlikely with a diffuse condition affecting the cerebellum. Dogs with these conditions primarily demonstrate cerebellar ataxia and significant vestibular signs are uncommon.

INVESTIGATION

Cerebrovascular Accident

There can be a high rate of clinical suspicion for stroke in a dog or cat that is middle-aged or older with a peracute onset of focal, asymmetric intracranial signs. Patients with risk factors for diseases that lead to hypercoagulability or vascular remodeling, as discussed above, provide additional reason for suspicion. Blood pressure should be performed and considered in any patient with an acute onset of intracranial signs. There is no definitive level of hypertension that is clearly associated with a risk for stroke, but due to patient stress in-hospital, the author typically assumes that significant hypertension when patients are at home is only likely in those with a systolic blood pressure of >180 mmHg in-hospital. Multiple readings should be taken with a goal to reduce apparent patient stress during or between readings when trying to confirm true hypertension. Oscillometric readings may be better tolerated in some patients since the paws are not handled, and appropriate cuff size selection is important, especially considering reduced accuracy with indirect blood pressure readings in veterinary patients. It is very important to avoid treating with anti-hypertensive medications in patients that are concerning for signs of increased intracranial pressure or have evidence of progressive intracranial disease, as hypertension can be a compensatory mechanism to maintain cerebral blood flow in such patients. In cases where it is difficult to determine what the most appropriate approach may be, administration of a single dose of mannitol (0.5 g/kg IV over 15 minutes) or hypertonic saline (4 mL/kg over 10 minutes in dogs) is likely to be safe and may reduce systolic blood pressure after 30–90 minutes in patients with increased intracranial pressure.

Ultimately, diagnosis of an ischemic stroke usually requires MRI since vascular studies of the brain are not readily available even to veterinary neurologists. MRI is capable of diagnosing lesions consistent with ischemic stroke, disclosing a focal, often well-defined region of T2-weighted hyperintensity confined to a region occupied by the involved artery. Such lesions lack significant contrast enhancement. Diffusion-weighted imaging (DWI) is an MRI technique used to assess the flow of water through tissues. Ischemic tissue displays "restricted diffusion," which creates a classic pattern observed on two comparative images (Figure 5.3.3). CT or MRI can identify significant hemorrhage in patients with hemorrhagic stroke, but this condition needs to be differentiated from hemorrhagic neoplasms, such as metastatic hemangiosarcoma, which is much more challenging with contrast CT than post-contrast MRI sequences. Cerebrospinal fluid (CSF) analysis can be performed but may have variable results, including either inflammatory or noninflammatory changes, often with an increase in protein content. In cases in which MRI is not possible, this condition can be assumed in patients that present with peracute, asymmetric intracranial signs and improve with only supportive care. It is important not to start corticosteroids in these patients, as that eliminates the ability to interpret improvement and will not affect clinical outcome for ischemic stroke. In dogs with confirmed or highly suspected stroke, evaluation for any contributing underlying condition should be performed, including CBC/Chemistry, urinalysis ± urine protein:creatinine ratio, thyroid testing and blood pressure evaluation. Any underlying disease must be treated to reduce the risk of recurrent stroke, and if the risk cannot be entirely resolved, anti-clotting medication such as clopidogrel is often used as part of long-term management.

Neoplasia

Neoplasms that are present in the hindbrain (caudotentorial or infratentorial location) can frequently be diagnosed with cross-sectional imaging. MRI is the preferred modality, though contrast CT can usually identify meningiomas, nerve sheath tumors and choroid plexus tumors due to their strong contrast enhancement. CSF analysis is occasionally beneficial in helping to differentiate

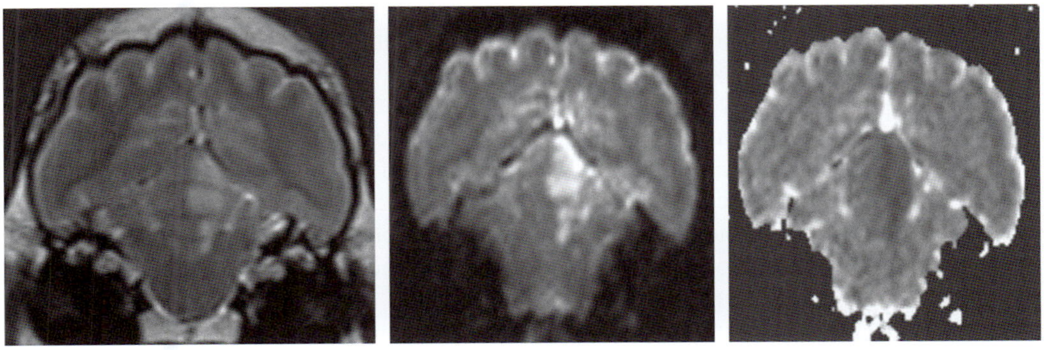

FIGURE 5.3.3 MRI of a dog with a left-sided rostral cerebellar artery territorial stroke. Note the sharply marginated region of T2-weighted hyperintensity in the left cerebellum (left image). Restricted diffusion is confirmed in this lesion by simultaneous evaluation of the middle and right images, which comprise diffusion-weighted imaging. The affected area is hyperintense on the trace image (middle) and hypointense on the apparent diffusion coefficient (ADC) map. This pattern is consistent with restricted movement of water molecules, since they are trapped intracellularly as cytotoxic edema.

malignant versus benign choroid plexus tumors, diagnosing lymphoma or helping to confirm that questionable neoplasms do not represent inflammatory/infectious granulomas instead, as most CSF samples in cases of neoplasia have no to minimal inflammatory change. Occasionally, external neoplasms, often involving the middle/internal ear, may also cause intracranial signs due to central extension. Diagnosis of these may be possible with cytology or biopsy if the mass can be adequately palpated or ultrasound guidance is possible. Ultimately, advanced imaging is still necessary in those cases to judge the extent of disease and guide realistic treatment options.

Trauma

Skull radiographs may occasionally be useful for diagnosing skull fractures, but these are challenging to obtain and interpret in many cases and tend to require general anesthesia in dogs with vestibular signs to position appropriately. CT is very sensitive for skull fracture, but may not be able to determine if trauma to the brain has occurred without evidence of fracture unless there is at least moderate hemorrhage present. MRI is very sensitive for trauma due to edema present in the brain tissue but is likely less sensitive for skull fracture than CT in most cases. Ultimately, it is rare to need surgical treatment in most cases of traumatic brain injury, so the presence of nondisplaced skull fracture is not of significant clinical importance in small animals and a displaced fracture should be visible on either CT or MRI. Many patients with known trauma are not subjected to advanced imaging if they are not declining neurologically or failing to improve somewhat within 1–2 days of onset of signs.

Infectious and Noninfectious Inflammatory Conditions

In patients where this is strongly suspected, MRI and CSF analysis should be performed promptly, prior to starting steroid therapy, if possible. If those tests are not available, contrast CT may be useful in evaluating for other diseases that can cause similar clinical signs such as a brain tumor and spinal fluid testing will usually indicate if inflammation is present. Infectious disease testing can be performed via titers for the most common conditions in the region where disease is occurring. For most dogs these would include testing for *Toxoplasma, Neospora,* and *Cryptococcus*. Other conditions can also be screened based on specific risk factors or concurrent bloodwork changes. It is much more challenging to diagnose most viral diseases of the nervous system in dogs and cats, including distemper and feline coronavirus without CSF, and rabies is only diagnosed post-mortem. Bacterial encephalitis can be suspected if CSF is available and shows neutrophilic inflammation, but a CSF culture positive for a specific bacterium is needed for a more definitive diagnosis. Bacterial encephalitis may have evidence of the area of extension of infection on advanced imaging (i.e., infection spread intracranially from otitis media/interna is particularly common). In cases where progressive intracranial signs are most concerning for an immune-mediated meningoencephalitis, but owners are unable to pursue advanced diagnostics, performing titers to rule out common infectious diseases is still recommended followed by immunosuppressive therapy. A positive response to treatment for >6 months would allow the reasonable assumption of a correct diagnosis of immune-mediated meningoencephalitis (referred to elsewhere as MUE or MUO).

Metronidazole Toxicity

Ultimately, if signs in this patient were less lateralized, discontinuing the medication ± treating with diazepam, which rapidly expedites recovery from metronidazole toxicity, would be the only likely way to "diagnose" the toxicity. Unless toxicity were extremely likely in a patient, it is strongly recommended to evaluate for other causes rather than making this assumption since certain intracranial diseases warrant urgent therapy to prevent death.

Storage Disease

Some storage diseases now have specific genetic tests, including NCL that leads to late-onset cerebellar dysfunction. When genetic testing is not available, but a neurodegenerative disease is suspected, metabolic panels performed on urine for inappropriate metabolite levels can help to diagnose a cause of clinical signs. MRI, if performed, is often normal or shows nonspecific parenchymal changes, but certain conditions may have more specific imaging changes. Typically, these degenerative diseases do not cause substantial MRI changes other than evidence of parenchymal atrophy, and CSF analysis is normal.

OUTCOME

Given the peracuity of the clinical signs, a stroke was prioritized as the top differential diagnosis. The owners declined diagnostic testing in favor of monitoring. Over a period of 2 weeks, the dog showed progressive improvement and was reportedly normal 3 months later. No additional episodes of dysfunction occurred for the remainder of the dog's life.

SUGGESTED READING

Altay, U.M., Skerritt, G.C., Hilbe, M. et al. (2011). Feline cerebrovascular disease: clinical and histopathologic findings in 16 cats. *J. Am. Anim. Hosp. Assoc.* 47 (2): 89–97. https://doi.org/10.5326/JAAHA-MS-5480.

Arnold, S.A., Platt, S.R., Gendron, K.P., and West, F.D (2020). Imaging ischemic and hemorrhagic disease of the brain in dogs. *Front. Vet. Sci.* 7: https://www.frontiersin.org/journals/veterinary-science/articles/10.3389/fvets.2020.00279. https://doi.org/10.3389/fvets.2020.00279.

Bosiack, A.P., Mann, F.A., Dodam, J.R. et al. (2010). Comparison of ultrasonic Doppler flow monitor, oscillometric, and direct arterial blood pressure measurements in ill dogs. *J. Vet. Emerg. Crit. Care* 20: 207–215. https://doi.org/10.1111/j.1476-4431.2010.00520.x.

Butterfield, S., Whittaker, D., Tabanez, J. et al. (2023). Bacterial meningitis secondary to otogenic infection in 10 French bulldogs: a retrospective case series. *Vet. Rec. Open* 10: e263. https://doi.org/10.1002/vro2.63.

Evans, J., Katz, M.L., Levesque, D. et al. (2005). A variant form of neuronal ceroid lipofuscinosis in American bulldogs. *J. Vet. Intern. Med.* 19: 44–51. https://doi.org/10.1111/j.1939-1676.2005.tb02657.x.

Evans, J., Levesque, D., Knowles, K. et al. (2003). Diazepam as a treatment for metronidazole toxicosis in dogs: a retrospective study of 21 cases. *J. Vet. Intern. Med.* 17: 304–310. https://doi.org/10.1111/j.1939-1676.2003.tb02452.x.

Garosi, L., McConnell, J.F., Platt, S.R. et al. (2005). Results of diagnostic investigations and long-term outcome of 33 dogs with brain infarction (2000–2004). *J. Vet. Intern. Med.* 19: 725–731. https://doi.org/10.1111/j.1939-1676.2005.tb02752.x.

Moore, S.A., Bentley, R.T., Carrera-Justiz, S. et al. (2019). Clinical features and short-term outcome of presumptive intracranial complications associated with otitis media/interna: a multi-center retrospective study of 19 cats (2009–2017). *J. Feline Med. Surg.* 21 (2): 148–155. https://doi.org/10.1177/1098612X18764582.

Phillipps, S., DeDecker, S., Gutierrez-Quintana, R. et al. (2022). Idiopathic generalised tremor syndrome in dogs. *Vet. Rec.* 191: e1734. https://doi.org/10.1002/vetr.1734.

Sande, A. and West, C. (2010). Traumatic brain injury: a review of pathophysiology and management. *J. Vet. Emerg. Crit. Care* 20: 177–190. https://doi.org/10.1111/j.1476-4431.2010.00527.x.

Skelly, B.J. and Franklin, R.J.M. (2002). Recognition and diagnosis of lysosomal storage diseases in the cat and dog. *J. Vet. Intern. Med.* 16: 133–141. https://doi.org/10.1111/j.1939-1676.2002.tb02344.x.

Snyder, J.M., Shofer, F.S., Van Winkle, T.J., and Massicotte, C. (2006). Canine intracranial primary neoplasia: 173 cases (1986–2003). *J. Vet. Intern. Med.* 20: 669–675. https://doi.org/10.1111/j.1939-1676.2006.tb02913.x.

Tauro, A., Beltran, E., Cherubini, G. et al. (2018). Metronidazole-induced neurotoxicity in 26 dogs. *Aust. Vet. J.* 96: 495–501. https://doi.org/10.1111/avj.12772.

Thomsen, B., Garosi, L., Skerritt, G. et al. (2015). Neurological signs in 23 dogs with suspected rostral cerebellar ischaemic stroke. *Acta Vet. Scand.* 58: 40. https://doi.org/10.1186/s13028-016-0219-2.

Troxel, M.T., Drobatz, K.J., and Vite, C.H. (2005). Signs of neurologic dysfunction in dogs with central versus peripheral vestibular disease. *J. Am. Vet. Med. Assoc.* 227 (4): 570–574. https://doi.org/10.2460/javma.2005.227.570. PMID: 16117064.

Whitney, M.S. and Coates, J.R. (2020). Cerebrospinal fluid analysis in the dog and cat. In: *Veterinary Cytology* (ed. L.C. Sharkey, M.J. Radin, and D. Seelig). https://doi.org/10.1002/9781119380559.ch48.

Whittaker, D.E., Drees, R., and Beltran, E. (2018). MRI and clinical characteristics of suspected cerebrovascular accident in nine cats. *J. Feline Med. Surg.* 20 (8): 674–684. https://doi.org/10.1177/1098612X17723775.

Abnormalities of Vision, Pupil Size, and Eye Position

Case 1—Dog with Dilated Unresponsive Pupil

CHAPTER 6.1

Joshua Warren

Head of Neurology and Neurosurgery, Triangle Veterinary Referral Hospital, Durham, NC, USA

CASE HISTORY

A 7-year-old neutered male English springer spaniel was presented for drooping of the right eyelid and dilated pupil (Figure 6.1.1). The owner first noticed the pupil was dilated 5 weeks prior to presentation and the eyelid was drooping 2 weeks later. The dog was otherwise healthy at home with no changes in behavior and no systemic signs. The dog was up to date on vaccinations and only receiving preventatives.

NEUROLOGICAL EXAMINATION

The dog was bright, alert, and responsive. He was ambulatory with no ataxia/paresis. Postural reactions and spinal reflexes, muscle mass and tone were all normal. Cranial nerve examination revealed anisocoria with a mydriatic pupil in the right eye as well as a narrowed palpebral fissure in that eye (Figure 6.1.2). There was a normal menace response and palpebral reflex in both eyes (oculus uterque = OU). The pupillary light reflex (PLR) was absent in the right eye when the light was shined OU, but normal in the left eye when the light was shined OU. No strabismus was noted but when evaluating the vestibulo-ocular reflex (VOR, normal/physiological nystagmus), there was reduced adduction of the right eye when the head was moved to the left. The rest of the neurological exam was normal.

Questions

1. **What is the neuroanatomic diagnosis?**
2. **What are the causes of a narrowed palpebral fissure?**
3. **What are the most likely causes of oculomotor neuropathy?**

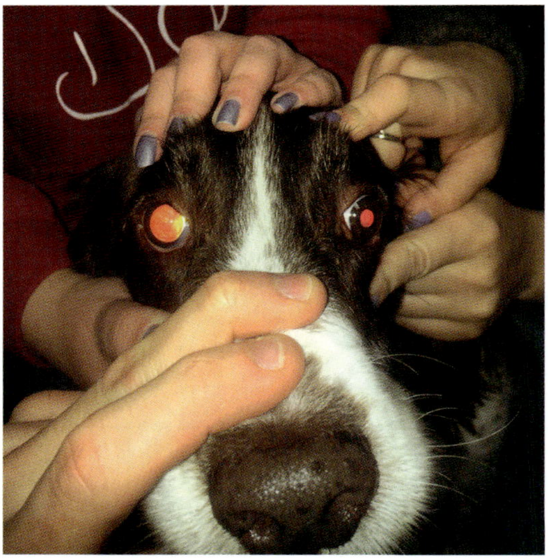

FIGURE 6.1.1 A 7-year-old neutered male English springer spaniel with a right-side dilated pupil.

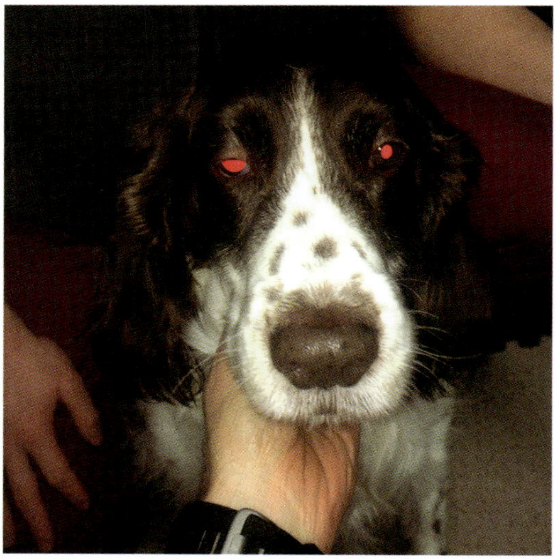

FIGURE 6.1.2 The dog in Figure 6.1.1 also has a right-sided ptosis associated with drooping of the upper eyelid.

NEUROANATOMIC DIAGNOSIS (Figure 6.1.3)

To be able to accurately localize the signs in this patient, both the afferent and efferent pathways for the PLR must be considered. The afferent component of the PLR is the retina, the optic nerve (more correctly termed the pre-chiasmatic optic tract as it is an extension of the CNS and myelinated by oligodendroglial cells), optic chiasm, post-chiasmatic optic tract, and the efferent component is the midbrain (mesencephalic) pretectal nucleus, parasympathetic motor nucleus of the oculomotor nerve (CN III), the parasympathetic neurons in the oculomotor nerve, as well as the iris constrictor muscle itself (Figure 6.1.4). Oculomotor nerve dysfunction should be differentiated from iris atrophy, which can cause mydriasis and reduced PLR in older animals. Iris atrophy generally will cause holes/spaces in the iris and irregular/scalloped pupillary margins (dyscoria) with secondary

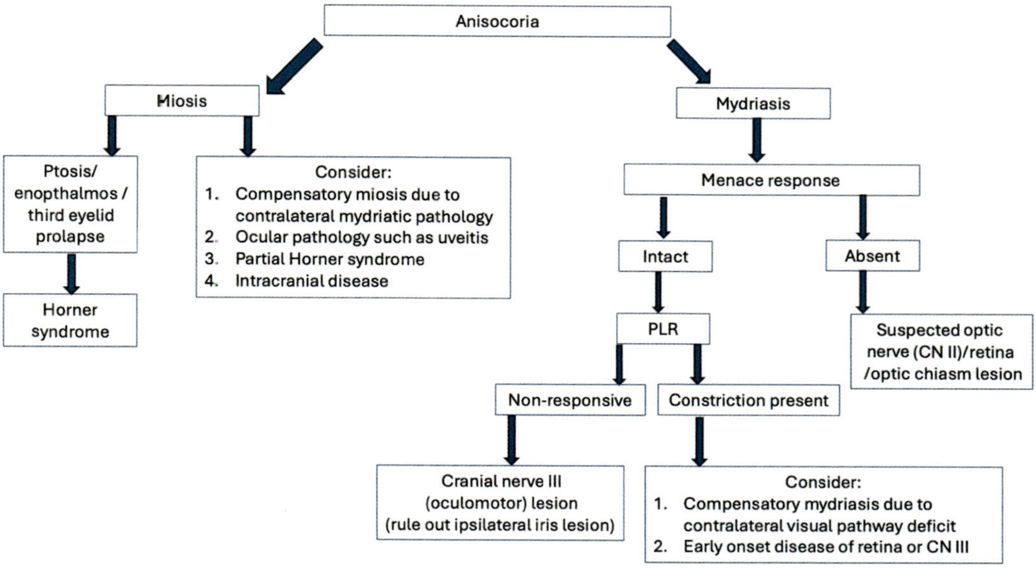

FIGURE 6.1.3 An algorithmic approach to lesion localization for anisocoria.

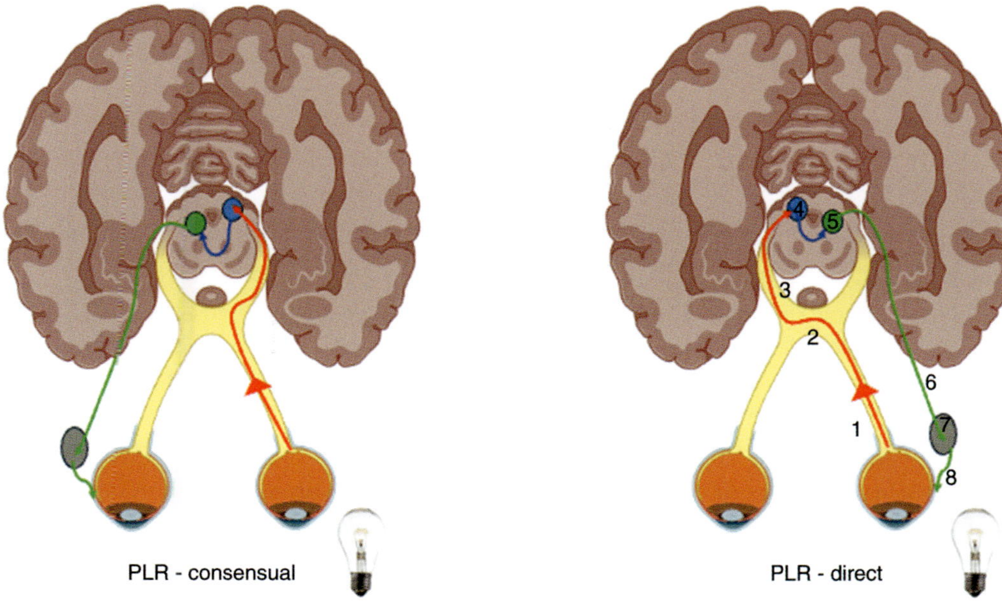

FIGURE 6.1.4 The neuroanatomic pathway for the pupillary light reflex (PLR) illustrating both the direct and consensual pathways following light stimulation of the left eye. The afferent component of the PLR is the retina and the optic nerve (pre-chiasmatic optic tract) (1), the optic chiasm (2), the post-chiasmatic optic tract (3); the efferent component consists of the midbrain (mesencephalic) pretectal nucleus (4), parasympathetic motor nucleus of the oculomotor nerve (CN III) (5), the parasympathetic neurons in the oculomotor nerve (6) that pass through the ciliary ganglion (7) to synapse with the post-ganglionic parasympathetic neurons (8) to the iris constrictor muscles. *Source:* Created with www.biorender.com.

anisocoria, mydriasis, and diminished or absent PLR. The oculomotor nerve also supplies motor innervation to the levator palpebrae superioris muscle of the upper eyelid and extraocular muscles (medial, dorsal, and ventral recti and ventral oblique muscles – also see Chapter 7 Case 5).

In this case, the afferent component of the PLR on the right side must be intact because a normal PLR is noted in the left eye when light is shined in the right eye (See Figure 1 – PLR – Consensual); additionally, there is a normal menace response in both eyes, which requires the same afferent pathway. Both the right-sided parasympathetic CN III innervation of the iris constrictor muscle and the motor CN III innervation of the levator palpebrae superioris muscle and extraocular muscles, specifically the medial rectus muscle, are affected in this dog:

- *Parasympathetic CN III innervation of the pupillary constrictor muscles in the iris* – dysfunction causes mydriasis or internal ophthalmoplegia.
- *Motor CN III innervation of the levator palpebrae superioris muscle* – dysfunction causes a narrowed palpebral fissure/ptosis.
- *Motor CN III innervation of the extraocular muscles, specifically the medial rectus muscle* – dysfunction causes decreased adduction during VOR; external ophthalmoparesis.

In some dogs with oculomotor nerve lesions, there will be a resting lateral or ventrolateral strabismus due to the loss of antagonism to the muscles innervated by trochlear (CN IV) and abducens (CN VI) nerves. Because of the superficial location of the parasympathetic pre-ganglionic neurons in the oculomotor nerve, mydriasis may be the first or only sign noted with a compressive extra-parenchymal mass in the middle cranial fossa, such as a meningioma.

CAUSES OF A NARROWED PALPEBRAL FISSURE

A narrowed palpebral fissure can be secondary to multiple neurogenic causes. Once squinting or blepharospasm have been ruled out by careful ophthalmological evaluation, then a neurogenic cause must be considered.

- Loss of innervation of the levator palpebrae superioris from the oculomotor nerve, as in this case, can be seen along with other clinical signs noted above.
- Horner syndrome secondary to sympathetic dysfunction to the eye can cause ptosis due to loss of innervation of the smooth muscles of the periorbita/orbitalis muscle. In addition to ptosis other signs associated with Horner syndrome include elevated third eyelid, enophthalmos, and miosis due to loss of innervation to the smooth muscles of the periorbita/eyelids and the dilator pupillae muscle, respectively.
- Enophthalmos and narrowed palpebral fissure can be seen with atrophy of the muscles of mastication (as seen with trigeminal nerve dysfunction or generalized muscle atrophy/cachexia seen in older animals) because they form a significant portion of the border of the periorbita. As a result of the atrophy, the globe will sink into the orbit, and the palpebral fissure narrows, resulting in passive elevation of the third eyelid. In contrast to Horner syndrome, pupil size will remain normal.
- Uncommonly in small animals, there will be a smaller palpebral fissure secondary to facial nerve paralysis/paresis due to denervation of the levator angularis oculi muscle or the orbicularis oculi muscle. Facial nerve tetanus is a unique disorder that may be preceded by facial nerve paralysis, resulting in sustained contraction of the mimetic muscles of the face innervated by the facial nerve. The result is a narrowed palpebral fissure as well as slight elevation of the ear, taut lips with the commissure of the lips drawn caudally, and the nose slightly deviated to the affected side.

DIFFERENTIAL DIAGNOSIS FOR OCULOMOTOR (CN III) NEUROPATHY

Oculomotor nerve dysfunction can be seen with lesions starting in the midbrain (affecting the motor nucleus of the oculomotor nerve and the parasympathetic nucleus of the oculomotor nerve) or anywhere along the pathway of the oculomotor nerve from its emergence on the ventral aspect of the midbrain to its terminal branches in the periorbita. Since the parasympathetic preganglionic axons are located superficially on the medial side of the nerve, they are susceptible to compressive lesions or disorders that cause the midbrain to swell or be displaced.

Neoplasia

Extra-parenchymal neoplasms arising in the middle cranial fossa (including suprasellar neoplasms in the region of the pituitary gland) can cause direct compression of either the midbrain or the oculomotor nerve. Differentials for tumors affecting this area include germ cell neoplasm, meningioma, lymphoma, craniopharyngioma, and pituitary tumors/macroadenomas. Retrobulbar neoplasms could also affect the oculomotor nerve in the periorbita. However, other signs would be expected, including exophthalmia, blindness, and reduced ability to manually retropulse the globe. Mass lesions affecting the cerebrum and causing increased intracranial pressure can cause herniation of the occipital lobes ventral to the tentorium cerebelli (caudal transtentorial herniation), thereby compressing or displacing the midbrain, oculomotor nerve(s), or both. Mydriasis may be seen due to parasympathetic dysfunction, but other neurogenic signs associated with the primary lesion would be expected with significantly increased intracranial pressure.

Inflammation

Meningoencephalitis of unknown origin (MUO) may affect the midbrain, causing oculomotor nerve dysfunction. However, often with MUO, signs are multifocal, and other neurological signs would be expected. Inflammatory or infectious granulomas in the middle cranial fossa (similar to neoplasms) could affect the midbrain or oculomotor nerves.

An infectious, retrobulbar abscess could also affect the oculomotor nerve, similar to a neoplasm; again, other signs would be expected related to the presence of this mass lesion.

Idiopathic

Idiopathic oculomotor neuropathy has been described more recently. These dogs display varying degrees of oculomotor dysfunction, from only internal ophthalmoparesis/ophthalmoplegia (mydriasis and absent PLR) to both internal ophthalmoplegia and external ophthalmoparesis/ophthalmoplegia (lateral strabismus, decreased adduction during VOR, ptosis). Magnetic resonance imaging findings in these dogs range from normal to variably enlarged (mild to marked) and contrast-enhancing (focal or diffuse) oculomotor nerve(s). Evaluation of cerebrospinal fluid is normal in most dogs, but mild elevations in protein or nucleated cell counts can be seen. Some dogs will have improvement in the clinical signs, but others will have no improvement, and corticosteroid therapy has not been shown to alter the clinical outcome. If improvements do occur, a mean recovery time of 5 weeks has been reported.

OUTCOME

Once the causative possibilities were explained to the owners, they decided not to pursue further investigation. Over the course of the next 2 months, the dog improved and was nearly back to normal without specific therapeutic intervention. An idiopathic cause of a CN III neuropathy was presumed.

SUGGESTED READING

Benito, M.B., Fuentes, M.P., Manso-Diaz, G. et al. (2022). Clinical signs, diagnostic imaging and histopathology in a dog with granulomatous meningoencephalitis manifested as a polyneuropathy. *Vet. Rec. Case Rep.* 10: e324.

Cook, L., Tensley, M., Drost, W.T. et al. (2018). MRI findings of suprasellar germ cell tumors in two dogs. *J. Am. Anim. Hosp. Assoc.* 54: 167–172.

De Lahunta, A., Glass, E., and Kent, M. (2021). *De Lahunta's Veterinary Neuroanatomy and Clinical Neurology*, 5e. Philadelphia: Elsevier.

Levitin, H.A., Lampe, R., and Hecht, S. (2020). Case report: meningoencephalomyelitis of unknown etiology manifesting as a bilateral cranial polyneuropathy in 3 dogs. *Front. Vet. Sci.* 7: 326.

Maggs, D.J., Miller, P.E., Ofri, R. et al. (ed.) (2008). *Slatter's Fundamentals of Veterinary Ophthalmology*, 4e. Philadelphia, Pa London: Elsevier Saunders.

Tetas Pont, R., Freeman, C., Dennis, R. et al. (2017). Clinical and magnetic resonance imaging features of idiopathic oculomotor neuropathy in 14 dogs. *Vet. Radiol. Ultrasound* 58 (3): 334–343.

Abnormalities of Vision, Pupil Size, and Eye Position

Case 2—Acute Bilateral Blindness in a Dog

CHAPTER 6.2

Joshua Warren

Head of Neurology and Neurosurgery, Triangle Veterinary Referral Hospital, Durham, NC, USA

CASE HISTORY

A 3-year-old female intact mini-Golden Doodle was presented for lethargy of 1-week duration. The dog initially experienced diarrhea, which was resolved with the administration of a probiotic and dewormer. Signs progressed to an abnormal gait affecting the left limbs with a subsequent onset of bumping into walls/furniture and tripping on objects. The owners felt that the dog was blind. The dog was otherwise healthy at home, was up to date on vaccinations, and was receiving routine parasitic preventatives.

NEUROLOGICAL EXAMINATION

The dog had a dull mentation and would bump into walls in the examination room (Video 6.2.1). She was ambulatory with dysmetria of the left limbs and mild vestibular ataxia, as well as titubation and swaying when standing still (Video 6.2.2). Cranial nerve examination revealed a mild right-sided head tilt, spontaneous and positional rotary nystagmus with fast phase changing from right to left, an absent menace OU with mydriasis (Figure 6.2.1), and an absent pupillary light reflex (PLR) OU. The rest of the cranial nerve examination was normal. Postural reactions revealed moderately delayed and "bursty" hopping (abnormal rate, range, and force of replacement of the limbs) in the left limbs and mildly delayed hopping in the right limbs.

VIDEO 6.2.1 Observation of the 3-year-old female intact mini-Golden Doodle wandering around the examination room identified several instances of walking into/bumping into the walls of the room.

VIDEO 6.2.2 Observation of the 3-year-old female intact mini-Golden Doodle's gait identified a left-sided stride length abnormality compatible with dysmetria and a vestibular ataxia.

Questions

1. **What is the neuroanatomic diagnosis of acute blindness with absent PLR OU?**
2. **What are the most common causes of acute blindness in the dog?**
3. **What diagnostics could be used to help determine the diagnosis?**
4. **What is the prognosis for optic neuritis?**

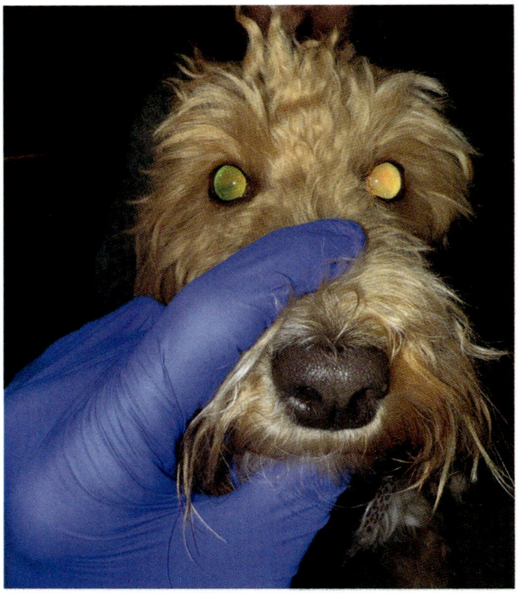

FIGURE 6.2.1 Bilateral mydriasis can easily be seen in this dog with the aid of the tapetal reflectivity.

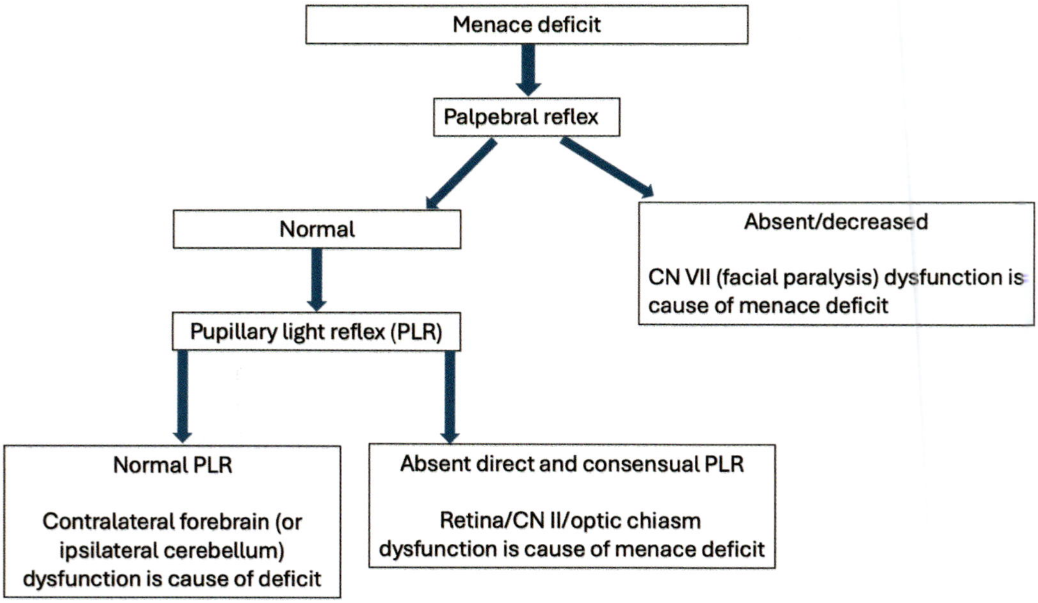

FIGURE 6.2.2 Localization of lesions responsible for a menace deficit.

NEUROANATOMIC DIAGNOSIS (Figure 6.2.2)

To accurately localize blindness in this patient, an understanding of the visual and PLR pathways is necessary. The visual pathway starts in the retina and traverses the optic nerve (prechiasmatic optic tract), optic chiasm, the contralateral post-chiasmatic optic tract, lateral geniculate nucleus, and optic radiation to the visual cortex in the occipital lobe of the cerebral hemisphere (Figure 6.2.3A and B). This is the afferent portion of the menace response (a learned behavioral response and not

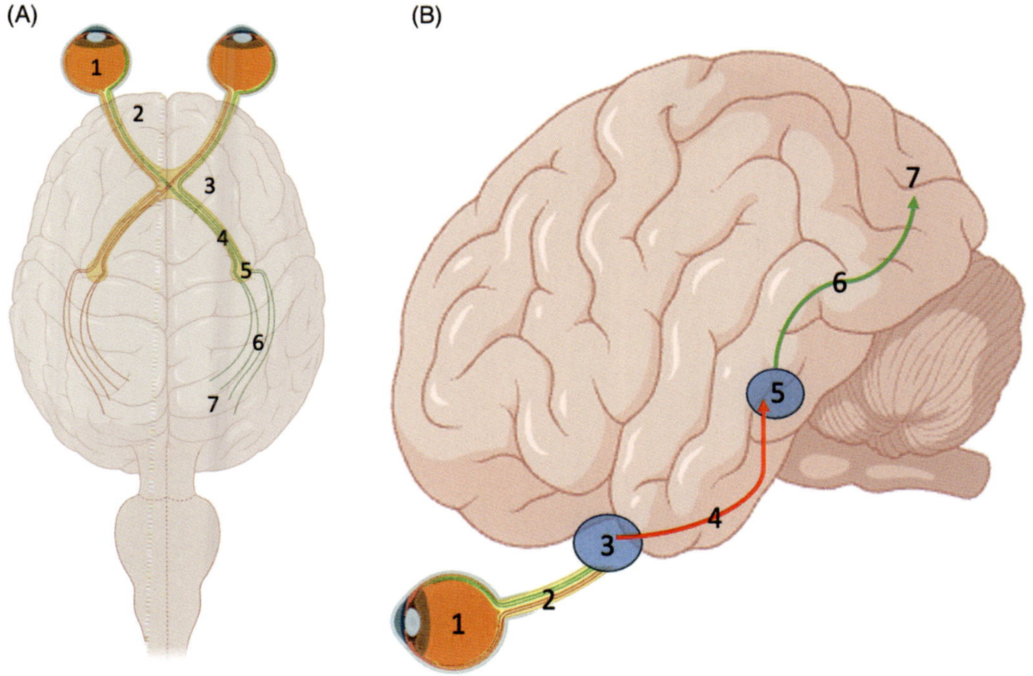

FIGURE 6.2.3 (A) Dorsal view and (B) Lateral view of the neuroanatomical visual pathway. (1) Retina, (2) optic nerve (pre-chiasmatic optic tract), (3) optic chiasm, (4) post-chiasmatic optic tract, (5) lateral geniculate nucleus, (6) optic radiation, and (7) occipital cortex. *Source:* Created with www.biorender.com.

a reflex), while the efferent portion is the medulla oblongata of the brainstem, facial nerve (CN VII), and the orbicularis oculi muscle (Figure 6.2.4).

The neuroanatomic diagnosis in this case for the blindness with mydriasis and absent PLR OU must be anywhere along the pathway bilaterally from the retina to the post-chiasmatic optic tract prior to the divergence of axons going to the PLR pathway (Figure 6.2.5). The PLR pathway diverges in the post-chiasmatic optic tract and synapses in the mesencephalic pretectal nucleus. Axons from the pretectal nucleus terminate in the parasympathetic motor nucleus of the oculomotor nerve (CN III) (Chapter 6 – Case 1; Figure 3). If either the visual or PLR pathways are affected beyond the divergence of the two pathways in the post-chiasmatic optic tract, there would be visual deficits with normal PLR or normal vision with abnormal pupil size and PLR, respectively, and the orbicularis oculi muscle (Figure 6.2.5).

DIFFERENTIAL DIAGNOSIS FOR ACUTE BLINDNESS

Once an anatomic diagnosis has been made, a differential diagnosis can be formulated. Acute blindness can be divided into ophthalmological and neurogenic causes (Figure 6.2.6 for dogs and Table 6.2.1 for cats).

Retina and optic nerve (pre-chiasmatic optic tract)

- Sudden acquired retinal degeneration syndrome (SARDS) is the most common ophthalmological cause of acute blindness. Patients with SARDS often have clinical signs similar to hyperadrenocorticism with polyphagia, polyuria/polydipsia, and weight gain, and may even have similar biochemical abnormalities, including elevations in serum alanine aminotransferase

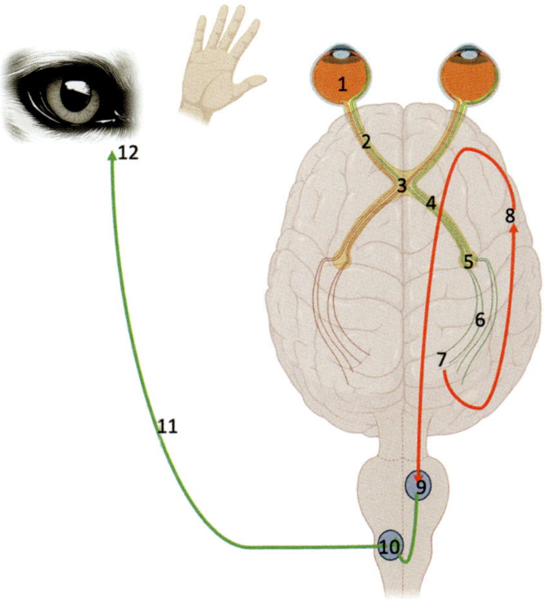

FIGURE 6.2.4 The menace response pathway. (1) Retina, (2) optic nerve (pre-chiasmatic optic tract), (3) optic chiasm, (4) post-chiasmatic optic tract, (5) lateral geniculate nucleus, (6) optic radiation, (7) occipital cortex, (8) motor cortex, (9) pontine nucleus, (10) facial nerve nucleus, (11) facial nerve, and (12) orbicularis oculi muscles. *Source:* Created with www.biorender.com.

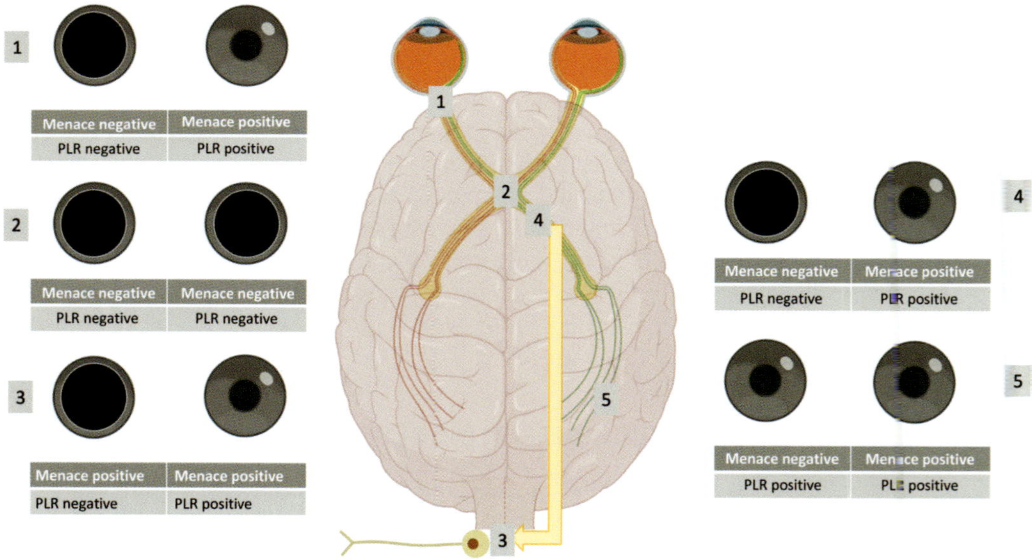

FIGURE 6.2.5 Localization of blindness and mydriasis. The pupillary light reflex (PLR) noted in the illustration refers to the direct PLR, or stimulation of the ipsilateral eye. (1) Retina and optic nerve (pre-chiasmatic optic tract), (2) optic chiasm, (3) oculomotor nerve (CN III), (4) post-chiasmatic optic tract, and (5) optic radiation and occipital cortex. *Source:* Created with www.biorender.com.

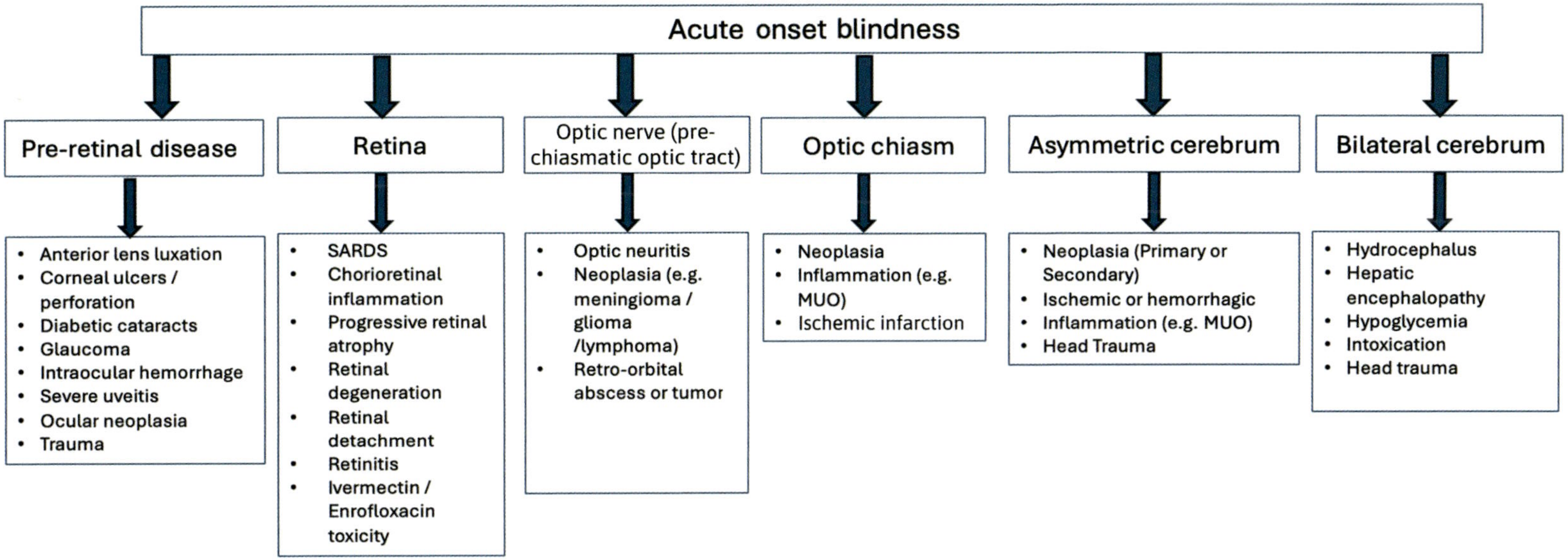

FIGURE 6.2.6 Lesion localization-based differential diagnosis for blindness in dogs.

Table 6.2.1 Common specific etiological considerations for blindness in cats; (PLR – pupillary light reflex).

Cause	Underlying disease	Expected signs/lesions
Systemic hypertension	Hyperthyroidism, renal disease, primary hypertension	Retinal detachment/hemorrhage and blindness with absent PLR
Global hypoxia/ ischemia	Anesthesia, mouth gag/maxillary artery occlusion	*Cerebral hypoxia* – blindness with normal pupil size and normal PLR ± vestibular ataxia, circling, proprioceptive deficits, mentation changes; *Retinal hypoxia* – blindness with dilated pupils and absent PLR
Thiamine deficiency	Fish diet consisting of species of fish containing thiaminase, diets with inadequate thiamine, food that is cooked destroying thiamine, or prolonged anorexia	Blindness with dilated pupils, cerebello-vestibular ataxia, seizures, head and neck flexion, coma, death
Infection	Feline infectious peritonitis virus (FIP), feline leukemia virus (FeLV), feline immunodeficiency virus (FIV), toxoplasmosis, cryptococcosis, etc.	Variable ocular (anterior uveitis, retinal lesions/detachment), systemic, and neurological signs
Neoplasia affecting eye, prechiasmiatic optic tracts, optic chiasm	Lymphoma, meningioma	Blindness with absent PLR ± ocular discomfort and other neurological signs
Taurine deficiency	Feeding diets deficient in taurine (including commercial dog food)	Retinal degeneration with blindness and absent PLR
Enrofloxacin toxicity	Administration of enrofloxacin >5 mg/kg q24h	Retinal degeneration with blindness and absent PLR
Retrobulbar lesions	Neoplasia, granuloma, abscess	Often unilateral blindness and absent PLR, exophthalmia, pain upon retropulsion

(ALT), serum alkaline phosphatase (ALP), and cholesterol. Decreased vision in dim light (nyctalopia) may be seen with SARDS prior to complete blindness.

- Optic neuritis is the most common neurogenic cause of acute blindness. Remember that the pre-chiasmatic optic tracts are an extension of the central nervous system (CNS) and are affected by diseases that affect the CNS. It is generally thought that optic neuritis is a focal form of meningoencephalitis of unknown origin (MUO – presumed immune-mediated disease), but optic neuritis can be seen with more diffuse or multifocal MUO. Dogs with acute blindness from optic neuritis, commonly have other neurological abnormalities ranging from mentation changes, seizures, vestibular signs, or other cranial nerve deficits. While optic neuritis is most often bilateral, 20–29% of dogs will present unilaterally. A diagnosis of MUO must not be assumed in patients with multifocal neurological signs because patients with focal optic neuritis may be diagnosed with other structural, incidental neurological diseases, including concurrent intervertebral disc herniation.

  Both optic neuritis and SARDS are progressive but subtle signs may be missed by owners and can appear to cause acute/sudden blindness. Vision is lost before the PLR with these disorders. While the PLR may be intact, the pupils are often too dilated in room light.

- Other ophthalmic causes of blindness include retinal detachment, progressive retinal atrophy/degeneration, glaucoma, uveitis, and corneal disease. Many of these will have more readily identifiable ophthalmic changes in the anterior or posterior segment of the globe.

Optic chiasm and cerebral hemispheres

- Chiasmatic causes for blindness include MUO, neoplasia (meningioma, lymphoma, pituitary tumors), microbial infection (tick-borne, fungal, bacterial, protozoal, viral), ischemia, and trauma.
    - Dogs with functional pituitary macroadenomas may have signs of hyperadrenocorticism. Uncommonly, compression of the optic chiasm from these tumors will cause blindness. It is important to consider this as a differential for SARDS. Advanced diagnostics will help differentiate the two.
- In bilateral cerebral hemisphere dysfunction, the patient may be bilaterally blind but with normal pupil size and PLRs and will usually have other neurological signs, including changes in sensorium or seizures. Considerations for bilateral disease include hypertension, metabolic diseases (hepatic encephalopathy, hypoglycemia), intoxication, inflammation (MUO and infections), malformations such as hydrocephalus, trauma, and multifocal neoplasia.
- Asymmetric cerebral hemisphere diseases affecting the visual pathways include ischemic/hemorrhagic stroke, inflammation, trauma, structural anomalies (e.g. porencephaly, asymmetrical hydrocephalus), and neoplasia (e.g. glioma, meningioma, metastasis).

DIAGNOSTIC TESTING

Thorough physical and neurological examinations are important in acutely blind patients.

- Fundoscopic examination is crucial in these patients. The most common fundic change seen with optic neuritis is optic nerve head swelling/elevation (papilledema), but peripapillary retinal edema or retinal detachment contiguous with the optic nerve head, optic disc or retinal hemorrhage, and dilation of retinal vasculature can be seen. Retrobulbar optic neuritis may present with normal fundic exam, making it harder to differentiate from SARDS. In early stages, patients with SARDS will have no fundoscopic changes, but can later develop hyperreflective tapeta lucida and retinal vascular attenuation. In rare instances with SARDS, the optic nerve head will be prominent due to pseudopapilledema, most commonly from excessive myelination in dogs.
- Chromatic PLR has been used in patients with blindness – in dogs with SARDS, blue light can elicit a PLR, whereas red light does not. Red light evaluates rod-cone PLR function that is lost in patients with SARDS. Blue light evaluates both rod-cone photoreceptors and retinal ganglion cell (melanopsin mediated) photoreceptors and therefore prechiasmatic optic tract function. Pupillary light reflex with blue and red light will be absent in dogs with optic neuritis with complete dysfunction. With end-stage retinal degeneration, PLR may be diminished/absent even with blue light stimulation.
- Electroretinography (ERG) can be considered, especially for cases in which the sole presenting complaint is blindness. Dogs with SARDS will have extinguished ERG. Dogs with normal ERG and without other neurological signs must not be assumed to have focal optic neuritis – up to 50–70% of dogs with blindness from neoplasia, infectious meningoencephalitis, and orbital cellulitis had no other neurological signs.
- MRI/CSF should always be considered, especially if ERG is normal (Figure 6.2.7). Of dogs diagnosed with optic neuritis, 11–68% without other neurological signs will have multifocal MRI lesions consistent with MUO. For cases in which other neurological abnormalities are present, MRI/CSF should be considered first. Changes on MRI consistent with optic neuritis include enlargement and/or enhancement of the pre-chiasmatic optic tracts/optic nerve head

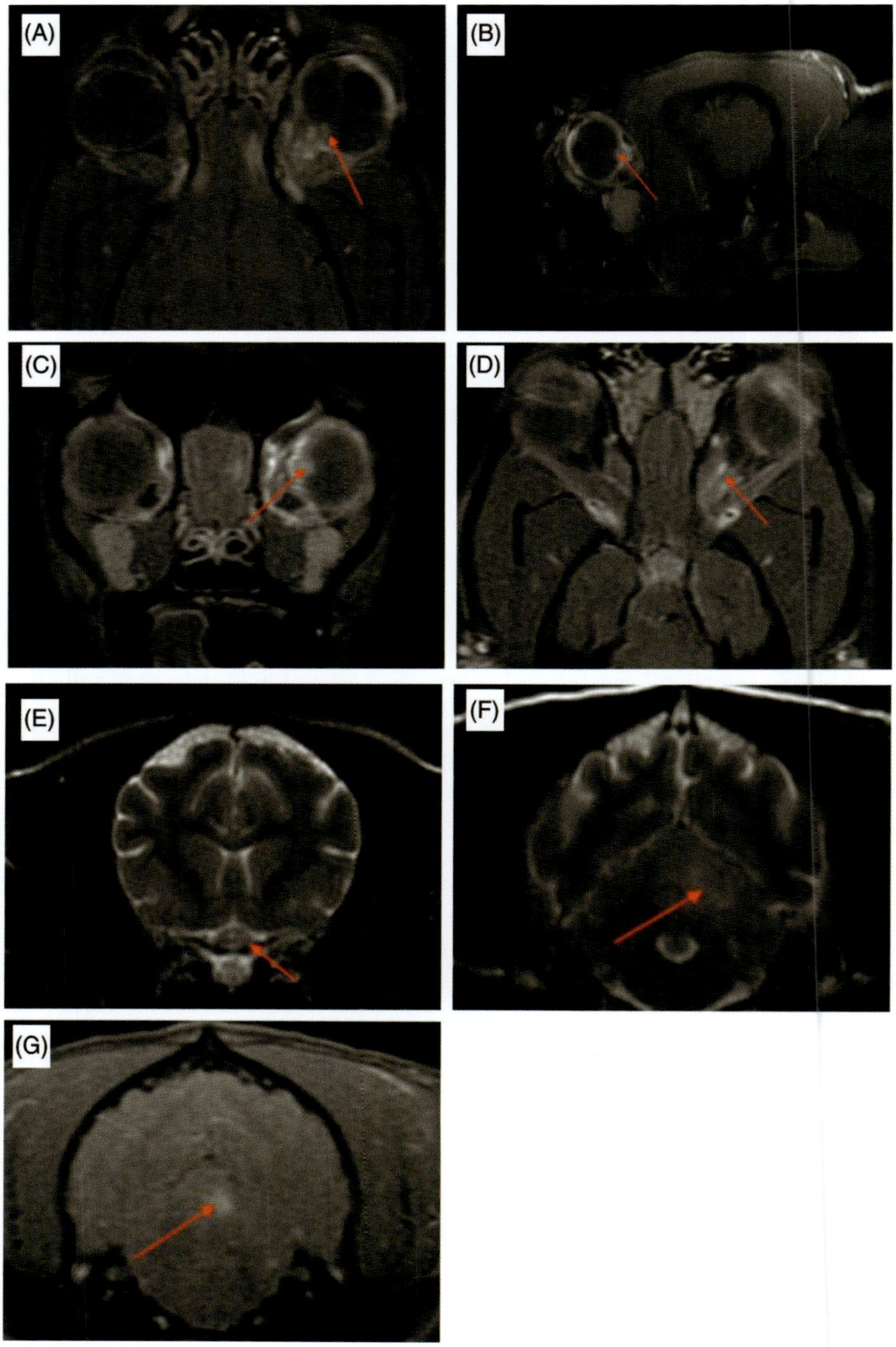

FIGURE 6.2.7 MRI study of the brain of the 3-year-old mini-Golden Doodle, revealing multifocal disease. T1W post-contrast (A) dorsal, (B) sagittal, and (C) transverse images demonstrating enlargement and enhancement of the optic disc of the dog's left eye. Contrast enhancement of the optic nerve (pre-chiasmatic optic tract) is seen on the dorsal T1W post-contrast image (D). T2W transverse view of optic chiasm shows mild enlargement and hyperintensity of the left side (E). T2W transverse view of the brain at the level of the cerebellum demonstrating an ill-defined and irregular intraparenchymal hyperintensity (F) with a focal region of contrast enhancement noted on the T1W post-contrast image at this level (G).

or optic chiasm. In the case of optic neuritis with MUO, MRI changes include multifocal T2W hyperintensities in the cerebrum, cerebellum, or brainstem with or without enhancement and thickening and/or enhancement of the meninges.

- CSF analysis – Mononuclear or mixed cell pleocytosis (elevated nucleated cell counts in CSF) is common in dogs with optic neuritis and MUO. Dogs with multifocal MUO are reported to have more significant pleocytosis than focal optic neuritis. In rare cases, MRI, CSF, or both may be normal with optic neuritis/MUO.

PROGNOSIS FOR OPTIC NEURITIS

The prognosis for regaining vision with optic neuritis is guarded to poor. Partial or complete recovery of vision (as assessed by the menace response) in the affected eye(s) may occur in 30–65% of cases treated with immunosuppressive medications. However, complete visual recovery is reported to be as low as 13.9–23%, up to 32%. The mainstay of treatment is a tapering course of immunosuppressive corticosteroids. Adjunct immunosuppressive medications are commonly used, including cytarabine, cyclosporine, azathioprine, mycophenolate, and leflunomide. Due to small case studies and lack of prospective clinical trials, it is unclear if additional immunosuppressive medications improve prognosis. However, for cases of MUO without optic neuritis, additional immunosuppressive medications have been shown to improve prognosis. In dogs with optic neuritis and MUO, other neurological signs can improve with treatment even if vision is not recovered. If recovery occurs, recurrence of both focal optic neuritis and MUO are possible. Improved prognosis for complete recovery of vision in one study was reported with lower CSF total nucleated cell counts, absence of fundoscopic lesions, presence of reactive (partial or complete) PLR, and younger age (median <2 years of age).

OUTCOME

In the present case, fundoscopic examination revealed moderate to severe optic nerve head swelling bilaterally (left > right). MRI revealed multifocal T2W hyperintensities in the cerebrum, brainstem, and cerebellum (left > right) with patchy contrast enhancement, mild leptomeningeal contrast enhancement, and enhancing and enlarged/T2W hyperintense left optic chiasm and pre-chiasmatic optic tract/optic nerve head. CSF revealed severe lymphocytic pleocytosis (total nucleated cell count 314/uL; normal range <5/uL). These findings are most consistent with optic neuritis as part of multifocal MUO.

SUGGESTED READING

Barton-Lamb, A.L., Martin-Flores, M., Scrivani, P.V. et al. (2013). Evaluation of maxillary arterial blood flow in anesthetized cats with the mouth closed and open. *Vet. J.* 196: 325–331.

Bedos, L., Tetas, R., Crespo, V., and Shea, A. (2020). Presumed optic neuritis of non-infectious origin in dogs treated with immunosuppressive medication: 28 dogs (2000-2015). *J. Small Anim. Pract.* 61: 676–683.

De Lahunta, A., Glass, E., and Kent, M. (2021). *De Lahunta's Veterinary Neuroanatomy and Clinical Neurology*, 5e. Philadelphia: Elsevier.

Gelatt, K.N., Van Der Woerdt, A., Ketring, K.L. et al. (2001). Enrofloxacin-associated retinal degeneration in cats. *Vet. Ophthalmol.* 4: 99–106.

Grozdanic, S.D., Matic, M., Sakaguchi, D.S. et al. (2007). Evaluation of retinal status using chromatic pupil light reflex activity in healthy and diseased canine eyes. *Invest. Ophthalmol. Vis. Sci.* 48: 5178.

Maggs, D.J., Miller, P.E., Ofri, R. et al. (ed.) (2008). *Slatter's Fundamentals of Veterinary Ophthalmology*, 4e. Philadelphia, Pa London: Elsevier Saunders.

Montgomery, K.W., Van Der Woerdt, A., and Cottrill, N.B. (2008). Acute blindness in dogs: sudden acquired retinal degeneration syndrome versus neurological disease (140 cases, 2000–2006). *Vet. Ophthalmol.* 11: 314–320.

Muñiz Moris, L., Cherubini, G.B., and Caine, A. (2021). Low-field magnetic resonance imaging findings in 18 dogs with presumed optic neuritis. *Front. Vet. Sci.* 7: 585828.

Posporis, C., Beltran, E., Dunning, M. et al. (2019). Prognostic factors for recovery of vision in canine optic neuritis of unknown etiology: 26 dogs (2003–2018). *Front. Vet. Sci.* 6: 415.

Smith, S.M., Westermeyer, H.D., Mariani, C.L. et al. (2018). Optic neuritis in dogs: 96 cases (1983–2015). *Vet. Ophthalmol.* 21: 442–451.

Stiles, J., Weil, A.B., Packer, R.A., and Lantz, G.C. (2012) Post-anesthetic cortical blindness in cats: twenty cases. *Vet. J.* 193: 367–373.

Abnormalities of Vision, Pupil Size, and Eye Position

Case 3—Horner Syndrome in a Cat

CHAPTER 6.3

Rose K. Peters

Veterinary Clinical Neurology, University of Illinois at Urbana-Champaign, Urbana, IL, USA

CASE HISTORY

A 10-year-old male neutered domestic shorthair cat was presented for evaluation of left-sided third eyelid elevation. The owner first noticed that the left eye looked "strange" about 2 weeks earlier. He was otherwise behaving normally, so the owner initially chose to monitor for progression. The problem persisted, so the cat presented for further evaluation. There was no resolution, but there had been no worsening or new concerns (Figure 6.3.1).

NEUROLOGICAL EXAMINATION

The cat was bright, alert, and responsive with a normal gait. Anisocoria could be appreciated with a relatively smaller left-sided pupil (miosis). There was drooping of the left upper eyelid (ptosis) with mild enophthalmos and protrusion of the third eyelid. When examined in dim light, the anisocoria was pronounced with minimal dilation of the left pupil. There was a moderate amount of dark brown ceruminous debris present in both ear canals, obstructing a clear view of the tympanic membranes. The physical examination was otherwise within normal limits.

1. **Where is the likely lesion localization?**
2. **What major disease processes should be considered?**
3. **What tests could you perform to help determine the diagnosis?**

LESION LOCALIZATION

The miosis, ptosis, and enophthalmos with third eyelid protrusion in the left eye are consistent with Horner syndrome. Horner syndrome reflects interruption of the sympathetic pathway to the eye and follows a complex course involving three neurons (Figure 6.3.2A).

- The first-order neuron originates in the hypothalamus and travels through the brainstem and lateral aspect of the cervical spinal cord before synapsing with the second-order neurons in the intermediolateral horn of the T1–3 spinal cord segments. (Figure 6.3.2B)
- The axons of the second-order neurons (also called "preganglionic neurons") pass from the intermediolateral horn of the spinal cord to exit the vertebral canal in the ventral nerve root

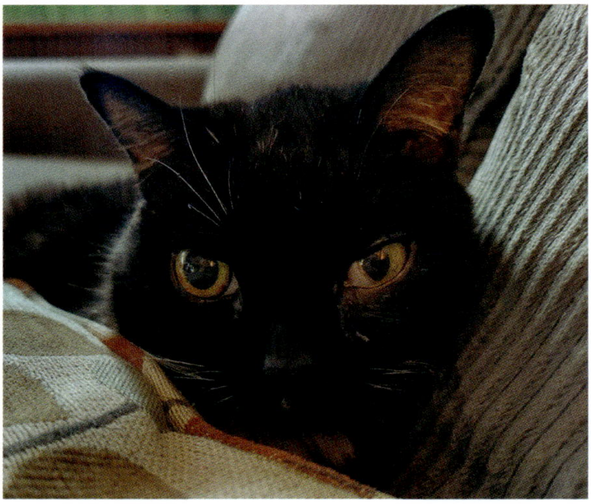

FIGURE 6.3.1 A 10-year-old male neutered domestic shorthair cat with left-sided third eyelid elevation, miosis, ptosis and mild enophthalmos.

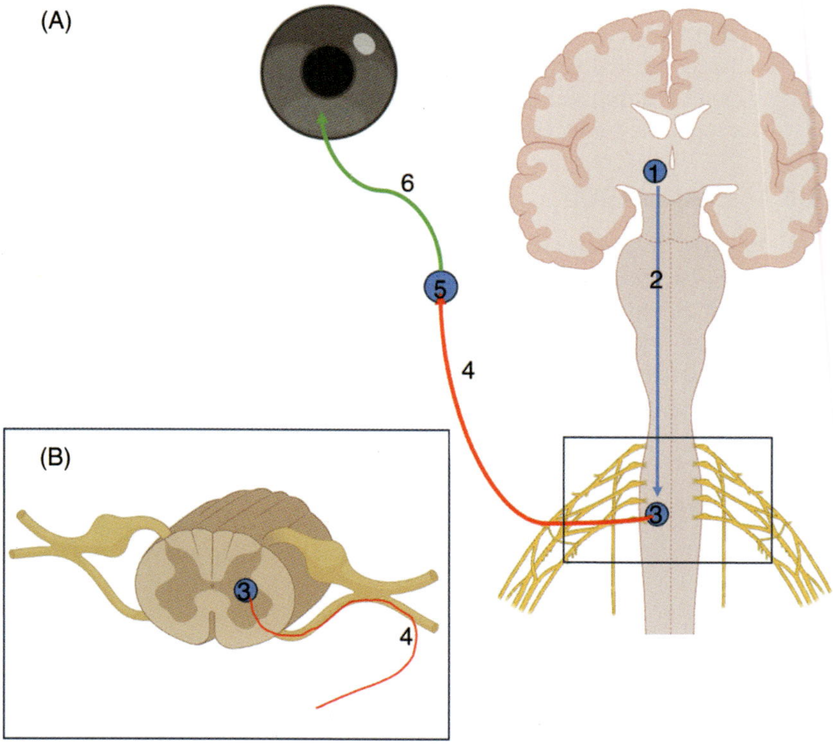

FIGURE 6.3.2 (A) Schematic representation of the neuroanatomy of the sympathetic nerve supply to the eye (Horner pathway). (1) Sympathetic cell bodies of the first-order neuron in the hypothalamus; (2) Lateral tectotegmental spinal tract; (3) Cell body of the second-order neuron within the intermediolateral horn of the T1–T3 spinal cord segments; (4) The second-order neuron exits the ventral nerve root via the Ramus communicans to become the vagosympathetic trunk; (5) Cranial cervical ganglion; (6) Post-ganglionic third-order neurons enter the middle ear and then the middle cranial fossa running to the orbit. (B) An expansion of the T1–T3 spinal cord segments illustrating the origin of the second-order neurons and their exit from the ventral nerve root to become the vagosympathetic trunk. Source: Created with www.biorender.com.

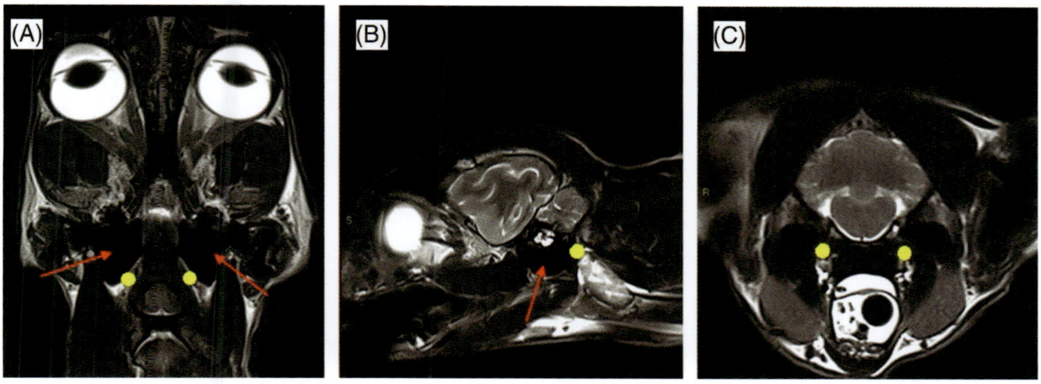

FIGURE 6.3.3 T2W dorsal (A), sagittal (B) and transverse (C) images of a cat head at the level of the tympanic bullae (arrows) illustrating the position of the cranial cervical ganglion (yellow circles) that is located immediately caudo-medial to the bulla.

before traversing into the sympathetic chain in the thoracic cavity via the ramus communicans. The axons continue to travel cranially through the mediastinum, passing through the cervicothoracic ganglion and middle cervical ganglion near the thoracic inlet without synapsing. These second-order neurons join the vagus nerve as the vagosympathetic trunk to travel cranially to the base of the cranium, Here, the sympathetic fibers divert from the vagus nerve to synapse in the cranial cervical ganglion, which is immediately caudo-medial to the tympanic bulla. (Figure 6.3.3)

- The axons of the third-order neurons (also called "post-ganglionic neurons") follow a path that is not well described. They are thought to pass from the soft tissues ventromedial to the tympanic bulla and run along the ventromedial surface of the bulla, through the petrosal portion of the temporal bone (the inner ear area) to enter the cranial cavity. The axons travel a short course through the ventrolateral aspect of the skull adjacent to the brain, then join the ophthalmic branch of the trigeminal nerve to exit the skull behind the eye through the orbital fissure. The fibers branch to innervate the iris, periorbital muscles, and eyelids; additional fibers travel with the internal carotid artery to influence arteries of the face and ears, as well as the regional sweat glands. Norepinephrine is the primary neurotransmitter acting on alpha-adrenergic receptors.

In animals with Horner syndrome, a lesion anywhere along this lengthy pathway can lead to the observed signs. The neurological exam helps to refine the localization. Examples of the clinical signs that can accompany Horner syndrome based on the responsible lesion localization are detailed in Table 6.3.1 and a clinical approach to the localization of a patient with anisocoria is detailed in Figure 6.3.4.

Tips: Make sure that you identify the correct "abnormal" eye when presented with a case of anisocoria. Pathological unilateral mydriasis can make the contralateral normal eye appear relatively miotic. Examine the patient in both well and dimly lit situations. With Horner syndrome, the smaller pupil will not dilate in the dark and the anisocoria will be enhanced. In pathological unilateral mydriasis, the smaller (normal) pupil will dilate appropriately in the dark and constrict in the light.

The most commonly confused condition with Horner syndrome is miosis and third eyelid protrusion caused by ocular pain and inflammation (uveitis). Look for evidence of conjunctivitis, corneal lesions, and aqueous flare to rule in ophthalmic causes of these signs.

Table 6.3.1 Neurological examination findings associated with Horner syndrome based on the responsible lesion localization.

Horner pathway segment	Neuroanatomic localization	Additional clinical findings (one or more of the following depending on the location, size, and nature of the lesion)
First order	Brainstem	Obtundation, stupor, coma
		Tetraparesis, proprioceptive ataxia, vestibular ataxia ± cerebellar ataxia
		Cranial nerve deficits (V, VI, VII, VIII ± III, IX, X, XII)
	C1–C5 myelopathy	Tetraparesis or hemiparesis/plegia, proprioception deficits in thoracic and pelvic limbs, normal to increased spinal reflexes in all four limbs, cervical pain
	C6–T2 myelopathy	Tetraparesis or hemiparesis/plegia, proprioception deficits in thoracic and pelvic limbs, normal to increased spinal reflexes in the pelvic limbs, reduced to absent reflexes in the thoracic limbs, cervical pain
Second order	Brachial plexus	Monoparesis/plegia, proprioception deficits in the affected limb, reduced to absent reflexes in the affected limb
		Axillary or caudal cervical pain
	Intrathoracic	No other clinical signs may be noted with this location - potential associated signs include: Changes in respiratory character, muffled heart or lung sounds, cough
	Extraspinal cervical	No other clinical signs may be noted with this location – if there is soft tissue trauma, the following clinical signs may be noted: Swelling, asymmetry, discoloration of the skin, cervical pain
Second or third order	Middle-inner ear	Head shaking, ear scratching, otitis externa, bulging or discolored tympanum, ruptured tympanum, ear pain
		Facial paresis/paralysis, vestibular syndrome
Third order	Middle cranial fossa (Cavernous Sinus) syndrome	Cranial nerves II, IV, V, and VI dysfunction
		± behavior changes, proprioceptive ataxia, tetra- or hemiparesis
	Retrobulbar	Eye irritation, exophthalmus, strabismus, CN II, III deficits, ophthalmic branch of cranial nerve V, ± changes in mental state, seizures, local myoclonus or myokymia, nasal congestion or discharge

In our cat, the only dysfunction detected on neurological examination were the changes consistent with Horner syndrome; this is insufficient information to narrow down the responsible localization beyond "the sympathetic pathway to the eye". This can also be supportive of an isolated vagosympathetic trunk lesion (second-order neurons).

DIFFERENTIAL DIAGNOSIS

Identifying the most likely differential diagnoses is easiest with a focal lesion localization. The list of possible diseases can be very different if the lesion localizes to the spinal cord, the brachial plexus, the vagosympathetic trunk or the middle-inner ear.

We can separate this into three main neuro-anatomical segments:

- **First-order neuron**

  This part of the pathway includes the brainstem and the cervicothoracic spinal cord to the level of T1–3. Any structural disease that can damage these neurons will cause Horner syndrome. The more common diseases include inflammatory disease (most commonly viral infections

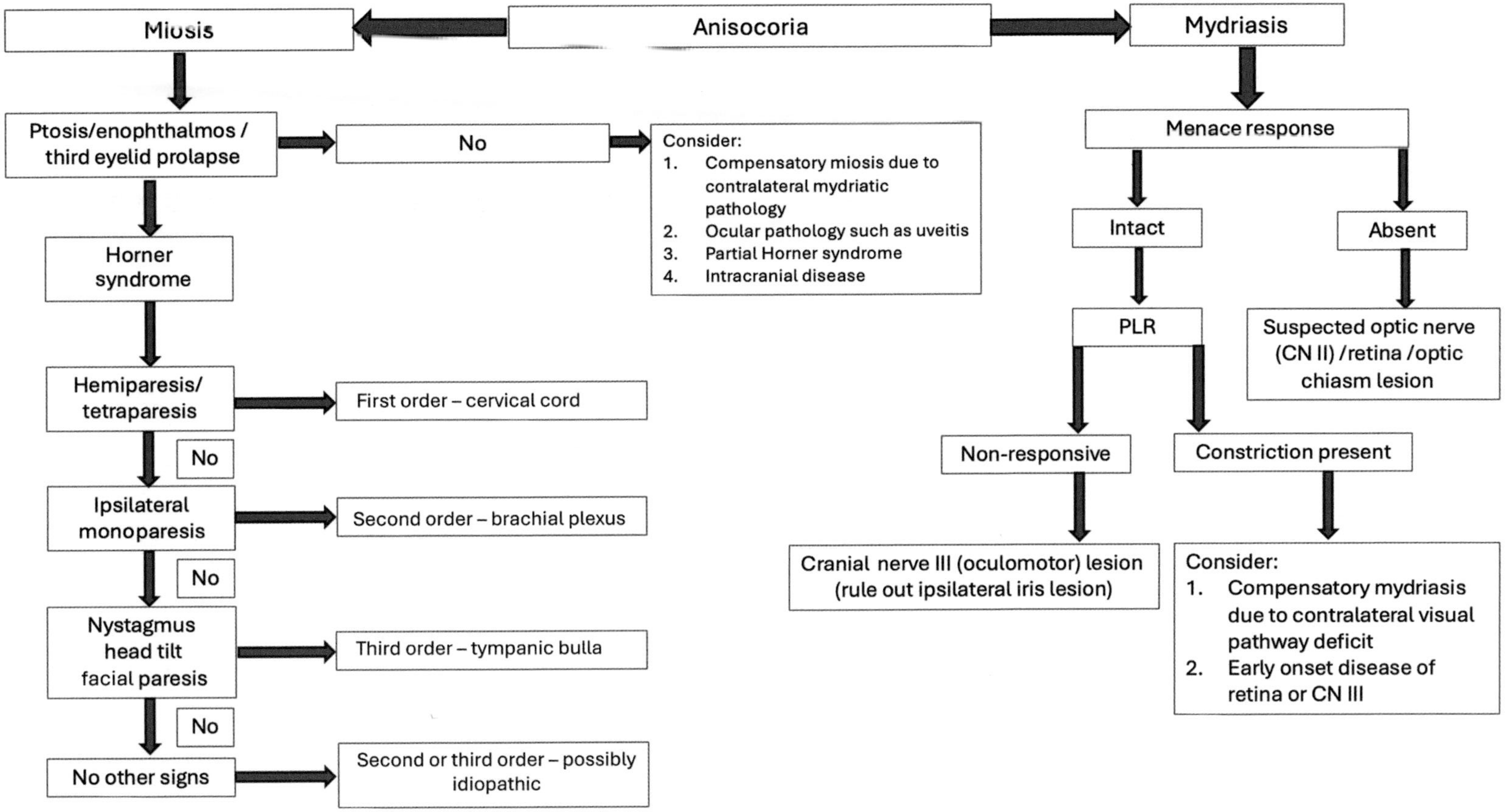

FIGURE 6.3.4 An algorithmic approach to the neuranatomic localization of anisocoria and Horner syndrome.

such as FIP in cats and sterile meningoencephalitis of unknown origin [MUO] in dogs) and neoplasia. These diseases can affect either the brainstem or the spinal cord. Additional common spinal cord diseases include fibrocartilaginous embolism (FCE) and intervertebral disc extrusions (IVDE). In one report reviewing a series of dogs with cervical myelopathy and Horner syndrome, 58% had non-compressive disease; 80% of those cases were diagnosed with FCE (Figure 6.3.5). In animals with compressive disease, 77% had some form of IVDE including Hanson type I, Hansen type II and hydrated nucleus pulposus extrusion (HNPE); 18% of these cases had an extramedullary tumor.

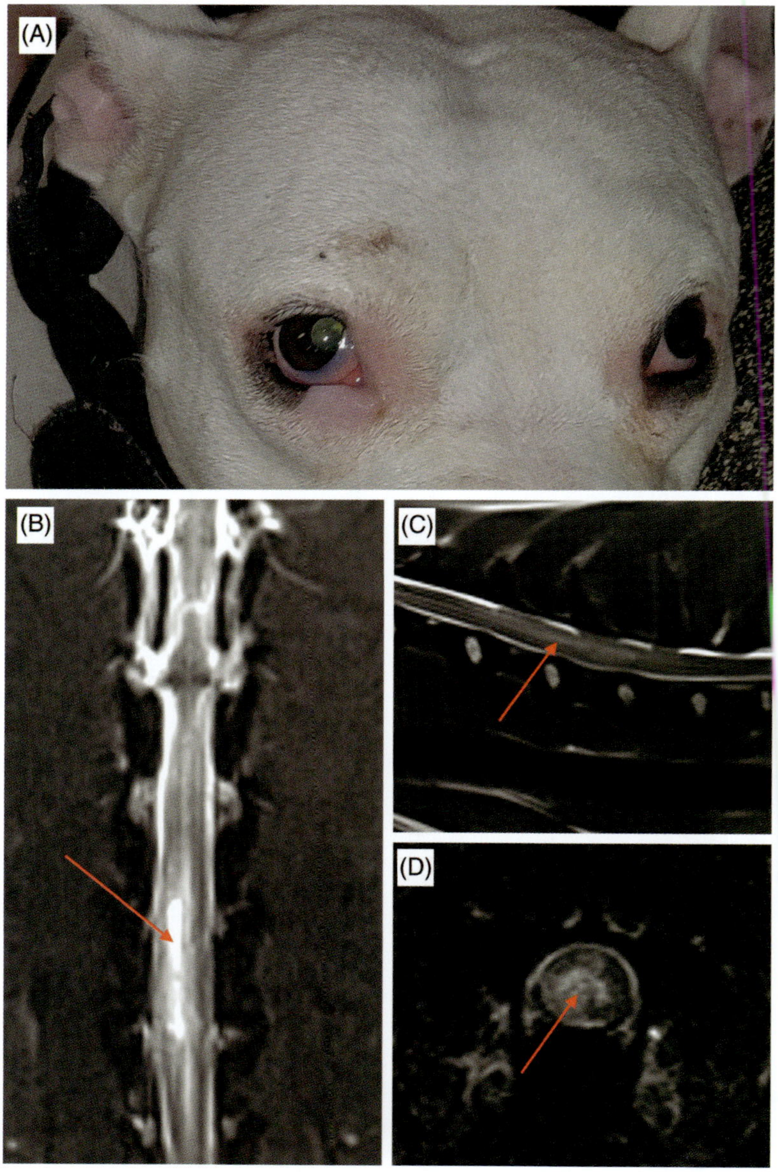

FIGURE 6.3.5 (A) An 8-year-old spayed female pit bull terrier presented with a history of acute onset of non-ambulatory tetraparesis that was worse on the right side. The dog's right eye exhibits miosis and third-eyelid protrusion compatible with Horner syndrome. (B) A T2W dorsal, (C) a T2W sagittal and (D) a T2W transverse MR image depicting an ill-defined and irregular right sided intramedullary lesion (arrows), centered over C5–C6, which is heterogeneously hyperintense to normal cord. The lesion is compatible with ischemic myelopathy likely secondary to fibrocartilaginous embolic myelopathy affecting the first-order sympathetic neuron.

- **Second-order (pre-ganglionic) neuron**

  This part of the pathway bilaterally includes the proximal nerve roots in the brachial plexus, the dorsal thoracic cavity, the cranial mediastinum, the thoracic inlet, the jugular groove, and the vicinity of the tympanic bulla. By far, the most common disease diagnosed with this localization is *Idiopathic Horner syndrome* followed by brachial plexus trauma. In a review of the available literature diagnosing Horner syndrome in small animals, 73% of cases localizing to the second-order neuron were determined to be an idiopathic Horner syndrome, 19% were caused by brachial plexus avulsions, and only 2% were caused by neoplasia (Video 6.3.1; Figure 6.3.6).

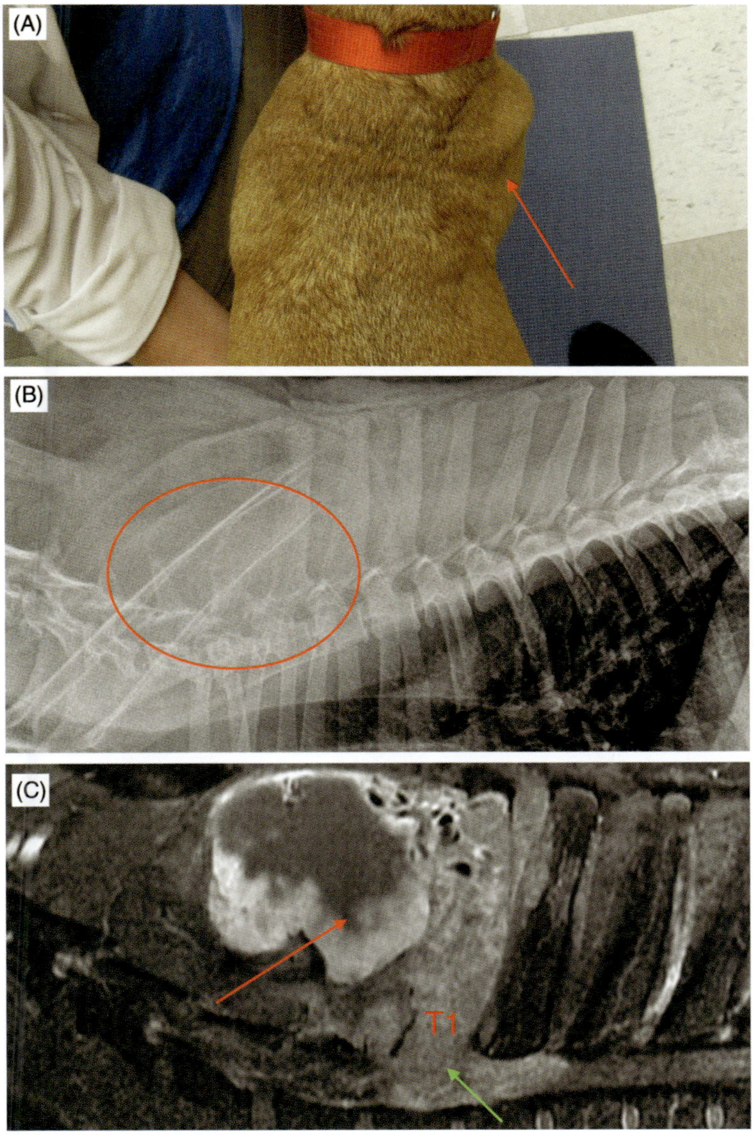

FIGURE 6.3.6 (A) Dorsal view of the shoulders of the 12-year-old neutered male mixed breed dog seen in Video 6.3.1. There is severe muscle wasting of the right shoulder (arrow). (B) A lateral radiograph of the cervicothoracic spine of this dog demonstrates near total lysis of the T1 spinous process and lytic changes also seen along the cranial edge of the T2 spinous process (red oval). (C) A T1-weighted, post-contrast sagittal image of the cervicothoracic spine of the same dog. A large mass (red arrow) is present extending from the level of the nuchal ligament ventrally to the level of the vertebral canal and nerve roots (green arrow) at the level of T1. Aspirate cytology was suggestive of a sarcoma tumor.

VIDEO 6.3.1 This is a 12-year-old male castrated mixed breed dog with a history of slowly progressing right thoracic limb lameness over 6 months. The dog started with subtle limping that progressed to periodic knuckling, then dragging the limb. For the last 2 weeks, he has been unable to use the limb at all. Note the global brachial plexus dysfunction with the inability to bear weight or lift the limb. See Figure 6.3.6.

- **Third-order (post-ganglionic) neuron**

  This part of the pathway includes the tympanic bulla area and the inner ear (in the segment of the skull immediately adjacent to the tympanic bulla), the middle cranial fossa (in the region of the cavernous sinus), and the retrobulbar space. The most common diseases that affect this part of the sympathetic pathway include infectious otitis media-interna (46%), iatrogenic (23%; secondary to otic surgeries or topical cleanings/medications), and idiopathic Horner syndrome (23%).

INVESTIGATION (Figure 6.3.7)

Diagnostic investigations might include two separate goals: confirming lesion localization and achieving a definitive disease diagnosis.

Three types of investigations address these goals:

1. Pharmacological testing to identify localization within the three-neuron pathway.
2. Targeted physical examination to confirm the broad neuroanatomic lesion location and look for evidence of underlying diseases.
3. Focused imaging and ancillary diagnostic tests to try to achieve a final disease diagnosis

- **Pharmacological testing**

  There are several drugs that have been reported for use in the evaluation of Horner syndrome including phenylephrine, cocaine, hydroxyamphetamine, and apraclonidine. Of these, only phenylephrine is used routinely in small animal patients owing to its easy access and lower chance of inconclusive test results. Phenylephrine is a sympathomimetic drug that can be used to try to distinguish between preganglionic (first and second-order neuron) and postganglionic (third order) lesions (Video 6.3.2). This test attempts to capitalize on a phenomenon called

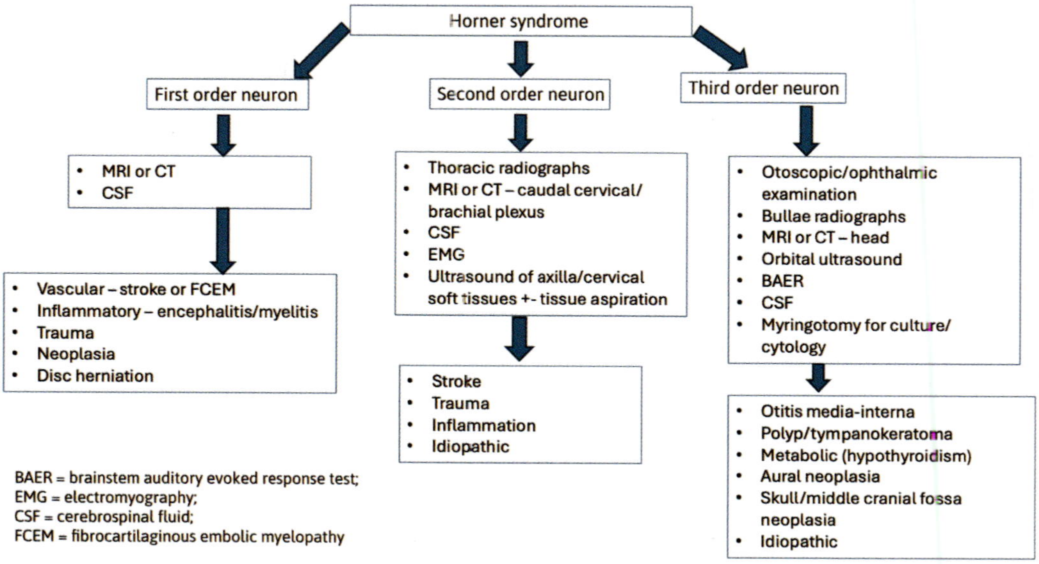

FIGURE 6.3.7 Diagnostic approach to Horner syndrome based on lesion localization. BAER = brainstem auditory evoked response test; EMG = electromyography; CSF = cerebrospinal fluid; FCEM = fibrocartilaginous embolic myelopathy.

"denervation hypersensitivity" that renders the postsynaptic muscle hyper-responsive to sub-physiological levels of the neurotransmitter. It is important to note that low doses of phenylephrine are required to highlight this phenomenon since higher doses will stimulate both abnormal and normal eyes and can be more difficult to interpret. Denervation hypersensitivity can take 2–3 weeks to develop in the average patient, so the duration of clinical signs must be taken into account when trying to interpret phenylephrine testing.

VIDEO 6.3.2 This 13-year-old neutered male Dalmatian presented with a 1-week history of bilateral Horner syndrome. He has a history of chronic mild protrusion of the right third eyelid due to "Cherry Eye" that was surgically corrected many years ago. Both eyelids are now very prominent along with classic miosis, ptosis, and enophthalmus. The signs of Horner syndrome resolved 18 minutes post-phenylephrine administration, supporting a third-order lesion. Advanced diagnostics could not be performed, so the underlying cause is unknown, though the signs did improve spontaneously in the next few weeks.

ESSENTIAL PROTOCOL

1. Perform the test in a room with controlled lighting (to ensure the same level of light stimulus at all times).
2. Ensure both eyes are clear and free from discharge or excessive tearing.
3. Use 0.5–1% phenylephrine ophthalmic solution.
4. Instill one drop into each eye at essentially the same time. In unilateral cases, you are using the "normal" eye as a timed control for comparison.
5. Within 1–2 minutes, instill a second drop into each eye to ensure adequate drug application.
6. Observe the eyes every 3–5 minutes for 60 minutes or until dilation is achieved. You should also see the resolution of ptosis, enophthalmos, and third eyelid elevation. Record the time at which pupil dilation is achieved for each eye.
7. If there is any question about the duration of clinical signs in the face of a negative or prolonged result on the phenylephrine test, the pet can return in 2–3 weeks to repeat the test. Cases that do not respond at the initial visit, then respond in less than 20 minutes at the second visit, can indicate a postganglionic lesion that needed more time to develop denervation hypersensitivity.

Please see Table 6.3.2 for a summary of expectations based on the concentration of phenylephrine and the duration of the disease.

Table 6.3.2 Pharmacological evaluation of Horner syndrome.

Drug	Normal eye	Horner eye
Phenylephrine 0.5–1% Tested in the ACUTE phase <2–3 weeks	No effect	No effect *May see dilation in >20 minutes in transition phase
Phenylephrine 0.5–1% Tested in the CHRONIC phase >2–3 weeks MOST USEFUL METHOD	No effect	• Third-order lesions dilate <20 minutes • No effect on first or second-order lesions
Phenylephrine 10%	Pupil dilates in 20–40 minutes *Note: Miosis due to other pathologies like uveitis will also dilate with this drug*	• Third-order lesions dilate <20 minutes • First- and second-order lesions dilate 20–40 minutes

Although phenylephrine is used to try to better distinguish lesion localization, there is some overlap in how an individual pet may respond to this test. This appears to be most relevant for third-order lesions that will sometimes have a delayed response despite a diagnosis confirming lesion location. The opposite does not appear to be true, so if a pet has a rapid response to dilute phenylephrine, then the pet likely has a true third-order, post-ganglionic lesion.

- **Targeted physical exam and careful history**

  As with most of our neurological patients, a multifaceted approach to diagnosis including a careful physical examination and detailed history is essential. In animals with Horner syndrome, special attention is paid to:

  1. The neurological exam to try to rule in evidence of pathology in the brain, spinal cord, or brachial plexus. Ask about any changes in strength, coordination, and mental state at home.
  2. The otic exam to try to rule in evidence of otitis or otic masses. Ask about any head shaking, ear scratching, or signs of ear pain.
  3. Palpating the cervical area to look for signs of diseases affecting the jugular groove. Ask about any recent blood draws or other recent cervical trauma.
  4. Respiratory character and auscultation to rule in evidence of intrathoracic disease.
  5. Examination of the eyes and face to rule in evidence of retrobulbar pathology.

- **Imaging and additional diagnostic tests**

  1. Thoracic radiographs to look for diseases like mediastinal masses.
  2. MRI of the brain, middle and inner ears, neck, and/or brachial plexus based on your neuroanatomic localization (Figure 6.3.8).

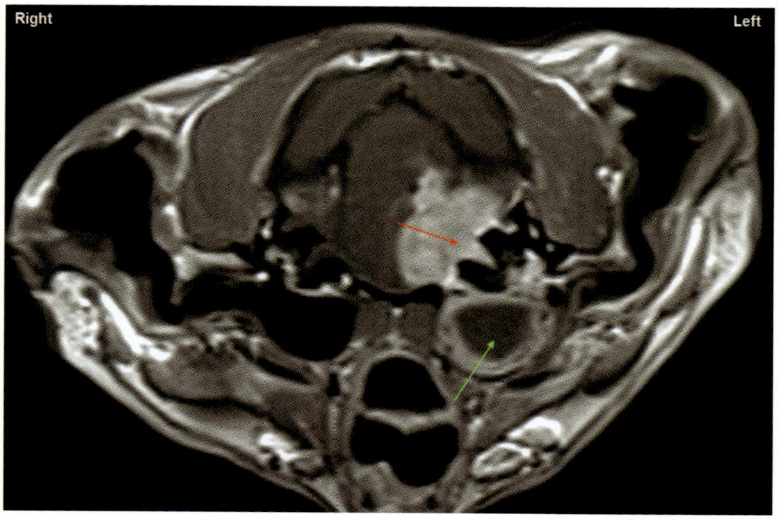

FIGURE 6.3.8 A T1W post contrast transverse MRI of a 6 year old spayed female domestic shorthaired cat with a history of chronic left ear infection that was not resolving with repeat courses of Clavamox. She became more dull 2 weeks prior to admission and acutely developed a left head tilt, stumbling gait, and horizontal nystagmus a week later with Horner syndrome in the left eye. There is obliteration of the left tympanic cavity with peripheral ring-enhancing material (green arrow) and extension of this material along the vestibulocochlear nerve into the cranial cavity to become a space occupying mass (red arrow). The MRI supports otitis media-interna with intracranial extension to abscessation and empyema.

3. Myringotomy with culture/cytology, CSF analysis, infectious disease testing, and biopsies as indicated based on imaging results

OUTCOME

In animals presenting with Horner syndrome in the absence of other neurological abnormalities, only 3–18% of cases will have an identifiable lesion on advanced diagnostics. The rest may achieve a "diagnosis by exclusion" of idiopathic Horner syndrome.

The patient in this case had a positive 1% phenylephrine test with dilation of the affected pupil at 14 minutes. Head MRI and CSF analysis were considered normal. The cat was diagnosed with presumed idiopathic Horner syndrome. Within 1 month, the cat's Horner syndrome spontaneously resolved (Figure 6.3.9).

The prognosis for idiopathic Horner syndrome is excellent. Most cases spontaneously resolve within 4 months. In those cases that do not resolve, the result is usually cosmetic without impacting quality of life.

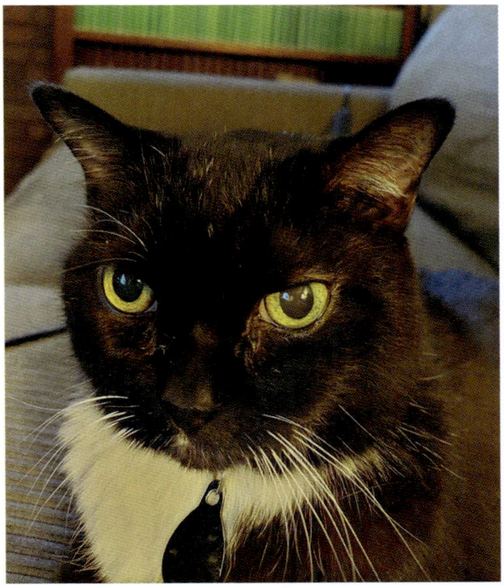

FIGURE 6.3.9 The 10-year-old neutered male domestic shorthaired cat in Figure 6.3.1, 1 month later, showing spontaneous resolution of the Horner syndrome in the left eye with mild residual miosis.

SUGGESTED READING

De Lahunta, A., Glass, E., and Kent, M. (2021). *Veterinary Neuroanatomy and Clinical Neurology*, 5e. Philadelphia: Elsevier.

Lockhart, R.L., Tzouganakis, I., Tsvetanova, A. et al. (2022) The diagnostic yield of advanced imaging in dogs with Horner's syndrome presenting with and without additional clinical signs: a retrospective study of 120 cases (2000–2018). *Vet. Ophthalmol.* 25 (Suppl. 1): 51–59.

Murthy, V., Phillips, K., Knipe, M. et al. (2023). Horner syndrome as a physiological biomarker of disease in canine cervical myelopathy. *J. Vet. Intern. Med.* 37: 598–605.

Simpson, K.M., Williams, D.L., and Cherubini, G.B. (2015). Neuropharmacological lesion localization in idiopathic Horner's syndrome in golden retrievers and dogs of other breeds. *Vet. Ophthalmol.* 18 (1): 1–5.

Zwueste, D.M. and Grahn, B.H. (2019). A review of Horner's syndrome in small animals. *Can. Vet. J.* 60: 81–88.

CHAPTER 6.4

Abnormalities of Vision, Pupil Size, and Eye Position

Case 4—Blindness and Depression in a Dog

Rose K. Peters

Veterinary Clinical Neurology, University of Illinois at Urbana-Champaign, Urbana, IL, USA

CASE HISTORY

A 6-month-old neutered male Yorkshire Terrier was presented for evaluation of lethargy and acute onset blindness. In the last several months, he has had episodes of reduced levels of consciousness that would usually resolve within a few hours. At one point, the owners found him standing facing a corner and he didn't seem to know where he was. One day prior to presentation, he was his normal, playful self with a great appetite. On presentation, he was much more sluggish than usual, and he was seen bumping into furniture.

One week ago, the owners started feeding him a homemade raw meat diet almost exclusively composed of chicken breast and steak. They tried mixing in carrots and green beans, but he ate around the vegetables. He is up to date on his vaccines and is not on any medications or supplements.

NEUROLOGICAL EXAMINATION

The dog was very dull with an element of confusion. When not being directly stimulated, he would fall asleep on the exam table. When placed on the floor, he would mechanically walk around the room without focus. He would bump into furniture and tried to head-press against a baby gate (Video 6.4.1). He had absent menace OU with normal pupil size and intact palpebral and pupillary light reflexes (PLR).

VIDEO 6.4.1 A 6-month-old castrated male Yorkshire Terrier that was presented for evaluation of lethargy and acute onset blindness. The video shows the dog with a reduced level of consciousness falling asleep on the exam table. When placed on the floor, he mechanically walks around the room without focus. He bumps into furniture and tries to head-press against a baby gate.

1. **Where is the likely lesion localization?**
2. **What major disease processes should be considered?**
3. **What tests could you perform to help determine the diagnosis?**

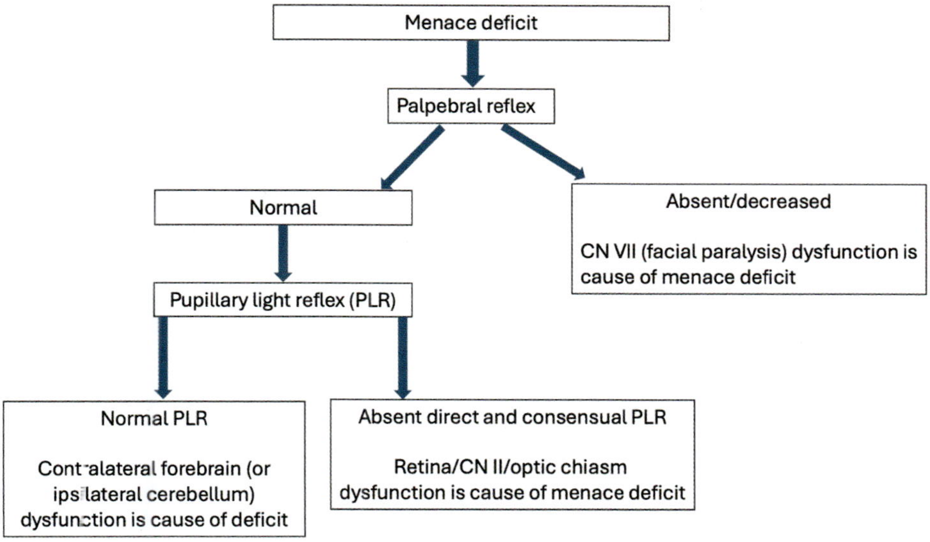

FIGURE 6.4.1 Localization algorithm for absent menace response.

LESION LOCALIZATION (Figure 6.4.1)

The dog appears to be blind based on difficulty navigating around objects. The lack of mydriasis or PLR deficits makes pre-chiasmal (ocular and optic nerve) diseases unlikely. Blindness with normal pupil function is consistent with "central blindness," which is also sometimes termed "cortical blindness" or "cerebral blindness." Central blindness occurs in association with pathology affecting the visual pathway components within the brain. Confusion and head-pressing behaviors are found with forebrain disease. These examination findings support bilateral occipital cortex dysfunction, which is the part of the brain responsible for conscious awareness of visual stimuli (see Chapter 6 Case 2 for an overview of the visual pathways).

> **Tips:** When trying to determine if an absent menace response indicates central blindness, don't assess unilateral visual function using dropped cotton balls, laser pointers on the floor, and similar stimuli. Animals with cerebellar disease might have a "visual menace deficit" in which the pet will not respond to a menace test but has no visual impairment (See Video 6.4.3).

VIDEO 6.4.2 Video of a 9-year-old spayed female mixed breed dog that was presented for recent onset seizures and lethargy. Note how the dog ignores the visual stimulus from the right side. This dog also adopts a leftward head and body turn (Figure 6.4.2) that supports a left-sided cerebrothalamic lesion.

VIDEO 6.4.3 Video of a 4-year-old neutered male pit bull terrier with slowly progressive cerebellar ataxia. The dog presented with normal navigation and no other outward signs of visual difficulty. Despite this, the dog is not demonstrating a normal menace response in either eye. The dog demonstrates intact visual function in both eyes by tracking dropped cotton balls. In cases with visual menace deficit, other signs of cerebellar dysfunction will be evident.

DIFFERENTIAL DIAGNOSIS

Differential diagnoses for this case should include diseases that can cause bilateral blindness with a "waxing and waning" nature based on the historical transient changes in level of consciousness:

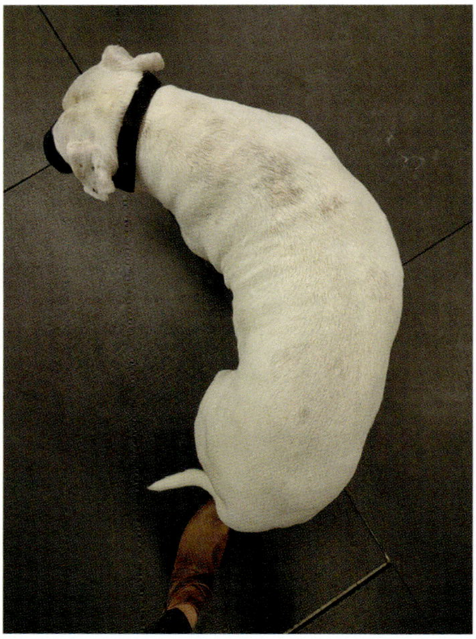

FIGURE 6.4.2 Central blindness – unilateral head turn. The dog seen in Video 6.4.2 periodically adopts a left head and body turn consistent with a left cerebrothalamic lesion.

Metabolic Disease – Portosystemic Shunt (PSS)

Portosystemic shunting is a condition in which portal blood from the gastrointestinal tract, pancreas, and spleen is allowed to bypass the liver and flow directly into systemic circulation via abnormal blood vessel formation. This results in toxins like ammonia, tryptophan, glutamine, aromatic amino acids, short-chain fatty acids, GABA, and endogenous benzodiazepines accumulating, which can result in hepatic encephalopathy. Hepatic encephalopathy signs can range from a mildly depressed mental state to seizures and coma (Table 6.4.1). Signs can be episodic and are often worse after meals.

Portosystemic shunts are categorized according to when the condition develops (congenital or acquired) and location (intrahepatic versus extrahepatic). This condition is more common in small and toy breed dogs, and one study reported that the Yorkshire Terrier is over 35 times more likely to be affected with an extrahepatic portosystemic shunt compared to all other breeds combined.

Anomalous Disease – Hydrocephalus

Hydrocephalus is a condition characterized by an abnormal accumulation of cerebrospinal fluid (CSF) in the cranial vault. Hydrocephalus is categorized in several ways. Most often, the disease is likely multifactorial with one or more of the characteristics detailed in Table 6.4.2.

Table 6.4.1 A clinical severity staging system proposed for hepatic encephalopathy.

Stages of hepatic encephalopathy	
Stage I	Mild lethargy and confusion, inappetence
Stage II	Lethargy, personality changes, mild ataxia, disorientation
Stage III	Stupor, pronounced ataxia, ptyalism, head pressing, blindness, circling
Stage IV	Recumbency, coma, seizures, death

Table 6.4.2 Overview of the classification and clinical characteristics of hydrocephalus.

Etiology	Congenital	Animals are born with hydrocephalus as part of an anomalous birth defect: E.g. stenosis of the mesencephalic aqueduct or lateral apertures.
	Acquired	Hydrocephalus may be acquired associated with any disease that develops later in life, obstructing CSF flow. E.g. neoplasia
Onset	Acute	Recent onset of actively accumulating CSF. This may be more common in cases of inflammatory disease or neoplasia.
	Chronic	Long-standing hydrocephalus that can have varying rates and degrees of progression.
Location of hydrocephalus	Internal	Accumulation of fluid inside the ventricular system with enlargement of the ventricles
	External	Accumulation of fluid outside the ventricular system with enlargement of the subarachnoid space
Nature of fluid accumulation	Obstructive	Accumulation of CSF due to obstruction of CSF outflow
	Non-obstructive	An example is "hydrocephalus ex-vacuo" in which CSF passively fills in empty space resulting from brain atrophy or other loss of normal brain parenchyma (E.g. post-inflammation).
Consequences of fluid accumulation	Hypertensive	Increased pressure within the ventricle.
	Non-hypertensive	Normal intracranial pressure.

Congenital internal hydrocephalus is one of the more common forms, which likely has a multifactorial cause, including congenital malformation of the mesencephalic aqueduct, that restricts CSF flow. As CSF accumulates in the lateral ventricles, progressive cerebral atrophy can occur secondarily. With ongoing loss of functional cerebral tissue, animals will develop progressive forebrain signs that can include varying degrees of obtundation, agitation, confusion and disorientation, pacing, circling, visual deficits, seizures, and head pressing (Video 6.4.4). If fluid accumulates within the fourth ventricle, it will compress the brainstem and cerebellum, and be associated with vestibular signs, paresis, and proprioceptive deficits.

Congenital hydrocephalus is more common in small and toy-breed dogs, including the Yorkshire Terrier; it can be accompanied by skull conformation changes that include a domed skull and malformations of the orbits leading to bilateral ventrolateral strabismus (Figure 6.4.3).

VIDEO 6.4.4 Video of a 4-month-old intact male Pug puppy presented for evaluation for circling, blindness, and incoordination secondary to hydrocephalus. Mild thoracic limb hypermetria, intermittent circling, and poor vision are appreciable.

Inflammatory Disease

Inflammatory disease affecting the brain is termed "encephalitis". Encephalitis is generally divided into two categories: infectious and sterile/immune-mediated inflammation.

Meningoencephalitis of unknown origin (MUO)

MUO is considered a noninfectious form of brain inflammation that is most likely immune-mediated in nature. Dogs of any breed and nearly any age can be affected. More specific syndromes within this category can include granulomatous meningoencephalitis (GME), necrotizing meningoencephalitis (NME), and necrotizing leukoencephalitis (NLE), which are based on a histopathological diagnosis. The Yorkshire Terrier breed is prone to NLE, which can manifest with signs of forebrain and/or brainstem pathology that progresses over several days to a few

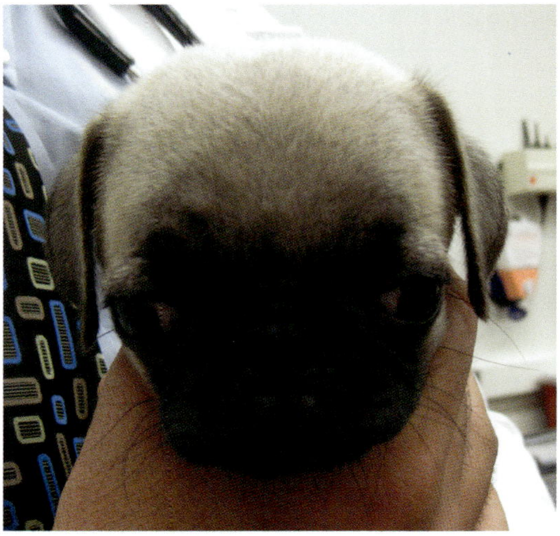

FIGURE 6.4.3 A 4-month-old male Pug puppy with a domed head and divergent strabismus that is supportive of congenital hydrocephalus.

weeks (Video 6.4.5). Animals affected with NME and NLE tend to be younger, averaging around 18 months of age. Animals with GME may have a later distribution of 4–8 years, though animals as young as 6 months of age have been reported to be affected. Across all forms of MUO, dogs as young as 11 weeks of age have been identified, so this disease cannot be ruled out due to age. In this case, the chronic, intermittent course makes MUO less likely.

Infection

Infectious agents that can cause inflammation in the brain more commonly include viral, bacterial, fungal, and protozoal diseases. Less frequent infections include parasitic, rickettsial, amoeboid, and algal organisms. Fewer than 20% of appropriately vaccinated dogs diagnosed with encephalitis using MRI and CSF analysis have an identifiable infection.

VIDEO 6.4.5 Video of a 7-year-old female spayed Yorkshire Terrier with MUO (suspected NLE) causing asymmetric cerebrothalamic signs inclusive of blindness.

> While not compatible with our patient's clinical history, an important cause of bilateral central blindness is an iatrogenic brain injury. This might be seen after anesthetic events in which there was substantial systemic hypotension and/or hypoxia. Cats are also prone to a form of brain ischemia, associated with the use of spring-loaded mouth gags for dental procedures. Excessive jaw retraction occludes the maxillary artery that contributes to the blood supply of the visual cortex in cats.
>
> Common causes of unilateral central blindness in dogs and cats include trauma, inflammatory disease, neoplasia, and infarction (hemorrhagic or ischemic stroke).

INVESTIGATION

Portosystemic Shunt

Blood and urine testing can often be suggestive in these cases:

1. **Complete blood count (CBC)**
   Mild non-regenerative anemia can be present, though this is seen more often in cases of intrahepatic PSS (31% versus 6% of extrahepatic shunts). Similarly, microcytosis, target cell formation, and hypochromia may also be noted. The CBC can also be very normal.

2. **Serum chemistry profile**
   Liver function parameters can be reduced from their normal values, including albumin, cholesterol, BUN, creatinine, and glucose. The liver enzymes, ALT and AlkP, can be increased or may be normal. Most animals with congenital PSS will have normal bilirubin levels.

3. **Urinalysis**
   Ammonium biurate crystals may be present in 26–57% of dogs with PSS. Over 50% of cases may exhibit isosthenuria or hyposthenuria.

4. **Bile acids and ammonia blood levels**
   Pre- and post-prandial bile acids and ammonia levels can also be elevated. Bile acid elevations higher than 100 umol/L are very suggestive of true functional pathology, though both bile acids and ammonia tests are at risk for false positive and false negative results.

Several imaging modalities can assist with the diagnosis of a portosystemic shunt, including contrast radiography, abdominal ultrasound, CT-angiography, nuclear scintigraphy, portograms, and MRI. Of these, abdominal ultrasound and CT-angiography are the most practical and commonly performed:

1. **Abdominal ultrasound**
   This is one of the more commonly used methods owing to the relative accessibility, affordability, and ease of performing the procedure. That being said, diagnostic utility is dependent on operator skill, contributing to sensitivity ranging from 74% to 95% and specificities of 67–100%. Ultrasound may identify microhepatica and anomalous intra- or extrahepatic vessels.

2. **Contrast computed tomography (CT)**
   Abdominal CT-angiography can provide a much more detailed view of the abdominal vascular anatomy compared to what can be appreciated on abdominal ultrasound. If there is not a readily identifiable abnormal vessel on ultrasound, then CT-angiography is the next best step for trying to identify the presence of (and number and nature of) any vascular anomalies.

Hydrocephalus

Some animals will exhibit compatible physical exam changes including a domed head, divergent ventrolateral strabismus, and may have a palpable open fontanelle. Definitive diagnosis is generally dependent on imaging the brain ventricles through one of the following methods:

1. **Ultrasound**
   If the pet has a large enough open fontanelle, a pediatric ultrasound probe can be gently used to identify ventricular enlargement and thinning of the cerebral cortex (Video 6.4.6).

2. **CT**
   A plain CT scan can show the size and shape of the ventricles (Figure 6.4.4), and can identify hydrocephalus, though soft tissue detail of the brain parenchyma is very limited, which can make it more difficult to identify other differentials for encephalopathy.

3. **MRI**
   MRI offers excellent soft tissue detail of the ventricular system as well as the rest of the brain (Figure 6.4.5). When an animal presents with neurological signs and the diagnosis of hydrocephalus is equivocal, MRI is the most informative imaging test, enabling the identification of other causative etiologies that include inflammatory disease, metabolic encephalopathies, and other congenital defects. Ventriculomegaly can be an incidental finding in some breeds, therefore a careful interpretation of results is required. The diagnosis of

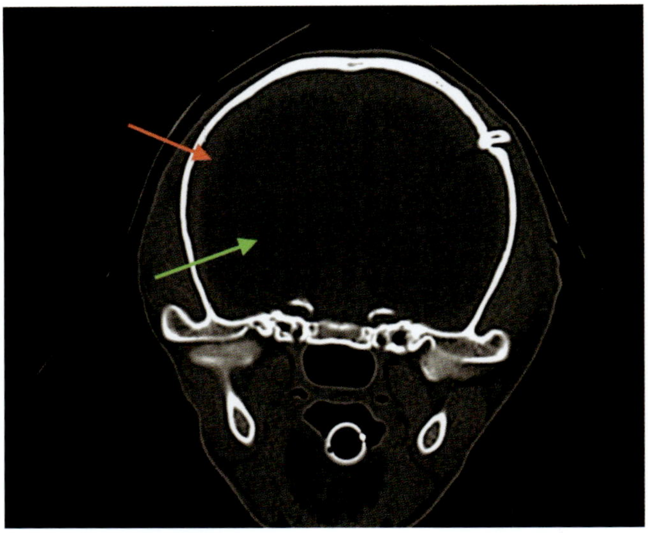

FIGURE 6.4.4 Transverse brain CT image of a dog with severe hydrocephalus (bilateral dilated and fused lateral ventricles [green arrow]), with near complete thinning of the cerebral cortex (red arrow).

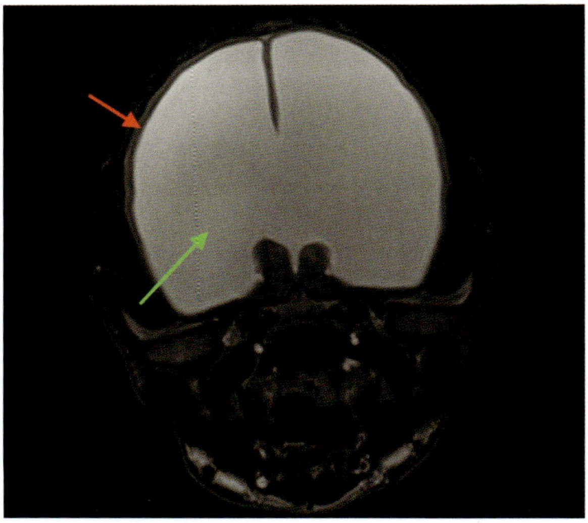

FIGURE 6.4.5 Transverse T2W MRI of a dog with severe hydrocephalus (bilateral dilated and fused lateral ventricles [green arrow]), with near complete thinning of the cerebral cortex (red arrow).

hydrocephalus rather than ventriculomegaly is supported in an animal with a ventricle, brain ratio of 0.6 or greater (indicating larger ventricles), and clinically compatible intracranial signs. Additional associated structural findings can include a dorsally deviated corpus callosum, dorsoventral flattening of the interthalamic adhesion, periventricular edema, dilation of the olfactory recesses, and thinning of the cortical sulci and subarachnoid space, and disruption of the internal capsule adjacent to the caudate nucleus.

VIDEO 6.4.6 Video of ultrasound through the fontanelle in a hydrocephalus puppy. Animals with an open fontanelle are candidates for ultrasound assessment of the ventricles. This patient has bilaterally dilated lateral ventricles consistent with hydrocephalus.

Inflammatory Disease

Inflammatory disease warrants a careful general physical and neurological examination as well as systemic health screening to answer the question: *Is this problem restricted to the nervous system, or is there multi-organ system involvement?* In cases in which there is multi-organ system involvement, infectious diseases or neoplasia (in an older pet) will be more likely. If the problem is restricted to the nervous system, both infectious and immune-mediated causes of CNS inflammation remain possible. Diagnostic testing includes:

1. **MRI**
   MRI of the brain provides the most informative detail of brain structure and any evidence of inflammatory-type lesions, which typically manifest as variably sized, ill-defined T2-weighted hyperintensities (Figure 6.4.6). Approximately 75% of these lesions display contrast enhancement. Up to approximately 25% of cases have a normal MRI despite obvious clinical neurological dysfunction. NME exclusively affects the cerebrum and will cause effacement of the gray-white matter distinction. NLE can cause lesions in both the cerebrum and brainstem and is localized in the white matter. GME and some other forms of MUO can be found in any part of the brain or spinal cord. These lesions may be difficult to distinguish from pathology caused by infection and some types of infarction and glial cell neoplasia without additional MRI sequences.

2. **CSF analysis**
   CSF analysis is performed in tandem with MRI imaging to help confirm inflammatory disease (Figure 6.4.7). In these cases, elevations in white blood cells (pleocytosis) and protein are used to support a diagnosis of CNS inflammation. Anywhere from 3% to 57% of dogs ultimately diagnosed with MUO can have relatively normal CSF parameters, which highlights the importance of utilizing MRI and CSF testing together. MRI might demonstrate inflammatory-type lesions with normal spinal fluid, or the spinal fluid might be quite inflammatory in the face of a normal MRI. Spinal fluid can also offer the opportunity for more sensitive infectious disease testing. For example, cats with neurological FIP will be more likely to have a positive FCoV-RT PCR CSF test compared to testing the blood.

3. **Regionally and individually appropriate infectious disease testing**
   When inflammatory CNS disease is suspected based on the results of MRI and CSF, infectious disease testing is pursued to rule in a readily identifiable infectious cause for the

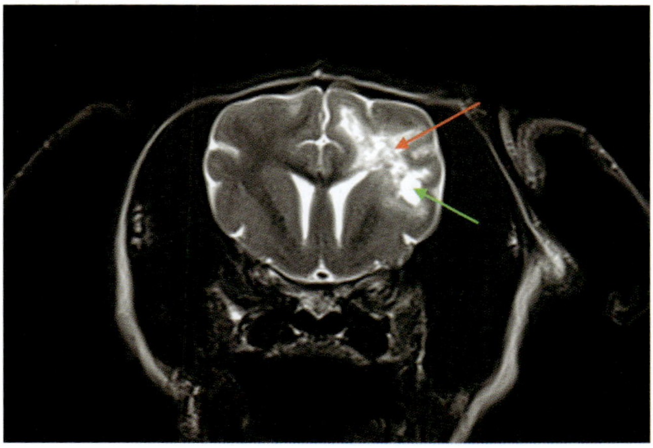

FIGURE 6.4.6 A T2-weighted transverse image of the brain from a 5-year-old female spayed Yorkshire Terrier with necrotizing leukoencephalopathy. There is extensive left-sided white matter hyperintensity (red arrow) with a suspect necrotic cavity (green arrow).

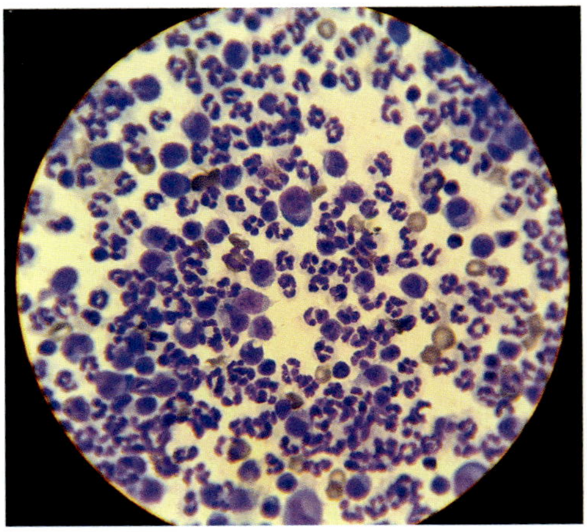

FIGURE 6.4.7 High-power field CSF cytology from a dog with granulomatous meningoencephalitis exhibiting a marked mixed-cell pleocytosis.

inflammation. Tests should be selected based on the clinical signs, species, lifestyle factors home region, any recent travel, recent exposure to any specific diseases, and the likelihood of achieving a useful result. In dogs, positive infectious test results are unusual, with fewer than 20% of inflammatory cases being attributed to an infection. In cats, the opposite is true, with the majority of cats suspected to have an infectious cause. In a review featuring cats with infectious CNS disease, 51% of cases were diagnosed with FIP, 35% were non-FIP viral diseases, 9% protozoal disease, 3% bacterial infection, 1% FIV, and 1% cryptococcus.

OUTCOME

The patient had elevated ALT (376 U/L) and AlkP (265 U/L), mildly low blood glucose (81 mg/dL), and elevated pre (78 umol/L) and post-prandial bile acids (126 umol/L). Ammonium biurate crystals were also seen in the urine sediment. Abdominal ultrasound confirmed a dilated vessel with blood flow in the left cranial quadrant between the liver and the stomach, which was consistent with a portosystemic shunt. The dog was treated overnight for hepatic encephalopathy with IV Norm-R fluids, IV metronidazole, and lactulose enemas. Video 6.4.7 is taken the next morning, demonstrating his return to normal attitude.

VIDEO 6.4.7 Video of the 6-month-old Yorkshire Terrier seen in Video 6.4.1, after medical management exhibiting barking and a normal mental state in the ICU cage.

SUGGESTED READING

Bach, F.S., Cray, C., Burgos, A.P. et al. (2023). A comparison between neurological clinical signs, cerebrospinal fluid analysis, cross-sectional CNS imaging, and infectious disease testing in 168 dogs with infectious or immune-mediated meningoencephalomyelitis from Brazil. *Front. Vet. Sci.* 10: 1239106.

Cornelis, I., Van Ham, L., Gielen, I. et al. (2019). Clinical presentation, diagnostic findings, prognostic factors, treatment, and outcome in dogs with meningoencephalomyelitis of unknown origin: a review. *Vet. J.* 244: 37–44.

Couture, Y., Keys, D., and Summers, S. (2024). Comparison of hematologic variables between dogs with congenital intrahepatic and extrahepatic portosystemic shunts. *J. Vet. Intern. Med.* 38: 1458–1464.

deLahunta, A., Glass, E., and Kent, M. (2021). *Veterinary Neuroanatomy and Clinical Neurology*, 5e. Philadelphia: Elsevier.

Falzone, C. and Lowrie, M. (2011). Blindness and behavioural changes in the cat: common neurological causes. *J. Feline Med. Surg.* 13: 863–873.

Farke, D., Olszewska, A., Buttner, K., and Schmidt, M.J. (2024). Association among raised intraventricular pressure, clinical signs, and magnetic resonance imaging findings in dogs with congenital internal hydrocephalus. *J. Vet. Intern. Med.* 38 (6): 3119–3128.

Galer, J., Forward, A., Hughes, J. et al. (2024). Clinical features, treatment, and outcomes of juvenile dogs with meningoencephalitis of unknown etiology. *J. Vet. Intern. Med.* 38: 2214–2220.

Goncalves, R., De Decker, S., Wamsley, G. et al. (2021). Inflammatory disease affecting the central nervous system in dogs: a retrospective study in England (2010-2019). *Front. Vet. Sci.* 8: 819945.

Goncalves, R., De Decker, S., Wamsley, G., and Maddox, T.W. (2024). Magnetic resonance imaging prognostic factors for survival and relapse in dogs with meningoencephalitis of unknown origin. *Front. Vet. Sci.* 11: 1370882.

Gunn-Moore, D. and Reed, N. (2011). CNS disease in the cat: current knowledge of infectious causes. *J. Feline Med. Surg* 13: 824–836.

Konstantinidis, A.O., Patsikas, M.N., Papazoglou, L.G., and Adamama-Moraitou, K.K. (2023). Congenital portosystemic shunts in dogs and cats: classification, pathophysiology, clinical presentation, and diagnosis. *Vet. Sci.* 10: 160.

Laubner, S., Ondreka, N., Failing, K. et al. (2015). Magnetic resonance imaging signs of high intraventricular pressure – comparison of findings in dogs with clinically relevant internal hydrocephalus and asymptomatic dogs with ventriculomegaly. *BMC Vet. Res.* 11: 181.

Lidbury, J.A., Cook, A.K., and Steiner, J.M. (2016). Hepatic encephalopathy in dogs and cats. *J. Vet. Emerg. Crit. Care* 26 (4): 471–487.

Ostrager, A., Bentley, T., Lewis, M., and Moore, G. (2024). Survival in dogs with meningoencephalomyelitis of unknown etiology with and without lesions detected by magnetic resonance imaging. *J. Vet. Intern. Med.* 38: 2204–2213.

Przyborowska, P., Adamiak, Z., and Zhalniarovich, Y. (2013). Hydrocephalus in dogs: a review. *Vet. Med.* 58 (2): 73–80.

Sarkar, S. and Tripathy, K. (2023). Cortical blindness. In: *StatPearls [Internet]*. Treasure Island, FL: StatPearls Publishing https://www.ncbi.nlm.nih.gov/books/NBK431128/.

Seruca, C., Rodenas, S., Leiva, M. et al. (2010). Acute postretinal blindness: ophthalmic, neurologic, and magnetic resonance imaging findings in dogs and cats (seven cases). *Vet. Ophthalmol.* 13 (5): 307–314.

Stiles, J., Weil, A.B., Packer, R.A., and Lantz, G.C. (2012). Post-anesthetic cortical blindness in cats: twenty cases. *Vet. J.* 193: 367–373.

Thomas, W.B. (2010). Hydrocephalus in dogs and cats. *Vet. Clin. Small Anim. Pract.* 40: 143–159.

Tobias, K. (2003). Determination of inheritance of single congenital portosystemic shunts in Yorkshire terriers. *J. Am. Anim. Hosp. Assoc.* 39 (4): 385–389.

Tobias, K.M. and Rohrbach, B.W. (2003). Association of breed with the diagnosis of congenital portosystemic shunts in dogs: 2,400 cases (1980-2002). *J. Am. Vet. Med. Assoc.* 223 (11): 1636–1639.

CHAPTER 7.1

Disorders of the Head and Face

Case 1—Acute Facial Paresis in a Dog

Amanda Brenna

Puget Sound Veterinary Specialty and Emergency, Gig Harbor, WA, USA

CASE HISTORY

A 7-year-old neutered male Boxer dog was presented for a 3-day history of left-sided facial drooping (Figure 7.1.1). The signs were first noted when the patient was at the food bowl, and the dog's owners noticed that occasionally food would drop out of the left side of his mouth. Later, the dog was observed to have an inability to blink in his left eye, although the third eyelid would elevate in response to motion near the eye. The dog did not seem to be in pain and was acting like his normal self at home. However, the owners had noticed some redness to the sclera of the left eye over the past day or so. The dog had a history of chronic, recurrent otitis externa in both ears and has been treated off and on with topical medications. Other than the history of chronic ear infections, the dog had no other health concerns and was up-to-date on vaccinations and flea, tick, and heartworm preventatives. He was not on any medications at the time of evaluation.

NEUROLOGIC AND PHYSICAL EXAMINATION

On neurologic examination, the dog was bright, alert, and responsive. He was ambulatory with no obvious ataxia or paresis in the thoracic or pelvic limbs. Postural reactions were normal based on proprioceptive positioning and hopping in all four limbs. Spinal reflexes were also normal (limited to flexor withdrawal and patellar reflexes). There was no evidence of pain or discomfort with deep palpation of the cervical and thoracolumbar vertebral columns. The dog's cranial nerve examination revealed an absent menace response and an absent palpebral reflex on the left side, though the third eyelid was observed elevating over the opened eye during these tests. Drooping of the left side of the muzzle and ear was noted, though sensation remained intact; saliva drooled out of this side. Mild crusting discharge was noted to be affecting the external perimeter of the left nare. The left pupil was noted to be mildly miotic, while the right remained mid-range. Pupillary light response (both direct and consensual) was normal in each eye. The Schirmer tear test was reduced on the left side but was normal on the right.

Key questions to consider

1. What is the likely lesion localization?
2. What are the most appropriate ranked differential diagnoses?
3. What are the best next diagnostic steps for this patient?

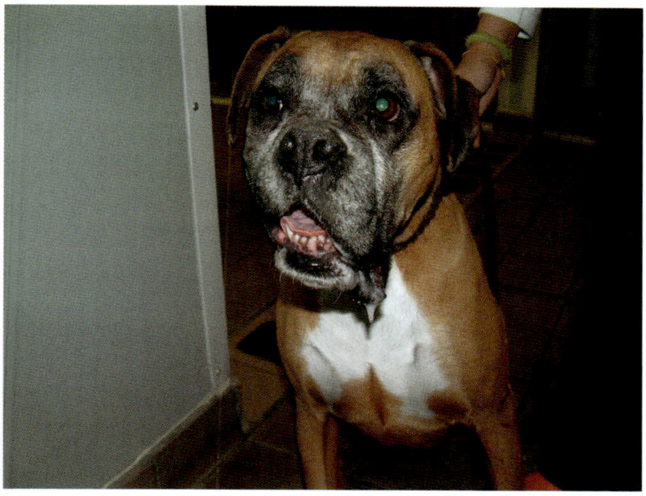

FIGURE 7.1.1 A Boxer dog with a left-sided facial droop and ipsilateral drooling of saliva.

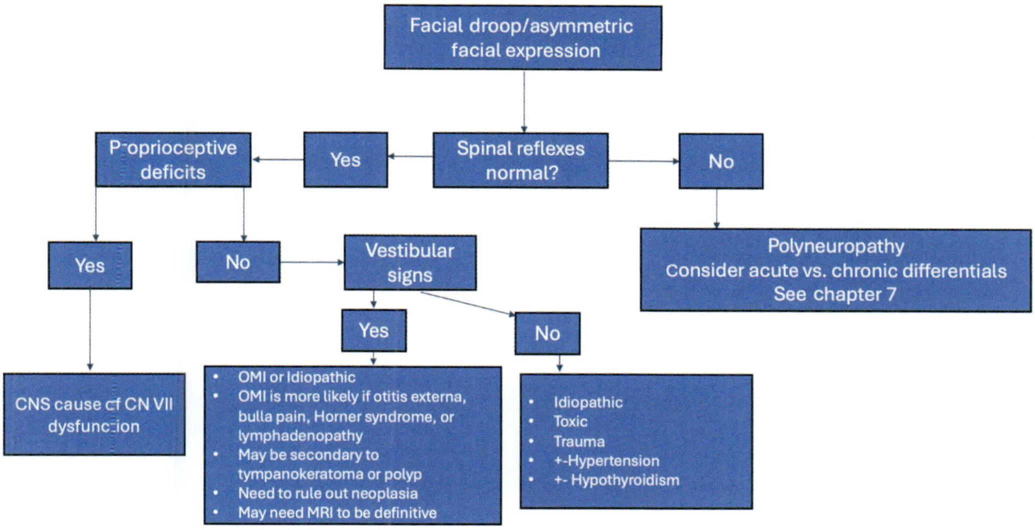

FIGURE 7.1.2 Algorithmic approach to localizing the lesion responsible for facial paresis. OMI = otitis media-interna.

LESION LOCALIZATION (Figure 7.1.2)

The most likely lesion localization for this patient is the left facial nerve (cranial nerve VII). The lesion is most likely to be a peripheral cranial neuropathy, given the lack of proprioceptive deficits, rather than a central cranial neuropathy or brainstem disease. However, it is important to note that intracranial disease can never fully be ruled out in the case of facial paresis. Normal spinal reflexes help to rule out a more diffuse polyneuropathy as the lesion localization, which can also result in proprioceptive deficits.

The miosis in the left pupil in this case could indicate concurrent Horner syndrome or involvement of the oculomotor nerve (cranial nerve III). However, given the history of facial paresis, reduced Schirmer tear test results, and scleral injection, the most likely cause for miosis in this patient is superficial corneal ulceration secondary to neurogenic keratoconjunctivitis sicca. Corneal

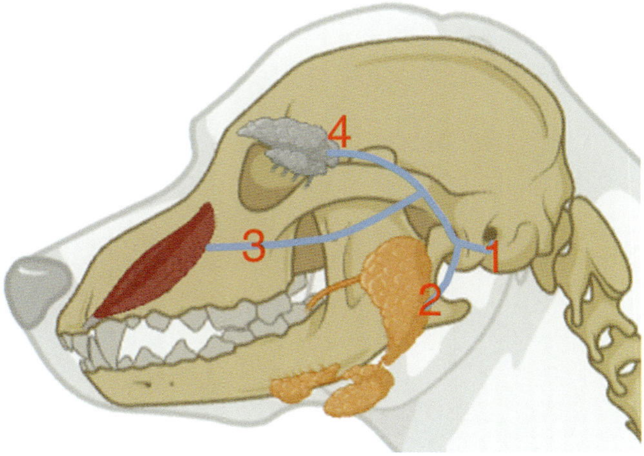

FIGURE 7.1.3 A schematic illustration of the structures innervated by the peripheral facial nerve. (1) The facial nerve exits the stylomastoid foramen of the skull to innervate the mandibular and sublingual salivary glands (2) and the muscles of facial expression (3). The greater petrosal nerve innervates the lacrimal gland (4) *Source:* Created with www.biorender.com.

ulceration is one of the leading causes of miosis in any patient and should be definitively ruled out before interpreting miosis as indicative of Horner syndrome or other neurologic dysfunction. Neurogenic keratoconjunctivitis sicca (KCS), however, is usually unilateral and occurs due to a failure of parasympathetic innervation to the lacrimal glands.

Crusting nasal discharge of the left nare can also be attributed to involvement of the autonomic contributions of the facial nerve. Parasympathetic denervation of the lateral nasal gland leads to unilateral desiccation and crusting called xeromycteria. See below for more details.

The neuroanatomy of the facial nerve responsible for these clinical signs is detailed below (Figure 7.1.3).

- The cell bodies of the motor neurons in the *facial nerve* are located in the facial nucleus in the rostral medulla.
- The axons of these cell bodies emerge from the brainstem ventral to the *vestibulocochlear nerve* (cranial nerve [CN] VIII). These nerves travel together through the internal acoustic *meatus* of the petrosal portion of the *temporal bone*, and then the facial nerve emerges to its extracranial location through the *stylomastoid foramen* [1].
- Branches of the facial nerve are distributed to the muscles of facial expression. These are the relatively thin muscles of the ear, eyelids, nose, cheeks, and lips. Dysfunction of this nerve results in clinical signs such as muzzle or ear droop, as well as menace response and palpebral reflex deficits. The menace response test involves the afferent branch (optic nerve, cranial nerve II) and the efferent branch (facial nerve, cranial nerve VII) (see Figure 4; Chapter 6, Case 2). The palpebral reflex involves the afferent, or sensory, path (trigeminal nerve, cranial nerve V) and the efferent branch (facial nerve, cranial nerve VII) (Figure 7.1.4). The clinician should be conscientious when performing a cranial nerve examination to always perform both menace and palpebral tests to avoid misinterpreting an absent menace response as blindness when the facial nerve dysfunction may be responsible.
- The facial nerve also innervates the caudal portion of the digastricus muscle, which belongs to the *muscles of mastication*, and this can be atrophied in association with CN VII dysfunction and identified on MR imaging (Figure 7.1.5) [2].

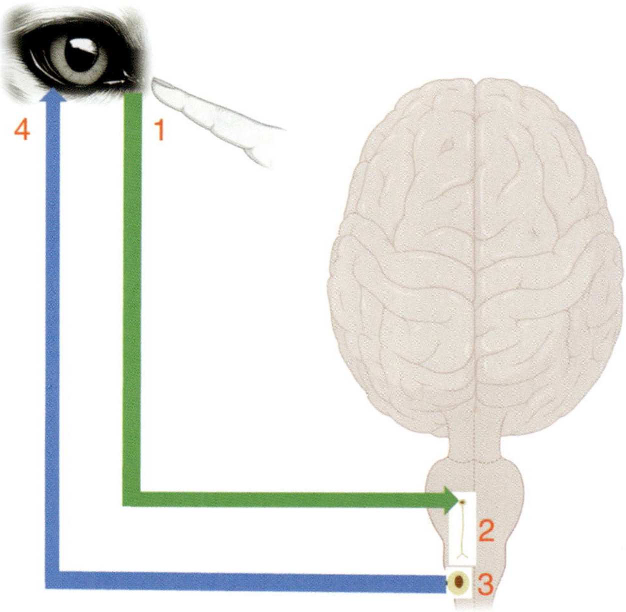

FIGURE 7.1.4 A schematic illustration of the neuroanatomy responsible for the palpebral reflex. (1) The afferent arm of the reflex involves sensory receptors and sensory components of the trigeminal nerve (maxillary and ophthalmic branches). (2) Sensory nucleus of the trigeminal nerve (CN V). (3) Motor nucleus of the facial nerve (CN VII) within the rostral aspect of the medulla oblongata of the brainstem. (4) The efferent arm of the reflex includes the motor branch of the facial nerve, which innervates the orbicularis oculi muscles, causing closure of the palpebral fissure. *Source:* Created with www.biorender.com.

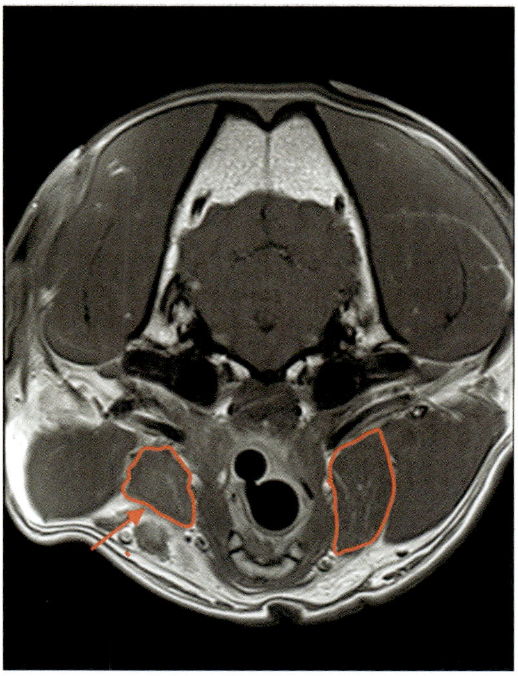

FIGURE 7.1.5 A transverse T1W post-contrast image of the head of a dog with right-sided facial paresis. The caudal digastricus muscle on the right (arrowed and outlined) is smaller than that seen on the left side.

- The sensory function of the rostral two-thirds of the tongue and palate (providing the sense of taste) and the inner part of the pinna is supplied by the sensory component of CN VII.
- The parasympathetic component of CN VII innervates the lacrimal glands the glands of the nasal mucosa, the palatine mucosa, and the mandibular and sublingual salivary glands. The parasympathetic fibers travel with the motor fibers of CN VII through the petrous temporal bone and split off at the geniculate ganglion. They travel from there via the pterygoid canal and pterygopalatine fossa to the lacrimal glands, eventually joining with the zygomaticotemporal nerve, which arises from the maxillary division of the trigeminal nerve (CN V).
- The facial nerve's greater petrosal nerve, through its connection with the pterygopalatine ganglion, indirectly influences nasal secretions by innervating the nasal mucosa. The pterygopalatine ganglion is a key relay point for these parasympathetic signals, which ultimately lead to mucus production in the nose.

DIFFERENTIAL DIAGNOSES

Idiopathic Facial Paresis/Paralysis

Idiopathic facial paresis/paralysis is one of the most common causes of unilateral or bilateral facial paresis in dogs. Certain breeds can be predisposed, such as the cocker spaniel, Cavalier King Charles spaniel, and the beagle [3]. For idiopathic facial paralysis to be considered as a differential diagnosis, there should be no evidence of central neurologic disease (such as proprioceptive deficits or other cranial nerve involvement). One notable exception to this rule is peripheral vestibular signs. A subset of dogs with idiopathic facial paralysis may also have concurrent idiopathic vestibular syndrome. Idiopathic facial paralysis (and idiopathic vestibular syndrome) is a diagnosis of exclusion, requiring a magnetic resonance imaging (MRI) and cerebrospinal fluid (CSF) analysis to rule out other conditions for a more definitive diagnosis [4]. MRI can sometimes reveal a hyperintensity of the facial nerve in post-contrast sequences [5].

Signs can present on one side of the face and sometimes progress to both sides. If clinical signs of facial paralysis persist, then over time, the development of contracture of the facial muscles may occur.

Inflammatory – Otitis Media/Interna

Otitis media/interna can often be a cause of facial paresis or paralysis on the affected side. The facial nerve exits the skull via the internal acoustic meatus, enters the facial canal, and exits at the stylomastoid foramen. This pathway allows the facial nerve to pass through the petrous temporal bone and adjacent to the tympanic bulla. In cases of severe otitis media/interna, reactive inflammation of the surrounding region can lead to inflammatory changes in the facial nerve and result in facial paresis. It is important to note that while otitis media/interna or other underlying causes may be effectively treated, facial paresis/paralysis can remain long term. Thus, it is difficult to use the resolution of facial paresis or paralysis as a monitoring tool to determine whether there has been resolution of underlying otitis media/interna. Patients with otitis media/interna may also display ipsilateral peripheral vestibular disease and Horner syndrome.

Metabolic – Hypothyroidism

Hypothyroidism has been linked to several neurologic conditions, including facial paralysis. However, the exact nature of the link between the two is poorly understood. If it is suspected that hypothyroidism may be the underlying cause in a canine patient, the clinical signs and laboratory results (TT4, fT4, thyroid stimulating hormone [TSH], cholesterol, etc.) should support this suspicion. Typically, patients experiencing facial paralysis secondary to hypothyroidism see satisfactory resolution of the clinical signs within about 1 month of starting appropriate thyroid supplementation, and the overall prognosis is considered good.

Idiopathic / Immune-Mediated – Myasthenia Gravis

One rare but important differential for weakness of facial muscles in canine patients is myasthenia gravis. The typical clinical picture of myasthenia gravis is an easily fatigable dog with a choppy gait, megaesophagus, and fatigable patellar reflexes. Focal myasthenia gravis most commonly presents as megaesophagus, but can also selectively affect muscles of the face, pharynx, and larynx. Paresis/paralysis may manifest as a waxing/waning deficit or may be inducible with repetition of the palpebral reflex.

Neoplasia

Neoplasia is an important consideration for patients with facial paralysis. Tumors affecting the soft tissues or bony structures of the skull, such as sarcomas, can produce deficits of facial nerve function. Infiltrative neoplasia such as lymphoma, histiocytic sarcoma, and other round cell tumors can have a predilection for nerves. While more commonly seen in the trigeminal nerve, nerve sheath tumors can occur in any cranial nerve. While not a neoplastic disease, space-occupying lesions such as cholesteatomas (tympanokeratomas) and nasopharyngeal polyps that disrupt the normal anatomy of the middle ear can produce signs similar to otitis media/interna [6].

NEXT DIAGNOSTIC STEPS FOR THIS PATIENT

- Testing for peripheral or extracranial causes of facial paralysis is important. Baseline lab work may prove helpful for identifying underlying evidence of inflammation, infection, or hypothyroidism. When considering hypothyroidism as a differential, it is important to rule out euthyroid sick syndrome prior to considering thyroid supplementation.
- While the middle and inner ear cannot be visualized during an otic examination, rupture, bulging, redness, or thickening of the tympanic membrane may increase suspicion for otitis media/interna. In cases where otitis media/interna is suspected, prolonged oral antibiotic therapy (6–8 weeks) may be indicated due to the difficulty of achieving adequate antibiotic concentrations in the bony labyrinth of the inner ear. Topical therapies for otitis externa should be limited to non-ototoxic medications in cases where the tympanic membrane cannot be visualized or is compromised, due to concerns about the induction of vestibular signs and deafness if fluid or exudates enter the middle ear.
- MRI is the modality of choice for evaluating brainstem and cranial nerve abnormalities, as it is better suited for imaging soft tissue structures. Facial nerve enhancement following contrast administration on the T1W sequence can be noted and is compatible with inflammation of the nerve associated with infection or an idiopathic neuropathy (Figure 7.1.6). Computed tomography (CT) is the preferred modality for evaluating bone and can help assess the integrity of the tympanic bullae and temporal bone. This is particularly helpful when trying to determine if otitis media/interna has resulted in reactive inflammation that extended into the cranial vault or the soft tissues surrounding the tympanic bullae. In cases where diagnostic cross-sectional imaging may not be possible for the client, radiographs of the skull may be performed to evaluate the bullae. However, this can be technically challenging and laborious, with many oblique views necessary to adequately visualize the bullae, making CT the preferred diagnostic method if available.

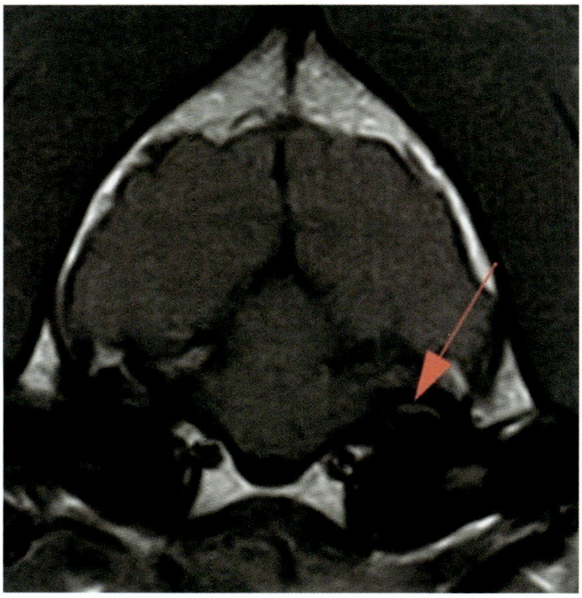

FIGURE 7.1.6 A transverse T1W post-contrast image of the head of a dog with left-sided facial paresis. There is enhancement and mild thickening of the intratemporal portion of the left-sided facial nerve (arrow).

- CSF analysis can help evaluate for infiltrative neoplasia, such as lymphoma or other round cell tumors, which may exfoliate tumor cells, or assess for inflammatory changes that may be consistent with immune-mediated, reactive, or infectious causes of meningoencephalitis or neuritis. It is expected to be normal with a peripheral disease.

OUTCOME

The owner requested a complete investigation for this dog, which included MRI and CSF. Blood work, infectious disease titers, and CSF analysis were normal. MRI revealed a left-sided intratemporal facial nerve enhancement following contrast on a T1W sequence. The intralabyrinthine structures were considered normal bilaterally, as were the intracranial structures. The findings were compatible with an idiopathic facial neuropathy. Supportive care was initiated for the neurogenic KCS. The owners reported moderate recovery of the dog's condition over the following 3 months.

SUGGESTED READING

Chan, M., Toribio, J.A., Podadera, J., and Child, G. (2020). Incidence, cause, outcome and possible risk factors associated with facial nerve paralysis in dogs in a Sydney population (2001–2016): a retrospective study. *Aust. Vet. J.* 98 (4): 140–147. https://doi.org/10.1111/avj.12906.

De Lahunta, A., Glass, E., and Kent, M. (2015). *Veterinary Neuroanatomy and Clinical Neurology*, 4e. Elsevier.

Dewey, C.W. and Da Costa, R.C. (2015). *Practical Guide to Canine and Feline Neurology*, 3e. Wiley.

Hardie, E.M., Linder, K.E., and Pease, A.P. (2008). Aural cholesteatoma in twenty dogs. *Vet. Surg.* 37 (8): 763–770.

Jeandel, A., Thibaud, J., and Blot, A. (2016). Facial and vestibular neuropathy of unknown origin in 16 dogs. *J. Small Anim. Pract.* 57 (2): 74–78. https://doi.org/10.1111/jsap.12428.

McGregor, O., Plested, M.J., and Beltran, E. (2021). Magnetic resonance imaging of the caudal portion of the digastric muscle in canine idiopathic facial neuropathy. *Vet. Radiol. Ultrasound* 62: 455–462. https://doi.org/10.1111/vru.12974.

Platt, S.R. and Olby, N.J. (2013). *Manual of Canine and Feline Neurology*, 4e. British Small Animal Veterinary Association.

Smith, P.M., Gonçalves, R., and McConnell, J.F. (2012). Sensitivity and specificity of MRI for detecting facial nerve abnormalities in dogs with facial neuropathy. *Vet. Rec.* 171 (14): 349.

Uemura, E.E. (2015). *Fundamentals of Canine Neuroanatomy and Neurophysiology*, 1e. Wiley.

CHAPTER 7.2

Disorders of the Head and Face

Case 2—Trismus in a Dog

Amanda Brenna

Puget Sound Veterinary Specialty and Emergency, Gig Harbor, WA, USA

CASE HISTORY

A 5-year-old neutered male Cavalier King Charles spaniel was presented with a 3-week history of difficulty eating and pain on opening the mouth. The owners first noticed signs when the dog would yelp while attempting to chew on his toys. They began to notice a decrease in appetite that progressively worsened. In the past 5 days, the dog became completely unable to open his mouth to eat. The owners reported that due to a history of dental disease and extractions, the dog protruded his tongue out of the left side of his mouth to lap up water and pureed food. Aside from the aforementioned dental extractions, previous medical history included surgical debridement of a ventral cervical abscess resulting from a migrating foreign body (stick ingestion) 5 weeks earlier. The dog has been systemically healthy and was up to date on all vaccinations. He also regularly takes flea, tick, and heartworm preventatives.

NEUROLOGICAL AND PHYSICAL EXAMINATION

On neurologic examination, the dog was bright, alert, and responsive. He was ambulatory, with no obvious ataxia or paresis in the thoracic or pelvic limbs. Postural reactions were normal based on proprioceptive positioning and hopping in all four limbs. Spinal reflexes were also normal (limited to withdrawal and patellar reflexes). There was no evidence of pain or discomfort with deep palpation of the cervical and thoracolumbar vertebral column. The dog's cranial nerve examination revealed normal palpebral and pupillary light reflexes, normal menace responses, and normal visual tracking. Facial sensation was intact. The patient had moderate, bilaterally symmetric swelling of the temporal muscles, which were painful on palpation. The eyes appeared buphthalmic, and the patient cried out when gentle retropulsion was attempted.

1. What is the lesion localization and the most appropriate ranked differential diagnoses for trismus or "lock-jaw"?
2. What are the best next diagnostic steps to consider for this patient?
3. What are the treatments and prognosis for these differentials?

LESION LOCALIZATION

Given the normal function of the ophthalmic and maxillary branches of the trigeminal nerve (evidenced by the normal palpebral reflex, corneal reflex, and facial sensation), as well as the bilaterally symmetric swelling and pain in the temporalis muscles, a primary myopathy should be considered more likely than a trigeminal nerve lesion for this patient. Diseases affecting the muscles of mastication should be considered as the leading cause for trismus in this patient, rather than trigeminal neuralgia, which has not been associated with trismus or temporal muscle swelling in the dog.

Temporomandibular joint diseases could also give rise to pain on opening the jaw, with restricted movement of the jaw. Rarely, central nervous system (CNS) disease can be responsible, particularly pseudorabies and tetanus.

DIFFERENTIAL DIAGNOSIS (Figure 7.2.1)

Masticatory Muscle Myositis

Masticatory muscle myositis (MMM) is an immune-mediated disease and the most common form of focal myositis seen in the dog. It is rare in the cat, though it has been reported.

Masticatory muscles contain a unique muscle fiber type (Type 2M) that differs both histochemically and biochemically from the fiber type present in limb muscles (Type I, IIa, IIx, and IIc), which explains the specific immune targeting of these muscles without involvement of the limb and trunk musculature.

The breeds of dog most susceptible to masticatory muscle myositis (MMM) are German shepherd dogs and Cavalier King Charles spaniels. There is no apparent sex predilection. The average age of onset is 3 years, although dogs as young as 4 months old have been reported with MMM.

Two stages of MMM exist: the acute form and the chronic form.

- In the acute form, patients have severe symmetric swelling of the temporalis and masseter muscles, which is incredibly painful. It is not recommended to attempt to open the mouth in these patients due to the severity of the pain they experience. In some cases, the swelling can be so severe that it causes the globe of the eye to protrude from its orbit, which can be appreciated as a "shocked" look in the affected patient. In the Cavalier King Charles spaniel, this can be harder to appreciate due to breed-related buphthalmia.
- The chronic form of MMM occurs in the late stage of the disease when the muscles undergo significant atrophy due to ongoing inflammation and necrosis and become fibrotic (Figure 7.2.2).

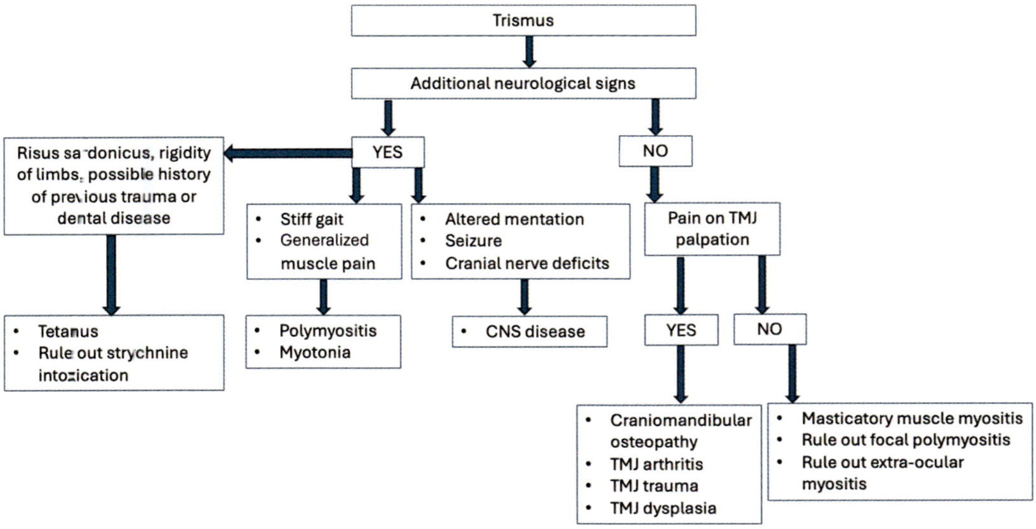

FIGURE 7.2.1 An algorithmic approach to the localization and differential diagnosis considerations for trismus.

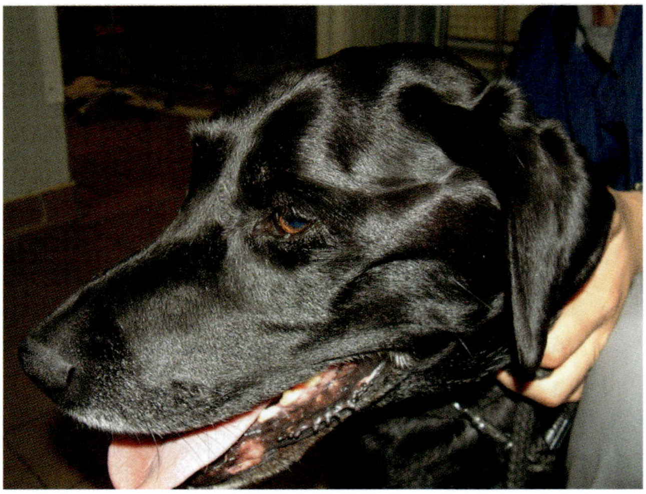

FIGURE 7.2.2 Severe masticatory muscle atrophy in a Labrador retriever with chronic masticatory muscle myositis.

This produces a mechanical inability to open the jaw due to scarification of the attachments of the temporal and masseter muscles to the ramus of the mandible.

Tetanus

One of the most well-known causes of trismus, or "lockjaw," is tetanus. Tetanus is caused by a neurotoxin (tetanospasmin) produced by the bacterium *Clostridium tetani*. Tetanospasmin gains access to the neurons at the neuromuscular junction and is retrogradely transported to the spinal cord, where it exits the motor neuron and enters the inhibitory neuron, preventing release of inhibitory neurotransmitters (glycine in the spinal cord and gamma-aminobutyric acid in the brain). This loss of inhibition results in excitation of the motor neurons, causing increased extensor rigidity and muscle spasms. Once bound to the interneuron, tetanospasmin may stay bound for upward of 3 weeks.

Typically, the clinical signs will begin in the area closest to the point of entry for the toxin. For instance, if the patient has stepped on a nail, it may first affect this specific limb. If the point of entry is a wound from chewing on a stick, signs may occur first in the head and neck. The onset of clinical signs is usually 5–10 days following a wound. Classic clinical signs that may accompany tetanus include trismus, rigid facial muscles and contracture (*risus sardonicus*), extreme extensor rigidity, a sawhorse gait, rarely seizures, and respiratory paralysis (Figure 7.2.3). A spastic retraction of the globe of the eye into the head due to spasming of the extraocular muscles may be observed. Patients with tetanus may exhibit worsening clinical signs associated with excitement or activity.

Immune-Mediated Polymyositis

Immune-mediated (also called idiopathic) polymyositis has been documented to affect muscles throughout the body, including hypaxial, epaxial, and masticatory muscles. Recent studies have documented immune-mediated polymyositis producing signs consistent with MMM in dogs. Therefore, in a patient who tests negative for serum 2M antibodies or histopathologic changes consistent with MMM (see below), immune-mediated polymyositis should be considered. Immune-mediated polymyositis can also be seen as a form of paraneoplastic syndrome.

Focal polymyositis of immune-mediated etiology has been described in several breeds, including Hungarian vizsla dogs, involving pharynx, larynx and tongue muscles as well as the masticatory muscles.

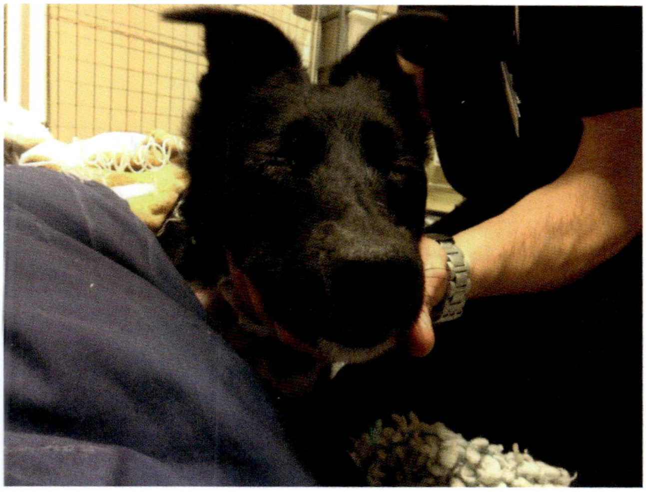

FIGURE 7.2.3 A mixed-breed dog with tetanus affecting the head and causing erect ears and palpebral fissure closure.

Extraocular myositis is a focal inflammatory myopathy observed in young, predominantly large- or giant-breed dogs, which typically causes exophthalmos but can be responsible for restrictive jaw movement.

Infectious Myositis

Several infectious organisms have been associated with myositis. The most prevalent organisms producing myopathies are protozoal *(Toxoplasma* and *Neospora)* and Leptospirosis. Other possible infectious agents include *Hepatozoon*, *Leishmania*, *Trypanosoma*, and rickettsial diseases. Unlike idiopathic polymyositis, the author is unaware of any reports in the literature of a systemic infectious myositis resulting in trismus in the dog. However, focal bacterial infections/abscesses within the masticatory muscles have been reported to produce clinical signs of severe pain and inability to open the mouth.

Diseases of the Temporomandibular Joint

Outside of tetanus and diseases of the masticatory muscles, disease of the temporomandibular joint needs to be considered, where clinically applicable. Primarily, ankylosis (articular) and pseudoankylosis (extra-articular) of the temporomandibular joint can occur secondary to maxillofacial trauma. Additionally, craniomandibular osteopathy, neoplasia, dysplasia, or osteoarthrosis are all possible considerations.

NEXT DIAGNOSTIC STEPS FOR THIS PATIENT

Masticatory Muscle Myositis

- The simplest test for MMM is the 2M serum antibody titer. This blood test assesses for circulating 2M antibodies, which are specific to the muscles of mastication. It is important to note that a subset of true positive cases will test negative for the 2M antibody, particularly if the antibody is primarily bound to the muscle and not circulating.
- Biopsy of the muscle allows direct staining of the muscle fibers to look for bound 2M antibodies and also provides information regarding the severity of the inflammation and necrosis in the muscle, which can help determine a prognosis for recovery of function.

- Testing for MMM should always be conducted before the initiation of any corticosteroid therapy. Corticosteroid therapy, particularly immunosuppressive doses or courses administered for longer than a week, has the potential to interfere with antibody production and can lead to false negatives in serum antibody and biopsy results.
- MRI in a patient with trismus can be useful in confirming inflammatory lesions within the temporalis and masseter muscles consistent with MMM (Figure 7.2.4), and ruling out other potential structural causes of jaw pain and muscle pain that may present as trismus. Imaging can also assist with targeted biopsies.
- Other helpful diagnostic tests include a serum creatine kinase (CK), which, if elevated, can be useful for monitoring clinical response to treatment. C-reactive protein has also been reported to be elevated in cases of MMM and is useful for clinical monitoring, though it is nonspecific to muscle.

Tetanus

There is no specific diagnostic test for tetanus. Diagnosis of tetanus is based on clinical suspicion and must incorporate a complete and thorough history and physical examination. The patient should be thoroughly examined for wounds, as even small puncture wounds can provide a point of entry for a potential bacterial infection. For veterinary patients, this can be particularly challenging and may require shaving of the animal in some cases. However, even in cases where the wound is not found, patients with clinical signs consistent with tetanus should be treated presumptively, as clinical signs can present after a wound may have healed. Fortunately, the clinical signs of tetanus are quite characteristic, so the astute clinician should be able to recognize when this differential presents itself.

TREATMENT AND PROGNOSIS

Masticatory Muscle Myositis

Treatment for MMM primarily centers around immunosuppressive therapy. If the disease is identified in the acute form of the disease, then expeditious diagnosis and treatment are essential for the prevention of scarring, fibrosis, and atrophy of the masticatory muscles. Once a chronic stage of the disease sets in, the prognosis for recovery of masticatory muscle mass and mandibular function is poor.

- Immunosuppressive corticosteroids (prednisone) at 1–2 mg/kg/day for 4 weeks, with a gradual taper (this author recommends a 25% taper every 4 weeks).

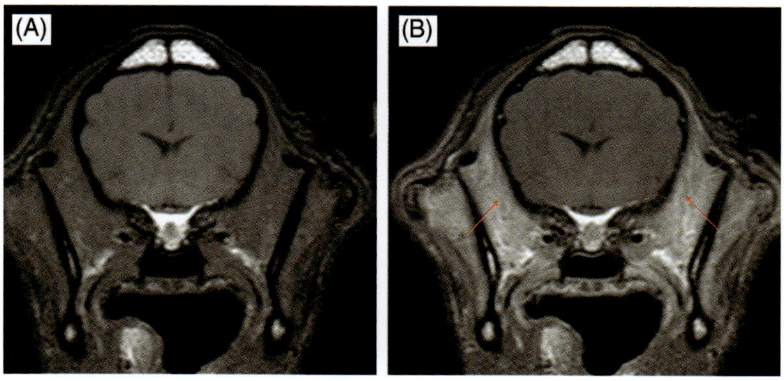

FIGURE 7.2.4 (A) T1W pre-contrast and (B) post-contrast of a 5-year-old mixed-breed dog with masticatory muscle myositis. Note the marked bilateral muscle atrophy and the contrast uptake (red arrows).

- Serum CK, jaw function, and occasionally serum antibody titers can be used to monitor treatment.
- The addition of other oral immunosuppressants, such as mycophenolate mofetil (10 mg/kg PO q12h), modified cyclosporine (5 mg/kg PO q12h), or even azathioprine and leflunomide, can be considered in cases where relapse of signs is observed with tapering of steroid therapy.
- Patients with severe trismus may require the support of a feeding tube to allow for adequate nutrition while waiting for clinical signs to regress.
- Multimodal pain control should also be provided for patients with the acute form, as this is a very painful disease.
- Once patients can open their mouths enough to allow some prehension and mastication of food, soft food should be provided to minimize discomfort to the patient.
- In patients with the chronic form of the disease who are suffering from significant muscle atrophy, chewing exercises (toys, hard food, etc.) can be encouraged to help stimulate muscle hypertrophy, once the pain has resolved. In chronic cases where contracture and fibrosis have caused permanent trismus, surgical release of the attachments of the temporalis and masseter muscles may be considered.

Tetanus

Treatment for tetanus, in large part, involves reducing patient stimulation and anxiety.

- The patient should be kept in a quiet, dark, calm environment for recovery.
- Plugging the patient's ears with cotton balls or headphones is recommended to reduce distraction, excitement, and auditory stimuli.
- Debridement of any wound that is found should be performed, and the patient should be treated with antibiotics both locally and systemically. Penicillin, ampicillin, metronidazole, and tetracyclines are all acceptable for the treatment of *Clostridium tetani* infections.
- Antitoxin will not have any effect on toxins that have already bound to the inhibitory interneurons. However, it may be successful in preventing further neurotoxins from entering the system. Antitoxin can be difficult to obtain in some clinical circumstances, and some patients may have a hypersensitivity reaction to it. A small amount (0.1 mL) should be given subcutaneously to monitor for any adverse reaction.
- Supportive care with recumbency care and appropriate hygiene to prevent urine and fecal scald is necessary. Urinary catheterization is preferable to bladder expression, given increased muscle tone and the desire to decrease stimulus to the patient.
- Nutritional supplementation is also needed, and often the placement of a feeding tube (a gastrostomy is preferred, since megaesophagus develops in some patients) allows for providing both nutritional and hydration needs, reducing the risk of aspiration pneumonia.
- Muscle relaxants, anxiolytics, and anticonvulsants can be helpful in managing patient anxiety, muscle spasms, and seizures (if indicated). Magnesium aspartate therapy has been reported recently in dogs, providing further muscle relaxation.

The prognosis for tetanus can be guarded to grave, depending upon the constellation and severity of clinical signs and the financial ability of the owner to hospitalize and provide the necessary supportive care. Complete recovery can take several weeks and even months in some patients. Most cats are focally affected, and the prognosis can be fair to good.

Patients who are recumbent and non-ambulatory may be nursed at home effectively with the placement of a feeding tube and a dedicated owner. However, if intravenous antibiotics, wound care, or respiratory support necessitate hospitalization, the cost of care can become exorbitant.

OUTCOME

A 2M serum antibody titer in this dog was markedly elevated. The owners elected not to confirm the diagnosis of masticatory myositis with muscle biopsy, and so immediate immunosuppressive treatment was initiated on a presumptive basis. The dog made a marked improvement and was considered almost normal after 3 months of tapering therapy; at that time, the corticosteroids were discontinued.

SUGGESTED READING

Arnold, S.A., Kent, M., Perlini, M. et al. (2020). What is your diagnosis? *J. Am. Vet. Med. Assoc.* 256 (6): 647–649. https://doi.org/10.2460/javma.256.6.647.

Blazejewski, S.W. and Shelton, G.D. (2018). Trismus, masticatory myositis and antibodies against type 2M fibers in a mixed breed cat. *JFMS Open Rep.* 4 (1): 2055116918764993.

Cauduro, A., Paolo, F., Asperio, R.M. et al. (2013). Use of MRI for the early diagnosis of masticatory muscle myositis. *J. Am. Anim. Hosp. Assoc.* 49 (5): 347–352.

De Lahunta, A., Glass, E., and Kent, M. (2015). *Veterinary Neuroanatomy and Clinical Neurology*, 4e. Elsevier.

Dewey, C.W. and Da Costa, R.C. (2015). *Practical Guide to Canine and Feline Neurology*, 3e. Wiley.

Di Tosto, M., Callegari, C., Matiasek, K. et al. (2022). Case report: atypical and chronic masticatory muscle myositis in a 5-month old Cavalier King Charles Spaniel. Clinical and diagnostic findings, treatment and successful outcome. *Front. Vet. Sci.* 9: 955758.

Dörfelt, S., Mayer, C., Wolf, G. et al. (2023). Retrospective study of tetanus in 18 dogs-causes, management, complications, and immunological status. *Front. Vet. Sci.* 10: 1249833.

Dussaux, A., Fuhrer, L., Dorner, M.B. et al. (2024). Clinical findings and outcome in feline tetanus: a multicentric retrospective study of 27 cases and review of the literature. *Front. Vet. Sci.* 11: 1425917.

Foreman, M. and Cherubini, G.B. (2021). Dexamethasone can be safely and effectively used for treatment of masticatory muscle myositis in dogs. *Top. Companion Anim. Med.* 44: 100538.

Han, J., Jang, K., Cho, S.B. et al. (2024). Successful diagnosis and treatment of canine polymyositis: utilizing MRI and immunohistochemistry for accurate detection. *BMC Vet. Res.* 20 (1): 560.

Haley, A.C., Platt, S.R., Kent, M. et al. (2011). Breed-specific polymyositis in Hungarian Vizsla dogs. *J. Vet. Intern. Med.* 25 (2): 393–397.

Jung, S., Park, J., Hong, Y.J., and Nom, A. (2024). Idiopathic polymyositis showing nonspecific clinical signs that mimicked masticatory myositis in a dog. *J. Vet. Clin.* 40 (1): 301–306. https://doi.org/10.17555/jvc.2024.41.5.301.

Papageorgiou, V., Kazakos, G., Anagnostou, T., and Polizopoulou, Z. (2021). The role of magnesium in the management of acute and long-term symptoms caused by tetanus in two dogs. *Top. Companion Anim. Med.* 44: 100535.

Platt, S.R. and Olby, N.J. (2026). *Manual of Canine and Feline Neurology*, 5e. British Small Animal Veterinary Association.

Schöniger, S., Klose, K., Werner, H. et al. (2012). Non-suppurative encephalitis in a dog. *Vet. Pathol.* 49 (4): 731–734.

Uemura, E.E. (2015). *Fundamentals of Canine Neuroanatomy and Neurophysiology*, 1e. Wiley.

Disorders of the Head and Face

Case 3—Dropped Jaw in a Dog

CHAPTER 7.3

Amanda Brenna

Puget Sound Veterinary Specialty and Emergency, Gig Harbor, WA, USA

CASE HISTORY

A 5-year-old neutered male Gordon setter presented with a 4-day history of being unable to close his mouth and difficulty eating. The owners first noticed signs when he had difficulty picking up his ball while playing outside. He began dropping food out of his mouth the following day. The owners also noticed copious amounts of water outside of the bowl and thick, "ropey" saliva drooling from his mouth anytime that he attempted to drink. The dog had been otherwise healthy with no significant clinical medical history. He was up-to-date on his vaccinations and was on flea, tick, and heartworm preventatives (Figure 7.3.1).

NEUROLOGICAL AND PHYSICAL EXAMINATION

On neurologic examination, the dog was quiet, alert, and responsive. He was ambulatory with no obvious ataxia or paresis in the thoracic or pelvic limbs. Postural reactions were normal based on proprioceptive positioning and hopping in all four limbs. Spinal reflexes were also normal (limited to flexor withdrawal and patellar reflexes). There was no evidence of pain or discomfort with deep palpation of the cervical and thoracolumbar vertebral column or over the head.

Mild atrophy of the muscles of mastication was noted. The dog's cranial nerve examination revealed a normal menace response, as well as normal pupillary light reflexes (direct and consensual) and palpebral reflexes in both eyes. The mandible was dropped and the patient struggled to pick up treats and drink (Video 7.3.1). The patient's gag reflex was normal, though thick saliva was noted to be present around the mouth and nose, and the patient had significant halitosis. No other cranial nerve or physical exam abnormalities were noted.

VIDEO 7.3.1 Gordon setter exhibiting a dropped jaw and difficulty prehending a treat and drinking water.

1. What is the likely lesion localization and the most appropriate ranked differential diagnoses?
2. What are the best next diagnostic steps for this patient?
3. What are the treatments and prognosis for these differentials?

LESION LOCALIZATION AND DIFFERENTIAL DIAGNOSES (Figure 7.3.2)

A dropped jaw inherently implies bilateral dysfunction of the mandibular motor branch of the trigeminal nerve. As such, diseases that are known to be diffuse or infiltrative and have a predilection for the trigeminal nerve should be prioritized when considering possible differentials for a

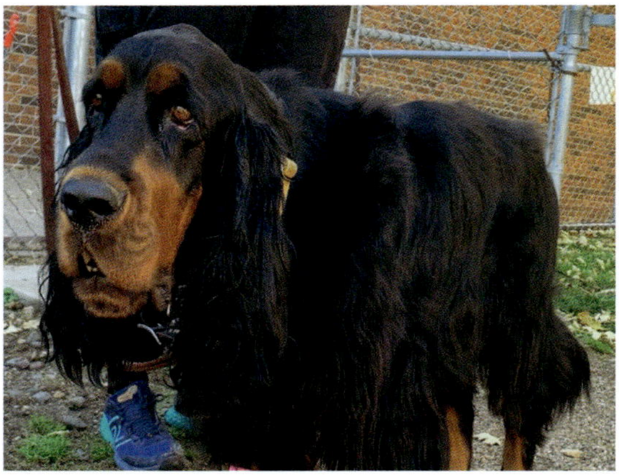

FIGURE 7.3.1 A 5-year-old male neutered Gordon setter with a mild dropped jaw.

patient with a dropped jaw. Diseases that cause bilaterally symmetric lesions of the motor nuclei of the trigeminal nerve (resulting in a pure, bilateral trigeminal neuropathy) are not typically seen in canines.

It is important to remember that an inability to close the mouth can also be due to non-neurological causes. The possibility of mechanical obstruction due to bilateral luxation of the temporomandibular joints, fracture of the mandible, or oral foreign bodies has to be considered in each patient.

Trigeminal Neuritis (Idiopathic Trigeminal Neuropathy)

The most common cause of a dropped jaw in canines is trigeminal neuritis (also known as idiopathic trigeminal neuropathy). This is an inflammatory condition of the trigeminal nerve that is thought to be immune-mediated in origin. Demyelination and axonal degeneration are prominent features of this disease and bear some resemblance to the lesions found in the ventral nerve roots of dogs suffering from polyradiculoneuritis. While involvement of the mandibular (motor) branch of the trigeminal nerve produces the most visibly obvious clinical signs, involvement of the maxillary and ophthalmic branches of the trigeminal nerve is possible and can result in the loss of sensation in some patients. Additionally, some patients may experience Horner syndrome, which occurs due to involvement of the postganglionic sympathetic neurons that join the ophthalmic branch near its origin from the trigeminal nerve to reach the smooth muscle of the eye, eyelids, and periorbita.

While thought to be immune-mediated in origin, the disease is self-limiting, and most patients make a full recovery within a few weeks. The degree of affectation can be gauged by the severity of dropped jaw and atrophy of the masticatory muscles.

Pachymeningitis

Pachymeningitis is defined as inflammation and thickening of the dura mater (and the inner periosteum of the skull), whereas leptomeningitis involves the subarachnoid and pia mater. Differentiating between pachymeningeal and leptomeningeal contrast enhancement is a critical part of determining the most likely differentials when evaluating inflammatory diseases of the central nervous system. Obtaining biopsies of central nervous system (CNS) tissue for histopathologic evaluation cannot only be harmful to the patient but is also technically challenging and financially untenable for some clients.

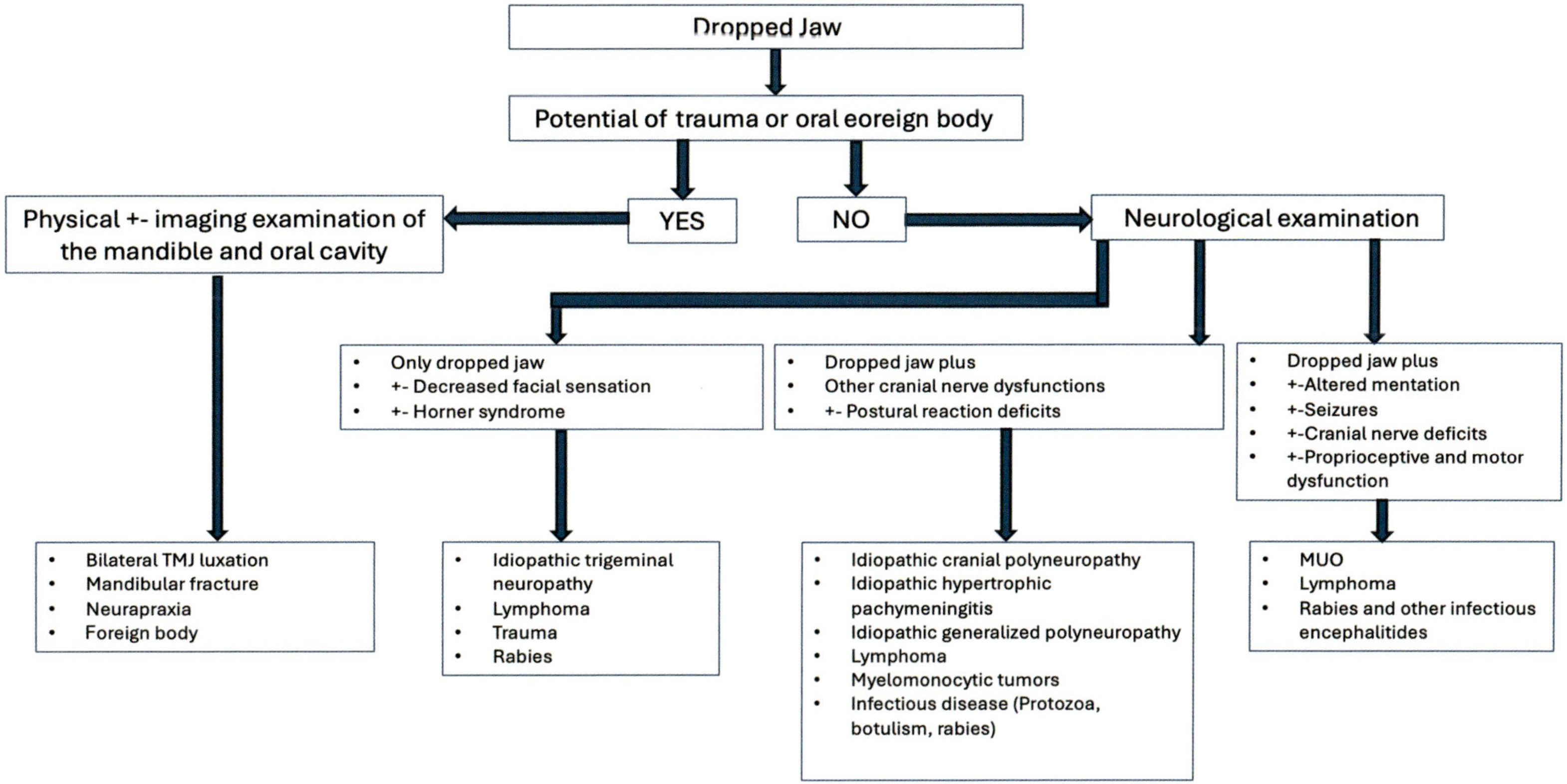

FIGURE 7.3.2 An algorithmic approach to the localization and differentials to consider for a case with a dropped jaw. (MUO – meningoencephalitis of unknown origin; TMJ – temporomandibular joint).

Both immune-mediated (idiopathic hypertrophic [chronic] pachymeningitis) and infectious forms of pachymeningitis exist and can affect the trigeminal nerves as they depart the brainstem and become enveloped within the pachymeninges. Top infectious etiologies that should be considered in the canine patient include fungal (*Aspergillus, Cryptococcus*), protozoal, and bacterial. Greyhounds and crossbreed sighthounds appear to be predisposed to the immune-mediated form, and most dogs exhibit other cranial nerve deficits.

CNS Lymphoma

Lymphoma can show a predilection for the trigeminal nerve, especially in cats. Bilateral infiltration of lymphoma into the mandibular branches of the trigeminal nerve can produce a dropped jaw and appear clinically identical to trigeminal neuritis, with involvement of the sensory branches of the trigeminal nerve. Other cranial nerve deficits may also be appreciated if the infiltrative changes spread beyond the trigeminal nerve.

Rabies

The prevalence of rabies has greatly diminished thanks to the vaccination of domesticated animals, wildlife vaccine programs, and its status as a reportable disease. However, rabies remains a clinical concern in patients who are unvaccinated and have had exposure to wildlife that may carry or be affected by the disease. Bats, raccoons, skunks, and foxes are the most common carriers in the United States. Dogs are still carriers in some countries where vaccination rates are low. The rabies virus is a rhabdovirus that is primarily spread via saliva through bites or scratches. The virus replicates at the site of the bite and infects peripheral nerves, where it undergoes retrograde axonal transport to the central nervous system. Clinical signs of rabies in dogs often begin with a "prodromal phase" of about 2–3 days of abnormal behavior, such as anxiousness/nervousness, observed by the owners. Fever may also be appreciated in this stage. Following this prodromal phase, two forms of rabies begin to emerge: the "furious" or psychotic form and the "dumb" or paralytic form. The furious form of rabies is characterized by erratic behavior, aggression, and hyperesthesia to stimuli (sight, sound, etc.), and eventually seizures. Signs can occur for around a week before death occurs. The "dumb" or paralytic form of rabies can appear 2–4 days after clinical signs set in and is characterized by flaccid paresis/paralysis. Dysphonia, dysphagia, and *dropped jaw* can all be seen, particularly if the site of viral inoculation occurs in the region of the head or neck. In unvaccinated animals, death uniformly occurs within seven days following the onset of clinical signs.

NEXT DIAGNOSTIC STEPS FOR THIS PATIENT

Trigeminal Neuritis (Idiopathic Trigeminal Neuropathy)

There is no definitive test for trigeminal neuritis, and diagnosis typically is based on recognition of clinical signs and monitoring for resolution of signs over the course of a few weeks. If the clinical signs are not resolving within the expected period of time, or other neurologic deficits are developing, a complete diagnostic workup, including magnetic resonance imaging (MRI) of the head and cerebrospinal fluid (CSF) analysis, is recommended at that time. MRI features of trigeminal neuritis are significant thickening and contrast enhancement of the trigeminal nerves bilaterally. Accumulation of fluid within the inner ear may also be notable due to dysfunction of the tensor veli palatini, which is innervated by the trigeminal nerve and regulates ventilation of the inner ear via opening of the eustachian tube.

Pachymeningitis and CNS Lymphoma

MRI of the head to evaluate the brain, brainstem, and trigeminal nerves as they course from the brainstem through the trigeminal canal into the various regions of the head is the most direct method of evaluating the trigeminal nerves. Thickening and contrast enhancement of the trigeminal nerves may be seen in cases of trigeminal neuritis or CNS lymphoma. These changes are severe enough to cause compression of the brainstem at the origin of the trigeminal nerve (Figure 7.3.3). Focal pachymeningeal contrast enhancement patterns may be observed surrounding the trigeminal nerves and coursing through the trigeminal canal, possibly extending cranially and caudally along the brainstem. Diffuse pachymeningeal enhancement is rarer and has been primarily reported in cases of immune-mediated disease and lymphoma. CSF analysis should be performed if no imaging characteristics of increased intracranial pressure are found. Infectious disease testing (fungal, protozoal, CSF culture) may be helpful. Baseline clinical laboratory work to evaluate for leukocytosis, hyperglobulinemia, or other clinical pathological findings consistent with infectious, inflammatory, or neoplastic disease may also prove useful.

Rabies

Unfortunately, there is no antemortem test for rabies, and postmortem testing is performed in cases where a rabies suspect patient dies following clinical suspicion or is euthanized either due to clinical decline or public health regulations. Direct antibody fluorescence is performed on brain tissues (primarily the brainstem and cerebellum) to confirm the presence of rabies virus.

TREATMENT AND PROGNOSIS

Trigeminal Neuritis (Idiopathic Trigeminal Neuropathy)

Treatment for trigeminal neuritis is aimed at supportive care and helping the patient to eat and maintain adequate caloric intake. Feeding soft meatballs and assisting with drinking by elevating the water bowl and adding water thickeners are tools that allow most patients with trigeminal neuritis to eat effectively, if not messily. However, some patients may benefit from the placement of a temporary feeding tube, such as an esophagostomy tube. The prognosis for trigeminal neuritis is excellent, with the majority of patients making a complete recovery within a few weeks.

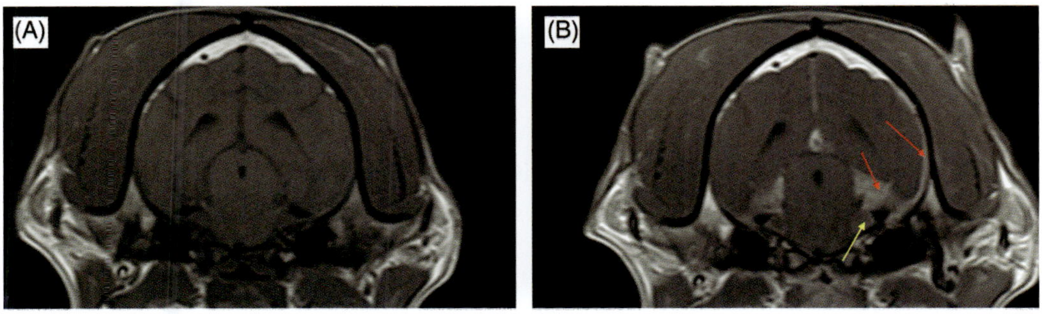

FIGURE 7 3.3 (A) T1W pre-contrast and (B) T1W post-contrast transverse MR image at the level of the midbrain and pons of a dog with idiopathic pachymeningitis. There is pachymeningeal thickening and contrast uptake (red arrows), which is in close proximity to the trigeminal nerve (cranial nerve V) (yellow arrow).

CNS Lymphoma and Pachymeningitis

Treatment for CNS lymphoma can involve immunosuppressive corticosteroid therapy, cytarabine arabinoside, and other chemotherapies (CHOP protocol). Clinically distinguishing lymphoma from immune-mediated neuritis can be challenging. A biopsy cannot be performed without the risk of severe and irreversible damage to the nerve. MRI changes for both disease processes can mirror one another. While large cell lymphoma may often exfoliate lymphoblasts into the cerebrospinal fluid, the finding of lymphocytic pleocytosis could be consistent with immune-mediated meningoencephalitis, small cell lymphoma, or reactivity to the presence of other neoplasia or even infectious disease. For this reason, incorporation of cytosine arabinoside therapy for treatment of pachymeningitis may be considered, as it is a fairly well-tolerated chemotherapy with few side effects. Other immunosuppressive therapies (cyclosporine, leflunomide, mycophenolate) may also be considered for immune-mediated pachymeningitis. The prognosis for CNS lymphoma is poor, while immune-mediated pachymeningitis has a fair prognosis. If an infectious etiology of pachymeningitis is found, appropriate antimicrobial therapy combined with anti-inflammatory steroids is recommended to prevent excessive inflammation due to the death of infectious organisms (particularly in the case of fungal disease). Prognosis for infectious CNS disease is guarded to poor, depending upon the etiologic agent.

OUTCOME

The dog in this report had a gradual improvement in jaw tone and ability to chew over the following 6 weeks with supportive care. Based on the diagnostic investigation results and the improvement noted, the dog was given a presumptive diagnosis of idiopathic trigeminal neuritis/neuropathy. At the 6-week mark, the dog was able to eat and drink normally with only mildly decreased jaw tone, attributed to the significant atrophy of the muscles of mastication. Owners report that the dog's muscle mass is beginning to improve now that he is more interested in his kibble and playing with his chew toys.

SUGGESTED READING

De Lahunta, A., Glass, E., and Kent, M. (2015). *Veterinary Neuroanatomy and Clinical Neurology*, 4e. Elsevier.

Dewey, C.W. and Da Costa, R.C. (2015). *Practical Guide to Canine and Feline Neurology*, 3e. Wiley.

Kent, M., Glass, E.N., de Lahunta, A. et al. (2013). Prevalence of effusion in the tympanic cavity in dogs with dysfunction of the trigeminal nerve: 18 cases (2004–2013). *J. Vet. Intern. Med.* 27: 1153–1158.

Kumar, A., Bhatt, S., Kumar, A., and Rana, T. (2023). Canine rabies: an epidemiological significance, pathogenesis, diagnosis, prevention, and public health issues. *Comp. Immunol. Microbiol. Infect. Dis.* 97: 101992.

Madden, M., Israeliantz, N., Malbon, A. et al. (2025). Meningeal null cell lymphoma causing diffuse pachymeningeal contrast enhancement in a dog. *J. Small Anim. Pract.* 66 (3): 209–213.

Mayhew, P.D., Bush, W.W., and Glass, E.N. (2002). Trigeminal neuropathy in dogs: a retrospective study of 29 cases (1991–2000). *J. Am. Anim. Hosp. Assoc.* 38 (3): 262–270.

Musso, C., Le Boedec, K., Gomes, E., and Cauzinille, L. (2020). Diagnostic values of clinical and magnetic resonance findings in presumptive trigeminal neuropathy: 49 dogs. *J. Am. Anim. Hosp. Assoc.* 56 (2): 106–113. https://doi.org/10.5326/JAAHA-MS-6997.

Pfaff, A.M., March, P.A., and Fishman, C. (2000). Acute bilateral trigeminal neuropathy associated with nervous system lymphosarcoma in a dog. *J. Am. Anim. Hosp.* Assoc. 36: 57–61.

Platt, S.R. and Olby, N.J. (2026). *Manual of Canine and Feline Neurology*, 5e. British Small Animal Veterinary Association.

Roynard, P., Behr, S., Barone, G. et al. (2012). Idiopathic hypertrophic pachymeningitis in six dogs: MRI, CSF and histological findings, treatment and outcome. *J. Small Anim. Pract.* 53 (9): 543–548. https://doi.org/10.1111/j.1748-5827.2012.01252.x.

Uemura, E.E. (2015). *Fundamentals of Canine Neuroanatomy and Neurophysiology*, 1e. Wiley.

Viswanathan, N., Sethuraman, S., Rajasekaran, R. et al. (2024). Probable paralytic rabies in a dog: ante-mortem clinical diagnosis implications in limited resource settings. *J. Infect. Dev. Ctries.* 18 (7): 1148–1151.

CHAPTER 7.4

Disorders of the Head and Face

Case 4—Unilateral Masticatory Muscle Atrophy in a Dog

Katherine Bibi

Blue Pearl Pet Hospital, Kirkland, WA, USA

CASE HISTORY

A 7-year-old neutered male Labrador retriever was presented for a 1-month history of progressive atrophy of the left-sided muscles of the head (Figure 7.4.1). The dog had been boarded for a week and upon pickup, was noted to have asymmetry of these muscles. This asymmetry progressed over the following 4 weeks. The dog had no other medical history, was up-to-date on vaccinations, and ate a commercial diet, with no travel history.

NEUROLOGIC EXAMINATION

Upon presentation, the dog was bright, alert, and responsive. He was ambulatory with no evidence of paresis or ataxia, and his posture was appropriate. Postural reactions were normal in all four limbs, as were spinal reflexes. Cranial nerve examination revealed atrophy of the muscles of mastication on the left side with subjectively normal jaw tone. The left eye was enophthalmic, and a mild anisocoria was observed, with the left pupil smaller than the right. This pupil responded somewhat to light, although given its relative miosis, the degree of response was considered to be less than normal. This pupil did not dilate significantly in the dark. All other cranial nerve (CN) reflexes and responses were normal. There was no evidence of discomfort upon vertebral palpation or cervical range of motion.

1. **What is the associated neuroanatomy?**
2. **Where is the likely lesion localization?**
3. **What major disease processes should be considered?**
4. **What tests could you perform to help determine the diagnosis?**
5. **What are the general treatments and prognoses associated with the main differentials?**

ASSOCIATED NEUROANATOMY

The muscles of mastication include the temporalis, masseter, rostral and caudal digastricus, and medial and lateral pterygoids (Figure 7.4.2). The temporalis, masseter, and medial and lateral pterygoids are responsible for closing the mouth, while the rostral and caudal bellies of the digastricus are responsible for opening the mouth. The temporalis and masseter muscles make up the majority of the muscular structure of the head, and loss of facial mass, as described by owners, is typically related to atrophy of these muscles.

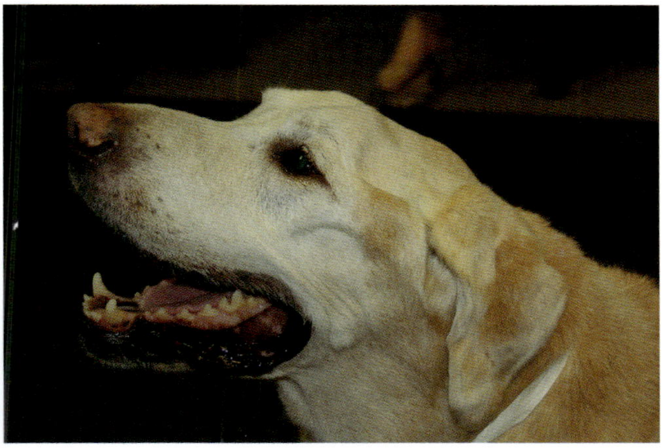

FIGURE 7.4.1 Atrophy of the left-sided masticatory muscles (temporalis and masseter) can be seen in this dog, with the underlying bony prominences such as the zygomatic arch now visible.

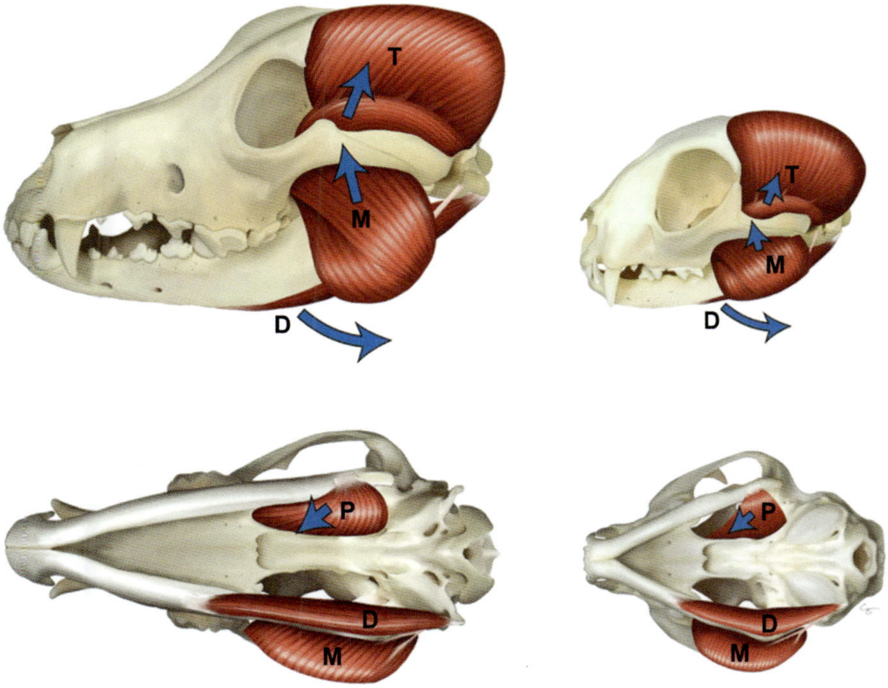

FIGURE 7.4.2 Masticatory muscles in the dog (left) and cat (right) – lateral view (top), ventral view (bottom). M, masseter muscle; T, temporal muscle; P, pterygoid muscle; and D, digastric muscles. Arrows indicate the direction of the "pull" of the muscles. *Source:* Figure reproduced with consent from Kim, Se & Arzi, Boaz & Garcia, Tanya & Verstraete, Frank. (2018). Bite Forces and Their Measurement in Dogs and Cats. Frontiers in Veterinary Science. 5. 10.3389/fvets.2018.00076. Copyright: © 2018 Kim, Arzi, Garcia, and Verstraete.

The mandibular branch of the trigeminal nerve (CN V) innervates the temporalis, masseter, rostral belly of the digastricus, and pterygoids. The caudal belly of the digastricus is innervated by the facial nerve (CN VII). The motor nucleus of CN V is located within the pons, and its axons emerge from the pons to travel through the canal for the trigeminal nerve within the petrosal portion of the temporal bone, pass through the trigeminal ganglion, join the mandibular nerve, and pass through the oval foramen to innervate the aforementioned muscles. Other branches of CN V include the ophthalmic and maxillary branches. All three branches carry sensory information from different parts of the face, but these fibers did not appear to be involved in this case based on this patient's clinically normal facial sensation.

LESION LOCALIZATION

Based on the visualized atrophy of the left-sided muscles of the face, there was clinical involvement of the temporalis and masseter muscles. Enophthalmos of the left eye was presumed to be secondary to atrophy of the pterygoids on that side. Involvement of the digastricus could not be proven clinically, but was suspected. Thus, the patient was localized to CN V, and more specifically the motor fibers of the mandibular branch of the left-sided trigeminal nerve. In addition, based on the relative miosis of the left eye and lack of significant dilation in the dark, involvement of the postganglionic sympathetic fibers on that side was suspected (see Chapter 6, Case 3). These fibers join the ophthalmic branch of the trigeminal nerve near its origin. Involvement of these fibers may also offer an alternative hypothesis for the cause of the enophthalmos.

DIFFERENTIAL DIAGNOSES

Neoplasia (Trigeminal Nerve Sheath Tumor, Skull Tumors Including Lymphoma)

Neoplasia of CN V is considered to be the most common cause of unilateral masticatory muscle atrophy in dogs. A trigeminal nerve sheath tumor (TNST) is the most common form of neoplasia affecting this nerve, and it is the most likely cause of muscle atrophy in this dog. Other neoplasias, such as lymphoma, are less prevalent. In one study, a presumptive TNST was the cause of unilateral masticatory muscle atrophy in 47.6% of included dogs, while other extra-parenchymal masses affected 20.6% of dogs; these could include histiocytic sarcoma, meningioma, or osteosarcoma.

Tumors of this nerve typically result in nerve dysfunction in the form of masticatory muscle atrophy, but additional signs of trigeminal involvement may be seen, including sensory deficits. When the maxillary and ophthalmic branches are involved, there may be a lack of sensation at the lateral and medial canthi (respectively), as well as the nasal septum and other aspects of the nare region. Isolated mandibular branch involvement would hypothetically result in loss of sensation over the lower jaw, but this is typically not clinically assessed. Neurogenic keratitis may also be seen if the ophthalmic branch of CN V is affected, as this branch contains the sensory component of the reflex arc involved in tear production (the motor component of this reflex arc to the lacrimal gland is transmitted via CN VII). When tumors become locally invasive and compress the pons, other CN deficits (facial [CN VII] and vestibulocochlear [CN VIII]), along with ipsilateral hemiparesis and postural reaction deficits, may be observed. In this author's experience, scratching or facial rubbing on the affected side is a common clinical finding in dogs that have concurrent sensory deficits.

> Interestingly, middle ear effusion may also be seen in cases of a TNST or other diseases affecting the mandibular branch of CN V, due to the innervation of the tensor veli palatini and its effect on the auditory tube function.

Idiopathic Trigeminal Neuropathy

Idiopathic trigeminal neuropathy (ITN), also known as trigeminal neuritis, is usually associated with bilateral involvement of CN V and most commonly results in a dropped jaw. Other less common signs include mild dysphagia, Horner syndrome, and deficits in facial sensation. This condition may occasionally affect the nerve unilaterally, although these cases may be missed because of more subtle signs. Neurogenic atrophy of the muscles of mastication may develop, and the degree of this atrophy is variable. The pathogenesis of this condition is unknown, but histopathology may reveal nonsuppurative inflammation of CN V with demyelination and rare axonal loss. Inflammatory findings support an immune-mediated cause, but steroids do not seem to hasten clinical improvement. In one study looking at dogs with unilateral masticatory muscle atrophy, 28.6% of included dogs had no observable magnetic resonance imaging (MRI) abnormalities, suggesting the possibility of ITN or a heterogeneous group of conditions that MRI lacked the sensitivity for diagnosis.

It is important to remember that ITN is most commonly associated with the abovementioned clinical presentation (dropped jaw due to bilateral CN V involvement), but the extent of the range of clinical and histologic presentations is somewhat unknown, especially since unilateral dysfunction would not result in a dropped jaw.

Other Differential Diagnoses

Other hypothetical differential diagnoses may include infectious diseases affecting CN V (infectious neuritis), focal immune-mediated, infectious, or vascular disease processes affecting the motor nucleus of CN V, primary diseases of the muscles of mastication (immune-mediated, neoplastic, or infectious myopathies), and traumatic injury, among other things.

INVESTIGATION

Investigation of patients with unilateral masticatory muscle atrophy may include both systemic work-up and advanced imaging, with systemic work-up including baseline blood work (complete blood count [CBC], serum chemistry), urinalysis, thoracic radiographs, and abdominal ultrasonography, as well as infectious disease testing for protozoal, tick-borne, viral, and fungal diseases that can affect the central nervous system (CNS). Systemic work-up typically does not reveal a primary disease diagnosis, and even when a disease process is identified, it still does not support cause and effect. However, it can identify systemic neoplasia and infectious disease processes, which can hypothetically involve the peripheral nervous system and CNS as well.

Magnetic resonance imaging (MRI) is the ideal method for diagnosing patients with unilateral masticatory muscle atrophy. When advanced imaging is not accessible, anesthetized dorsoventral radiographs of the head may reveal an enlarged oval foramen on the ipsilateral side of the atrophy in patients with a TNST. Computed tomography (CT) imaging may also demonstrate enlargement of the oval foramen, in addition to CN V pathology if it is significant, but subtle pathology of the nerve may be missed. Thus, based on the superior contrast resolution of MRI for nerve imaging, this method would be preferred over CT if it is accessible.

MRI of patients with presumptive TNSTs will reveal ipsilateral muscle atrophy, which appears as decreased muscle mass with hyperintensity on T2-weighted (T2W) images, fluid-attenuated inversion recovery (FLAIR), and T1-weighted (T1W) images. There will be mild to marked trigeminal nerve enlargement on the ipsilateral side; the majority of lesions are iso- to hyperintense on T2W images and hypo to isointense on T1W images. There can be mild to marked contrast enhancement, but it is important to remember that a degree of contrast enhancement (similar to that of the pituitary) of the trigeminal nerves and ganglia is considered normal. There may be a mass effect on the adjacent brainstem parenchyma, and enlargement of the oval foramen may also be noted on MRI. MR images from this case are included below (Figure 7.4.3).

With other types of neoplasia, MRI may reveal extra-parenchymal lesions that are contrast-enhancing, which may be consistent with a meningioma or histiocytic sarcoma. MRI may also reveal extra-parenchymal lesions affecting the petrosal portion of the temporal bone, possibly consistent with osteosarcoma. Although CT imaging may not be sensitive for subtle CN V pathology, it is useful for the diagnosis of skull neoplasms.

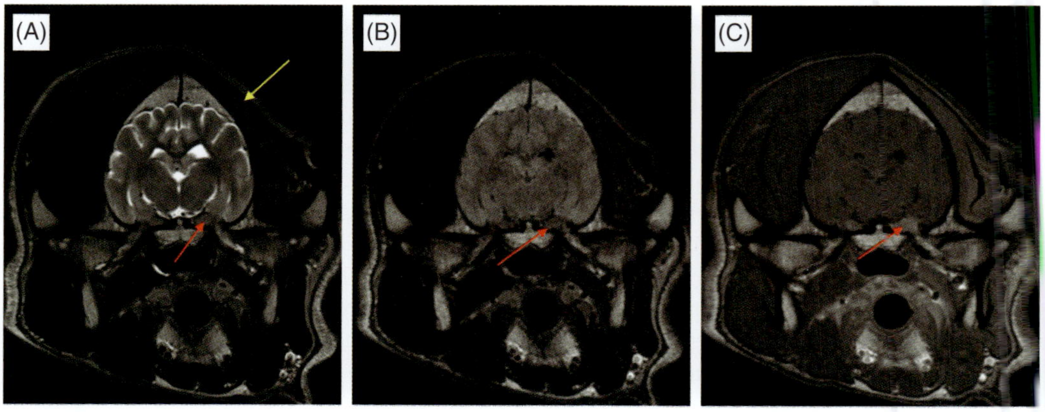

FIGURE 7.4.3 Transverse MR images at the level of the trigeminal nerve from a 7-year-old neutered male Labrador retriever. All images confirm pronounced atrophy of the left temporalis muscles (yellow arrow). In addition, the images show a more pronounced left-sided trigeminal nerve as it exits the brainstem (red arrow), which is hyperintense on T2W images (A), does not suppress with FLAIR (B), and has homogeneous contrast enhancement on TW1 + C (C). This nerve had a more discrete region of focal enlargement rather than being diffusely enlarged along its entirety, consistent with a neoplastic lesion.

MRI is also useful in patients with non-neoplastic conditions. Dogs with ITN may have diffuse nerve enlargement without a specific mass lesion. One study documented that these patients had nerves that were iso- to hyperintense on T2W images, isointense on T1W images, isointense on proton-density-weighted images, and had contrast enhancement.

MRI can also reveal changes consistent with prior trauma or an active infectious process originating within the muscles of mastication or involving the central nervous system primarily. In this author's experience, coccidioidomycosis was diagnosed in a case of masticatory muscle atrophy based on MRI findings and cytology with fungal culture of the affected muscles; serologic testing was negative.

Cerebrospinal fluid (CSF) assessment is unlikely to be of high yield in cases where the trigeminal nerve is affected in isolation, but if the adjacent brainstem is affected, CSF assessment is suggested. Electromyography and muscle biopsy of the affected muscles may be consistent with denervation atrophy in patients with ITN and other trigeminal nerve pathologies, such as TNST. Muscle biopsy may be useful in other disease processes as well.

As shown above, this patient had MRI findings consistent with a presumptive TNST, and CSF analysis was unremarkable.

TREATMENT AND PROGNOSIS

Patients with suspected TNSTs are typically treated with steroids and/or radiation therapy. Surgical removal is difficult because of the disease's location. Variable median survival times are reported in patients undergoing conservative medical therapy, but a recent study documented a median survival time of 5 months, with a range of 1 day to 21 months. In another study, patients treated with stereotactic radiation therapy had a median disease-specific survival of 745 days, and no statistically significant difference in survival was identified in patients with features including an extracranial component, enlarged oval foramen, or tumor shrinkage at 3 months. Radiation therapy typically does not resolve the muscle atrophy observed. A different study determined that there was no significant difference in median survival times between dogs that underwent stereotactic radiation and those that did not; there was also no statistically significant difference in survival between dogs with and without intracranial signs. Of note, it may be difficult to distinguish late radiation side effects from tumor progression clinically, on MRI, or both.

In dogs with other types of extra-parenchymal neoplasia, one study found that almost 50% were euthanized at the time of assessment due to diagnosis and severity of clinical signs. Of the remaining dogs, overall survival time ranged from 6 days to 25 months following diagnosis, with a median of 2.5 months. Treatment included supportive care, corticosteroid therapy, chemotherapy, radiation therapy, or a combination of therapies.

In patients with ITN, there is no evidence to suggest that the use of corticosteroids, such as prednisone, is clinically useful. Recovery time may be associated with the degree of axonal damage, but the majority of patients recover within 2–3 weeks. Recurrence is possible but not commonly documented. Dogs that are bilaterally affected may require assistance eating and drinking, but those that are unilaterally affected should not require this help.

With other causes of unilateral muscle atrophy, treatment should be directed at specific findings, and prognosis is variable depending on the underlying disease process.

OUTCOME

The patient in this chapter underwent an MRI investigation, with the results reported in Figure 7.4.3. Supportive care was provided; anti-inflammatory corticosteroids were initiated 8 weeks later at a recheck when the dog exhibited a mild paresis and proprioceptive deficits in the thoracic and pelvic limbs on the left side. The dog was euthanized on humane grounds 3 months later, with progressive weakness and perceived onset of neck pain.

SUGGESTED READING

Bagley, R.S., Wheeler, S.J., Klopp, L. et al. (1998). Clinical features of trigeminal nerve-sheath tumor in 10 dogs. *J. Am. Anim. Hosp. Assoc.* 34 (1): 19–25.

De Lahunta, A. et al. (2015). *Veterinary Neuroanatomy and Clinical Neurology*. Elsevier.

Dewey, C.W and Da Costa, R.C. (ed.) (2015). *Practical Guide to Canine and Feline Neurology*. Wiley.

Hansen, K.S., Zwingenberger, A.L., Théon, A.P. et al. (2016). Treatment of MRI-diagnosed trigeminal peripheral nerve sheath tumors by stereotactic radiotherapy in dogs. *J. Vet. Intern. Med.* 30: 1112–1120.

Kent, M., Glass, E.N., de Lahunta, A. et al. (2013). Prevalence of effusion in the tympanic cavity in dogs with dysfunction of the trigeminal nerve: 18 cases (2004-2013). *J. Vet. Intern. Med.* 27: 1153–1158.

Mayhew, P.D., Bush, W.W., and Glass, E.N. (2002). Trigeminal neuropathy in dogs: a retrospective study of 29 cases (1991-2000). *J. Am. Anim. Hosp. Assoc.* 38: 262–270.

Milodowski, E.J., Amengual-Batle, P., Beltran, E. et al. (2019). Clinical findings and outcome of dogs with unilateral masticatory muscle atrophy. *J. Vet. Intern. Med.* 33: 735–742.

Pettigrew, R., Rylander, H., and Schwarz, T. (2009). Magnetic resonance imaging contrast enhancement of the trigeminal nerve in dogs without evidence of trigeminal neuropathy. *Vet. Radiol. Ultrasound* 50 (3): 276–278.

Schultz, R.M., Tucker, R.L., Gavin, P.R. et al. (2007). Magnetic resonance imaging of acquired trigeminal nerve disorders in six dogs. *Vet. Radiol. Ultrasound* 48 (2): 101–104.

Swift, K.E., McGrath, S., Nolan, M.W. et al. (2017). Clinical and imaging findings, treatments, and outcomes in 27 dogs with imaging diagnosed trigeminal nerve sheath tumors: a multi-center study. *Vet. Radiol. Ultrasound* 58: 679–689.

CHAPTER 7.5

Disorders of the Head and Face

Case 5—Ophthalmoplegia and Strabismus in a Cat

Katherine Bibi

Blue Pearl Pet Hospital, Kirkland, WA, USA

CASE HISTORY

A 12-year-old spayed female domestic shorthair cat was presented for an acute onset of ocular changes. A few days prior, the owner was teaching the cat how to walk on a harness and leash outdoors. When in the bright sun, the cat's left eye seemed very dark compared to the right. Upon closer inspection, the left pupil was much larger than the right. This eye didn't seem to move normally like the right eye, and the owner compared it to a "glass eye." Over the previous 2 weeks, the cat had been observed to eat less than normal, and she seemed to be less alert than was normal for her. The cat was adopted at 6 months of age from a local shelter in the Northeastern United States; she was indoor-only, with the exception of the recent leash walks outside; she was up-to-date on vaccinations; and she had no other medical history.

NEUROLOGIC EXAMINATION

Upon evaluation, the cat was dull and resisted walking in the examination room. Postural reactions were normal in all four limbs, as were spinal reflexes. Cranial nerve (CN) examination revealed anisocoria, with the left pupil larger than the right. Direct pupillary light reflexes of the left eye were absent, but they were normal in the right eye. When the left eye was stimulated with light, the right pupil normally constricted; when the right eye was stimulated with light, the left pupil did not constrict. There was a very subtle ptosis of the left eye, as reflected by a narrowed palpebral fissure. The vestibulo-ocular reflex was absent in the left eye, and this eye appeared unable to move in any direction. Facial sensation was normal with the exception of the left-sided cornea and the medial nasal planum on the left. The remainder of the neurologic examination was clinically unremarkable.

1. **What is the associated neuroanatomy?**
2. **Where is the likely lesion localization?**
3. **What major disease processes should be considered?**
4. **What tests could you perform to help determine the diagnosis?**
5. **What are the general treatments and prognoses associated with the main differentials?**

ASSOCIATED NEUROANATOMY

The cavernous sinus is a paired venous sinus that is located on the floor of the middle cranial fossa and is responsible for venous drainage from the frontal sinus and nasal cavity. It extends from the orbital fissure rostrally to the petrooccipital canals caudally. This sinus contains the internal carotid artery, the middle meningeal artery, and the external ophthalmic artery. Several cranial nerves course adjacent to this sinus and are thus considered closely related to it, including the oculomotor nerve (CN III) and its associated parasympathetic fibers, the trochlear nerve (CN IV), the abducens nerve (CN VI), and the ophthalmic and maxillary branches of the trigeminal nerve (CN V), along with the postganglionic sympathetic fibers. CN III, IV, and VI are all involved with ocular movement (See Chapter 1, Figure 1.5).

CN III – the oculomotor nerve

- The motor fibers of CN III supply the medial, dorsal, and ventral recti muscles, the ventral oblique, and the levator palpebrae superioris.
- The autonomic fibers of the parasympathetic preganglionic neurons run with this nerve and innervate the iris constrictor muscle, responsible for pupil constriction.

CN IV – the trochlear nerve

- The motor fibers of CN IV innervate the contralateral dorsal oblique; i.e. the left trochlear nerve originates from the right-sided brainstem (midbrain).

CN VI – the abducens nerve

- The motor fibers of CN VI innervate the lateral rectus and retractor bulbi muscles.

With the exception of the iris constrictor, all of the aforementioned muscles are responsible for ocular movement: the medial rectus adducts the eyeball, the dorsal rectus elevates the eyeball, the ventral rectus depresses the eyeball, the ventral oblique rotates the dorsal eye ventrolaterally from midline, the levator palpebrae superioris widens the ocular fissure, the dorsal oblique rotates the dorsal aspect of the globe ventromedially toward midline, the lateral rectus abducts the eye, and the retractor bulbi retracts the globe.

CN III, IV, and VI are connected via the medial longitudinal fasciculus (MLF), which is essential for conjugate ocular movements.

CN V – the trigeminal nerve

- The ophthalmic branch of CN V carries sensory information from the cornea, nasal septum mucosa, and medial canthus to the nucleus of the spinal tract of the trigeminal nerve. Loss of this corneal innervation can sometimes result in neurotrophic keratitis.
- The maxillary branch of CN V carries sensory information from the upper lip (lateral to the canine tooth) and the lateral canthus, as well as the nasal mucosa and outer nare.

LESION LOCALIZATION

Based on the lack of pupillary light reflex of the left eye with normal consensual right eye constriction, involvement of the left sided parasympathetic fibers of CN III was suspected. The mild ptosis affecting this eye could also be explained by the involvement of ipsilateral CN III due to its innervation of the levator palpebrae superioris. The absent vestibulo-ocular reflex on the left was consistent with a lesion affecting both CN III and VI on that side, given the loss of innervation of the lateral and medial rectus muscles of that eye. However, the complete lack of eye movement with normal globe position indicated that all three nerves responsible for innervating the extraocular muscles were involved. It is important to remember that the vestibulo-ocular reflex may be subtle in the cat, and rarely, it may not be present at all in the normal cat. We might expect to see the dorsal aspect of the pupil rotated laterally with an isolated CN IV lesion, but this was not seen in this case, likely because of other cranial nerve involvement. The lack of corneal reflex in the presence of an intact palpebral reflex, and the lack of nasal sensation, indicate involvement of the ophthalmic branch of CN V. This combination of deficits is considered to be consistent with "cavernous sinus syndrome," more appropriately termed middle cranial fossa syndrome. The general anatomic location would also explain this patient's dull mentation. Of note, the cat's mentation may have also played a role in the lack of response to the assessment of nasal sensation.

> The autonomic motor axons of CN III are typically first affected by compressive lesions over the somatic motor axons. Therefore, anisocoria may be the first sign of a compressive disease affecting this nerve.

DIFFERENTIAL DIAGNOSES

Middle cranial fossa syndrome (MCFS) is a relatively uncommon presentation documented in the cat. In general, unilateral signs of disease are much more common than bilateral signs; external ophthalmoplegia or ophthalmoparesis and/or mydriasis (internal ophthalmoplegia) and/or decreased corneal sensation are the most common examination findings.

General differential diagnoses for MCFS may include:

- Neoplasia – A mass lesion within the middle cranial fossa is typically considered the most common cause of MCFS in dogs and cats. In published reports of cats with MCFS related to intracranial neoplasia, lymphoma is the most commonly reported diagnosis. Aside from lymphoma, other types of neoplasia that have been reported in cats with MCFS include adenosquamous carcinoma.
- Infectious disease – Bacterial disease (empyema or abscessation), protozoal disease (toxoplasmosis), fungal disease (cryptococcus), viral disease (feline infectious peritonitis) [2, 5]. Ascending otogenic meningoencephalitis should also be considered as a differential for cats with bacterial causes of MCFS.
- Trauma
- Anomalous conditions – Specifically osteochondromatosis is also been diagnosed in cats with MCFS.

Although lymphoma can be a primary central nervous system (CNS) cancer, it can also be identified in the CNS associated with extranodal forms (such as renal lymphoma). In addition, direct extension from local anatomy or extension via destruction of bone has also been documented. In one case report, magnetic resonance imaging (MRI) suggested direct communication between nasopharyngeal lymphoma and the middle cranial fossa in two cats. Communication was hypothesized via a foramen, lymph drainage pathways, or the craniopharyngeal canal (rather than spread via destruction of bone). The CNs III, IV, V, and VI have also been affected by lymphoma at the site of their exit from the calvaria via the orbital fissure. Thus, isolated masses even outside the calvaria should be considered when diagnosing these cats. Technically, retrobulbar neoplasia may also involve one or more of the cranial nerves discussed above, thus presenting as MCFS when not necessarily involving the region adjacent to the cavernous sinus.

Hematogenous spread of neoplasia has also been hypothesized. Given the direction of venous drainage from the frontal sinus and nasal cavity, it is possible that such diseases could spread from these regions to the middle cranial fossa.

INVESTIGATION

Systemic workup: Blood pressure evaluation, baseline blood work (complete blood count [CBC], serum chemistry), urinalysis, thoracic radiographs, and abdominal ultrasonography.

as well as infectious disease testing for protozoal, tick-borne, viral, and fungal diseases that can affect the CNS, should all be considered. Infectious disease titers indicate disease exposure, and not necessarily active disease. Acute and convalescent titers showing an increase in titer levels can increase suspicion of active infection. Systemic work-up may indicate abnormalities that could point to a primary disease process but not necessarily identify the disease itself. For example, chemistry may reveal elevated muscle enzymes, including alanine aminotransferase (ALT), which can be seen in cats with toxoplasma, an infectious disease that can affect the middle cranial fossa.

Imaging: MRI is the ideal method for diagnosing patients with MCFS. However, other imaging modalities are also options.

- Radiographs have been documented to evaluate cats with MCFS; osteolysis was found in a cat with MCFS secondary to lymphoma, while a soft tissue density around the zygomatic arch and axilla was identified in a cat with metastatic anaplastic adenocarcinoma. However, it is important to note that radiographs may also be normal.
- Computed tomography (CT) imaging may demonstrate osseous abnormalities of the middle cranial fossa, but subtle pathologies of the nerves may be missed.

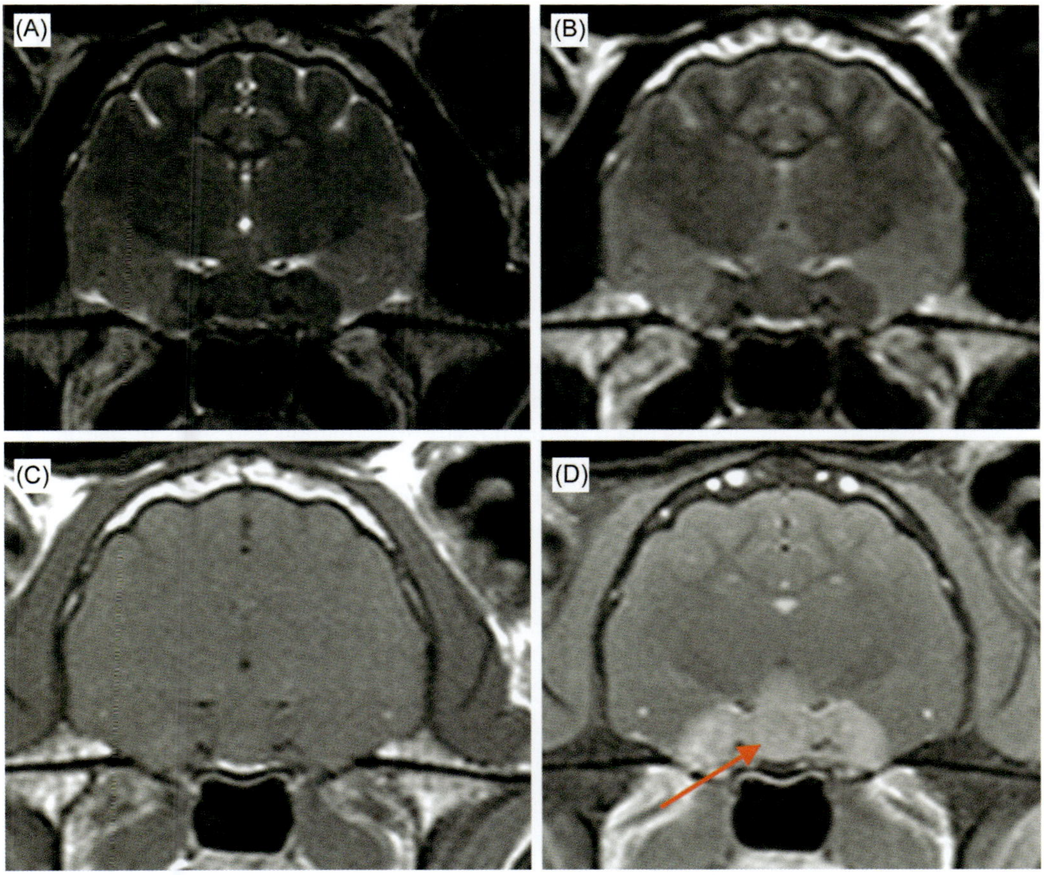

FIGURE 7.5.1 A transverse MRI of the brain of a 5-year-old male neutered cat with a slow progressive onset of middle cranial fossa syndrome. (A) T2W, (B) FLAIR, (C) T1W pre-contrast, and (D) T1W post-contrast images confirm the presence of a relatively well-defined, multilobulated extradural lesion on the base of the cranial vault within the middle cranial fossa. The lesion was confirmed to be lymphoma.

- MRI exhibits superior contrast and spatial resolution for soft tissues, enabling identification of the nerves within the middle cranial fossa and pathologies affecting them (Figure 7.5.1). This method is preferred over CT (and radiographs), if feasible.

Cerebrospinal fluid (CSF): CSF assessment may be useful when diagnosing underlying infectious diseases. Thus, CSF analysis should always be considered in these cases. In one study, two cats with MCFS were diagnosed with *Cryptococcus neoformans* identified in spinal fluid, and a cat with positive toxoplasmosis titers had a mixed pleocytosis with a prominent eosinophilic component (although convalescent titers were not performed).

CSF analysis may not be as useful in neoplastic cases, but should still be performed when neoplasia is suspected. In a cat with lymphoma affecting the cavernous sinus, CSF revealed albuminocytologic dissociation. However, in a separate study, a cat with large granular lymphoma was diagnosed on CSF evaluation.

TREATMENTS AND PROGNOSES

The clinical outcome in patients with MCFS is determined by the underlying cause. Time of presentation may play a role, and it is hypothesized that many cases already have advanced disease by the time of presentation, which may affect outcome. It is important to remember that some conditions (such as FIP) may now be considered more treatable because of more recent scientific advances, so newer studies are necessary.

Most prognostic information seems to be available for cats with MCFS secondary to lymphoma. In a paper summarizing general response to chemotherapy and survival in 110 cats with extranodal lymphoma, 15/110 cats were diagnosed with CNS lymphoma, and these cats had the shortest median survival time (70 days). These patients were either treated with the COP protocol (cyclophosphamide, vincristine, and prednisolone) or the Wisconsin-Madison protocol (vincristine, L-asparaginase, cyclophosphamide, prednisolone, doxorubicin, and methotrexate), or other protocols. Not necessarily specific to lymphoma, but radiation therapy does not seem to be a reported treatment for cats with MCFS, although it does seem to improve survival time in dogs with MCFS.

Without treatment, it is a reasonable assumption that the prognosis for these cats is poor. The study that documented two cats with MCFS secondary to intracranial neoplasia (lymphoma, adenosquamous carcinoma) that did not receive treatment had a median survival time of 14 days. In the case of the cat with MCFS due to osteochondromatosis, the cat was euthanized following a CT scan due to the diffuse lesions identified on physical examination and signs of discomfort. There was no reasonable treatment option for this cat.

Ultimately, prognosis should be dependent upon the clinician's ability to diagnose a definitive condition and pursue appropriate treatment.

OUTCOME

The family of the cat in this case could not proceed with advanced neurologic testing, and radiographs of the head were normal. The cat was ultimately euthanized, but a necropsy was performed. This revealed a mass lesion of the middle cranial fossa, which was consistent with lymphoma on histopathology.

SUGGESTED READING

British Small Animal Veterinary Association (2013). *BSAVA Manual of Canine and Feline Neurology, (with DVD-ROM)* (ed. S.R. Platt and N.J. Olby). Wiley.

Chang, Y., Thompson, H., Reed, N., and Penderis, J. (2006). Clinical and magnetic resonance imaging features of nasopharyngeal lymphoma in two cats with concurrent intracranial mass. *J. Small Anim. Pract.* 47: 678–681.

DeLahunta, A., Glass, E., and Kent, M. (2015). *Veterinary Neuroanatomy and Clinical Neurology*. Elsevier.

Dewey, C.W. and Da Costa, R.C. (ed.) (2015). *Practical Guide to Canine and Feline Neurology*. Wiley.

Evans, H.E. and DeLahunta, A. (2013). *Miller's Anatomy of the Dog* (ed. H., E. Evans and A. DeLahunta). Elsevier Saunders.

Guevar, J., Gutierrez-Quintana, R., Peplinski, G. et al. (2014). Cavernous sinus syndrome secondary to intracranial lymphoma in a cat. *J. Feline Med. Surg.* 16 (6): 513–516.

Jones, A.M., Bentley, E., and Rylander, H. (2018). Cavernous sinus syndrome in dogs and cats: case series (2002-2015). *Open Vet. J.* 8 (2): 186–192.

Lorenz, M.D., Coates, J., and Kent, M. (2011). *Handbook of Veterinary Neurology*. Elsevier/Saunders.

Osinchuk, S.C., Zwueste, D.M., and Grahn, B.H. (2019). Peripheral cranial neuropathies consistent with cavernous sinus syndrome caused by extracranial nasopharyngeal lymphoma in a cat. *Can. Vet. J.* 60 (11): 1156–1160.

Perazzi, A., Bernardini, M., Mandara, M.T. et al. (2013). Cavernous sinus syndrome due to osteochondromatosis in a cat. *J. Feline Med. Surg.* 15 (12): 1132–1136.

Taylor, S.S., Goodfellow, M.R., Browne, W.J. et al. (2009). Feline extranodal lymphoma: response to chemotherapy and survival in 110 cats. *J. Small Anim. Pract.* 50: 584–592.

Theisen, S.K., Podell, M., Schneider, T. et al. (1996). A retrospective study of cavernous sinus syndrome in 4 dogs and 8 cats. *J. Vet. Intern. Med.* 10 (2): 65–71.

CHAPTER 8.1

Tremors, Shakes, and Involuntary Movement

Case 1—Generalized Tremors and Ataxia in a Cat

Georgina Stewart

Neurology Department, ARC – Animal Referral Centre, Auckland, New Zealand

CASE HISTORY

A 4-month-old (16-week) intact male domestic shorthaired kitten was presented for evaluation of ataxia and tremors following adoption from a shelter. The kitten was reported to be abnormal from the time of arrival at the shelter, at approximately 4 weeks old, and the signs have been stable. The kitten is otherwise bright and playful and has always had a good appetite, although it has occasionally struggled to prehend food. The queen was a stray found with a litter of kittens and brought to the shelter. His vaccination status is unknown. Two other kittens in the litter have similar signs.

NEUROLOGIC EXAMINATION (Video 8.1.1)

VIDEO 8.1.1 A kitten exhibiting an intention tremor.

The kitten was bright, alert, and responsive on presentation. He was ambulatory with marked ataxia, often falling equally toward one side or the other. All four limbs exhibited a hypermetric gait along with a wide-based stance. When stationary, a truncal sway that worsened when attempting to play or eat was observed, along with a marked head tremor when attempting to prehend food or drink water. Postural reactions were present in all four limbs but were delayed and subsequently exaggerated (hypermetric). Spinal reflexes were normal in all four limbs. Cranial nerve examination revealed a bilaterally absent menace response with all other tests being normal. The kitten interacted with people and objects in a way that suggested he was visually oriented. There was no pain on palpation of the vertebral column or with cervical range of motion.

1. What is the most likely lesion localization?
2. What major disease processes should be considered?
3. What tests could you perform to help determine the definitive diagnosis?
4. What is the treatment and prognosis?

LESION LOCALIZATION

Hypermetria, intention tremors, and truncal sway are highly suggestive of a problem with the cerebellum. In health, the cerebellum regulates movement, essentially dampening down and fine-tuning movements. In the absence of cerebellar modulation, exaggerated movements develop and lead to hypermetria, intention tremors, and truncal sway. The gait dysfunction observed in patients with cerebellar lesions is characterized as cerebellar ataxia, which manifests as dysmetric limb movements. Most often, this dysmetria manifests as hypermetria, in which patients display excessive limb flexion while walking. Hypermetria is sometimes described as a "goose stepping" or high-stepping gait, particularly in dogs. Head tremors associated with cerebellar dysfunction are often referred to as "intention tremors" as they worsen with goal-oriented movement, such as playing or trying to eat, and are often more noticeable in the head. Truncal sway occurs due to a lack of fine-tuning of reciprocal epaxial muscle activation and inhibition of one side of the trunk versus the other. Postural reaction testing in animals with cerebellar dysfunction often discloses delayed responses. When these patients are hopped, this delay may be followed by an exaggerated or overcompensated hop. Notably, animals with isolated cerebellar dysfunction will display a normal level of mentation. The menace response can be absent as well because the menace pathway courses through the cerebellum. However, vision is maintained in animals with purely cerebellar lesions. Keep in mind when examining pediatric patients that the menace response typically develops between 12 and 16 weeks of age.

WHAT MAJOR DISEASE PROCESSES SHOULD BE CONSIDERED? DIFFERENTIAL DIAGNOSES

INFLAMMATION–FELINE PARVOVIRUS-ASSOCIATED CEREBELLAR HYPOPLASIA

Feline parvovirus (FPV) is a small non-enveloped single-stranded DNA virus that infects domestic cats and other Felidae, as well as some non-felid species.

The virus replicates in mitotically active tissues such as lymphoid tissue, bone marrow, and intestinal mucosa. In late prenatal and early neonatal infection, viral replication can occur in the central nervous system, including the cerebrum, cerebellum, and retina. Most commonly, the virus destroys the external germinal layer of the cerebellum. This destruction prevents the formation of the granular layer (aka granuloprival hypoplasia), leading to diffuse cerebellar hypoplasia. Depending on when the infection occurs, affected cats may also have varying degrees of concurrent hydrocephalus and hydranencephaly. Clinical signs of cerebellar hypoplasia are apparent from the time that kittens start to walk (between 2 and 4 weeks of age). Mild vestibular signs may also be seen, including nystagmus and head tilt, due to the cerebellum's role in modulating the vestibular system. Signs are typically static over the lifetime of the cat after peaking around 3-4 months of age.

Due to the early onset of nonprogressive cerebellar signs in a kitten born to a (likely) unvaccinated queen, FPV-related cerebellar hypoplasia is considered an extremely likely differential diagnosis for this patient.

INFECTION

Infectious disease should always be a primary differential diagnosis for central nervous system dysfunction in a young animal, especially one under 6 months old, where the immune system is still developing, and full vaccination has not occurred. The most common infectious causes of neurological dysfunction include feline coronavirus, *Toxoplasma*, feline immunodeficiency virus (FIV), and feline leukemia virus (FeLV). Similar to storage diseases, cerebellar signs are common, but most affected animals will have multifocal neurological signs along with evidence of systemic illness such as fever, malaise, and bloodwork changes.

Feline infectious peritonitis (FIP), resulting from the virulent mutant of feline coronavirus, is the most common infectious disease of the central nervous system in cats, typically affecting animals <3 years of age. The virus causes a marked immune-mediated inflammatory reaction leading to multisystemic pyogranulomatous vasculitis. Common neurological signs include vestibulocerebellar dysfunction, ataxia, seizures, and mentation change.

Clinical toxoplasmosis, caused by the coccidian parasite *Toxoplasma gondii*, is uncommon in cats, as they are the definitive host of this organism. *T. gondii* has been reported to cause a wide variety of neurological signs in cats, including focal intracranial granulomas, multifocal central nervous system dysfunction, and neuromuscular signs. A thorough ophthalmic evaluation should be performed if toxoplasmosis is suspected due to the potential for multisystemic disease.

Due to the nonprogressive cerebellar signs and lack of other abnormalities, infection is considered less likely for this patient.

DEGENERATIVE – (1) CEREBELLAR CORTICAL DEGENERATION

Cerebellar cortical degeneration (historically called cerebellar abiotrophy) is a postnatal syndrome where there is premature loss of fully differentiated cells due to genetic or metabolic defects. Purkinje cells are predominately affected, with the granular layer affected to a lesser extent. This condition is differentiated from cerebellar hypoplasia, where there is failure of complete neuronal development. Cerebellar cortical degeneration can be divided into three forms – early onset (first few weeks of life), mid-onset (first few months of life), and late-onset (adult). There are numerous reports of cerebellar cortical degeneration in cats, with most cases developing signs in the first 6–12 months of life. Clinical signs are progressive over months to years, with the speed of progression varying. Clinical signs may include cerebellar and proprioceptive ataxia, hypermetria, tremor, absent menace response, blindness and retinal lesions, postural reaction deficits, and nystagmus.

Due to the early onset of nonprogressive cerebellar signs, cerebellar cortical degeneration is considered less likely for this patient, but cannot be ruled out completely.

(2) FELINE NEUROAXONAL DYSTROPHY

Feline neuroaxonal dystrophy is a neurodegenerative disease seen in cats less than 1 year of age, occasionally linked to coat color dilution. Affected cats have progressive ataxia, hypermetria, head tremor, proprioceptive deficits, and paralysis.

Due to the early onset of nonprogressive cerebellar signs, neuroaxonal dystrophy is considered less likely for this patient.

(3) STORAGE DISEASE

Storage diseases are a large group of inherited neurodegenerative diseases caused by the deficiency of one or more enzymes required for normal cell metabolism. This enzyme deficiency disrupts a given catabolic pathway, leading to the accumulation of storage material within the cell and subsequent cell dysfunction and death. Many storage diseases lead to lysosomal accumulation but others lead to cytosolic accumulation.

Cerebellar signs, including ataxia and tremor, are common in storage diseases; however, they often have multifocal neurological signs reflecting more global brain dysfunction. Clinical signs typically occur before the age of 1 year and are progressive. Many diseases are breed-specific and have characteristic clinical signs and examination findings.

Due to the early onset of nonprogressive cerebellar signs and lack of other abnormalities, a lysosomal storage disease is considered less likely for this patient.

WHAT TESTS COULD YOU PERFORM TO HELP DETERMINE THE DEFINITIVE DIAGNOSIS?

The starting point of any neurological investigation should be a thorough physical and neurological examination. In this case, investigation for other signs of illness, including fever, uveitis, retinal dysfunction, enlarged abdominal organs, and abnormalities of skeletal development is important.

Labwork

Blood tests may include a complete blood count, biochemistry, and infectious disease screening, including FIV, FeLV, and *Toxoplasma* titers. Elevated globulins should raise concern for FIP. Storage diseases can lead to vacuolation and inclusion bodies in circulating white blood cells, so a clinical pathologist should closely examine the white blood cells for these abnormalities. In FPV-related cerebellar hypoplasia, cerebellar cortical degeneration, and neuroaxonal dystrophy, labwork will be normal as there is no systemic illness.

Advanced Imaging

Advanced imaging (computed tomography (CT) and magnetic resonance imaging (MRI)) is often required for full evaluation of the central nervous system. MRI offers superior soft tissue resolution, making it ideal for central nervous system imaging. CT of the brain, in particular of the brainstem and cerebellum, has limitations due to beam hardening artifact secondary to the bony anatomy of the caudal fossa.

FPV-related cerebellar hypoplasia:

- MRI of affected cats shows a reduction in the size of the cerebellum with increased CSF visualized between the cerebellar folia. Other CNS abnormalities may also be seen, such as hydrocephalus.

Cerebellar cortical degeneration:

- MRI of affected cats shows normal to slightly decreased cerebellar size.

Other conditions:

- Additional brain abnormalities found on MRI can help point in the direction of other conditions, such as white matter abnormalities and reduced corpus callosum volume seen in cases of lysosomal storage disease; ventriculomegaly and ependymal contrast enhancement with FIP; and meningeal contrast enhancement or granuloma formation with toxoplasmosis.

Cerebrospinal Fluid Analysis

Cerebrospinal fluid (CSF) collection and analysis are complementary to advanced imaging. Most commercial laboratories can perform polymerase chain reaction (PCR) screening for *Toxoplasma*, FPV, FIP, FIV, and FeLV. The presence of an elevated nucleated cell count or protein level can further support an infectious etiology. In cerebellar hypoplasia and cerebellar cortical degeneration, CSF will be normal.

Histopathology

Ultimately, in many neurodegenerative conditions, a definitive diagnosis cannot be reached without histopathological evaluation of brain tissue, and cerebellar sampling is not recommended. Many of these disorders have been well described and have characteristic histopathological findings.

Cerebellar hypoplasia: profound granuloprival hypoplasia

Cerebellar cortical degeneration: profound loss of Purkinje cells, with varying degrees of granular cell loss. Purkinje cells are typically replaced by astrocytes, a finding known as "Bergmann gliosis."

Neuroaxonal dystrophy: characteristic swelling of the distal axons (spheroids) within the central nervous system, including ballooning and loss of Purkinje cells, white matter vacuolation and spheroids in the granular layer of the cerebellum.

Storage disease: widespread vacuolation within cells throughout the body, varying with particular syndromes. Further characterized by special stains.

TREATMENT AND PROGNOSIS

There is no treatment for cerebellar hypoplasia. The cerebellar dysfunction of these kittens remains static for life. Most cats affected by cerebellar hypoplasia have an excellent quality of life and should be kept as indoor-only pets. Feline neuroaxonal dystrophy and lysosomal storage disorders similarly do not have any treatment but are progressive diseases that ultimately lead to poor quality of life due to immobility and systemic derangements. Feline infectious peritonitis was historically a nearly universally fatal condition, but many cases can now be treated successfully with antiviral medications, including GS-441524 and remdesivir. Toxoplasmosis treatment consists primarily of clindamycin and occasionally other antimicrobials; prognosis is variable.

OUTCOME

The kitten was monitored at home for several months, and no change in the signs was observed. Thus, cerebellar hypoplasia was presumptively diagnosed. The cat enjoyed an excellent quality of life, other than being unable to jump on and off furniture.

SUGGESTED READING

Barone, G., Foureman, P., and deLahunta, A. (2002). Adult onset cerebellar cortical abiotrophy and retinal degeneration in a domestic shorthair cat. *J. Am. Anim. Hosp. Assoc.* 38 (1): 51–54. https://doi.org/10.5326/0380051.

Biolatti, C., Gianella, P., Capucchio, M.T. et al. (2010). Late onset and rapid progression of cerebellar abiotrophy in a domestic shorthair cat. *J. Small Anim. Pract.* 51 (2): 123–126. https://doi.org/10.1111/j.1748-5827.2009.00852.x.

Carmichael, K.P., Howerth, E.W., Oliver, J.E. Jr., and Klappenbach, K. (1993). Neuroaxonal dystrophy in a group of related cats. *J. Vet. Diagn. Invest.* 5 (4): 585–590. https://doi.org/10.1177/104063879300500414.

Crawford, A.H., Al, S., Sanchez-Masian, D. et al. (2017). Clinicopathologic features and magnetic resonance imaging findings in 24 cats with histopathologically confirmed neurologic feline infectious peritonitis. *J. Vet. Intern. Med.* 31 (5): 1477–1486. https://doi.org/10.1111/jvim.14791.

Dickinson, P.J., Bannasch, M., Thomasy, S.M. et al. (2020). Antiviral treatment using the adenosine nucleoside analogue GS-441524 in cats with clinically diagnosed neurological feline infectious peritonitis. *J. Vet. Intern. Med.* 34 (4): 1587–1593. https://doi.org/10.1111/jvim.15780.

Dubey, J.P., Cerqueira-Cezar, C.K., Murata, F.H.A. et al. (2020). All about toxoplasmosis in cats: the last decade. *Vet. Parasitol.* 283: 109145. https://doi.org/10.1016/j.vetpar.2020.10.145.

Giron, C., Helie, P., Parent, J. et al. (2024). Clinical, imaging and histopathological characterization of a series of three cats with cerebellar cortical degeneration. *BMC Vet. Res.* 20 (1): 263. https://doi.org/10.1186/s12917-024-04127-3.

Gunn-Moore, D.A. and Reed, N. (2011). CNS disease in the cat: current knowledge of infectious causes. *J. Feline Med. Surg.* 13 (11): 824–836. https://doi.org/10.1016/j.jfms.2011.09.004.

Hasegawa, D., Tamura, S., Nakamoto, Y. et al. (2013). Magnetic resonance findings of the corpus callosum in canine and feline lysosomal storage diseases. *PLoS One* 8 (12): e83455. https://doi.org/10.1371/journal/pone.0083455.

Kent, M. (2009). The cat with neurological manifestations of systemic disease. Key conditions impacting on the CNS. *J. Feline Med. Surg.* 11 (5): 395–407. https://doi.org/10.1016/j.jfms.2009.03.007.

Negrin, A., Bernadini, M., Baumgartner, W., and Castagnaro, M. (2016). Late onset cerebellar degeneration in middle aged cat. *J. Feline Med. Surg.* 8 (6): 424–429. https://doi.org/10.1016/j.jfms.2006.04.007.

Partridge, B. and Rossmeisl, J.H. Jr. (2020). Companion animal models of neurological disease. *J. Neurosci. Methods* 331 (331): 108484. https://doi.org/10.1016/j.jneumeth.2019.108484.

Penderis, J. (2009). The wobbly cat. Diagnostic and therapeutic approach to generalized ataxia. *J. Feline Med. Surg.* 11 (5): 349–359. https://doi.org/10.1016/j.jfms.2009.03.003.

Pfohl, J.C. and Dewey, C.W. (2005). Intracranial Toxoplasma gondii granuloma in a cat. *J. Feline Med. Surg.* 7 (6): 369–374. https://doi.org/10.1016/j.jfms.5.03.004.

Rodríguez, F., Espinosa de los Monteros, A., Morales, M. et al. (1996). Neuroaxonal dystrophy in two siamese kitten littermates. *Vet. Rec.* 138 (22): 548–549. https://doi.org/10.1136/vr.138.22.548.

Scott, E.Y., Woolard, K.D., Finno, C.J., and Murray, J.D. (2018). Cerebellar abiotrophy across domestic species. *Cerebellum* 17 (3): 372–379. https://doi.org/10.1007/s12311-017-0914-1.

Shamir, M., Perl, S., and Sharon, L. (1999). Late onset of cerebellar abiotrophy in a Siamese cat. *J. Small Anim. Pract.* 40 (7): 343–345. https://doi.org/10.1111/j.1748-5827.1999.tb03095.x.

Sharp, N.J., Davis, B.J., Guy, J.S. et al. (1999). Hydranencephaly and cerebellar hypoplasia in two kittens attributed to intrauterine parvovirus infection. *J. Comp. Pathol.* 121 (1): 39–53. https://doi.org/10.1053/jcpa.1998.0298.

Skelly, B.J. and Franklin, R.J.M. (2002). Recognition and diagnosis of lysosomal storage diseases in the cat and dog. *J. Vet. Intern. Med.* 16 (2): 133–141. https://doi.org/10.1111/j.1939-1676.2002.tb02344.x.

Stuetzer, B. and Hartmann, K. (2014). Feline parvovirus infection and associated diseases. *Vet. J.* 201 (2): 150–155. https://doi.org/10.1016/j.tvjl.2014.05.027.

Woodard, J.C., Collins, G.H., and Hessler, J.R. (1974). Feline hereditary neuroaxonal dystrophy. *Am. J. Pathol.* 74 (3): 551–566. PMID: 4814900.

CHAPTER 8.2

Tremors, Shakes, and Involuntary Movement
Case 2—Dyskinesia in a Dog

Georgina Stewart

Neurology Department, ARC – Animal Referral Centre, Auckland, New Zealand

CASE HISTORY

A 3-year-old spayed female Norwich terrier was presented for having two neurological episodes. During an episode, the dog would become distressed, develop stiffness in all four limbs, sit down and lift one thoracic limb into the air for ~10–20 seconds. This was repeated several times. The dog remained conscious throughout the episode, but her owner felt she was distressed and slightly disoriented. Both episodes occurred during the day and lasted approximately 2–5 minutes. The dog was adopted from a breeder approximately 1 month prior. She had been used as a breeding bitch prior to adoption and had recently been spayed.

Please see the associated video (Video 8.2.1) of one of the episodes.

VIDEO 8.2.1 A dog with paroxysmal dyskinesia.

NEUROLOGIC EXAMINATION

The dog was bright, alert, and responsive on presentation, although slightly anxious. Her physical and neurological examinations were normal.

Questions

1. What are your main differential diagnoses for this case?
2. What additional history questions would you ask the owner of this dog?
3. What tests would you carry out?
4. What are the treatment options and prognosis for the most likely diagnosis in this case?

WHAT ARE YOUR MAIN DIFFERENTIAL DIAGNOSES FOR THIS CASE?

Focal Seizure

The International Veterinary Epilepsy Task Force defines epileptic seizures as "manifestations of excessive synchronous, usually self-limiting epileptic activity of neurons in the brain. This results in transient occurrence of signs which may be characterized by short episodes with convulsions of focal motor, autonomic or behavioral features and due to abnormal excessive or synchronous epileptic neuronal activity in the brain."

Focal seizures are characterized by lateralized or regional signs with a consistent ictal onset. The abnormal electrical activity associated with focal seizures arises within one hemisphere of the brain. Focal seizures may include motor signs (such as facial twitching or jerking, rhythmic blinking, or repeated rhythmic jerks of one extremity), autonomic signs (such as dilated pupils, hypersalivation, or vomiting), and behavioral signs (such as transient anxiousness, restlessness, fear, or attention-seeking behavior). Consciousness may be partially impaired in a focal seizure, but animals do not lose consciousness as occurs in a generalized epileptic seizure. There are currently no reports on a genetic or suspected genetic epilepsy in Norwich terriers, although epilepsy can occur in any dog.

Movement Disorder

Movement disorders are a group of conditions characterized by involuntary movements without loss of or changes in consciousness. They include tremors, peripheral nerve hyperexcitability (which includes fasciculations, myokymia, neuromyotonia, myotonia, cramps, and tetany/tetanus), myoclonus, dystonia, and paroxysmal dyskinesia.

Paroxysmal dyskinesias (PDs) are a type of movement disorder characterized by recurrent self-limiting episodes of abnormal involuntary movements without changes in consciousness. Episodes are painless, autonomic signs are absent, consciousness is not impaired, and abnormal post-ictal signs are not observed. Episodes can last seconds to hours with an abrupt beginning and end. There is marked variation in presentation between different dogs.

PDs are the result of dysfunction of the basal nuclei along with other central nervous system structures such as the cerebellum. Causes of PDs include both genetic or suspected genetic, reactive (i.e. drug-induced, toxic), structural (neoplasia, inflammatory brain disease), and unknown.

Norwich terriers display a suspected autosomal recessive hereditary PD. Affected dogs will display episodes of sustained muscular hypertonicity in the pelvic limbs, trunk, and thoracic limbs that impair posture and locomotion. Dogs often lift a limb off the ground or have sustained flexion of a limb. There is no loss of consciousness. The mean age of onset is 3 years old. Episode duration ranges from 2 to 30 minutes and triggers include stress, anxiety, and excitement.

There are many other breed-associated and individual reports of movement disorders in dogs. A selection of such conditions includes:

- Episodic falling in Cavalier King Charles spaniels
- "Scottie cramp" in Scottish terriers
- Gluten-sensitive paroxysmal dyskinesia in Border terriers (previously called epileptoid cramping syndrome or Spike's disease)

Based on the description of the episode, lack of "red-flag" behaviors for seizures (such as pre/post-ictal signs and autonomic dysfunction) as well as the known breed-associated movement disorder, Norwich terrier PD is considered the most likely differential diagnosis for this patient.

WHAT ADDITIONAL HISTORY QUESTIONS WOULD YOU ASK THE OWNER OF THIS DOG?

a. Were the episodes associated with exercise, excitement, stress, or rest?

- Identifying triggers can help with narrowing down the nature of the episode. Seizures are typically associated with rest, while some PDs may be associated with exercise, stress, or excitement.

b. Were there any autonomic signs noticed?

- If autonomic signs are noticed during an episode, it should raise suspicion for a seizure disorder. Autonomic signs are not reported with PDs.

c. Did the dog display any abnormal behaviors/signs either immediately before or immediately after the episode?

- Pre- and post-ictal signs are classically associated with seizure disorders, whereas PDs are characterized by an abrupt start and finish.

d. Do any of the other dogs in the family or any of the puppies of this dog exhibit similar episodes?

- Many breed-associated PDs will have strong family histories of similar episodes. If other immediate family members have similar episodes, it should raise concern for a genetic or inherited condition. However, some forms of epilepsy are also inherited, so this may not help you differentiate. Online searches should clarify if there is documented genetic cause in a specific breed.

WHAT TESTS WOULD YOU CARRY OUT?

The diagnostic approach for neurological episodes where there is concern for both PD and focal seizures should start with a clear description of the episodes, along with a complete physical and neurological examination. In both epilepsy and genetic/suspected genetic PD, neurological examination will be normal. In reactive and structural PDs and seizure disorders, neurological examination may be abnormal.

Labwork

A minimum database including a complete blood count and chemistry evaluation should be performed to exclude reactive causes such as electrolyte abnormalities (such as hypocalcemia), hypoglycemia, hepatic encephalopathy, and endocrine disturbances (such as hypoadrenocorticism).

There is recent evidence that Border terriers with epileptoid cramping syndrome, as well as sporadic reports in other breeds, have a gluten-sensitive form of PD with affected dogs having elevated levels of anti-transglutaminase 2 and anti-gliadin antibodies. These antibody tests are not widely available in commercial laboratories and elevated antibody levels can also occur in normal dogs.

Advanced Imaging

Magnetic resonance imaging (MRI) can be pursued to investigate structural causes of epilepsy and PD. If no abnormalities are found on MRI, then a presumptive diagnosis of genetic/suspected genetic PD can be made. It is important to keep in mind that even in breeds with well-described PDs and genetic forms of epilepsy, structural abnormalities of the brain can occur. Cerebrospinal fluid evaluation following MRI will help to rule out infectious and non-infectious inflammatory brain conditions.

Electrodiagnostics

When available, electroencephalography (EEG) can be a valuable tool to differentiate a potential paroxysmal dyskinesia from focal seizures, although inter-ictal evaluations can be normal in some seizure dogs.

Medication Trial

An alternative diagnostic tool, if EEG is unavailable, is a treatment trial with an anticonvulsive medication. Using a medication with a rapid onset of action, such as levetiracetam, rather than a drug that requires a several week buildup period such as phenobarbital, can speed this process along. Keep in mind that if the episodes are infrequent, a treatment trial may not yield a meaningful response.

WHAT ARE THE TREATMENT OPTIONS AND PROGNOSIS FOR THE MOST LIKELY DIAGNOSIS IN THIS CASE?

There are many potential treatment options available for dogs with PDs, although the response to these treatments appears to be very variable, even among individual dogs with the same breed-specific condition. The most commonly reported successful medication is acetazolamide, with additional sporadic reports of success using clonazepam, fluoxetine, and phenobarbital.

Another treatment option to consider is a gluten-free diet, as there are reports of success not only in Border terrier PD but also in other affected dogs (in particular, Maltese dog PD).

However, as many PDs are benign, self-limiting, and even improve over time, it is reasonable to consider monitoring these patients for several months after diagnosis to see if treatment is justified. Many of the reported medications have side effects, and their use may not be worth the expense of the medication and the risk of side effects.

Overall, the prognosis for this dog is likely to be very good. Norwich terrier PD is reported to be either unchanged or improved in 50–75% of dogs over their lifetime. Generally, PDs are considered not to negatively affect the quality of life in the majority of affected dogs.

OUTCOME

No abnormalities were observed on lab work, and an MRI of the brain was normal. The dog was presumptively diagnosed with paroxysmal dyskinesia based on the episode phenotype and these normal findings. She continued to have episodes sporadically every 3–4 months. Given the infrequency of the episodes, which typically only lasted 15–20 minutes, treatment was not considered necessary.

SUGGESTED READING

Berendt, M., Farquhar, R.G., Mandigers, P.J.J. et al. (2015). International veterinary epilepsy task force consensus report on epilepsy definition, classification and terminology in companion animals. *BMC Vet. Res.* 11: 182. https://doi.org/10.1186/s12917-015-0461-2.

Cerda-Gonzalez, S., Packer, R.A., Garosi, L. et al. (2021). International veterinary canine dyskinesia task force ECVN consensus statement: terminology and classification. *J. Vet. Intern. Med.* 35: 1218–1230. https://doi.org/10.1111/jvim.16108.

De Risio, L., Forman, O.P., Mellersh, C.S., and Freeman, J. (2016). Paroxysmal dyskinesia in Norwich Terrier dogs. *Mov. Disord. Clin. Pract.* 3 (6): 573–579. https://doi.org/10.1002/mdc3.12334.

Hulsmeyer, V.I., Fischer, A., Mandigers, P.J.J. et al. (2015). International veterinary epilepsy task force's current understanding of idiopathic epilepsy of genetic or suspected genetic origin in purebred dogs. *BMC Vet. Res.* 11: 175. https://doi.org/10.1186/s12917-015-0463-0.

Jenkins, C.A., De Risio, L., Dietschi, E. et al. (2024). A preliminary genome-wide association study of paroxysmal dyskinesia in the Norwich Terrier. *Anim. Genet.* 55 (6): 914–917. https://doi.org/10.1111/age.13479.

Lowrie, M. and Garosi, L. (2016). Classification of involuntary movements in dogs: tremors and twitches. *Vet. J.* 214: 109–116. https://doi.org/10.1016/j.vjl.2016.05.011.

Lowrie, M. and Garosi, L. (2017). Classification of involuntary movements in dogs: paroxysmal dyskinesias. *Vet. J.* 220: 65–71. https://doi.org/10.1016/j.tvjl.2016.12.017.

Mandigers, P.J.J., Santifort, K.M., Lowrie, M., and Garosi, L. (2024). Canine paroxysmal dyskinesia – a review. *Front. Vet. Sci.* 11: 1441332. https://doi.org/10.3389/fvets.2024.1441332.

Marioni-Henry, K., Rusbridge, C., and Volk, H.A. (2016). Clinical features in border terrier dogs with paroxysmal involuntary movements. *Mov. Disord. Clin. Pract.* 3: 73–79. https://doi.org/10.1002/mdc3.12232.

Packer, R.A., Wachowiak, I., Thomovsky, S.A. et al. (2021). Phenotypic characterization of PIGN-associated paroxysmal dyskinesia in soft-coated wheaten terriers and preliminary response to acetazolamide therapy. *Vet. J.* 269: 105606. https://doi.org/10.1016/j.tvjl.2021.105606.

Polidoro, D., Van Ham, L., Santens, P. et al. (2020). Phenotypic characterization of paroxysmal dyskinesia in Maltese dogs. *J. Vet. Intern. Med.* 34: 1541–1545. https://doi.org/10.1111/jvim.15804.

Stassen, Q.E.M., Koskinen, L.L.E., van Steenbeek, F.G. et al. (2017). Paroxysmal dyskinesia in border terriers: clinical, epidemiological and genetic investigations. *J. Vet. Intern. Med.* 31: 1123–1131. https://doi.org/10.1111/jvim.14731.

Tremors, Shakes, and Involuntary Movement

Case 3—Tremor and Ataxia in a Dog

CHAPTER 8.3

Vivian Lau

Sage Veterinary Centers, Redwood City, CA, USA

CASE HISTORY

A 9-year-old neutered male Norfolk terrier was presented for the acute onset of ataxia and generalized tremors within the past 24 hours. He was normal in the morning, but by the afternoon, was noted to be lethargic and having a difficult time walking. His owner noted some foreign material in some stool in the dog run. He lives on an acreage with two other dogs and goes to the neighborhood park, but has no known toxin exposure. The other dogs in the home were acting normally.

NEUROLOGICAL AND PHYSICAL EXAMINATION

The dog was quiet but responsive and was unable to stand and bear weight on all four limbs. He had generalized tremors and a low head carriage. On postural reaction testing, he had absent placing and moderately delayed hopping in all four limbs. Spinal reflexes were all intact. The cranial nerve exam was within normal limits, and the dog was comfortable on paravertebral palpation and cervical manipulation.

1. **Where is the likely lesion localization?**
2. **What major differential diagnoses should be considered?**
3. **What tests could you perform to help determine the diagnosis?**

LESION LOCALIZATION

With the generalized tremors and proprioceptive deficits, we would be most suspicious of a diffuse myelin disorder, either in the central nervous system, the peripheral nervous system, or both. Generalized tremors are often erroneously attributed to cerebellar dysfunction. However, if the cerebellum is exclusively affected, the only tremor that occurs is an intention tremor. Diffuse tremors do not originate from cerebellar dysfunction.

DIFFERENTIAL DIAGNOSES

Neurotoxicity

Bromethalin toxicity: Bromethalin is a non-anticoagulant rodenticide that works by uncoupling oxidative phosphorylation in mitochondria. This leads to deficient levels of adenosine triphosphate production and failure of cellular membrane sodium-potassium pumps, causing a loss of cellular osmotic equilibrium. In the central nervous system, this osmotic dysregulation leads to intracellular and intramyelinic fluid accumulation, resulting in severe cerebral edema and neurologic dysfunction. Clinical signs of toxicity vary depending on the dosage ingested. Cats are even more sensitive to this toxin, with lethal dosages being less than half of those reported in dogs. For patients exposed to lower dosages, clinical signs will develop on a slower timeline within hours to days of exposure. Signs of low-dose toxicity include vomiting, generalized tremors, ataxia, and paresis, potentially progressing to paralysis. In cases of higher dosage exposure, clinical signs are primarily related to severe cerebral edema and can include dramatic mentation change (severe dullness or hyperesthesia), seizures, circling, hyperthermia, and death. Initial treatments after recent exposure should include decontamination with induction of emesis and the administration of activated charcoal. There is evidence to support the use of intravenous lipid emulsion therapy for this toxin, which tends to deposit in fatty tissues in the body. Other supportive treatments include corticosteroids, mannitol, anticonvulsants, muscle relaxers, and sedatives. While clinical signs can improve and abate after a few weeks in lower-dosage exposures, cases with clinical signs related to severe cerebral edema (presumably from higher-dosage exposure) are usually fatal.

Molluscicides: Metaldehyde is a substance found in snail bait, which can cause severe neurologic signs. Lethal doses in dogs are reported to be about 100 mg/kg, with clinical signs ranging from vomiting and salivation to generalized tremors, seizures, and respiratory distress. There is no known specific antidote, and treatments usually include early decontamination with induction of emesis and activated charcoal administration. Supportive therapies can include constant rate infusion of anesthetics, muscle relaxants, anticonvulsant therapies, and intravenous lipid emulsion infusion. The tremors can result in severe, life-threatening hyperthermia if left untreated With supportive care and lower toxin exposure, many cases of metaldehyde can survive with resolution of clinical signs. As with other toxins, exposure to larger dosages and cases with more severe clinical signs may result in death or humane euthanasia.

Tremorgenic mycotoxins: Ingestion of compost or spoiled foods can result in exposure to tremorgenic mycotoxins such as roquefortine and penitrem A contained in *Penicillium* species and various mold species. While the exact mechanism of action is unknown, the tremorgenic mycotoxins have effects on neurotransmitter levels at both peripheral synapses and, in indole-containing mycotoxins that cross the blood-brain barrier, at central synapses. These alterations of neurotransmitters cause clinical signs ranging from vomiting and ataxia to severe generalized tremors and even seizures. Early treatment involves induction of emesis and repeated doses of activated charcoal (the toxins undergo enterohepatic recirculation). Supportive care is initiated with muscle relaxants, benzodiazepine therapy, and anticonvulsants if seizures are noted. Active cooling and fluid therapy are indicated when hyperthermia develops, and in some cases, the heavy sedation and anesthetics required to improve generalized tremors or seizure activity may require the need for intubation and ventilatory support Intravenous lipid emulsion therapy has been attempted since the mycotoxins are lipid-soluble, with good anecdotal outcomes. With early and aggressive treatments, the prognosis after tremorgenic mycotoxin ingestion can be good.

Methylxanthine toxicities: Methylxanthines are compounds contained in common household foods such as chocolate, coffee, and tea. Theobromine and caffeine, the methylxanthines contained in these foods, are generally considered stimulants. Their primary mechanism of action is through inhibition of cellular adenosine receptors, leading to diuresis, stimulation of the central nervous system, and tachycardia. Methylxanthines can also compete for benzodiazepine receptors within the central nervous system, leading to further excitability. They have also been shown to increase intracellular calcium levels, resulting in increased muscle contractility. By inhibiting phosphodiesterase, methylxanthines also increase intracellular cyclic adenosine monophosphate (c-AMP), mimicking a sympathetic nervous system fight or flight response in the patient, which also raises epinephrine and norepinephrine levels. The combination of these effects can cause signs in dogs (and cats) ranging from vomiting and tremors to hypertension, tachycardia, and generalized seizures. Early treatment is through decontamination with induction of emesis and repeated doses of activated charcoal (methylxanthines undergo enterohepatic recirculation). Supportive treatment with sedatives and anticonvulsants should be initiated in cases of severe tremors, hyperexcitability, or seizures. Beta-blockers (metoprolol) may be indicated for severe tachycardia. IV fluid therapy and urinary catheterization to avoid bladder reabsorption of caffeine can also be helpful. Prognosis is usually good with early and aggressive treatment, although ingestion of large quantities of methylxanthines, especially found in dark chocolate and baking chocolate, can be fatal.

Organophosphates: Organophosphates or carbamates, found in many insecticides and some flame-retardant fabric treatments, can cause severe neurologic signs in dogs and cats. The primary mechanism of action is inhibition of anticholinesterase, resulting in a cholinergic crisis. Clinical signs of toxicity can range from miosis, excessive salivation, vomiting, and diarrhea to generalized tremors, ataxia, muscle weakness, and seizures. Initial treatments involve decontamination, with gastric lavage being shown to improve outcomes. Specific therapies for organophosphate toxicity include atropine and pralidoxime (2-PAM). Supportive therapy with IV fluid therapy, sedatives, and anticonvulsants can be helpful. In cases with severe weakness or that require heavy sedation, intubation for ventilatory support is indicated, although these cases tend to have a worse prognosis.

Immune-Mediated Inflammatory Brain Disease

Inflammatory diseases of the brain can be divided into infectious versus noninfectious etiologies. In North America and Europe, noninfectious inflammatory diseases of the dog brain, specifically Meningoencephalitis of Unknown Etiology (MUE) or Meningoencephalitis of Unknown Origin (MUO), are far more common than infectious diseases. MUE and MUO are generally considered umbrella terms to describe the immune-mediated group of inflammatory encephalitides found in dogs, including granulomatous meningoencephalitis (GME), necrotizing leukoencephalopathy (NLE), and necrotizing meningoencephalitis (NME), among others.

The specific subtypes of inflammatory disease are generally histopathologic diagnoses, and many of these cases do not undergo histopathology of brain tissues until postmortem examination. While specific etiologies have not been identified, a combination of genetics and environmental factors is suspected. The disease was originally described in young, small-breed dogs such as Maltese Terriers, Yorkshire terriers, Chihuahuas, and pug dogs, but it is now well known that it can affect breeds of all sizes. Clinical signs vary depending on the areas where inflammation is focused, and neurolocalization is often multifocal. GME in particular can have an optic nerve form, a focal form, or more commonly, a multifocal form. NME often affects the cerebral grey matter, with many patients presenting with seizures. Biopsies of affected tissue for histopathology would offer a definitive diagnosis, but because it is quite invasive, it is rarely performed.

Diagnosis is usually through a combination of brain MRI and spinal fluid analysis. Neurologic infectious diseases should be ruled out through serology and antigen testing on peripheral blood or spinal fluid. The first line of treatment for MUE is high-dose corticosteroids, often in combination with other immunosuppressive agents (cyclosporine, mycophenolate, leflunomide, cytarabine arabinoside, etc.). Prognosis is variable, with necrotizing forms of the disease generally carrying a worse prognosis than non-necrotizing types. While a majority of patients will respond to initial therapies, a small subset do not survive beyond the first week of diagnosis. Patients can experience repeated relapses of the disease, requiring lifelong immunosuppressive therapy.

Canine Idiopathic generalized tremor syndrome

Canine Idiopathic Generalized Tremor Syndrome (IGTS) is also known as steroid-responsive tremor syndrome, "Little White Shaker Dog Syndrome," and idiopathic cerebellitis. As the name suggests, a hallmark feature of this disease is generalized full-body tremors (Video 8.3.1). Other signs can include cerebellar or vestibular dysfunction. The syndrome was first described in young small white dog breeds such as the West Highland white terrier and Maltese, hence the previous moniker of Little White Shaker Dog Syndrome. The condition has now been described in a variety of different breeds of all colors and sizes, making IGTS a more appropriate term for the condition, although smaller breeds are still overrepresented. A specific etiology for the disease is unknown, although, similar to MUE, IGTS is believed to be an immune-mediated inflammatory disease. In contrast to MUE, however, IGTS cases often have minimal changes on MRI and either no evidence of inflammation or only mild pleocytosis on spinal fluid analysis. A mild diffuse lymphocytic inflammation has been described on necropsy, with the cerebellum being most affected. The disease is also known as corticosteroid-responsive tremor syndrome, and the first line of treatment is steroids. A combination of steroids and other immunomodulatory medications (cyclosporine, mycophenolate, etc.) has been described for treatment of this condition at dosages and durations similar to those used for MUE. Again, in contrast to MUE cases, however, patients tend to have better responses and long-term outcomes with IGTS, rarely succumbing to this disease.

VIDEO 8.3.1 Four-year-old neutered male mixed breed dog with diffuse tremors secondary to idiopathic generalized tremor syndrome.

Degenerative Disorders

Several degenerative and hereditary conditions can cause demyelination and signs of tremors and ataxia over time:

(1) Inborn errors of metabolism

Many of these are due to inborn errors of metabolism, causing either abnormal function or a lack of key enzymes that break down cellular products. Over time, this leads to abnormal cellular product accumulation within cells throughout the body. These disorders include encephalopathies related to organic aciduria and lysosomal storage diseases. In the central nervous system, abnormal cellular product accumulation can cause signs that may include cerebellar/vestibular dysfunction, mentation change, and seizures. Globoid leukodystrophy (Krabbe's disease) is a well-characterized storage disease of both humans and animals that has been reported in several breeds, including Cairn terriers and West Highland white terriers. In this condition, an autosomal recessive genetic mutation results in a deficiency of the galactosylceramidase (galactocerebrosidase) enzyme, leading to accumulation of psychosine in the brain. Psychosine is a neurotoxic compound affecting oligodendrocytes and Schwann cells, causing demyelination. The globoid cells noted on histopathology in these cases are macrophages, which are swollen with phagocytized myelin and other white matter cellular breakdown products.

Clinical signs in affected dogs can vary between an early onset pelvic limb paresis and paralysis or gradually progressive cerebellar signs (ataxia and dysmetria, intention tremors) with later stages causing severe mentation changes, seizures, and death. Another example of a storage disease is neuronal ceroid lipofuscinosis (NCL), in which various lipopigments accumulate within the neurons. A variety of subtypes of NCL associated with mutations in different genes have been characterized in various breeds and humans. For many of the affected breeds (dachshunds, herding breeds, American bully breeds, etc.), commercially available genetic testing is available. The onset of clinical signs can vary slightly between different subtypes, but generally, onset is in older puppies and young dogs, with signs progressing and worsening over months or a few years. Clinical signs of NCL can include loss of learned behaviors, ataxia, tremors, and vision change progressing to severe mentation change, seizures, incontinence, and loss of independent ambulation.

Unfortunately, storage diseases generally carry a grave prognosis with no current commercially available therapies, and most patients are expected to succumb to their disease at a young age. Where genetic testing is available, responsible breeders should test potential mating pairs before breeding to minimize the genetic perpetuation of these diseases. Genetic testing developed for L-2-hydroxyglutaric aciduria, an inborn error of metabolism that can cause ataxia, dysmetria, tremors, and dyskinesia/seizures in Staffordshire bull terriers, has been utilized by breeders in the UK to help reduce the frequency of this disease.

(2) Leukoencephalomyelopathies

Degenerative leukoencephalomyelopathies have been described in Leonbergers, Rottweilers, Danoodles (Great Dane-Poodle mixes), and Great Danes, which can affect the white matter tracts of the central nervous system, causing progressive ataxia and tremors. The disorder in these breeds has been traced to different genetic mutations in the *NAPEPLD* gene involved in myelin homeostasis. Affected dogs begin showing clinical signs at 1–3 years old of progressive ataxia and paresis affecting all four limbs. Clinical signs generally progress over months to severely affect the ability for independent ambulation, typically resulting in humane euthanasia. These patients have well-described MRI changes with symmetrical signal change in the crus cerebri, pyramidal tracts, and the dorsal portion of the lateral funiculi of the spinal cord corresponding to areas of demyelination on histopathology of necropsy samples. Spongiform leukoencephalomyelopathies of varying kinds have also been described in several dog breeds, including Labrador retrievers, Shetland sheepdogs, Samoyeds, and border terriers. While most of these dogs displayed signs of seizures and opisthotonus, the border terriers and Samoyeds displayed progressive tremors, titubation, and cerebellar ataxia corresponding to a higher distribution of spongiform changes in the cerebellar white matter tracts. Genetic causes of these spongiform leukoencephalomyelopathies have not been identified.

(3) Neuraxonal dystrophy

Rottweilers can also develop a neuroaxonal dystrophy, which can cause similar signs of progressive ataxia and head tremors. More often than in Rottweilers with leukoencephalomyelopathy, these patients can also develop nystagmus and vestibular signs with a slower course of clinical progression over years rather than months. Signs are due to axonal degeneration within the spinal cord and brainstem nuclei, as well as a loss of Purkinje cells within the cerebellum. An autosomal recessive mode of inheritance of a mutation in the *VPS11* gene is associated with this disease.

(4) Canine multiple system degeneration

Canine Multiple System Degeneration (CMSD) is a disorder that has been described in Kerry blue terriers, Chinese crested dogs, and Ibizan hounds. Signs are noted in puppies under a year of age and consist of progressive cerebellar signs (ataxia, tremors, truncal sway, absent menace response) that worsen over months, resulting in humane euthanasia usually before 2 years of age. On necropsy, affected animals are found to have severe degeneration affecting the cerebellum, olivary nuclei, substantia nigra, and caudate nuclei of the brain. An autosomal recessive inheritance pattern related to the *SERAC1* gene has been identified in the Kerry blue terriers and Chinese crested dogs.

Alexander Disease-like Disorders

Alexander disease is a well-described neurodegenerative disorder associated with astrocyte dysfunction in humans. Histopathology of affected tissues typically reveals characteristic intracellular inclusions within astrocytes called Rosenthal fibers, which consist of glial fibrillary acidic protein (GFAP), ubiquitin, vimentin, and other proteins. Mutations in the GFAP gene are associated with the disease.

A similar condition causing Rosenthal fiber accumulation in the central nervous system has been described in several dog breeds, including the Bernese mountain dog, Labrador retriever, Scottish terrier, and miniature poodle. Affected dogs began showing clinical signs at a few months of age, which include progressive ataxia, tetraparesis, generalized tremors, and altered mentation. Rosenthal fibers can be found throughout the central nervous system on necropsy, with minimal to mild demyelination noted within the white matter. There is no known treatment, and worsening neurologic status typically results in humane euthanasia within a few months.

(5) Spinocerebellar ataxia

Russell group terriers (consisting of Jack Russell terriers, Parson Russell terriers, and Russell terriers) can develop a hereditary ataxia known as spinocerebellar ataxia. Histopathology of affected animals shows axonal loss, myelin degeneration, and gliosis in the dorsolateral and ventromedial spinal cord white matter of the cervical spinal cord. Myelin and axonal degeneration with diffuse gliosis are also described in the auditory pathways of the brainstem, with spongy degeneration of the cortical white matter and cerebellar granular layer. The age of onset and array of signs associated with the ataxia can vary greatly between individuals, and it is theorized that several subtypes of spinocerebellar subtypes exist in the Russell group terriers. Mutations in *KCNJ10*, a gene for voltage-gated potassium channels, are associated with an earlier onset of spinocerebellar ataxia (at 2–10 months of age) with affected animals potentially displaying other signs such as myokymia (fine rippling muscular tremors described as vermicular or "worm-like" in nature), neuromyotonia, and seizures.

Signs gradually progress over months to years. This mutation and subtype of spinocerebellar ataxia has also been described in a number of other breeds, including a dachshund, smooth haired fox terriers, Belgian Malinois, Patterdale terriers, and Bouvier des Ardennes. Larger breeds tend to be euthanized at younger ages due to difficulty managing them as their ataxia and mobility decline. Mutations in the *CAPN1* gene seem to be associated with a later onset of spinocerebellar ataxia (between 6 and 12 months of age), which is not associated with other neurologic signs. Signs of progress over time, leading to severe mobility issues in later stages. A separate late-onset spinocerebellar degeneration is described in Brittany spaniels with progressive cerebellar signs (ataxia, hypermetria, and intention tremors) developing between 5 and 10.7 years. Necropsy in affected individuals shows neuron loss and axonal degeneration within the cerebellum, medulla oblongata, and spinal cord. The genetic cause of this condition is unknown.

NEXT DIAGNOSTIC STEPS FOR THIS PATIENT

- In cases of suspected neurotoxicity, ingesta, vomitus, or fecal matter can be analyzed for the suspected toxic compounds such as mycotoxins, methylxanthines, and metaldehyde.
- Serum and fat samples can be analyzed for desmethylbromethalin levels.
- Brain MRI and spinal fluid analysis can be helpful for diagnosing or ruling out inflammatory brain disease. In cases of suspected bromethalin toxicity, a distinctive pattern of white matter edema can be detected on brain MRI. Similar distinctive patterns of structural change can be noted in cases of specific demyelinating disorders or storage diseases.
- Urine organic acid screening may be helpful in diagnosing some of the encephalopathies associated with organic acidurias.
- Genetic testing is available through various genetic testing labs for known demyelinating disorders in specific breeds like Rottweilers, Jack Russell terriers, and Kerry blue terriers. Similarly, for many of the storage diseases like NCL and globoid leukodystrophy, genetic testing is available through commercial laboratories.

OUTCOME

In this case, brain MRI revealed diffuse white matter changes concerning for bromethalin toxicity, and on further investigation, bromethalin exposure was confirmed (Figure 8.3.1). Despite aggressive supportive care, the patient declined neurologically to severe obtundation, generalized tremors, vision loss, and severe tetraparesis. Humane euthanasia was ultimately elected.

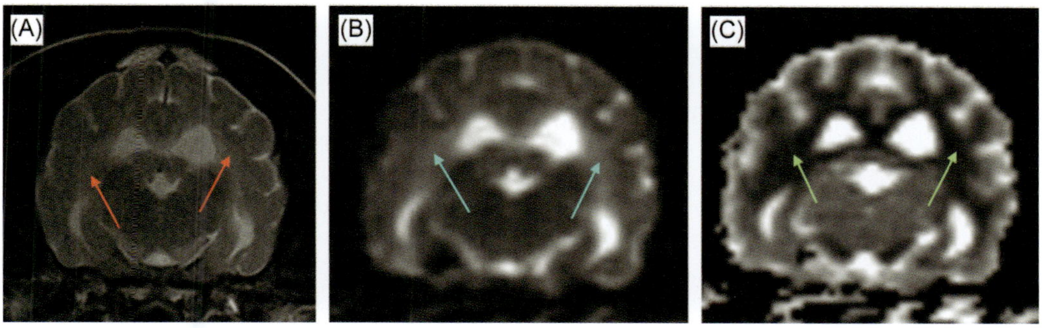

FIGURE 8.3.1 Magnetic resonance images of bromethalin toxicosis in a dog. (A) T2-weighted transverse image showing the diffuse hyperintensity of the white matter (red arrows), which is due to intramyelinic edema. Intramyelinic edema is observed in the cerebral white matter as hyperintense on the diffusion-weighted trace image (B) (blue arrows) and hypointense (green arrows) on the apparent diffusion coefficient map (C).

SUGGESTED READING

Alemañ, N., Marcaccini, A., Espino, L. et al. (2006). Rosenthal fiber encephalopathy in a dog resembling alexander disease in humans. *Vet. Pathol.* 43 (6): 1025–1028. https://doi.org/10.1354/vp.43-6-1025.

Chrisman, C.L. (1992). Neurological diseases of Rottweilers: neuroaxonal dystrophy and leukoenceph- alomalacia. *J. Small Anim. Pract.* 33 (10): 500–504. https://doi.org/10.1111/j.1748-5827.1992.tb01033.x.

Coates, J.R. and OBrien, D.P. (2004). Inherited peripheral neuropathies in dogs and cats. *Vet. Clin. N. Am. Small Anim. Pract.* 34 (6): 1361–1401. https://doi.org/10.1016/j.cvsm.2004.05.011.

Cox, N.R., Kwapien, R.P., Sorjonen, D.C., and Braund, K.G. (1986). Myeloencephalopathy resembling Alexanders disease in a Scottish terrier dog. *Acta Neuropathol.* 71 (1): 163–166. https://doi.org/10.1007/BF00687980.

Forman, O.P., Risio, L.D., and Mellersh, C.S. (2013). Missense mutation in CAPN1 is associated with spinocerebellar ataxia in the Parson Russell terrier dog breed *PLoS One* 8 (5): e64627. https://doi.org/10.1371/journal.pone.0064627.

Gill, J.L., Tsai, K.L., Krey, C. et al. (2012). A canine BCAN microdeletion associated with episodic falling syndrome. *Neurobiol. Dis.* 45 (1): 130–136. https://doi.org/10.1016/j.nbd.2011.07.014.

Gilliam, D., O'brien, D.P., Coates, J.R. et al. (2014). A homozygous KCNJ10 mutation in Jack Russell terriers and related breeds with spinocerebellar ataxia with myokymia, seizures, or both. *J. Vet. Intern. Med.* 28 (3): 871–877. https://doi.org/10.1111/jvim.12355.

Lucot, K.L., Dickinson, P.J., Finno, C.J. et al. (2018). A missense mutation in the vacuolar protein sorting 11 (*VPS11*) gene is associated with neuroaxonal dystrophy in Rottweiler dogs. *G3 (Bethesda)* 8 (8): 2773–2780. https://doi.org/10.1534/g3.118.200376.

Richardson, J.A., Tang, K., and Burns, D.K. (1991). Myeloencephalopathy with rosenthal fiber formation in a miniature poodle. *Vet. Pathol.* 28 (6): 536–538. https://doi.org/10.1177/030098589102800612.

Sigurdson, C.J., Basaraba, R.J., Mazzaferro, E.M., and Gould, D.H. (2002). Globoid cell-like leukodystrophy in a domestic longhaired cat. *Vet. Pathol.* 39 (4): 494–496. https://doi.org/10.1354/vp.39-4-494.

St. Jean, S.C., Jortner, B.S., Doan, R.N. et al. (2022). Pathologic characterization of canine multiple system degeneration in the Ibizan hound. *Vet. Pathol.* 59 (1): 132–137. https://doi.org/10.1177/03009858211043088.

Stee, K., Van Poucke, M., Lowrie, M. et al. (2023). Phenotypic and genetic aspects of hereditary ataxia in dogs. *J. Vet. Intern. Med.* 37 (4): 1306–1322. https://doi.org/10.1111/jvim.16742.

Urkasemsin, G., Linder, K.E., Bell, J.S. et al. (2010). Hereditary cerebellar degeneration in Scottish terriers: cerebellar degeneration in Scottish terriers. *J. Vet. Intern. Med.* 24 (3): 565–570. https://doi.org/10.1111/j.1939-1676.2010.0499.x.

Urkasemsin, G. and Olby, N.J. (2014). Canine hereditary ataxia. *Vet. Clin. North Am. Small Anim. Pract.* 44 (6): 1075–1089. https://doi.org/10.1016/j.cvsm.2014.07.005.

Van Ham, L., Vandevelde, M., Desmidt, M. et al. (1994). A tremor syndrome with a central axonopathy in Scottish terriers. *J. Vet. Intern. Med.* 8 (4): 290–292. https://doi.org/10.1111/j.1939-1676.1994.tb03235.x.

Van Poucke, M., Martlé, V., Van Brantegem, L. et al. (2016). A canine orthologue of the human GFAP c.716G>A (p.Arg239His) variant causes Alexander disease in a Labrador retriever. *Eur. J. Hum. Genet.* 24 (6): 852–856. https://doi.org/10.1038/ejhg.2015.223.

Vanhaesebrouck, A.E., Bhatti, S.F.M., Franklin, R.J.M., and Van Ham, L. (2013). Myokymia and neuromyotonia in veterinary medicine: a comparison with peripheral nerve hyperexcitability syndrome in humans. *Vet. J.* 197 (2): 153–162. https://doi.org/10.1016/j.tvjl.2013.03.002.

Vanhaesebrouck, A., Van Poucke, M., Stee, K. et al. (2023). Generalized myokymia, or neuromyotonia, or both in dogs with or without spinocerebellar ataxia. *J. Vet. Intern. Med.* 37 (6): 2310–2314. https://doi.org/10.1111/jvim.16892.

Wessmann, A., Goedde, T., Fischer, A. et al. (2004). Hereditary ataxia in the Jack Russell terrier–clinical and genetic investigations. *J. Vet. Intern. Med.* 18 (4): 515–521. https://doi.org/10.1111/j.1939-1676.2004.tb02577.x.

Wood, S.L. and Patterson, J.S. (2001). Shetland sheepdog leukodystrophy. *J. Vet. Intern. Med.* 15 (5): 486–493. https://doi.org/10.1111/j.1939-1676.2001.tb01580.x.

Tremors, Shakes, and Involuntary Movement
Case 4—Phantom Scratching in a Dog

CHAPTER 8.4

Vivian Lau

Sage Veterinary Centers, Redwood City, CA, USA

CASE HISTORY

A 2-year-old spayed female Cavalier King Charles spaniel was presented for exhibiting odd scratching behavior during walks outside (Video 8.4.1). The scratching started about 6 months ago and has been steadily increasing in frequency. It was primarily noted along the left side and was most noticeable when the dog was walking outside, although the behavior could be induced by touching the neck area. Examination with a veterinary dermatologist did not reveal any dermatologic cause for pruritus. The dog would intermittently vocalize when touched around the neck area, but otherwise seemed comfortable and was still interested in playing. She had a somewhat sensitive digestive system but had otherwise been healthy and was not on any medications.

VIDEO 8.4.1 A dog scratching in the region of the neck.

NEUROLOGICAL EXAMINATION

The dog had a normal mentation and body posture. No lameness, paresis, or ataxia was noted during gait analysis. Postural reactions and spinal reflexes were normal in all four limbs. Intermittent air-scratching behavior with the left pelvic limb was elicited with palpation along the left thorax or cervical area. The dog consistently tensed on palpation of the cervical vertebral column and near the thoracolumbar junction. Cranial nerve examination was within normal limits.

1. **Where is the likely lesion localization?**
2. **What major disease processes should be considered?**
3. **What tests could you perform to help determine the diagnosis?**

LESION LOCALIZATION

Cervical and thoracolumbar myelopathies causing neuropathic pain syndromes would be the main neurolocalization for this patient. The air-scratching behavior is reminiscent of phantom scratching, which is observed with paresthesia in the cervical region.

DIFFERENTIAL DIAGNOSIS

Chiari-like malformation (CM) with syringomyelia (SM) is the primary differential diagnosis for this patient. CM is a congenital anomaly commonly seen in the Cavalier King Charles spaniel breed, among many other brachycephalic and toy breeds (Pomeranian, Griffon Bruxellois, Yorkshire terrier, Maltese, etc.). In affected animals, the occipital bone is malformed with a rostral curvature, causing crowding of structures in the caudal fossa. This can be associated with varying degrees of craniofacial hypoplasia, rostrotentorial crowding of the forebrain and multiple craniocervical junction deformations, including a shortened basicranium, medullary kinking (medullary elevation), and rostral displacement of the dens and atlas. The severity of the malformation varies between patients and, in more severe cases, causes alterations in the flow dynamics of cerebrospinal fluid (CSF), primarily via an outflow obstruction at the level of the foramen magnum. This can lead to hydrocephalus (abnormal CSF accumulation within the brain) and contribute to syringomyelia (abnormal fluid distension of the central canal of the spinal cord). Syringomyelia can be associated with varying amounts of discomfort or neurologic dysfunction for the patient. Syrinxes that extend into the superficial dorsal horn of the mid cervical spinal cord have been linked to more signs of phantom scratching (air scratching or scratching toward the shoulder area) and cervical torticollis. Other signs of discomfort may include random vocalizing, restless sleep, aversion to touch, and crying out when being picked up under the sternum. The syrinx is hypothesized to progress in size over time, although this is not believed to be a linear progression with age.

Intervertebral Disc Disease (IVDD): Cavalier King Charles spaniels can develop intervertebral disc disease (IVDD), making them prone to intervertebral disc extrusions. Cervical disc extrusions could certainly cause lateralized pain, but are not typically associated with phantom scratching behavior. IVDD is described in more detail in Chapters 10, 12, and 13.

Inflammatory disease (Meningomyelitis of Unknown Etiology/Origin – MUE/MUO): The distribution of inflammation within the central nervous system can vary with MUE/MUO, and if the superficial dorsal horn of the cervical spinal cord is affected, signs like phantom scratching can be appreciated. Inflammation both within the brain and spinal cord can contribute to neck pain. MUE/MUO is described in more detail in Chapter 5, Case 3.

NEXT DIAGNOSTIC STEPS FOR THIS PATIENT

MRI of the brain and cervical spinal cord would be most helpful in the diagnosis of CM/SM and IVDD. Note that the syrinx in some CM patients can be quite extensive, and additional imaging through the thoracolumbar spinal cord may be needed to assess the full extent of the syrinx. CSF analysis is helpful for ruling out or diagnosing an inflammatory disease. For patients with severe CM, high intracranial pressure, or other craniocervical junctionopathies, the foraminal cistern may not be safely accessible, and a spinal tap may not be possible. Refer to other chapters for details about diagnostic steps for IVDD and MUE/MUO.

TREATMENT AND PROGNOSIS

Chiari-like Malformation and Syringomyelia

Treatment for CM and syringomyelia can be either surgical or nonsurgical. Surgical treatments include foramen magnum decompression (where the supraoccipital bone and rostral dorsal lamina of C1 are removed) with or without implantation of titanium mesh, ventriculoperitoneal shunting (more appropriate for cases with hydrocephalus), and syringopleural shunting (more appropriate for cases where other surgeries are not good options). While the surgeries can be helpful in reducing signs of acute pain, they are not as successful in resolving the syrinx, and signs of phantom scratching may persist. For many of the patients undergoing foramen magnum decompression, fibrous scar tissue and adhesions can lead to recurrence of clinical signs within months to years. Shunting surgeries are usually less invasive than a foramen magnum decompression but can be fraught with complications such as shunt blockage, infection, subdural hematomas, overshunting, and hemispheric collapse.

Because of the high rate of complications and recurrence of clinical signs, medical (nonsurgical) treatment of CM/SM is a more common practice. Medications used for this condition largely consist of analgesics and medications theorized to reduce CSF production. The most commonly used analgesics are pregabalin and gabapentin. Other pain medications include amantadine and topiramate. Maropitant is being investigated as a potential treatment for phantom scratching since it is an NK-1 receptor antagonist (NK-1 receptors are found in the superficial dorsal horn of the spinal cord). Carprofen was not shown to improve signs of pain when used alone, but may have some effect if used in combination with gabapentin or pregabalin. Medications hypothesized to reduce CSF production include corticosteroids (prednisone/prednisolone), acetazolamide, and antacids (omeprazole, cimetidine). The ability of omeprazole to reduce spinal fluid production is controversial, with newer studies detecting no effect from this drug on CSF in dogs. The prognosis for full resolution of clinical signs related to CM/SM is poor, but the majority of affected patients can achieve an acceptable quality of life long-term with medical management.

OUTCOME

The patient in this case underwent brain and cervical MRI, which revealed moderate hydrocephalus and syringomyelia secondary to CM (Figure 8.4.1). Her syrinx was 4 mm in diameter and extended into the thoracic spinal cord. There was no evidence of intervertebral disc extrusion or protrusion. She was started on a regimen of gabapentin and omeprazole. Clinical signs were improved but still present on recheck several years later. Omeprazole was eventually stopped with no clinical change appreciated.

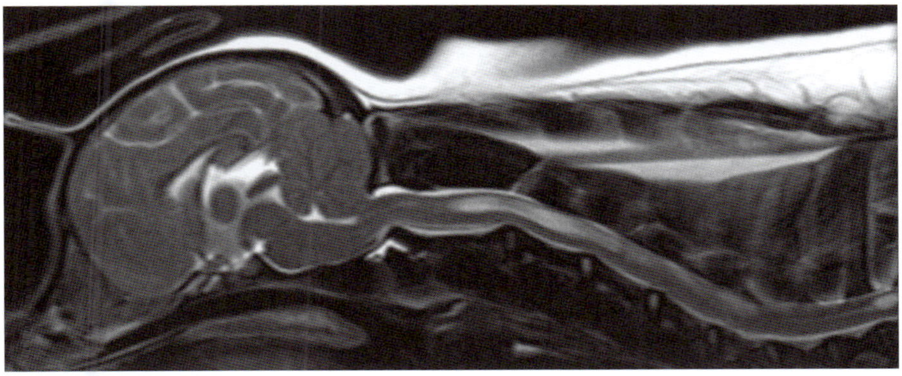

FIGURE 8.4.1 An MRI showing features of Chiari-like malformation. Note the coning of the cerebellum due to crowding of the caudal fossa, and hyperintensity in the cervical spinal cord. This cervical spinal cord hyperintensity is a syrinx.

SUGGESTED READING

Cerda-Gonzalez, S., Olby, N.J., and Griffith, E.H. (2015). Medullary position at the craniocervical junction in mature cavalier King Charles spaniels: relationship with neurologic signs and syringomyelia. *J. Vet. Intern. Med.* 29 (3): 882–886. https://doi.org/10.1111/jvim.12605.

Girod, M., Allerton, F., Gommeren, K. et al. (2016). Evaluation of the effect of oral omeprazole on canine cerebrospinal fluid production: a pilot study. *Vet. J.* 209: 119–124. https://doi.org/10.1016/j.tvjl.2015.10.045.

Javaheri, S., Corbett, W.S., Simbartl, L.A. et al. (1997). Different effects of omeprazole and Sch 28080 on canine cerebrospinal fluid production. *Brain Res.* 754 (1): 321–324. https://doi.org/10.1016/S0006-8993(97)00175-3.

Mortensen, D., Thoefner, M.S., Agerholm, J.S. et al. (2022). Dorsal horn volume loss and pain pathway changes in cavalier King Charles spaniels with syringomyelia, signs of pain, and phantom scratching. *Pain* 163 (12): 2365–2379. https://doi.org/10.1097/j.pain.0000000000002630.

Nalborczyk, Z.R., McFadyen, A.K., Jovanovik, J. et al. (2017). MRI characteristics for "phantom" scratching in canine syringomyelia. *BMC Vet. Res.* 13 (1): 340. https://doi.org/10.1186/s12917-017-1258-2.

Rusbridge, C. (2007). Chiari-like malformation with syringomyelia in the cavalier King Charles spaniel: long-term outcome after surgical management. *Vet. Surg.* 36 (5): 396–405. https://doi.org/10.1111/j.1532-950X.2007.00285.x.

Rusbridge, C. (2020). New considerations about Chiari-like malformation, syringomyelia and their management. *In Pract.* 42 (5): 252–267. https://doi.org/10.1136/inp.m1869.

Rusbridge, C., Stringer, F., and Knowler, S.P. (2018). Clinical application of diagnostic imaging of Chiari-like malformation and syringomyelia. *Front. Vet. Sci.* 5: 280. https://doi.org/10.3389/fvets.2018.00280.

Santifort, K.M., Carrera, I., and Mandigers, P.J.J. (2024). Longitudinal assessment of syringomyelia in pomeranians. *Front. Vet. Sci.* 11: 1364464. https://doi.org/10.3389/fvets.2024.1364464.

Exercise-Related Weakness and Collapse

Case 1—Acute Collapse in a Dog with Loss of Reflexes

CHAPTER 9.1

Koen Santifort

IVC Evidensia Small Animal Hospital Arnhem, Arnhem, The Netherlands and IVC Evidensia Small Animal Hospital Hart van Brabant, Waalwijk, The Netherlands

CASE HISTORY

A 14-week-old male Stabyhoun (Friese Stabij) was presented for acute collapse in all four limbs. The dog had been left mainly unsupervised for about 1.5 days. The neighbors reported that the dog did not come to greet them, and they had to pick up the dog to have it go outside, where it urinated and defecated, barely standing and dragging its pelvic limbs. It ate and drank well and wagged its tail at that time. The following morning, when the owners returned home, the dog was unable to walk. No previous health concerns were reported, the rest of the litter and parents were healthy, and the dog was not receiving any medications. The dog was fed a raw meat diet. It was vaccinated and treated with anti-parasitics according to the veterinarian's vaccination schedule. The general clinical examination was unremarkable, except for a shallow and slightly abdominal breathing pattern.

NEUROLOGICAL EXAMINATION (Video 9.1.1)

VIDEO 9.1.1 A 14-week-old puppy with signs of diffuse neuromuscular disease.

The neurological examination revealed that the dog was bright, alert, and responsive. Non-ambulatory lower motor neuron tetraparesis with only minor voluntary movement in the pelvic limbs. More tail function was observed than limb function. The dog exhibited more voluntary motor activity in the thoracic limbs. There was generalized decreased muscle tone. Postural reactions were abnormal, but with adequate support, hopping was evident in all four limbs. Spontaneous knuckling and buckling occurred in all four limbs, even with support. Spinal reflexes were abnormal in all four limbs, including extremely weak to absent withdrawal reflexes, absent patellar reflexes bilaterally, and absent cutaneous trunci reflexes. The perineal reflex was normal. A mild laryngeal stridor and dysphonia were noticeable as well. Mild diffuse paraspinal hyperesthesia was noticed as apparent discomfort while putting manual pressure in the region of the thoracolumbar vertebrae. Nociception was intact in all extremities, including the tail.

1. **What differential diagnoses should be considered?**
2. **What tests could you perform to help determine the diagnosis?**
3. **What are the treatment and prognostic considerations for such patients?**

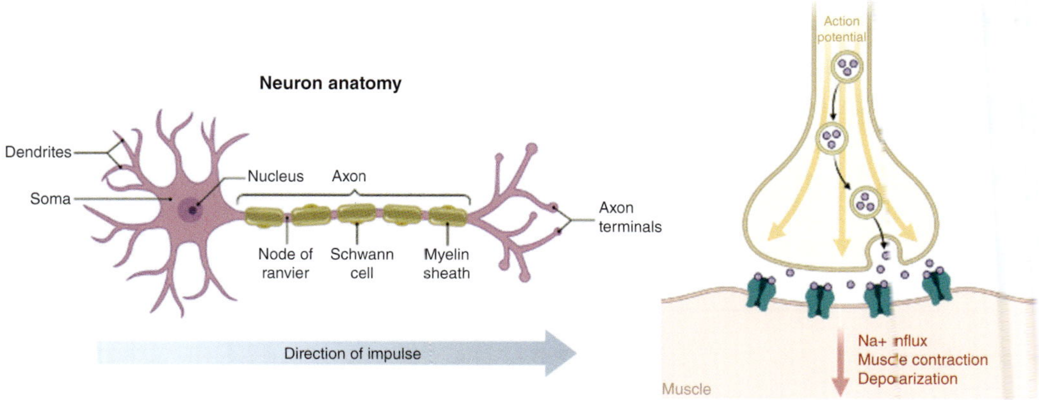

FIGURE 9.1.1 An illustration of the anatomic components of the neuromuscular system. The left panel shows a neuron. Neuronal cell bodies are found in the ventral horn of the spinal cord. Their axons exit the spinal cord and continue as parts of named nerves through the peripheral nervous system to reach their effector muscles. Axons have variable degrees of myelination, which increases the rate of action potential impulse. The right panel shows the components of the neuromuscular junction. The action potential conducted along the axon reaches the terminus, where it leads to a series of intracellular changes that result in the passage of synaptic vesicles to the presynaptic membrane. These vesicles contain neurotransmitters. At the somatic neuromuscular junction, the neurotransmitter that is released is acetylcholine. Acetylcholine is released into the synaptic cleft, where it binds with acetylcholine receptors on the myocyte membrane. This binding leads to sodium ion influx, which subsequently results in muscle contraction.

DIFFERENTIAL DIAGNOSES

For the diffuse neuromuscular signs in this case, disorders of the peripheral nervous system (i.e. the nerve roots, brachial/lumbosacral plexus, cranial and spinal nerves), the neuromuscular junction, and muscles should be considered (Figure 9.1.1 and Figure 9.4.2). Four major differential diagnoses should be considered in any patient with acute flaccid tetraparesis or tetraplegia. These are discussed in turn below.

Polyradiculoneuritis (PRN)/Coonhound Paralysis/Polyradiculoneuropathy

PRN is a (suspected) autoimmune disorder that can affect dogs of all breeds at any age. Generally, affected patients show signs in the pelvic limbs first. The thoracic limb and cervical muscle involvement follow later on. Loss of spinal reflexes with a retained perineal reflex is typical. Laryngeal paresis to paralysis, leading to dysphonia and stridor, is frequently observed. Many animals retain the ability to move their tails. Regurgitation and dysphagia due to pharyngeal and esophageal involvement are much less common, and even uncharacteristic, as are other cranial nerve deficits. Respiratory difficulties due to laryngeal paresis/paralysis and involvement of diaphragmatic and intercostal muscles occur in severe cases. Clinical severity varies greatly, as do the onset and duration of signs. Most often, clinical signs develop over the span of a few days to 1–2 weeks. Research results implicate *Campylobacter* spp. in the development of autoimmune responses. Eating raw chicken is a risk factor. Guillain-Barré syndrome in humans has similar clinical characteristics, and *Campylobacter* infections have been implicated as a causative or triggering factor as well. The nickname “Coonhound paralysis” comes from the occurrence of PRN after contact with saliva (often through bite trauma) of raccoons, mostly in the United States of America but also in other parts of the world. *Toxoplasma gondii* has been implicated in possibly triggering PRN as well.

Botulism

Ingestion of preformed toxin (type C most commonly, B and D also reported) created by *Clostridium botulinum* is the most common cause of botulism in dogs. Spoiled food, cadavers, or buried and dug-up organic materials are relatively common sources. The toxin is a metalloprotease that targets proteins needed for the release of neurotransmitter (acetylcholine) at the neuromuscular junction. Clinical signs of botulism usually occur within less than a day of toxin ingestion and include motor as well as autonomic signs. Flaccid muscle paralysis involves all skeletal muscles, including pharyngeal, facial, esophageal, and masticatory muscles. Autonomic signs include dysuria, alterations of heart rate (bradycardia or tachycardia), xeromycteria, gastrointestinal dysfunction, and mydriasis with weak pupillary light reflexes. Respiratory insufficiency and/or aspiration pneumonia is a frequent cause of death.

Tick Paralysis/Snake or Spider Envenomation

In geographically predisposed areas (e.g. the United States of America, Australia, Africa, and South Korea), these occur much more commonly than in other parts of the world, although climate change and improved diagnostic efforts and scientific reporting render some knowledge on these phenomena useful even for veterinarians in, for example, Europe. *Ixodes holocyclus* (Australia), *Dermacentor variabilis* (the United States of America), and *Dermacentor andersoni* (the United States of America) are most commonly incriminated for tick paralysis. In the United States of America, coral snake envenomation and black widow spider envenomation can also cause diffuse neuromuscular disease. With these envenomations, non-motor neurological signs can be seen but are variable for different species. The most important part of the treatment of tick paralysis, aside from supportive treatment, is the removal of offending ticks. Antidotes for snake and spider envenomation are crucial for the survival of patients bitten by toxic species for which antidotes are available. The reader is referred to the suggested readings on this topic for further details.

Fulminant Myasthenia Gravis (MG)

MG is discussed in more detail in Case 3 in this chapter. Fulminant MG carries a much graver prognosis than focal or generalized MG in general, and clinical signs resemble PRN, botulism, and tick paralysis/snake envenomation more than focal or generalized MG. A loss of muscle tone and spinal reflexes can be seen. Severe dysphagia and regurgitation are typical, as is palpebral hypo-/areflexia.

Other Polyneuropathies and Myopathies

Polyneuropathies in general are expected to result in clinical findings as in this case. An example is a toxic polyneuropathy, such as that induced by organophosphate intoxications. Exposure to toxins should be excluded where possible, but a diagnosis of toxic polyneuropathy would otherwise be based mainly on other signs (e.g. previous cholinergic crisis in the acute phase of organophosphate intoxication prior to intermediate syndrome). Paraneoplastic syndromes could, like PRN, result in acute progressive signs. Excluding or confirming paraneoplastic syndromes is fraught with difficulties, though. Finding neoplasia in a patient with acute neuromuscular signs may be coincidental.

A variety of other underlying causes should be considered for polyneuropathies, including endocrine disorders (e.g. hypothyroidism and diabetes mellitus), degenerative disorders (e.g. genetic and breed-related), and infectious diseases (e.g. Neospora caninum). All of these would not be expected to result in such a severe clinical manifestation within 1.5 days.

Acute, severe myopathies (toxin- or exercise-induced rhabdomyolysis) may result in acute tetraplegia, but flaccidity is not expected, and those patients would be expected to show clear signs of pain. Polymyositis, an immune-mediated disease, can cause animals to be non-ambulatory secondary to myalgia, but spinal and cranial nerve reflex testing is expected to be normal in these cases. Polymyositis also causes a severe elevation in serum creatine kinase secondary to myolysis.

WHAT TESTS COULD YOU PERFORM TO HELP DETERMINE THE DIAGNOSIS?

Hematology and Biochemistry

A complete blood count and biochemistry, including electrolytes (e.g. to exclude hypokalemia) should be performed in any patient presented with acute lower motor neuron tetraplegia or collapse. Assessments of leukograms and C-reactive protein may help to diagnose complications related to neuromuscular disorders, such as aspiration pneumonia.

Serology

Studies have found increased levels of anti-GM2 antibodies in dogs with PRN. This test is not commercially available at the time of writing. Infectious disease testing (e.g. *Neospora caninum*) is recommended, especially when dogs are fed a raw meat diet. Positive serology tests do not confirm that such an infection is the actual cause of the clinical signs. Still, treatment could be considered prudent. An acetylcholine receptor antibody titer should be performed to rule out fulminant acquired myasthenia gravis.

Fecal Analysis

Polymerase chain reaction or cultures aiming to identify *Campylobacter* spp. could help to assess causality, but there is no evidence for treatment approaches based on outcomes thereof (e.g. antibiotic, probiotic, or other), nor is there a proven prognostic value.

CSF Analysis

Increased protein levels without increased total nucleated cell counts are commonly reported for those cases where CSF was taken. A lumbar puncture is preferable. While increased total nucleated cell counts are not expected, the nerve roots are at least partially bathed in CSF, and histological specimens have shown inflammatory cells in the subarachnoid space of the spinal cord. Therefore, some increase in cell count and mononuclear pleocytosis might be present and should not be considered inconsistent with PRN. For all other differentials, CSF analysis is expected to be normal.

Searching for Ticks, Snake Bites, and Spider Bites (or Local Skin Reactions)

Finding ticks on a patient in predisposed geographical areas forms a large part of the diagnosis, especially if clinical signs start to resolve afterward.

Electrodiagnostic Testing

The major downside of electrodiagnostic testing in veterinary patients is the need for general anesthesia. Such procedures in neuromuscular patients carry risks of complications, including hypoventilation, specifically in the recovery phase when weaning off mechanical ventilation. Also, anesthetic agents may further exacerbate clinical signs. However, part of the examination may be performed with only analgesia in patients with flaccid tetraplegia, such as needle electromyography (EMG).

1. Needle EMG can determine if there are any signs of spontaneous activity in muscles when the patient is under general anesthesia. If such activity is found, this would suggest a primary muscle and/or nerve disorder. However, for all four major differentials, EMG abnormalities would not typically be expected after only 1.5 days of clinical signs, though studies have found abnormalities in dogs with PRN in which EMG was performed within 1–6 days.

Nerve conduction studies can assess the function of peripheral nerves, as well as the neuromuscular junction and muscles.

2. Motor nerve conduction velocity and compound muscle action potential (CMAP) assessments are valuable to characterize neuropathies in general. Decreased velocities and CMAP amplitudes/areas can be expected in PRN.
3. F-waves, cord dorsum potentials, and/or H-reflexes (as parts of nerve conduction studies) can be valuable to assess nerve root function, the primary pathological site in PRN.
4. Repetitive nerve stimulation (RNS), a specific form of nerve conduction study where nerves are repeatedly stimulated, can reveal a decrement (at low frequency stimulation) or an increment (at high frequency stimulation). High-frequency RNS has the potential to identify true facilitation (i.e. increased CMAP area) in the case of botulism.
5. Single-fiber EMG is a very sensitive test for neuromuscular junction dysfunction, but it requires even more expertise and specific equipment than the other tests. This can be useful to diagnose MG.

Pharmacological Testing

Edrophonium chloride or neostigmine, both acetylcholinesterase inhibitors, have been reported to be of use to evaluate improvement of signs in a clinical setting when MG is considered a differential diagnosis. This test is discussed in more detail in Case 3 in this chapter. Of note, in fulminant MG cases, the result of this test may be negative (i.e. no improvement) as most or all of the acetylcholine receptors are disabled.

Diagnostic Imaging

Thoracic radiographs to identify aspiration pneumonia and megaesophagus, among other abnormalities, or abdominal ultrasound and computed tomographic imaging studies (e.g. to identify neoplasia or complications) can be considered on a case-by-case basis (Figure 9.1.1).

WHAT ARE THE TREATMENT AND PROGNOSTIC CONSIDERATIONS?

The section below refers to the treatment of PRN in dogs. The reader is encouraged to consult other resources for treatment recommendations for the other diseases.

Supportive Treatment

Supportive treatment is most important in all flaccid tetraplegic dogs. This includes basic care (e.g. comfortable positioning, frequent turning/repositioning to prevent ulceration, hygiene, bladder care) as well as respiratory support (e.g. flow-by oxygen supplementation or mechanical ventilation). Physiotherapy can help to retain muscle strength and regain motor function during long-term recovery. Nutritional support is vital for debilitated patients, taking care to reduce the chances of aspiration pneumonia by placing dogs in upright positions during and shortly after feeding. Placing nasal tubes or esophageal tubes provides a way to administer food straight into the stomach, reducing regurgitation and the odds of aspiration pneumonia (Figure 9.1.2).

Medical Treatment

The use of corticosteroids or other immunosuppressive treatments has not been shown to improve outcomes in dogs with PRN. Use of human IV immunoglobulin and manual therapeutic plasma exchange may be indicated, as promising results have been described. Complications, such as aspiration pneumonia and urinary tract infections, should be addressed promptly.

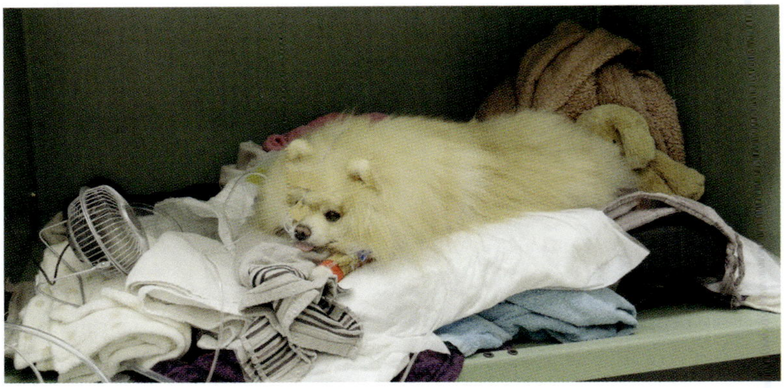

FIGURE 9.1.2 Another dog with polyradiculoneuritis supported in sternal recumbency with a nasal oxygen supplementation tube in place.

Prognosis

Dogs that develop respiratory insufficiency or aspiration pneumonia tend to have poor outcomes compared to dogs that only develop motor signs and tetraparesis rather than tetraplegia. That being said, each individual case has the chance of improvement despite severe clinical signs. Even when long-term mechanical ventilatory support is necessary, the patient may recover. Therefore, owner and staff dedication, as well as discussions on quality of life, will play a major role in outcomes of such cases.

CAUTION: Respiratory muscle weakness or complications (e.g. aspiration pneumonia) are major reasons for death or euthanasia in neuromuscular patients.

OUTCOME

The complete blood count and blood chemistry panel were unremarkable. An acetylcholine receptor antibody titer was performed, which was negative. No ticks were observed on the dog, but a tick product was applied nonetheless without associated clinical improvement. Presumptively, the dog was diagnosed with PRN and was treated with supportive care for 8 weeks. The dog made a complete recovery.

SUGGESTED READING

PRN

Añor, S. (2014). Acute lower motor neuron tetraparesis. *Vet. Clin. North Am. Small Anim. Pract.* 44 (6): 1201–1222. https://doi.org/10.1016/j.cvsm.2014.07.010.

Calero Rodriguez, A., van Oostrom, H., and de Grauw, J. (2022). Long-term mechanical ventilation of an 8-week-old dog with idiopathic polyradiculoneuritis. *Vet. Rec. Case Rep.* 10 (2): e292.

Cuddon, P.A. (1998). Electrophysiologic assessment of acute polyradiculoneuropathy in dogs: comparison with Guillain-Barré syndrome in people. *J. Vet. Intern. Med.* 12 (4): 294–303. https://doi.org/10.1111/j.1939-1676.1998.tb02125.x.

Cummings, J.F. and Haas, D.C. (1972). Animal model for human disease: idiopathic polyneuritis,

Guillain-Barré Syndrome. Animal model: coonhound paralysis, idiopathic polyradiculoneuritis of coonhounds. *Am. J. Pathol.* 66 (1): 189–192.

Czerwik, A., Jarešová, T., Olszewska, A. et al. (2023). Manual therapeutic plasma exchange for treatment of a dog with suspected acute canine polyradiculoneuritis. *Acta Vet. Scand.* 65 (1): 14. https://doi.org/10.1186/s13028-023-00675-0.

Halstead, S.K., Gourlay, D.S., Penderis, J. et al. (2022). Serum anti-GM2 and anti-GalNAc-GD1a IgG antibodies are biomarkers for acute canine polyradiculoneuritis. *J. Small Anim. Pract.* 63 (2): 104–112. https://doi.org/10.1111/jsap.13439.

Hirschvogel, K., Jurina, K., Steinberg, T.A. et al. (2012). Clinical course of acute canine polyradiculoneuritis following treatment with human IV immunoglobulin. *J. Am. Anim. Hosp. Assoc.* 48 (5): 299–309. https://doi.org/10.5326/JAAHA-MS-5651.

Holt, N., Murray, M., Cuddon, P.A., and Lappin, M.R. (2011). Seroprevalence of various infectious agents in dogs with suspected acute canine polyradiculoneuritis. *J. Vet. Intern. Med.* 25 (2): 261–266. https://doi.org/10.1111/j.1939-1676.2011.0692.x.

Laws, E.J., Harcourt-Brown, T.R., Granger, N., and Rose, J.H. (2017). An exploratory study into factors influencing development of acute canine polyradiculoneuritis in the UK. *J. Small Anim. Pract.* 58 (8): 437–443. https://doi.org/10.1111/jsap.12683.

Martinez-Anton, L., Marenda, M., Firestone, S.M. et al. (2018). Investigation of the role of campylobacter infection in suspected acute polyradiculoneuritis in dogs. *J. Vet. Intern. Med.* 32 (1): 352–360. https://doi.org/10.1111/jvim.15030.

Porcarelli, L., Cauduro, A., Bianchi, E. et al. (2024). Early neurophysiological abnormalities in suspected acute canine polyradiculoneuropathy. *Vet. Sci.* 11 (4): 178. https://doi.org/10.3390/vetsci11040178.

Rupp, A., Galban-Horcajo, F., Bianchi, E. et al. (2013). Anti-GM2 ganglioside antibodies are a biomarker for acute canine polyradiculoneuritis. *J. Peripher. Nerv. Syst.* 18 (1): 75–88. https://doi.org/10.1111/jns5.12011.

Rutter, C.R., Rozanski, E.A., Sharp, C.R. et al. (2011). Outcome and medical management in dogs with lower motor neuron disease undergoing mechanical ventilation: 14 cases (2003–2009). *J. Vet. Emerg. Crit. Care (San Antonio)* 21 (5): 531–541. https://doi.org/10.1111/j.1476-4431.2011.00669.x.

BOTULISM

Bruchim, Y., Steinman, A., Markovitz, M. et al. (2006). Toxicological, bacteriological and serological diagnosis of botulism in a dog. *Vet. Rec.* 158 (22): 768–769. https://doi.org/10.1136/vr.158.22.768.

Fischer, A. (2020). Tetanus and botulism. In: *Clinical Small Animal Internal Medicine*, 967–970.

Sykes, J.E. and Creedon, J.M.B. (2021). Tetanus and botulism. In: *Greenes Infectious Diseases of the Dog and Cat*, 893–904. WB Saunders.

Uriarte, A., Thibaud, J.L., and Blot, S. (2010). Botulism in 2 urban dogs. *Can. Vet. J.* 51 (10): 1139–1142.

TICK PARALYSIS & SNAKE AND SPIDER ENVENOMATION

Atwell, R.B., Campbell, F.E., and Evans, E.A. (2001). Prospective survey of tick paralysis in dogs. *Aust. Vet. J.* 79 (6): 412–418. https://doi.org/10.1111/j.1751-0813.2001.tb12986.x.

Atwell, R. and Vankan, D. (2024). Prospective study of 506 dogs with tick paralysis: investigating measures of severity and clinical signs as predictors of mortality and assessing the benefits of different therapeutics. *Animals (Basel)* 14 (2): 188. https://doi.org/10.3390/ani14020188.

Gilliam, L.L. and Brunker, J. (2011). North American snake envenomation in the dog and cat. *Vet. Clin. North Am. Small Anim. Pract.* 41 (6): 1239–1259. https://doi.org/10.1016/j.cvsm.2011.08.008.

Hardy, M.C., Cochrane, J., and Allavena, R.E. (2014). Venomous and poisonous Australian animals of veterinary importance: a rich source of novel therapeutics. *Biomed. Res. Int.* 2014: 671041. https://doi.org/10.1155/2014/671041.

Heller, J., Mellor, D.J., Hodgson, J.L. et al. (2007). Elapid snake envenomation in dogs in New South Wales: a review. *Aust. Vet. J.* 85 (11): 469–479. https://doi.org/10.1111/j.1751-0813.2007.00194.x.

Khan, S.A. (2018). Common reversal agents/antidotes in small animal poisoning. *Vet. Clin. North Am. Small Anim. Pract.* 48 (6): 1081–1085. https://doi.org/10.1016/j.cvsm.2018.07.004.

Khan, S.A. (2018). Differential diagnosis of common acute toxicologic versus nontoxicologic illness. *Vet. Clin. North Am. Small Anim. Pract.* 48 (6): 1069–1079. https://doi.org/10.1016/j.cvsm.2018.07.003.

Lee, J.M., Song, J.H., and Song, K.H. (2022). A retrospective evaluation of snake envenomation in dogs in South Korea (2004–2021). *Toxins (Basel)* 14 (8): 565. https://doi.org/10.3390/toxins14080565.

Leister, E., Morton, J., Atwell, R., and Webster, R. (2018). Clinical presentations, treatments and risk factors for mortality in cats with tick paralysis caused by Ixodes holocyclus: 2077 cases (2008–2016). *J. Feline Med. Surg.* 20 (6): 465–478. https://doi.org/10.1177/1098612X17733628.

Lobetti, R.G. and Joubert, K. (2004). Retrospective study of snake envenomation in 155 dogs from the Onderstepoort area of South Africa. *J. S. Afr. Vet. Assoc.* 75 (4): 169–172. https://doi.org/10.4102/jsava.v75i4.477.

Morris, C.A.D. and Donaldson, R.E. (2023). Mechanical ventilation in snake envenomation of dogs and cats. *Front. Vet. Sci.* 10: 1071257. https://doi.org/10.3389/fvets.2023.1071257.

OKeeffe, T. and Donaldson, R.E. (2023). Mechanical ventilation in dogs and cats with tick paralysis. *Front. Vet. Sci.* 10: 1071191. https://doi.org/10.3389/fvets.2023.1071191.

Padula, A.M., Leister, E.M., and Webster, R.A. (2020). Tick paralysis in dogs and cats in Australia: treatment and prevention deliverables from 100 years of research. *Aust. Vet. J.* 98 (1–2): 53–59. https://doi.org/10.1111/avj.12891.

Pérez, M.L., Fox, K., and Schaer, M. (2012). A retrospective evaluation of coral snake envenomation in dogs and cats: 20 cases (1996–2011). *J. Vet. Emerg. Crit. Care (San Antonio)* 22 (6): 682–689. https://doi.org/10.1111/j.1476-4431.2012.00806.x.

Peterson, M.E. (2006). Black widow spider envenomation. *Clin. Tech. Small Anim. Pract.* 21 (4): 187–190. https://doi.org/10.1053/j.ctsap.2006.10.003.

Valenza, L., Allavena, R., Haworth, M. et al. (2021). Diagnosis and treatment of snake envenomation in dogs in Queensland, Australia. *Vet. Sci.* 8 (2): 14. https://doi.org/10.3390/vetsci8020014.

OTHER

Klainbart, S., Kelmer, E., Chai, O. et al. (2022). Prevalence, clinical manifestations, laboratory findings, treatment, and outcome of intermediate syndrome in anticholinesterase pesticide intoxication of dogs: a retrospective study. *Vet. J.* 287: 105883. https://doi.org/10.1016/j.tvjl.2022.105883.

Spinella, G., Bettella, P., Riccio, B., and Okonji, S. (2022). Overview of the current literature on the most common neurological diseases in dogs with a particular focus on rehabilitation. *Vet. Sci.* 9 (8): 429. https://doi.org/10.3390/vetsci9080429.

Exercise-Related Weakness and Collapse

Case 2—Acute Weakness and Ventroflexion in a Cat

CHAPTER 9.2

Koen Santifort DVM, PhD, Dip. ECVN

IVC Evidensia Small Animal Hospital Arnhem, Arnhem, The Netherlands and IVC Evidensia Small Animal Hospital Hart van Brabant, Waalwijk, The Netherlands

CASE HISTORY

A 10-year-old neutered male domestic shorthaired cat was presented for exercise intolerance and exercise-induced collapse. Owners started noticing weakness in his pelvic limbs a week ago. Since then, signs had progressed to inability to jump, inactivity, and a stiff, short-strided gait. After walking short distances, the cat would drop into lateral recumbency. It was kept indoors, fed a complete feline diet, and no health issues were reported leading up to the clinical signs. Vaccination and anti-parasitic treatment were performed according to standard veterinary recommendations.

NEUROLOGICAL EXAMINATION

Neurological examination revealed that the cat was ambulatory with a short-strided gait in all four limbs (Video 9.2.1). Cervical ventroflexion was continuously present, and bilateral mild scapula protrusion was noticed. The cat demonstrated a positioning head tilt to the left and right. Intermittently, the cat would suddenly assume (drop into) a lateral recumbent position. The limbs and digits were extended in that position for a short while afterward. Palpation revealed decreased muscle tone, though the tone increased after palpation, eliciting signs consistent with myalgia (hissing, struggling). Spinal reflexes of all four limbs were weak. The rest of the neurological examination was normal.

VIDEO 9.2.1 A 10-year-old neutered male domestic shorthaired cat demonstrating tetraparesis and cervical ventroflexion.

1. **Where is the likely lesion localization?**
2. **What differential diagnoses should be considered?**
3. **What tests could you perform to help determine the diagnosis?**

LESION LOCALIZATION

A diffuse neuromuscular disorder explains the findings in this case.

Neuromuscular disorders include disorders of the peripheral nervous system (i.e. the nerve roots, brachial/lumbosacral plexus, cranial and spinal nerves), the neuromuscular junction, and muscles (See Figure 9.4.2). The type of gait, with short strides and intermittent collapse into lateral recumbency exemplified in the video, can also be referred to as a "lower motor neuron" type of paresis. Although the term "lower motor neuron" suggests that the neuron itself must be involved, it is frequently used to refer to dysfunction of any of the above anatomical structures.

Although decreased muscle tone is expected in most neuromuscular disorders, primary myopathies can present as an inability to support weight, exercise intolerance, intermittent collapse, and muscle stiffness, as well as myalgia. In this patient, there is a clear stiffness to the gait and limbs, which could still be seen when the cat assumed lateral recumbency. This failure of muscle relaxation is not reflective of upper motor neuron dysfunction. It rather reflects the inability of the muscle fibers themselves to relax (i.e. cramping). Indeed, the presence of myalgia is consistent with a neuroanatomical localization to the muscles.

CAUTION: Myopathies may clinically manifest as weakness, exacerbated by exercise, together with stiffness of the limbs and joints. The description "flaccid" paresis does not really describe this clinical picture well, though it is often used synonymously with neuromuscular or lower motor neuron paresis.

WHAT DIFFERENTIAL DIAGNOSES SHOULD BE CONSIDERED?

Hypokalemic Myopathy

Hypokalemic myopathy is a major differential diagnosis for clinical signs of acute onset and progressive generalized weakness, especially including cervical ventroflexion, in cats of any age. Myalgia may be a clinical feature in some cases. The peculiar clinical sign of positioning head tilt has been described in hypokalemic cats; the head is in a level position when the animal looks forward, however, the head tilts to the opposite side when the animal turns its head. Potassium supplementation and addressing underlying disturbances or disorders are the mainstay of treatment. This very common cause of neuromuscular weakness in cats usually carries a good short-term prognosis, while the long-term prognosis is dependent on the underlying cause. A temporary cause usually implies a very good long-term prognosis.

Polymyositis

Infectious (e.g. *Toxoplasma gondii*) or immune-mediated polymyositis can result in identical clinical signs as hypokalemic myopathy. Differentiation is based on showing consistently normal potassium levels in blood samples, markedly increased creatine kinase (CK) activity levels, as well as response to immunosuppressive treatment or anti-inflammatory and anti-infectious treatments (e.g. clindamycin for *Toxoplasma gondii* infections). The diagnosis of polymyositis is furthermore based on the identification of inflammatory cell infiltrates in multiple muscle biopsies.

Thiamine Deficiency

The clinical sign of ventroflexion is specifically reported for thiamine deficiency in cats. However, the ventroflexion is of a different nature. While ventroflexion in neuromuscular patients is due to loss of muscle tone, cervical muscle tone in thiamine deficiency patients is increased. Vestibular signs, obtundation, and pupillary abnormalities are often seen concurrently with ventroflexion in these cases. Concurrent hypokalemia and thiamine deficiency could be due to nutritional or gastrointestinal issues; concurrent thiamine deficiency and hypokalemic myopathy are possible and have been reported in a cat.

Myasthenia Gravis (MG)

MG is a differential diagnosis for generalized neuromuscular weakness, worsening during or after exercise, and often includes the clinical sign of ventroflexion in cats. MG is discussed in more detail for the dog in Case 3 in this chapter, including specific considerations for feline patients.

Polyneuropathy

Feline polyneuropathy could be due to infection, (para)neoplastic syndromes, degenerative disorders, or, more commonly, it is suspected to be immune-mediated. The latter is a very common cause for acute progressive generalized neuromuscular signs and clinically includes reduced or absent spinal reflexes. Electrodiagnostic testing shows prominent abnormalities on electromyography (EMG) as well as motor nerve conduction studies. Histopathological examinations are consistent with primary nerve pathology and secondary (neurogenic) myopathy.

WHAT TESTS COULD YOU PERFORM TO HELP DETERMINE THE DIAGNOSIS?

Exercise Test

Cats often do not want to move much in veterinary clinics. The wheelbarrow exercise stress test (WEST) has been suggested to evaluate exercise-related exacerbation of clinical signs of neuromuscular disease in cats with myopathies or MG.

Hematology and Biochemistry

A complete blood count and biochemistry (e.g. to look for elevated CK activity levels), including electrolytes (e.g. potassium) and thyroid function tests, should be performed in any neuromuscular feline patient. Elevated CK activity levels in conjunction with or isolated decreased potassium levels are highly suggestive of hypokalemic myopathy. Sometimes, especially in patients who have already improved clinically, potassium levels may have normalized, and CK activity levels are on their way back to normal (e.g. only mildly elevated). This is especially relevant for patients who may have been malnourished, leading to nutritional deficiency of potassium, who subsequently have eaten and restored levels back to normal. Hypokalemia and acute muscle weakness may be associated with hyperthyroidism. Differentials for hypokalemia include chronic or acute kidney disease, renal tubular acidosis, metabolic alkalosis, nutritional deficiency, gastrointestinal disorders, post-urethral obstruction excretion, toxicity/drug-related (e.g. loop diuretics, beta-adrenergic agonists, insulin treatment [diabetes mellitus patients], or thiazides), genetic mutation (Burmese), and primary hyperaldosteronism. These may all require additional tests.

Genetic Testing

In Burmese (and related) cats, a WNK4 gene mutation has been reported as a causative variant for what is called "hypokalemic periodic polymyopathy."

Serology

Testing for infectious diseases such as *Toxoplasma gondii,* especially in outdoor cats, is valuable for including or excluding *Toxoplasma* as a likely causative factor in clinical signs of a patient with neuromuscular disease. Immunoglobulin M (IgM) as well as immunoglobulin G (IgG) levels should be tested, preferably at least 2 weeks apart, as an acute onset of signs would be expected to result in increased IgM levels and seroconversion. Acetylcholine receptor antibody titers should also be performed to investigate MG.

Electrodiagnostic Testing

For the identification of myopathies, as well as for the evaluation of peripheral nervous system disorders, electrodiagnostic testing is useful. However, if blood work has already shown increased CK activity levels and/or hypokalemia, EMG offers little more than confirmation of suspicions, and the lack of EMG abnormalities does not exclude myopathy or neuropathy in any case. Nerve conduction tests can help to rule out polyneuropathy nonetheless.

Muscle and Nerve Biopsy

Muscle biopsy would not be recommended in strongly suspected cases of hypokalemic myopathy, but it is the only way to acquire confirmation of the diagnosis of polymyositis. Nerve biopsies are required for the confirmation of neuropathies, although electrodiagnostic testing provides adequate clinical information for a presumptive diagnosis, along with clinical development.

Pharmacological Testing

Edrophonium chloride or neostigmine, both acetylcholinesterase inhibitors, have been reported to be of use to evaluate improvement of signs when MG is suspected. False-positive test results are possible and reported in feline patients with myopathies. This test is discussed in more detail in this chapter in Case 3.

OUTCOME

A complete blood count was generally unremarkable. A blood chemistry panel showed severe hypokalemia along with moderately increased blood urea nitrogen and creatinine. Urinalysis disclosed a urine specific gravity of 1.012. Total T4 was normal. The cat was presumptively diagnosed with chronic renal disease resulting in hypokalemia. The cat was started on a renal diet, subcutaneous fluid supplementation, and oral potassium gluconate supplementation. The cat's weakness responded to potassium supplementation, and the renal disease was well-managed for 2 years before progressing.

SUGGESTED READING

Brough, A. and Duchaussoy, A.C. (2021). A novel hypokalaemic polymyopathy and subsequent unrelated nutritional thiamine deficiency in a young Burmese cat. *J. Feline Med. Surg. Open Rep.* 7 (2): 20551169211041930. https://doi.org/10.1177/20551169211041930.

DiBartola, S.P. (2001). Management of hypokalaemia and hyperkalaemia. *J. Feline Med. Surg.* 3 (4): 181–183. https://doi.org/10.1053/jfms.2001.0147.

Dickinson, P.J. and LeCouteur, R.A. (2002). Muscle and nerve biopsy. *Vet. Clin. North Am. Small Anim. Pract.* 32 (1): 63–102. vi. https://doi.org/10.1016/s0195-5616(03)00080-9.

Kolb, N., Matiasek, K., van Renen, J. et al. (2022). Biopsy characteristics, subtypes, and prognostic features in 107 cases of feline presumed immune-mediated polyneuropathy. *Front. Vet. Sci.* 9: 928309. https://doi.org/10.3389/fvets.2022.928309.

Malik, R., Musca, F.J., Gunew, M.N. et al. (2015). Periodic hypokalaemic polymyopathy in Burmese and closely related cats: a review including the latest genetic data. *J. Feline Med. Surg.* 17 (5): 417–426. https://doi.org/10.1177/1098612X15581135.

Nemzek, J.A., Kruger, J.M., Walshaw, R., and Hauptman, J.G. (1994). Acute onset of hypokalemia and muscular weakness in four hyperthyroid cats. *J. Am. Vet. Med. Assoc.* 205 (1): 65–68.

Nghiem, P., Platt, S., and Schatzberg, S. (2009). The weak cat. Practical approach and common neurological differentials. *J. Feline Med. Surg.* 11 (5): 373–383. https://doi.org/10.1016/j.jfms.2009.03.005.

van Renen, J., Fischer, A., Kolb, N. et al. (2022). Clinical course and diagnostic findings of biopsy controlled presumed immune-mediated polyneuropathy in 70 European cats. *Front. Vet. Sci.* 9: 875657. https://doi.org/10.3389/fvets.2022.875657.

Tamura, S., Nakamoto, Y., and Tamura, Y. (2023). Reversible positioning head tilt observed in 14 cats with hypokalaemic myopathy. *J. Feline Med. Surg.* 25 (6): 1098612X231175761. https://doi.org/10.1177/1098612X231175761.

Van Caenegem, N., Arti, L., Troupel, T. et al. (2023). Immune-mediated polyneuropathy in cats: clinical description, electrodiagnostic assessment, and treatment. *J. Vet. Intern. Med.* 37 (3): 1088–1099. https://doi.org/10.1111/jvim.16701.

Volk, H.A., Shihab, N., and Matiasek, K. (2011). Neuromuscular disorders in the cat: clinical approach to weakness. *J. Feline Med. Surg.* 13 (11): 837–849. https://doi.org/10.1016/j.jfms.2011.09.005.

CHAPTER 9.3

Exercise-Related Weakness and Collapse

Case 3—Activity Intolerance/ Generalized Weakness in a Dog

Koen Santifort DVM, PhD, Dip. ECVN

IVC Evidensia Small Animal Hospital Arnhem, Arnhem, The Netherlands and IVC Evidensia Small Animal Hospital Hart van Brabant, Waalwijk, The Netherlands

CASE HISTORY

A 6-year-old spayed female American pitbull terrier was presented for exercise intolerance and exercise-induced collapse. Exercise intolerance had been noticed approximately 3 weeks earlier and had progressed over time. During walks, the dog tended to slow down, started trembling in the pelvic limbs, and frequently sat down. After a period of rest, the dog was able to resume ambulation. However, during the last few days, the dog also collapsed in all four limbs after walking a few dozen strides. The owners had also noticed the dog tended to take longer to finish a meal, seemed to choke intermittently, and sometimes dropped food from its mouth (interpreted as regurgitation after careful questioning). No previous health concerns were reported, and the dog was not receiving any medications. The dog had not been vaccinated for 2 years, and the use of antiparasitics was inconsistent. The general clinical examination was unremarkable.

NEUROLOGICAL EXAMINATION

Neurological examination at rest was unremarkable aside from a weak palpebral reflex of both eyes when tested repeatedly. After two minutes of exercise outdoors, the dog started to show a weak gait in the pelvic limbs with tremors in those limbs when standing still, progressing to obvious paraparesis and eventually tetraparesis without ataxia and a tendency to assume sternal recumbency (Video 9.3.1). Sometimes, the dog would stumble and suddenly collapse in all four limbs, hitting the ground with its nose. After collapsing, withdrawal reflexes were weak in all four limbs.

VIDEO 9.3.1 A six-year-old spayed female American pitbull terrier exhibiting exercise intolerance.

1. **Where is the likely lesion localization?**
2. **What differential diagnoses should be considered?**
3. **What tests could you perform to help determine the diagnosis?**

LESION LOCALIZATION

A diffuse neuromuscular disorder explains the findings in this case.

Neuromuscular disorders include disorders of the peripheral nervous system (i.e. the nerve roots, brachial/lumbosacral plexus, and cranial and spinal nerves), the neuromuscular junction, and muscles (See Figures 9.1.1 and 9.4.2). The type of gait, with short strides and difficulty bearing weight, exemplified in the video, can also be referred to as a "lower motor neuron" type of paresis. Although the term "lower motor neuron" suggests that the neuron itself must be involved, it is frequently used to refer to dysfunction of any of the above anatomical structures. Additionally, the neuronal cell body of the peripheral nervous system, in the case of motor neurons, is located in the central nervous system (e.g. spinal cord in the case of cell bodies of the motor neuron innervating muscles of the limbs).

Looking closely at the video, one can appreciate that the dog does not seem to exhibit any form of ataxia, which is supportive of a neuromuscular disorder in a case with generalized weakness. As the dog continues to walk, the stride lengths of the limbs become increasingly shorter, especially in the pelvic limbs. The thoracic limbs are affected to a lesser degree. This activity-related exacerbation of weakness is again compatible with a neuromuscular disorder.

The palpebral reflexes weaken upon repeat testing, which, if related to the same condition affecting the limbs, denotes either a multifocal or diffuse disease process. Weakening of spinal reflexes upon repeat testing can also be noticed, but is even more evident after inducing weakness through exercise, as in this case. A weak palpebral reflex itself neuroanatomically localizes to the motor part (facial motor nucleus, nerve roots, facial nerve, neuromuscular junction, and orbicularis oculi muscles), the sensory part [receptors, sensory fibers of the trigeminal nerve (ophthalmic for medial and maxillary for lateral canthus), trigeminal ganglion, trigeminal nerve roots, and the (nucleus of the) spinal tract of the trigeminal nerve], or the interneurons of this reflex arc.

A diffuse localization is furthermore corroborated by the fact that owners noted the dog tended to take longer to finish a meal and exhibited signs of dysphagia and regurgitation, which is consistent with involvement of the tongue, pharyngeal, or esophageal musculature. Megaesophagus is a common finding in dogs with MG and results in regurgitation and risk of aspiration pneumonia. In more subtle cases, clinically determining dysfunction of these latter muscles is very difficult.

CAUTION: Exercise-induced weakness may be associated with the potential for respiratory and/or cardiovascular dysfunction. A thorough general clinical examination is necessary to evaluate these systems. Evaluating the patient during activity to witness the clinical signs and examine them during an episode should be done after assessing the risks of acutely exacerbating the clinical signs.

WHAT DIFFERENTIAL DIAGNOSES SHOULD BE CONSIDERED?

Myasthenia Gravis

The presentation of the dog in this case is typical for a generalized form of myasthenia gravis (MG). MG has been called "the great imitator" because the clinical presentation can be highly variable. Nonetheless, the hallmark of this disorder is exercise-induced muscle weakness, which alleviates, in most cases, after variable periods of rest.

MG is a neuromuscular disorder that affects dogs, as well as humans, cats, and other animals. It was formerly classified as acquired MG and congenital MG, but the term MG should refer only to the acquired form related to an autoimmune response to proteins of the neuromuscular junction. Congenital myasthenic syndrome is the preferred term for what was previously called congenital MG.

MG leads to muscle weakness, which can manifest in clinical signs such as exercise intolerance, difficulty chewing, difficulty swallowing and regurgitation, laryngeal paresis/paralysis, respiratory muscle weakness, and drooping eyelids. Focal, generalized, and acute fulminating variants are recognized in veterinary medicine. All these are further subcategorized as thymoma-associated or non-thymoma-associated. For the generalized form in dogs, a subcategory of "seronegative" is included. Canine patients with the seropositive variant are positive for acetylcholine receptor (AChR) autoantibodies and account for about 98% of cases, reportedly. Cases with the seronegative variant, which do not show a positive result for AChR autoantibody titer testing, account for the minority. Some other autoantibodies (muscle-specific kinase, titin, and ryanodine receptor autoantibodies) have been found in canine cases of (AChR autoantibody) seronegative MG. The possibility of spontaneous clinical remission in dogs with MG has been reported in up to 31–88.7% of cases, occurring between a median of 6.4–7.3 months from the start of treatment. Relapse can subsequently occur in a minority of patients.

In MG, antibodies affect the ability of the postsynaptic (muscle) membrane to reach the threshold for development of an activation potential by blocking the receptors. The severity of clinical signs can, at least theoretically, be linked to the number of receptors that are still functional. A pivotal part of the treatment of MG patients is to enhance neuromuscular transmission by increasing the amount and duration of (the presence of) acetylcholine in the synaptic cleft. Acetylcholinesterase inhibitors (AchE-I) such as pyridostigmine and neostigmine can be employed to this effect. These medications are used diagnostically as well as therapeutically.

Notes on Feline MG

1. A smaller proportion of cats have dysphagia and/or regurgitation as clinical signs compared to dogs, as the esophageal musculature of cats largely consists of smooth muscle. For this reason, prednisolone could be considered part of standard treatment, as the risk of aspiration pneumonia and complications thereof is lower than in dogs.
2. Feline MG patients (non-thymoma-associated) may have a very good prognosis, even without treatment.
3. Thymoma-associated MG is more common in cats than in dogs.
4. Genetic tests for congenital myasthenic syndromes are available for the Devon Rex and Sphynx cat breeds.

Polymyopathies

Polymyopathies should be strongly considered as a possibility for a patient with a presentation similar to this case. Myopathies can be focal, multifocal, or diffuse. Underlying etiologies are highly variable, including infection (e.g. *Neospora caninum*), immune-mediated disease (e.g. immune-mediated polymyositis), metabolic disorders (e.g. hypokalemia in cats), endocrine disease (e.g. hyperadrenocorticism), degenerative disorders (e.g. muscular dystrophy), neoplastic disease (e.g. lymphoma), or paraneoplastic syndromes. Exertional or necrotizing rhabdomyolysis can also occur, but typically lead to a single, severe bout of clinical signs with a possibly fatal outcome. Over time, however, polymyopathies often lead to severe muscle atrophy in a fairly short period of time, a feature that would be inconsistent with MG. Degenerative disorders are mostly breed-related, for which some genetic causes have been identified. These disorders usually affect younger patients. Nevertheless, polymyopathies or indeed focal myopathies can affect the pharyngeal muscles, laryngeal muscles, and esophageal muscles as well as appendicular and core muscles, which can lead to clinical signs identical to MG, including dysphagia, dysphonia, and exercise-related weakness, until they begin to show muscle atrophy, which is not seen with MG.

Polyneuropathies (Chronic or Acute)

This is an unlikely differential diagnosis for this patient, based mostly on the neurological examination findings. Polyneuropathies would be expected to result in consistent cranial and/or spinal reflex deficits, and not just after exercise. Moreover, the patellar reflex was normal in this case, while this particular reflex is often abnormal in polyneuropathy cases.

In patients with laryngeal dysfunction (laryngeal paralysis), focal MG should be included in the differential diagnosis list alongside polyneuropathies, such as geriatric onset laryngeal paralysis/polyneuropathy (GOLPP).

A variety of underlying causes should be considered for polyneuropathies, including endocrine disorders (e.g. hypothyroidism and diabetes mellitus), degenerative disorders (e.g. genetic and breed-related), infectious diseases (e.g. *Neospora caninum*), (suspected) immune-mediated disorders (e.g. polyradiculoneuritis, "Coonhound paralysis"), and paraneoplastic syndromes. While polyneuropathies present broadly as a diffuse neuromuscular problem, they would typically not be exercise-induced. The inability to perform exercise is what the owners may report. However, it should be considered that polyneuropathies may concurrently be diagnosed in dogs with MG.

Metabolic, Upper Airway, Pulmonary, and Cardiovascular Disease

Several non-neurological or neuromuscular disorders need to be considered in patients presented for exercise intolerance and collapse. Precisely for this reason, it is vital to consider the signalment and history, perform a thorough general clinical examination, and acquire a minimum database including hematology, biochemistry, and electrolytes.

- Abdominal palpation may reveal masses (e.g. hemangiosarcoma) or abdominal effusion. The author has been presented with patients suspected of having neurological disorders that instead had recurrent intra-abdominal hemorrhages leading to acute collapse. On numerous occasions, these collapses may occur during activity, suggesting to owners that it was exercise-induced.
- Hypoglycemia due to any cause, but particularly in older dogs, secondary to insulinoma (pancreatic beta islet cell tumors), can often result in weakness, and exercise may trigger or exacerbate signs.
- Brachycephalic obstructive airway syndrome, tracheal collapse, pulmonary fibrosis, pericardial effusion and aortic thrombosis are among the numerous reasons for cardiorespiratory causes of weakness or collapse associated with exercise. Especially in the latter, clinical presentation may be remarkably similar to that shown in the video of this case.

WHAT TESTS COULD YOU PERFORM TO HELP DETERMINE THE DIAGNOSIS?

Exercise Test

Clinically, it is very valuable to be able to witness the signs reported by owners, especially if the owner cannot provide a video in which the signs are included. Most patients who exhibit exercise-induced weakness can therefore be examined before and after exercise, after careful weighing of the risks that can be associated with exercising the patient in question (see word of caution above).

Hematology and Biochemistry

A complete blood count (e.g. to exclude anemia) and biochemistry (e.g. to look for elevated creatine kinase activity levels or hypoglycemia), including electrolytes (e.g. to exclude hypokalemia), should be performed in any patient presented with exercise-related weakness and/or collapse. Moreover, assessments of leukograms and C-reactive protein may help to diagnose complications related to neuromuscular disorders, such as aspiration pneumonia.

Serology

The most reliable test for the diagnosis of MG in dogs is radioimmunoassay (RIA) for the presence of AChR autoantibodies. A positive test confirms the diagnosis, though a negative test does not exclude the diagnosis. A diagnosis of seronegative MG is based on the following criteria. Dogs should have undergone a general and neurological examination with findings consistent with MG; have a response to pharmacologic testing (e.g. neostigmine test) consistent with MG; have electrophysiologic test findings consistent with MG; show normalization of clinical signs after AChE-I treatment; and have at least two negative serum AChR autoantibody tests by RIA with an interval of 1–2 months.

Electrodiagnostic Testing

For the identification of myopathies, as well as for the evaluation of peripheral nervous system disorders, electrodiagnostic testing is useful.

1. Needle electromyography (EMG) can determine if there are any signs of spontaneous activity in muscles when the patient is under general anesthesia. If such activity is found, this would suggest a primary muscle and/or nerve disorder. Neuromuscular junctionopathies often do not lead to abnormal EMG results.
2. Nerve conduction studies can assess the function of nerves, as well as the neuromuscular junction and muscles. In dogs or cats with MG, both EMG and nerve conduction studies are often normal.
3. Repetitive nerve stimulation (RNS), a specific form of nerve conduction study where nerves are repeatedly stimulated (at low frequency, e.g. 3 Hz), can reveal a decrement of >10% between successive compound muscle action potential amplitudes and/or areas in cases with MG.
4. Single-fiber EMG is a very sensitive test for neuromuscular junction dysfunction, but requires even more expertise and specific equipment than the other tests.
   The major downside of electrodiagnostic testing in veterinary patients is the need for general anesthesia. Such procedures in neuromuscular patients carry risks of complications, including hypoventilation, specifically in the recovery phase when weaning off mechanical ventilation. Also, anesthetic agents may further exacerbate clinical signs.

Pharmacological Testing

Edrophonium chloride or neostigmine, both AChE inhibitors, have been reported to be of use in evaluating the improvement of signs in a clinical setting. Neostigmine (0.02–0.04 mg/kg IM/IV) is more commonly employed in countries where edrophonium chloride (a very short-acting AChE-I) is no longer available. Within minutes after administration of neostigmine, improvement in muscle strength and ambulation is expected in MG cases. Some authors have reported responses to the neostigmine test as negative (no effect), weak positive (some effect), and strong positive (clearly effective). It is recommended to assess the effect from the moment of administration until at least 30 minutes later. Though longer-acting than edrophonium chloride, neostigmine plasma concentrations drop rapidly after IV administration. This means that the clinical benefit of administration of this drug is short-term. However, results are highly variable between individual dogs, both in effect and duration of effect. While these pharmacological tests have their merits, false-positive and false-negative results are also possible. Also, acute cholinergic crises may result from overdosing on these medications. Having atropine at hand is recommended to counter cholinergic side effects, including salivation, lacrimation, urination, gastrointestinal upset, dyspnea, and emesis (±0.02 mg/kg, dose depending on severity of side effects).

Diagnostic Imaging

- **Thoracic radiographs**
  Orthogonal or three-view thoracic radiographs are recommended in patients suspected of having MG or esophageal dysfunction (Figure 9.3.1). In MG patients, they serve at least three main goals: (1) diagnosis of megaesophagus, (2) diagnosis of (aspiration) pneumonia, and (3) diagnosis of cranial mediastinal mass lesions (specifically thymoma).

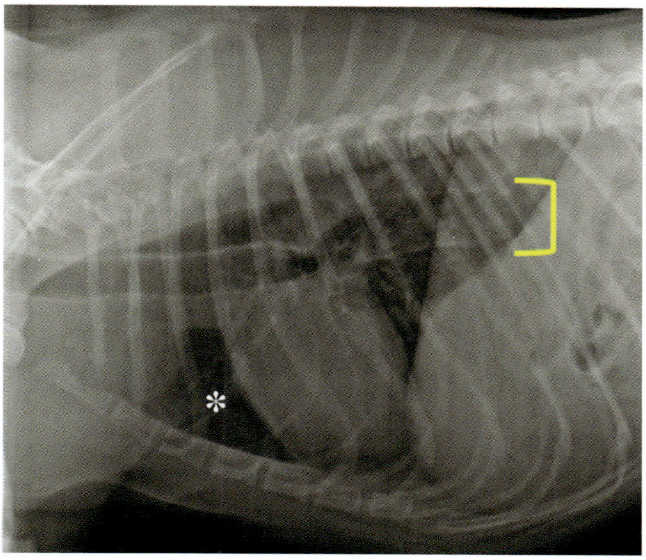

FIGURE 9.3.1 Lateral thoracic radiograph of a dog with megaesophagus, indicated by the yellow bracket. The patient also has a cranial mediastinal mass lesion (thymoma)*.

Aspiration pneumonia deserves specific attention, as this is the primary cause of death or euthanasia for MG patients. The presence of esophageal dysfunction or megaesophagus, as clinically evidenced by regurgitation in most cases of MG in dogs, is negatively associated with clinical remission.

- **CT-scan/abdominal ultrasound**
  In addition to confirming radiographical abnormalities, equivocal radiographic results and staging patients with masses in the cranial thoracic region/mediastinum can be accomplished with CT, or abdominal ultrasound.

OUTCOME

Thoracic radiographs confirmed megaesophagus with mild aspiration pneumonia observed in the right middle lung lobe. Amoxicillin-clavulanic acid was prescribed to treat aspiration pneumonia. Given the megaesophagus, the owners were instructed to feed the dog upright and to keep the dog upright for 15 minutes following meal completion. An AChR antibody titer was positive, confirming the diagnosis of myasthenia gravis. The dog was started on pyridostigmine (initially 0.25 mg/kg every 8 hours to reach a final dose of 0.7 mg/kg every 8 hours). The dog showed a strong response to pyridostigmine but experienced several bouts of aspiration pneumonia secondary to megaesophagus. Three months after initiating therapy, an AChR antibody titer was performed and was more elevated than at the time of diagnosis. Thoracic radiographs were repeated, raising suspicion for the presence of a cranial mediastinal mass which was later confirmed (via CT and fine-needle aspiration biopsies) to be a thymoma. The dog underwent a thymectomy via median sternotomy. Pyridostigmine was continued postoperatively until antibody levels dipped below the diagnostic cutoff. At this point, the pyridostigmine was slowly discontinued, and the dog was clinically normal until its death from unrelated issues 4 years later.

SUGGESTED READING

Baker, P.R., Calvey, T.N., Chan, K. et al. (1978). Plasma clearance of neostigmine and pyridostigmine in the dog. *Br. J. Pharmacol.* 63 (3): 509–512. https://doi.org/10.1111/j.1476-5381.1978.tb07805.x.

Cridge, H., Little, A., José-López, R. et al. (2021). The clinical utility of neostigmine administration in the diagnosis of acquired myasthenia gravis. *J. Vet. Emerg. Crit. Care (San Antonio)* 31 (5): 647–655. https://doi.org/10.1111/vec.13043.

Cuddon, P.A. (2002). Electrophysiology in neuromuscular disease. *Vet. Clin. North Am. Small Anim. Pract.* 32 (1): 31–62. https://doi.org/10.1016/S0195-5616(03)00072-8.

Dewey, C.W., Bailey, C.S., Shelton, G.D. et al. (1997). Clinical forms of acquired myasthenia gravis in dogs: 25 cases (1988–1995). *J. Vet. Intern. Med.* 11 (2): 50–57. https://doi.org/10.1111/j.1939-1676.1997.tb00073.x.

Forgash, J.T., Chang, Y.M., Mittelman, N.S. et al. (2021). Clinical features and outcome of acquired myasthenia gravis in 94 dogs. *J. Vet. Intern. Med.* 35 (5): 2315–2326. https://doi.org/10.1111/jvim.16223.

Hague, D.W., Humphries, H.D., Mitchell, M.A., and Shelton, G.D. (2015). Risk factors and outcomes in cats with acquired myasthenia gravis (2001–2012). *J. Vet. Intern. Med.* 29 (5): 1307–1312. https://doi.org/10.1111/jvim.13596.

Mignan, T., Garosi, L., Targett, M., and Lowrie, M. (2020). Long-term outcome of cats with acquired myasthenia gravis without evidence of a cranial mediastinal mass. *J. Vet. Intern. Med.* 34 (1): 247–252. https://doi.org/10.1111/jvim.15655.

Mignan, T., Targett, M., and Lowrie, M. (2020). Classification of myasthenia gravis and congenital myasthenic syndromes in dogs and cats. *J. Vet. Intern. Med.* 34 (5): 1707–1717. https://doi.org/10.1111/jvim.15855.

Ruehl, M., Lynch, A.M., O'Toole, T.E. et al. (2020). Outcome and treatments of dogs with aortic thrombosis: 100 cases (1997–2014). *J. Vet. Intern. Med.* 34 (5): 1759–1767. https://doi.org/10.1111/jvim.15874.

Ryan, D., Pérez-Accino, J., Gonçalves, R. et al. (2021). Clinical findings, neurological manifestations and survival of dogs with insulinoma 116 cases (2009–2020). *J. Small Anim. Pract.* 62 (7): 531–539. https://doi.org/10.1111/jsap.13318.

Shelton, G.D. (2002). Myasthenia gravis and disorders of neuromuscular transmission. *Vet. Clin. North Am. Small Anim. Pract.* 32 (1): 189–206. https://doi.org/10.1016/S0195-5616(03)00085-6.

Shelton, G.D. (2010). Routine and specialized laboratory testing for the diagnosis of neuromuscular diseases in dogs and cats. *Vet. Clin. Pathol.* 39 (3): 278–295. https://doi.org/10.1111/j.1939-165X.2010.00250.x.

Shelton, G.D., Ho, M., and Kass, P.H. (2000). Risk factors for acquired myasthenia gravis in cats: 105 cases (1986–1998). *J. Am. Vet. Med. Assoc.* 216 (1): 55–57. https://doi.org/10.2460/javma.2000.216.55.

Shelton, G.D. and Lindstrom, J.M. (2001). Spontaneous remission in canine myasthenia gravis: implications for assessing human MG therapies. *Neurology* 57 (11): 2139–2141. https://doi.org/10.1212/WNL.57.11.2139.

Shelton, G.D., Schule, A., and Kass, P.H. (1997). Risk factors for acquired myasthenia gravis in dogs: 1,154 cases (1991–1995). *J. Am. Vet. Med. Assoc.* 211 (11): 1428–1431. PMID: 9364307.

Shelton, G.D., Skeie, G.O., Kass, P.H., and Aarli, J.A. (2001). Titin and ryanodine receptor autoantibodies in dogs with thymoma and late-onset myasthenia gravis. *Vet. Immunol. Immunopathol.* 78 (1): 97–105 https://doi.org/10.1016/S0165-2427(01)00237-3.

Williams, T.P., Shaw, S., Porter, A., and Berkwitt, L. (2017). Aortic thrombosis in dogs. *J. Vet. Emerg. Crit. Care (San Antonio)* 27 (1): 9–22. https://doi.org/10.1111/vec.12527.

Exercise-Related Weakness and Collapse

Case 4—Chronic Weakness/Plantigrade Posture in a Cat

CHAPTER 9.4

Koen Santifort DVM, PhD, Dip. ECVN

IVC Evidensia Small Animal Hospital Arnhem, Arnhem, The Netherlands and IVC Evidensia Small Animal Hospital Hart van Brabant, Waalwijk, The Netherlands

CASE HISTORY

A 12-year-old neutered male domestic shorthaired cat was presented for progressive weakness, inactivity, and difficulty jumping. Owners had also noticed polydipsia and polyuria. The cat had outdoor access. The cat had been obese just a year before, but a reduction in weight was accomplished swiftly over time, though poor muscle condition had been noticed. The cat was not receiving any medications. The cat was vaccinated according to recommended schemes, and the use of anti-parasitics was inconsistent. General clinical examination yielded a heart murmur (2/6 systolic, mitral valve punctum maximum), poor fur condition, and low body condition score (3/9) with generalized appendicular muscle atrophy.

NEUROLOGICAL EXAMINATION

Neurological examination showed bilaterally symmetrical ambulatory tetraparesis with difficulty supporting weight (Video 9.4.1). The cat tended to sit down after a few strides and needed prompting to evaluate ambulation. When standing, all four limbs buckled in the distal joints, with a complete plantigrade and palmigrade posture, including the tarsi and carpi touching the floor (Figure 9.4.1). The limb stride length was normal to increased, with a "throwing" quality to limb protraction in the thoracic limbs and a "skating" type of gait with scuffing of the paws and inward rotation of the tarsi. Spinal reflexes were abnormal, including weak to absent withdrawal reflexes in all limbs, absent patellar reflexes bilaterally, and absent cutaneous trunci reflexes. Thoracolumbar kyphosis could be appreciated as well. Proprioceptive placement tests of the pelvic and thoracic limbs were considered abnormal, as the cat would not correct the position of the paws when carefully knuckled over. Muscle tone was decreased in all four limbs, especially distally. Severe distal limb muscle atrophy and moderate proximal limb muscle atrophy were noticed. The rest of the neurological examination was considered normal.

VIDEO 9.4.1 Video of a tetraparetic 12-year-old domestic shorthaired cat with difficulty bearing weight.

1. **Where is the likely lesion localization?**
2. **What is the primary differential diagnosis?**
3. **What tests could you perform to help determine the diagnosis?**

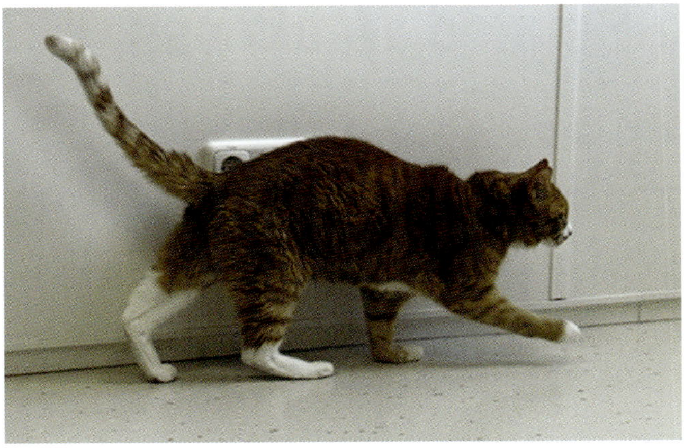

FIGURE 9.4.1 Plantigrade and palmigrade stance (weight-bearing right pelvic limb and left thoracic limb)

LESION LOCALIZATION

A diffuse motor and sensory peripheral nervous system disorder (mainly affecting distal appendicular neuromuscular structures) explains the findings in this case.

Neuromuscular disorders include disorders of the peripheral nervous system (i.e. the nerve roots, brachial/lumbosacral plexus, cranial and spinal nerves), the neuromuscular junction, and muscles (Figure 9.4.2). Sensory receptors, nerves, spinal ganglia, and dorsal nerve roots should be considered to be involved in cases with proprioceptive and sensory abnormalities. Although our clinical ability to assess the function of this system is limited, in severe cases, such as this one, failure of the sensory peripheral nervous system component can result in confusing signs, including proprioceptive deficits or decreased nociception. The lack of short-stridedness in the gait in this neuromuscular patient, which is usually seen with this localization, is most likely a reflection of the preferential involvement of the distal neuroanatomy, leading to weakness distally with largely retained muscle strength proximally. There is involvement of the truncal and proximal limb musculature, but to a lesser degree. As such, thoracic limbs are thrown forward and the distal part "flops" (carpal flaccidity). The tarsi are poorly flexed and extended, also contributing to the overall "floppy" nature (flaccid tetraparesis; distal limbs most severely affected).

This peculiar type of gait is often confused for generalized upper motor neuron tetraparesis and proprioceptive ataxia, prompting consideration of spinal disorders and diagnostic imaging studies such as magnetic resonance imaging (MRI). As some of these cats indeed show proprioceptive deficits, this can contribute to the suspicion of central nervous system lesions. Recognition of the three main features of neuromuscular disease (i.e. hyporeflexia, muscle atrophy, and decreased muscle tone) should be given preference in such a case, explaining the other findings by involvement of the sensory peripheral nervous system. Indeed, the retained ability to extend the stifle with an absent patellar reflex is a clear sign of involvement of the sensory arc of this reflex pathway. Although the cranial nerve examination is often normal in such patients, this does not mean that the pathogenesis underlying the appendicular signs does not affect the cranial nerves and their targets.

CAUTION: Involvement of sensory components of the peripheral nervous system can lead to confusing clinical signs and neurological examination findings. Looking for the three main signs of neuromuscular disease helps to reach a correct neuroanatomical localization in such patients: hyporeflexia, muscle atrophy, and decreased muscle tone.

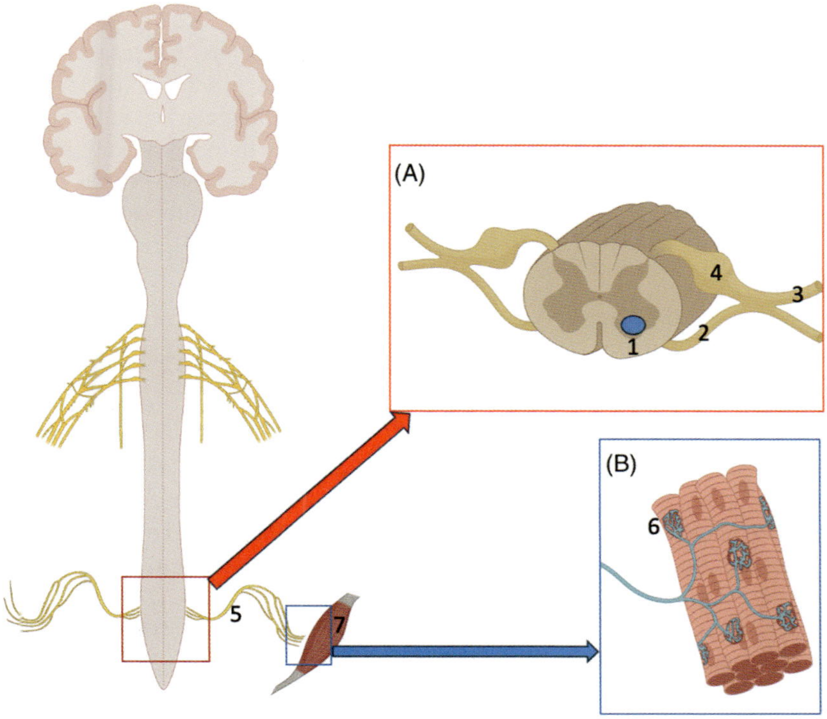

FIGURE 9.4.2 An illustrated overview of the neuromuscular system. Inset (A) depicts a cross-section of the spinal cord at the level of the lumbar intumescence and the origin of the lower motor neuron. (1) Ventral horn cell; (2) ventral nerve root; (3) dorsal nerve root; (4) dorsal nerve root ganglion. The nerve roots form spinal nerves which combine to form specific peripheral nerves extending into neuromuscular junctions (6) as shown in inset (B) innervating specific muscles (7).

WHAT IS THE PRIMARY DIFFERENTIAL DIAGNOSIS?

Diabetic Polyneuropathy (DP)

The presentation of the cat in this case is classical for DP.

A plantigrade stance is either due to mechanical issues (e.g. tendinopathies) or lower motor neuron disorders that include the spinal cord segments (L6–S1/2) where the motor neuron cell bodies are, nerve roots, plexus, peripheral nerves, neuromuscular junction, or muscles. Other metabolic conditions, paraneoplastic syndromes, toxins, myasthenia gravis (MG), degenerative polyneuropathies and myopathies, immune-mediated neuropathies and myopathies, as well as infectious diseases and lymphoma, could theoretically lead to combinations of the various features seen in this patient. Still, all of these are less likely than DP, especially taking into account the main features of the history that included (a) chronic progression, (b) polydipsia and polyuria, and (c) neurological examination findings (e.g. reduced spinal reflexes, inconsistent with MG).

WHAT TESTS COULD YOU PERFORM TO HELP DETERMINE THE DIAGNOSIS?

The diagnosis of DP relies on confirming the diagnosis of diabetes mellitus in a cat with consistent clinical findings. Additional tests, including cardiac ultrasound (in this case, a heart murmur was reported), abdominal ultrasound, and serology for infectious diseases and myasthenia gravis, should be considered on a case-by-case basis.

Hematology and Biochemistry

A complete blood count and biochemistry, including electrolytes, fructosamine levels, feline pancreatic lipase, and thyroid function, should be performed. Fructosamine levels can help to differentiate stress-induced hyperglycemia. Hyperglycemia is often marked in DP patients, leaving little doubt that the hyperglycemia reflects true diabetes rather than stress. Polyendocrine disease can occur, which is one of the reasons not to just measure glucose levels for the diagnosis of DP. Diabetic ketoacidosis is a risk in cats that are unmanaged or managed for diabetes mellitus.

Urinalysis

Since polyuria/polydipsia is reported, urinalysis is key in the diagnosis of DP as well as excluding or diagnosing concurrent diseases such as renal disorders or urinary tract infections.

Electrodiagnostic Testing and Muscle and Nerve Biopsies

For further characterization of DP, electromyography (EMG), nerve conduction studies, and muscle and nerve biopsies may all be considered. However, they should not be considered a necessity in cases where blood and urinary tests have already confirmed a diagnosis of diabetes mellitus. Studies describing these tests and the results thereof have shown involvement of motor and sensory nerves.

MRI or CT

Although imaging studies are not part of the workup of a DP patient in general, MRI or CT of the head in cats suspected or shown to have hypersomatotropism is to be considered, especially if surgical treatment is contemplated.

Other notes: Importantly, treatment of DM in cats can result in significant improvement of neurological signs over time. Neuropathic pain may occur, and treatment should be considered in cases that exhibit signs of allodynia or hyperesthesia.

OUTCOME

Diabetes mellitus was confirmed via persistent hyperglycemia. The cat was transitioned to a high-protein, low-carbohydrate diet, and insulin therapy was initiated. Neurological function improved over the course of the next months.

SUGGESTED READING

Blois, S.L., Dickie, E.L., Kruth, S.A., and Allen, D.G. (2010). Multiple endocrine diseases in cats: 15 cases (1997–2008). *J. Feline Med. Surg.* 12 (8): 637–642. https://doi.org/10.1016/j.jfms.2010.03.017.

van Bokhorst, K.L., Galac, S., Kooistra, H.S. et al. (2021). Evaluation of hypophysectomy for treatment of hypersomatotropism in 25 cats. *J. Vet. Intern. Med.* 35 (2): 834–842. https://doi.org/10.1111/jvim.16047.

Cuddon, P.A. (2002). Electrophysiology in neuromuscular disease. *Vet. Clin. North Am. Small Anim. Pract.* 32 (1): 31–62. https://doi.org/10.1016/S0195-5616(03)00072-8.

Dickinson, P.J. and LeCouteur, R.A. (2004). Feline neuromuscular disorders. *Vet. Clin. North Am. Small Anim. Pract.* 34 (6): 1307–1359. https://doi.org/10.1016/j.cvsm.2004.05.012.

Epstein, M.E. (2020). Feline neuropathic pain. *Vet. Clin. North Am. Small Anim. Pract.* 50 (4): 789–809. https://doi.org/10.1016/j.cvsm.2020.02.004.

Estrella, J.S., Nelson, R.N., Sturges, B.K. et al. (2008). Endoneurial microvascular pathology in feline diabetic neuropathy. *Microvasc. Res.* 75 (3): 403–410. https://doi.org/10.1016/j.mvr.2007.12.002.

Fleeman, L. and Gostelow, R. (2020). Updates in feline diabetes mellitus and hypersomatotropism. *Vet. Clin. North Am. Small Anim. Pract.* 50 (5): 1085–1105. https://doi.org/10.1016/j.cvsm.2020.06.005.

Gilor, C. and Graves, T.K. (2023). Diabetes mellitus in cats and dogs. *Vet. Clin. North Am. Small Anim. Pract.* 53 (3): xiii–xiv. https://doi.org/10.1016/j.cvsm.2023.02.018.

Kramek, B.A., Moise, N.S., Cooper, B., and Raffe, M.R. (1984). Neuropathy associated with diabetes mellitus in the cat. *J. Am. Vet. Med. Assoc.* 184 (1): 42–45.

Mizisin, A.P., Nelson, R.W., Sturges, B.K. et al. (2007). Comparable myelinated nerve pathology in feline and human diabetes mellitus. *Acta Neuropathol.* 113 (4): 431–442. https://doi.org/10.1007/s00401-006-0163-8.

Mizisin, A.P., Shelton, G.D., Burgers, M.L. et al. (2002). Neurological complications associated with spontaneously occurring feline diabetes mellitus. *J. Neuropathol. Exp. Neurol.* 61 (10): 872–884. https://doi.org/10.1093/jnen/61.10.872.

Mizisin, A.P., Shelton, G.D., Wagner, S. et al. (1998). Myelin splitting, Schwann cell injury and demyelination in feline diabetic neuropathy. *Acta Neuropathol.* 95 (2): 171–174. https://doi.org/10.1007/s004010050783.

Rusbridge, C. (2024). Neuropathic pain in cats: mechanisms and multimodal management. *J. Feline Med. Surg.* 26: https://doi.org/10.1177/1098612X241246518.

Volk, H.A., Shihab, N., and Matiasek, K. (2011). Neuromuscular disorders in the cat: clinical approach to weakness. *J. Feline Med. Surg.* 13 (11): 837–849. https://doi.org/10.1016/j.jfms.2011.09.005.

Xenoulis, P.G. and Fracassi, F. (2022). Feline comorbidities: clinical perspective on diabetes mellitus and pancreatitis. *J. Feline Med. Surg.* 24 (7): 651–661. https://doi.org/10.1177/1098612X221106355.

CHAPTER 10.1

Spinal Pain

Case 1—Thoracolumbar Pain in a Dog

Fred Wininger[1] and Susan A. Arnold[2]

[1] *The Animal Neurology Center, Saint Louis, MO, USA*

[2] *Department of Veterinary Clinical Sciences, University of Minnesota St. Paul, MN, USA*

CASE HISTORY

A 5-year-old neutered male mixed-breed dog was presented with a 10-day history of progressive spinal pain. The owner reported that the dog had become increasingly reluctant to jump on furniture, seemed painful when picked up, and vocalized occasionally during movement. Appetite, urination, defecation, and activity levels were otherwise unchanged. No prior illnesses, traumas, or systemic diseases were reported, and the dog was up to date on vaccinations and receiving monthly parasite prevention.

The dog had no recent travel history, had not been kenneled, and had not undergone any recent surgical or dental procedures. The patient had no history of previous back problems or systemic infections.

GENERAL PHYSICAL EXAMINATION

The dog was bright, alert, and responsive. His body temperature was 103.3 °F, his pulse was 126 beats per minute, and his respiratory rate was 44 breaths per minute. The physical examination was unremarkable, with normal body condition, hydration status, and no signs of external trauma, lymphadenopathy, or orthopedic abnormalities. No palpable abdominal masses or abdominal pain were noted.

NEUROLOGICAL EXAMINATION

The dog's mentation was normal, but he was reluctant to be touched. The patient needed to be coaxed to walk, and despite no overt abnormalities noted, the stride length seemed shorter than expected. Postural reaction testing was normal. Segmental reflexes and tone were normal. Cranial nerve examination was normal. Marked spinal hyperesthesia was evident upon palpation over the thoracolumbar junction (T12–L1 region).

Key questions to consider

1. What is the likely lesion localization and the most appropriate ranked differential diagnoses?
2. What are the best next diagnostic steps for this patient?
3. What are the treatments and prognosis for these differentials?

LESION LOCALIZATION AND DIFFERENTIAL DIAGNOSES

The localization in this case is focal to the vertebral column at the thoracolumbar junction. In the absence of neurologic deficits, neurolocalization based on spinal hyperesthesia is appropriate. In this case, the dog would be considered "neurologically normal with thoracolumbar junction hyperesthesia." Despite being the conduit and perception center of pain, the spinal cord and neuroparenchyma have a paucity of nociceptors. For this reason, animals with primary nervous tissue disease can be nonpainful, and pain generally emanates from surrounding structures, including the vertebrae and periosteum, meninges and perineural tissues, epaxial musculature, and intervertebral discs themselves.

Since animals cannot describe their discomfort, pain is generally a term reserved for human medicine, as patients can verbalize their symptoms. Hyperesthesia is considered a more appropriate term, as it is an observation indicating increased sensitivity or responsiveness to palpation.

Meningomyelitis

This condition leads to inflammation of the spinal cord and surrounding meninges. Meningomyelitis can be either infectious or noninfectious. Noninfectious meningomyelitis is more common in dogs than infectious meningomyelitis. Though considered for this case, the focal thoracolumbar nature of the condition without neurologic deficits makes it less likely than other differential diagnoses. Typically, immune-mediated disease of the central nervous system more commonly affects the brain than the spinal cord. Nonetheless, the diagnostic and treatment approaches are the same for both locations. For more information on central nervous system inflammation, refer to Chapter 3 and Chapter 5.

Inflammation – Discospondylitis

This is an infectious disease of the intervertebral disc and adjacent vertebral endplates. Hyperesthesia without neurologic deficits is the most common presentation for discospondylitis. Hyperesthesia results from inflammation and lysis of the vertebral endplates. Rarely, proliferative inflammatory tissue and epidural empyema can cause spinal cord compression and secondary neurological deficits. Catastrophic vertebral pathologic fracture is also possible and can lead to both contusive and lacerative injury to the spinal cord as well as vertebral column instability. The presence of a low-grade fever and slight lethargy in this case is consistent with this diagnosis.

Discospondylitis is more common in large male breed dogs than in others. The most common sites are the lumbosacral junction, followed by the thoracolumbar junction and then the caudal cervical vertebral column. It is distinct from both physitis and vertebral osteomyelitis, which affect the vertebral endplates alone or the vertebra, respectively. There are several routes of infection. The most common route of infection is hematogenous spread from other locations, including the urogenital tract, heart (endocarditis), and potentially the skin. It has been hypothesized that many infections spread from the urinary bladder during periods of high intra-abdominal pressure when the venous drainage shares the vertebral plexus. Less commonly, direct extension or local infection occurs secondary to a migrating foreign body, such as a grass awn that traverses caudally from the lungs into the abdomen and lodges into the retroperitoneal space and hypaxial muscles. Interestingly, steroid use has been associated with an increased risk of progressive neurologic dysfunction.

The most common infections are bacterial, often *Staphylococcus pseudintermedius*. However, other bacteria may be implicated. Although less common, *Brucella canis* can cause canine discospondylitis and carries a zoonotic risk. Less common than bacteria but perhaps more serious are fungal causes, particularly *Aspergillus* species (with a German shepherd breed predisposition), *Blastomyces dermatitidis, Coccidioides immitis,* and *Cryptococcus neoformans.*

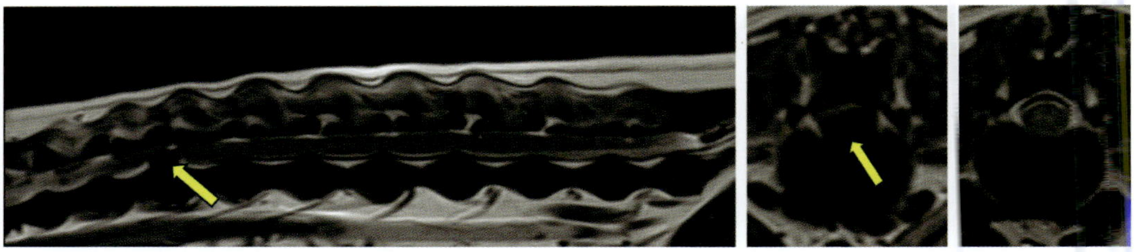

FIGURE 10.1.1 An MRI showing an intervertebral disc extrusion associated with marked spinal cord compression in a 7-year-old Corgi whose only clinical sign was hyperesthesia. The middle image is a transverse image at the level of the disc extrusion, causing marked compression of the spinal cord. The right-sided image is a transverse image at an unaffected area, showing the normal appearance of the spinal cord.

Degenerative – Intervertebral Disc Disease (IVDD)

Hansen type I or II intervertebral disc disease (IVDD) may present with hyperesthesia only. The magnetic resonance imaging (MRI) in Figure 10.1.1 is a study of a 7-year-old Pembroke Welsh Corgi with a 2-month history of spinal hyperesthesia over the mid-lumbar vertebral column and an otherwise normal neurologic examination. The MRI demonstrates a high degree of compression, greater than 50% of the vertebral canal. The anatomic degree of spinal cord compression and the severity of sensorimotor dysfunction often do not correlate. For more details regarding Hansen type I IVDD, refer to Chapter 12, Case 1. For more details regarding Hansen type II IVDD, refer to Chapter 12, Case 2.

Neoplasia

Neoplasms of the vertebral column/spinal cord are often differentiated into extradural, intradural, extramedullary, and intramedullary. Extradural tumors are often primary or metastatic tumors of the vertebrae that erode bone and produce pain. Intradural/extramedullary tumors are those that occur between the spinal cord meninges and the spinal cord. Intramedullary tumors are those that occur in the spinal cord itself. Intramedullary tumors occur but rarely cause spinal hyperesthesia in the absence of neurologic deficits. Overall, neoplasia is an important differential diagnosis to consider in a patient that displays vertebral column hyperesthesia, especially if the patient is older.

- Examples of extradural tumors:
  - Primary tumors:
    - Osteosarcoma
    - Fibrosarcoma
    - Chondrosarcoma
    - Plasma cell tumor or multiple myeloma
    - Myxosarcoma
  - Metastatic tumors:
    - Lymphoma
    - Hemangiosarcoma and other round cell neoplasms, including mast cell tumors and melanomas
    - Various carcinomas (mammary adenocarcinoma, prostatic adenocarcinoma, transitional cell carcinoma, thyroid adenocarcinoma, among others)

- Examples of intradural/extramedullary tumors:
  - Meningioma
  - Nerve sheath tumor
  - Lymphoma
  - Nephroblastoma (rare, affects young dogs in the thoracolumbar region)
- Examples of intramedullary tumors:
  - Glioma
  - Lymphoma
  - Ependymoma
  - Metastasis

WHAT ARE THE BEST NEXT DIAGNOSTIC STEPS FOR THIS PATIENT?

Discospondylitis

Radiography remains the most accessible and widely used first-line imaging modality for evaluating discospondylitis. Typical radiographic signs include disc space narrowing, endplate irregularity or lysis, reactive sclerosis, and periosteal new bone formation (Figure 10.1.2). However, it is important to note that radiographic changes may lag behind clinical disease by as much as 2–4 weeks. In the early stages of infection, radiographs may appear normal or subtly abnormal, and serial imaging may be necessary if clinical suspicion remains high. Computed tomography (CT) and MRI provide superior anatomic detail and increased sensitivity and specificity for the diagnosis of discospondylitis.

Identifying the underlying infectious agent in canine discospondylitis is a critical step in directing appropriate therapy, assessing zoonotic risk, and guiding prognosis. Despite extensive diagnostic efforts, a causative organism remains unidentified in 25–50% of cases for a variety of possible reasons. Blood and urine cultures can be obtained and are more sensitive in conjunction with fever. Image-guided fine-needle aspiration (FNA) or CT-guided biopsy of the affected disc space and vertebral endplates may be pursued, but sensitivity is poor when compared to urine and blood cultures. In cases requiring surgery for decompression or stabilization, open surgical biopsy and culture provide the highest yield, with specificities exceeding 80–95%.

Special attention must be given to *Brucella canis*, a zoonotic cause of discospondylitis increasingly recognized in rescue and imported dogs. Initial screening typically includes a rapid slide agglutination test (RSAT), which offers high sensitivity but limited specificity. Positive RSATs

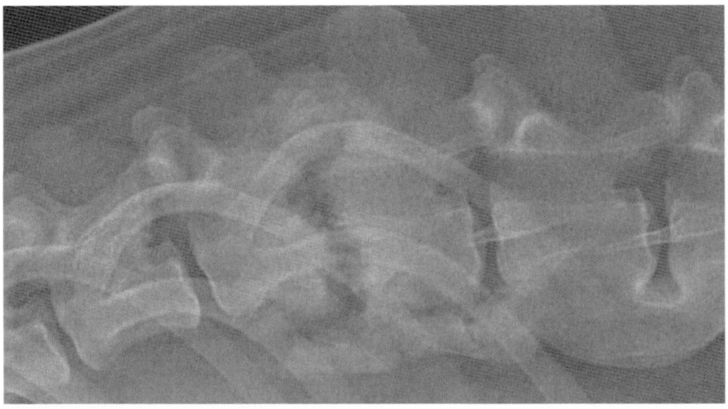

FIGURE 10.1.2 Vertebral column radiograph showing the radiographic appearance of discospondylitis.

should be followed by a 2-mercaptoethanol (2-ME) test or agar gel immunodiffusion (AGID) to improve diagnostic confidence. Culturing *Brucella* from blood or bone requires prolonged incubation (up to 6 weeks) and biosafety level-3 containment due to zoonotic risk. Newer polymerase chain reaction (PCR)-based assays show promise for early and accurate diagnosis but are not yet widely available in routine practice.

Intervertebral Disc Disease

Vertebral column radiographs have some utility in investigating IVDD but have limited sensitivity. Radiographic signs of IVDD include intervertebral disc space narrowing, in situ disc mineralization, and mineral opacity in the region of the intervertebral foramen. Patients with IVDD may not have lesions that are radiographically apparent, and patients with radiographic changes consistent with IVDD may have other active causes of their pain and myelopathy. CT and MRI are both superior to radiography in the diagnosis of IVDD.

Neoplasia

Vertebral column radiographs are an important screening tool for neoplasia in patients with vertebral column hyperesthesia (with or without accompanying myelopathy), especially in older animals. However, both intradural/extramedullary and intramedullary tumors are unlikely to be visible on radiographs. Extradural neoplasms in which there is vertebral lysis are more likely to be visible on radiographs, but at least 50% of bone mineralization must be lost before radiographic pathology is noted (Figure 10.1.3). Both CT and MRI have higher sensitivity and specificity for extradural neoplasms, and MRI is the best imaging modality for identifying intradural/extramedullary and intramedullary neoplasms. Depending on the tumor location and degree of vertebral bony lysis, fine needle aspiration or core biopsy can be performed for histopathologic evaluation, but if the neoplasm is not exfoliative, these biopsy techniques are typically low-yield. In cases in which surgical debulking is pursued, surgical biopsies are generally highly sensitive and specific for tumor type and grade.

Meningomyelitis

As this is a disease of the spinal cord and meninges, radiographs and CT have limited utility in diagnosing this condition. MRI typically discloses changes consistent with inflammation and variable contrast enhancement of the spinal cord and meninges. Cerebrospinal fluid (CSF) analysis typically discloses an increased concentration of CSF white blood cells and elevated total protein. Noninfectious meningomyelitis is typically associated with either a lymphocytic, mononuclear, or mixed pleocytosis. Infectious meningomyelitis may be associated with these patterns but may also be associated with neutrophilic pleocytosis or eosinophilic pleocytosis. Occasionally, dogs with meningomyelitis have normal CSF analysis results. For more details on the diagnostic path for meningomyelitis, please refer to Chapter 10 and Chapter 3.

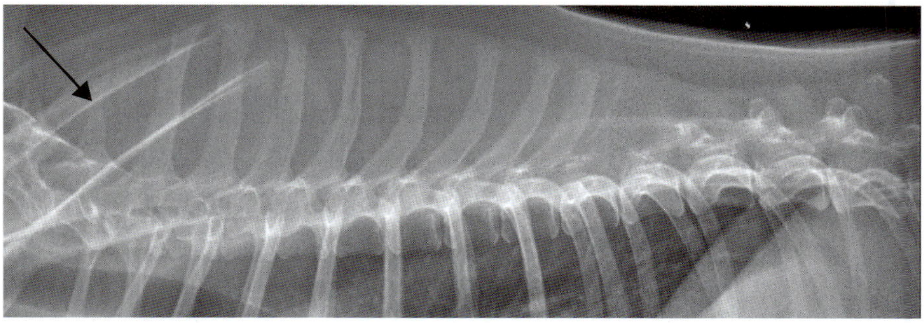

FIGURE 10.1.3 Vertebral column radiograph showing the radiographic appearance of a lytic extradural neoplasm affecting the T9 vertebra.

WHAT ARE THE TREATMENTS AND PROGNOSIS FOR THESE DIFFERENTIALS?

Discospondylitis

Treatment of discospondylitis in dogs relies on the selection of appropriate antimicrobials, careful monitoring, and patience, as the resolution of infection often lags behind clinical improvement. The majority of cases are bacterial in origin, and therefore, long-term antimicrobial therapy remains the cornerstone of treatment. When no organism is identified through blood, urine, or tissue cultures, empirical treatment is typically initiated based on the most common causative agents: *Staphylococcus pseudintermedius*, *Streptococcus* spp., *E. coli*, and *Proteus* spp.

Cephalexin is widely accepted as a suitable first-line agent for empirical treatment due to its activity against most gram-positive cocci, including *Staphylococcus pseudintermedius*, which is the most commonly isolated pathogen. Its safety profile, affordability, and favorable pharmacokinetics – particularly its ability to penetrate infected bone and disc spaces – make it a rational choice. Doses of 22–30 mg/kg are administered orally every 8–12 hours. Clinical improvement is typically observed within 5–7 days of initiating therapy, particularly when combined with a short course of initial nonsteroidal anti-inflammatory drugs. Concurrent analgesics, such as gabapentin or pregabalin, should be considered. A failure to improve within this window should prompt reconsideration of the diagnosis or organism, including the possibility of resistant bacteria, atypical organisms, or fungal etiologies, particularly in predisposed breeds such as German shepherds.

When cephalexin fails, broader-spectrum antibiotics, such as amoxicillin-clavulanate or fluoroquinolones, may be indicated, ideally guided by culture and sensitivity results. In cases of suspected fungal discospondylitis, antifungal agents such as itraconazole or fluconazole may be trialed, though success is limited and often requires months of treatment.

Surgery may be necessary to treat discospondylitis. Indications for surgery would include epidural empyema to lavage and decompress the neuroparenchyma, instability of the vertebral column, intractable pain secondary to radicular compromise, or worsening neurologic deficits. An added surgical benefit is a higher likelihood of achieving a definitive diagnosis. Care should be taken to use bioinert stabilization constructs when possible. The recent availability of poly-axial rod-screw systems is likely preferable to polymethylmethacrylate techniques.

A significant challenge in managing discospondylitis lies in determining the appropriate duration of therapy. Despite its frequency, there is poor evidence-based guidance on this topic. Historically, antibiotics have been continued for at least 4 weeks beyond resolution of clinical signs and radiographic changes, but more recent literature suggests that this approach may underestimate the true duration required for complete resolution. In one multi-institutional study, the average treatment duration was approximately 54 weeks, with many dogs requiring 9–12 months of therapy to achieve resolution on imaging. In clinical practice, some cases may require therapy that exceeds 1 year.

Radiography is commonly used to monitor the response to therapy, with serial imaging performed every 4–8 weeks. Classic radiographic features – lysis of the vertebral endplates, narrowing of the disc space, and eventual sclerosis or bony bridging – may take months to normalize, and radiographic improvement often trails clinical signs. Furthermore, radiographs are relatively insensitive, particularly in the early or healing phases of disease. Studies have shown poor correlation between radiographic changes and clinical status. In a recent comparative study, MRI and CT were found to be significantly more sensitive than radiography for both diagnosis and monitoring. For example, MRI may reveal persistent paraspinal inflammation, epidural granulation tissue, or nonunion of vertebral endplates, even long after radiographs appear stable. CT may also reveal subtle lysis or bridging that is not yet radiographically evident.

Given these limitations, treatment decisions should not rely on radiographs alone. A combination of clinical assessment, owner observations, and, when needed, advanced imaging provides a more complete picture. The cessation of therapy should only be considered when the patient is pain-free, systemically well, and imaging supports the resolution – or, at the very least, stabilization – of the lesion.

Long-term monitoring is essential. Relapses can occur, particularly when treatment is prematurely discontinued. Cases with incomplete resolution on imaging but clinical stability may require continued low-dose or pulse therapy or close follow-up. Adjunctive therapies, including pain management, rest, and physical therapy, are often necessary to support patient comfort and functional recovery during the prolonged treatment window.

Intervertebral Disc Disease

IVDD can be managed with conservative management or surgical management. The treatment route depends on numerous factors, including the severity of signs, the degree of progression, and various patient- and client-specific considerations. For more details on treatment options for IVDD, see Chapter 12.

Neoplasia

Neoplasia can be managed either with definitive treatment options (surgical resection, radiation therapy, and, in some cases, chemotherapy) or palliative treatment options (typically steroids and adjunct analgesics). These treatment options depend on the tumor location, tentative or definitive diagnosis, and various patient- and client-specific considerations. For more details on treatment options for vertebral column neoplasia, see Chapter 12.

Meningomyelitis

Treatment of meningomyelitis depends on if it is determined to be infectious or noninfectious. For more details on meningomyelitis treatment, please refer to Chapter 10 and Chapter 3.

OUTCOME

Survey radiographs of the thoracolumbar vertebral column in the patient in this case were obtained under light sedation in both lateral and ventrodorsal projections. These images revealed hallmark changes consistent with discospondylitis: specifically, irregular lysis of the vertebral endplates at T12–T13, narrowing of the associated intervertebral disc space, and surrounding sclerosis of the vertebral bodies (Figure 10.1.2). Mild ventral spondylosis was also evident, likely a reflection of chronic inflammation and reactive bone remodeling. Taken together with the patient's clinical signs and laboratory findings, the radiographic abnormalities were considered diagnostic. Blood and urine cultures were obtained but did not reveal a putative organism. The dog was started on cephalexin (22 mg/kg by mouth every 12 hours) and a 7-day course of carprofen (2.2 mg/kg by mouth every 12 hours). Four days into treatment, the owner reported that the dog's signs of discomfort had improved, and this improvement was sustained even after the carprofen was discontinued. Eight weeks after starting therapy, the dog returned for follow-up radiographs. Signs of active discospondylitis were still present, so the dog remained on cephalexin. The owner declined further radiographs due to cost. After a total of 6 months of treatment, the cephalexin was discontinued. The dog remained pain-free. The owner was counseled to monitor for signs of recurrent hyperesthesia and to contact their veterinarian should these signs return.

SUGGESTED READING

Platt, S, Olby, N, and Beltran, E. (2026). BSAVA Manual of Canine and Feline Neurology. 5e.

Spinal Pain

Case 2—Neck Pain in a Dog

CHAPTER 10.2

Fred Wininger[1] and Susan A. Arnold[2]

[1] *The Animal Neurology Center, Saint Louis, MO, USA*

[2] *Department of Veterinary Clinical Sciences, University of Minnesota, St. Paul, MN, USA*

CASE HISTORY

A 3-year-old neutered male beagle was presented for a 3-day history of severe neck pain, low head carriage, and reluctance to move his head. The owner described the dog as holding his neck stiffly, often with a "shortened neck" posture, and noted that he appeared to be moving his eyes to track objects rather than moving his neck. Frequent episodes of muscle twitching (fasciculations) in his neck were noted, and the dog cried out when approached or handled, especially when attempts were made to move his head. He had been intermittently lifting one thoracic limb at a time, holding it in the air for seconds before replacing it. Additional signs included reluctance to eat or drink, decreased activity, and the owner thought that the dog felt warmer to the touch than normal. The dog was fully vaccinated, not on any medications, and had no recent history of trauma, illness, or travel. He had been previously healthy.

VITAL PARAMETERS

Temperature: 104.1 °F

Heart Rate: 112 bpm

Respiratory Rate: 32 bpm

NEUROLOGICAL AND PHYSICAL EXAMINATION

The dog was bright and alert but subjectively appeared uncomfortable. His gait was normal aside from low head carriage and mild right thoracic limb lameness (Video 10.2.1). Postural reactions in all four limbs were normal. Segmental reflexes were normal in all limbs. Cranial nerve examination was normal. However, attempts to flex, extend, or laterally move the head were met with resistance or vocalization.

VIDEO 10.2.1 A dog demonstrating cervical hyperesthesia and a mild right thoracic limb nerve root signature.

Key questions to consider

1. **What is the likely lesion localization?**
2. **What are the most appropriate ranked differential diagnoses?**
3. **What are the next best diagnostic steps for this patient?**

LESION LOCALIZATION

The clinical signs – marked cervical hyperesthesia without neurologic deficits – localize the lesion to the cervical musculature, vertebrae, meninges of the cervical spinal cord, or nerve roots. The intermittent lifting of a thoracic limb may represent a nerve root signature, suggestive of lateralized cervical vertebral column/radicular (nerve root) pain.

DIFFERENTIAL DIAGNOSIS

Inflammatory – (1) Steroid-Responsive Meningitis-Arteritis (SRMA)

SRMA, also referred to historically as beagle pain syndrome, is the most likely diagnosis in a young beagle with acute cervical pain, low head carriage, general malaise, and a normal neurologic examination. This immune-mediated disease is characterized by necrotizing arteritis of the cervical spinal arteries and leptomeninges, leading to significant neck pain and systemic illness. Affected dogs are typically between 6 months and 4 years of age and belong to medium- or large-sized breeds, with beagles, boxers, Bernese Mountain dogs, and Nova Scotia duck tolling retrievers being overrepresented.

Clinically, dogs exhibit reluctance to move the neck, low head posture, stiffness, muscle fasciculations, fever, and often behavioral withdrawal. Some may also display limb lifting or trembling due to pain rather than true motor dysfunction. The condition is generally considered to be a type III hypersensitivity reaction involving IgA-mediated immune complex deposition in the meningeal vasculature.

(2) Infectious Meningoencephalitis/Meningomyelitis

Though less common, infectious causes of meningoencephalitis or meningomyelitis should be considered, particularly when systemic signs such as fever, lethargy, or gastrointestinal upset accompany neurologic complaints.

Toxoplasma gondii is an intracellular protozoan that can invade the central nervous system (CNS), causing a multifocal meningoencephalomyelitis. Neurologic signs range from cervical hyperesthesia and altered mentation to seizures or vestibular dysfunction. Diagnosis is based on cerebrospinal fluid (CSF), polymerase chain reaction (PCR), IgM/IgG serologic titers, and supportive imaging findings.

Neospora caninum, closely related to *T. gondii*, can cause polyradiculoneuritis and encephalitis, particularly in young dogs. It often presents with pelvic limb rigidity or paresis, but in disseminated cases can cause neck pain and CNS inflammation. Diagnosis is similar to toxoplasmosis and includes serologic testing and CSF analysis.

Cryptococcus neoformans and *Cryptococcus gattii* are fungal organisms capable of hematogenous or direct CNS invasion, often presenting with cervical pain, cranial nerve deficits, or vestibular signs. Diagnosis is aided by CSF cryptococcal antigen testing, India ink staining, or fungal culture. Additional fungal infections, including *Blastomyces dermatitidis, Histoplasma capsulatum*, and *Coccidioides immitis,* may affect the CNS in endemic regions. Although less commonly presenting with neck pain, systemic fungal disease should be considered in dogs from relevant geographic locations.

Bacterial meningoencephalitis is substantially rarer in dogs compared to people, who develop meningococcal infections from *Neisseria meningitidis*. Dogs with bacterial meningitis can develop it by hematogenous dissemination, local extension, and most commonly otogenic extension from otitis media/interna. Recent reports suggest that brachycephalic breeds may be at greater risk. In addition to cervical hyperesthesia, dogs with this form of infection may have systemic clinical signs, including vomiting and malaise.

Degenerative – Cervical Intervertebral Disc Disease (IVDD)

IVDD, particularly in early or noncompressive forms, can cause focal neck pain in the absence of paresis. Type I disc extrusion or Type II protrusion at the cervical level may irritate nerve roots or the annulus without creating significant spinal cord compression. Pain is typically localized, and patients may be reluctant to move the head, cry out when touched, or exhibit tension in the cervical muscles. Beagles are one of the most common breeds to develop cervical IVDD. This wouldn't explain the dog's body temperature in this instance.

Neoplasia

While possible, this is considered less likely given the acute onset of the condition and the dog's young age.

NEXT DIAGNOSTIC STEPS FOR THIS PATIENT

Given that the dog has an elevated core body temperature and is showing signs of systemic illness, a complete blood count, blood chemistry panel, and urinalysis are the first recommended diagnostic tests. Dogs with SRMA often develop an inflammatory leukogram. Magnetic resonance imaging (MRI) of the cervical region is indicated to evaluate the vertebrae, nerve roots, meninges, and spinal cord. Cerebrospinal fluid (CSF) analysis is useful for investigating evidence of inflammation, either infectious or noninfectious (Figure 10.2.1). If CSF analysis increases suspicion for an inflammatory etiology, then serologic testing for the infectious diseases listed above is recommended.

TREATMENT AND PROGNOSIS

SRMA

SRMA is a highly treatable, immune-mediated disease – with prednisone (or prednisolone) as the traditional foundation of therapy. In clinically typical cases, rapid clinical improvement is expected within 24–72 hours of initiating an immunosuppressive dose of prednisone. Typically, 2 mg/kg/day is sufficient to achieve an immunosuppressive level. Prednisone dose, duration, and tapering

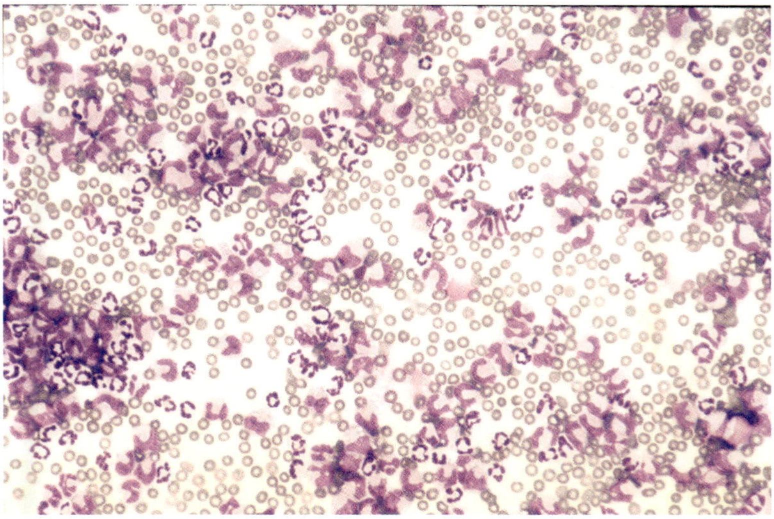

FIGURE 10.2.1 Cerebrospinal fluid from a dog with steroid-responsive meningitis-arteritis. In addition to red blood cell contamination, there is an abundance of neutrophils, leading to a neutrophilic pleocytosis. Nondegenerate neutrophilic pleocytosis without evidence of infectious organisms is the most common finding in cerebrospinal fluid analysis of dogs with steroid-responsive meningitis-arteritis.

protocols are highly variable among clinicians, but in general, prednisone therapy is the mainstay of SRMA treatment.

While prednisone alone controls most SRMA cases, relapse occurs in ~30–40% of cases, often associated with tapering. In these cases, adjunctive immunomodulators may be added to prednisone therapy to improve clinical response and disease control.

Monitoring therapeutic response includes regular physical exams, temperature checks, and pain assessments. Repeat CSF analysis is typically unnecessary unless relapse or treatment failure occurs. Inflammatory biomarkers such as C-reactive protein (CRP) or serum IgA may be helpful in tracking disease activity. The prognosis for SRMA remains favorable, particularly in dogs without significant relapses or complications.

Infectious Meningoencephalitis or Meningomyelitis

Treatment for infectious meningoencephalitis or meningomyelitis consists of antimicrobial medication, sometimes coupled with anti-inflammatory medication. For protozoal cases, clindamycin is the most commonly used antimicrobial, with the recommended dosage of 10–12.5 mg/kg by mouth every 12 hours in dogs and 25–50 mg/kg by mouth every 12 hours in cats for 3–4 weeks. Trimethoprim-sulfa is sometimes also used to address the acute stage of disease in which active parasite multiplication is occurring, but it typically does not eradicate the infection.

Cervical Intervertebral Disc Disease (IVDD)

Treatment of cervical IVDD consists broadly of either conservative or surgical management. For more information regarding the treatment of cervical IVDD, see Chapter 13.

Neoplasia

Treatment of neoplasia affecting the vertebral column, nerve roots, or spinal cord depends on the tumor location and suspected cellular origin. For more information regarding the treatment of neoplasia, see Chapter 13, Case 2.

CASE OUTCOME

In this case, a full diagnostic workup was recommended, including cervical MRI and CSF analysis. However, due to financial constraints, the client elected to forgo advanced imaging. As an alternative, and in line with a pragmatic diagnostic pathway, a CSF tap was performed under a propofol constant rate infusion following appropriate preanesthetic screening and stabilization.

Cerebrospinal fluid was collected from the cerebellomedullary cistern using an aseptic technique. The analysis revealed a total nucleated cell count (TNCC) of 1,480 cells/μL, with 92% nondegenerate neutrophils on differential cell count – indicating a marked neutrophilic pleocytosis (Figure 10.2.1). The protein concentration was elevated at 138 mg/dL, further supporting active inflammation of the meninges. No infectious organisms were identified on cytology, and the bacterial culture of the CSF was negative. This cytologic pattern – marked neutrophilic inflammation with elevated protein but absent intracellular organisms – is highly characteristic of acute SRMA.The dog was placed on prednisone (2 mg/kg by mouth every 24 hours). Within 2 days of starting prednisone the dog's fever, pain, inappetence, and lethargy had resolved. The prednisone dose was decreased to 1 mg/kg every 24 hours after 7 days, and the dog remained on this dose for 6 weeks The prednisone dose was decreased by 25% every month. The owner was instructed to monitor for signs of relapse. No signs of relapse occurred at any point through treatment. Prednisone therapy was completely discontinued 6 months after the onset of therapy and the dog did not show evidence of relapse.

SUGGESTED READING

Merck Veterinary Manual [Internet]. [cited 2025 Sept 25]. (2025). Toxoplasmosis in Animals - Generalized Conditions. Available from: https://www.merckvetmanual.com/generalized-conditions/toxoplasmosis/toxoplasmosis-in-animals

Platt, S. Olby, N. and Beltran, E. (2026). BSAVA Manual of Canine and Feline Neurology. 5e.

CHAPTER 10.3

Spinal Pain

Case 3—Lumbosacral Pain in a Dog

Fred Wininger[1] and Susan A. Arnold[2]

[1] The Animal Neurology Center, Saint Louis, MO, USA

[2] Department of Veterinary Clinical Sciences, University of Minnesota St. Paul, MN, USA

CASE HISTORY

An 8-year-old neutered male German Shepherd was presented for evaluation of a 3-week history of reluctance to jump, painful defecation, and progressive signs of pelvic limb weakness. The owner described low tail carriage, vocalization during bowel movements, and avoidance of physical activities. There was no known trauma, and no history of incontinence. The dog had otherwise been healthy.

NEUROLOGIC AND PHYSICAL EXAMINATION

The dog was bright, alert, and responsive on presentation. Vital parameters were within normal limits. On physical examination, low tail carriage was noted. The dog exhibited marked discomfort at tail elevation and digital pressure over the sacrum. Mild bilateral cranial tibial muscle atrophy was present, more severe on the right. Neurologic examination revealed the dog was ambulatory but with a mildly crouched pelvic limb posture and a mildly plantigrade stance that was more prominent in the right pelvic limb. There was minimal ataxia. Proprioception was intact in all limbs. Spinal reflexes were present, but the withdrawal reflexes at the hock were subjectively diminished bilaterally, worse in the right pelvic limb compared to the left (Video 10.3.1). Thoracic limb proprioception/segmental reflexes and cranial nerves were normal.

VIDEO 10.3.1 Patient demonstrating mild lameness associated with lumbosacral pain.

Key questions to consider

1. What is the likely lesion localization?
2. What are the most appropriate ranked differential diagnoses?
3. What are the best next diagnostic steps for this patient?

LESION LOCALIZATION

The constellation of clinical signs in this patient localizes the lesion to the L6 to caudal spinal cord segments or nerve roots that emerge from this region. Collectively, the nerve roots that emerge at the termination of the spinal cord are called the cauda equina and are the lower motor neurons to the pelvic limbs, tail, and external urethral and anal sphincters (Figure 10.3.1). Several key examination findings support this anatomical localization. First, the patient exhibits pain during tail manipulation and on digital pressure applied over the sacrum, both of which are classic

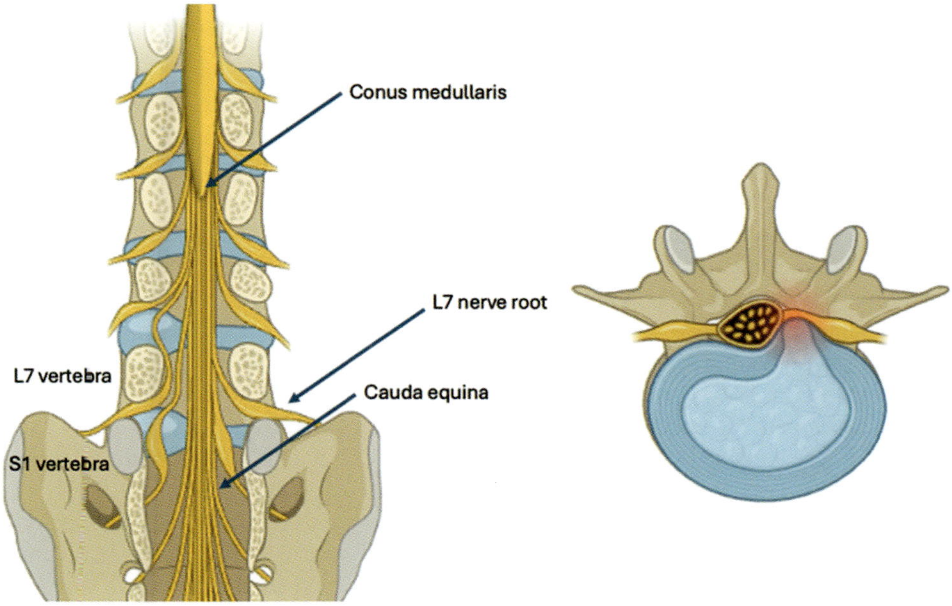

FIGURE 10.3.1 Left image: Illustration of the caudal end of the spinal cord (conus medullaris), from which the nerve roots emerge to form the cauda equina. The L7 nerve root exits the vertebral canal through the L7–S1 intervertebral foramen. This region is particularly susceptible to stenosis, which causes discomfort and neurological deficits. Right image: Illustration showing protrusion of the L7–S1 intervertebral disc, leading to compression of the cauda equina and the L7 nerve root, which is inflamed.

indicators of irritation or compression of the caudal nerve roots or associated meninges in the lumbosacral region.

Additionally, the low tail carriage and apparent reduction in tail tone further support involvement of the caudal spinal nerves and roots, which control tail elevation and movement. These signs imply that motor innervation to the tail is compromised, likely due to direct impingement on the caudal aspect of the cauda equina.

Muscular atrophy noted in the cranial tibial muscles, especially when coupled with diminished withdrawal reflexes at the level of the hock, suggests sciatic nerve dysfunction. The sciatic nerve is formed by fibers from the L6, L7, and S1 nerve roots, all of which exit the vertebral canal in the lumbosacral region. In this case, the bilateral but asymmetric atrophy, combined with reduced reflex strength, implies a chronic, progressive insult to the sciatic components – more pronounced on the right.

The preservation of normal patellar reflexes is diagnostically useful, as it indicates that the femoral nerve, which originates from the L4–L6 nerve roots, remains functionally intact. This observation helps to refine the localization further caudally, suggesting that the pathology spares the cranial lumbar spinal segments and is primarily confined to the L7–S1 region and associated roots.

Finally, the absence of urinary or fecal incontinence, along with normal perineal reflexes, suggests that the S2–S3 nerve roots, which contribute to the pudendal nerve, are either not significantly affected or are only in the early stages of involvement. As such, while sphincter tone appears currently preserved, progression of disease at this location may lead to incontinence if left untreated.

Taken together, these findings present a cohesive picture of a lesion localized to the cauda equina at the lumbosacral junction, most prominently affecting the L7 and S1 roots, with partial involvement of caudal and possibly sacral nerve roots.

DIFFERENTIAL DIAGNOSES

Degenerative – (1) Degenerative Lumbosacral Stenosis (DLSS)

DLSS is a progressive neurologic and orthopedic condition arising from structural degeneration at the lumbosacral junction, most commonly the L7–S1 articulation. This region, which serves as the transition between the mobile lumbar spine and the rigid sacrum, is subject to significant biomechanical stress, especially in large-breed and working dogs. Over time, chronic mechanical strain can result in a combination of degenerative lesions, including intervertebral disc protrusion, ligamentous hypertrophy, osteoarthritis, and vertebral malalignment. These changes collectively narrow the vertebral canal and intervertebral foramina, placing increasing pressure on the exiting nerve roots of the cauda equina. The L7 nerve roots are particularly vulnerable in DLSS. They emerge through the L7–S1 intervertebral foramina, which are particularly at risk for stenosis. The L7 nerve roots are also positioned between the intervertebral disc ventrally and the hypertrophied ligamentum flavum dorsally.

With continued degenerative change, compression of these roots impairs both motor and sensory function, leading to the hallmark clinical signs of DLSS: reluctance to jump, difficulty rising, pain during tail elevation or defecation, low tail carriage, and weakness or ataxia of the pelvic limbs. The neurological deficits in DLSS are predominantly lower motor neuron in nature. Sciatic nerve dysfunction – arising from compression of the L6–L7 roots – often leads to decreased withdrawal reflexes, proprioceptive deficits, and atrophy of the cranial tibial and other distal pelvic limb muscles. Involvement of the sacral nerve roots, especially those contributing to the pudendal nerve, results in pain during defecation, changes in sphincter tone, and, in some cases, urinary or fecal incontinence. Compression of the caudal (coccygeal) nerves may further contribute to tail flaccidity or hyperesthesia.

The clinical signs may be exacerbated by movement or posture, as extension of the lumbosacral joint during activities such as jumping or climbing can further narrow the canal and increase nerve root impingement. In this way, DLSS can behave as a dynamic condition – more than just a static anatomic narrowing. The slow and progressive nature of this disease also allows time for compensatory neural plasticity and variable pain expression, which may lead to intermittent or subtle signs that are easily misattributed to orthopedic conditions such as hip dysplasia or stifle disease. In cases of severe compression or secondary inflammation, patients may exhibit severe lameness secondary to nerve root irritation and compression (called a nerve root signature) that can also be mistaken for orthopedic conditions (Video 10.3.2). Colloquially, this neurogenic pain is referred to as "sciatica."

VIDEO 10.3.2 Right pelvic limb nerve root signature secondary to compression of the L7 nerve root.

As compression persists, inflammatory neuropathy and axonal injury may develop in the affected roots. This chronic neural insult contributes not only to the progression of neurologic dysfunction but also to the variability in patient response to medical versus surgical management. In advanced cases, neurogenic muscle atrophy and functional impairments may become irreversible.

(2) Hansen Type II Intervertebral Disc Disease

Type II intervertebral disc disease (IVDD) at L7–S1 is another consideration, especially in older dogs. These chronic, fibroid disc protrusions can contribute to nerve root compression, often indistinguishable from DLSS on history alone. MRI is often required to differentiate isolated disc protrusion from broader stenosis. For more details regarding Hansen type II IVDD refer to Chapter 12, Case 2.

Inflammation – Discospondylitis

Discospondylitis is an infectious disease that can also cause lumbosacral pain and reluctance to jump and is often accompanied by systemic signs such as fever, malaise, or leukocytosis.

Radiographs or magnetic resonance imaging (MRI) may reveal lytic lesions of the vertebral endplates and disc space narrowing. See Chapter 10, Case 1.

Neoplasia

Given this dog's age, breed, and the clinical progression, a neoplasm that is causing either bony lysis or nerve root compression is an important differential to explain this dog's discomfort and neurological deficits. A list of various neoplasms that affect the vertebral column and spinal cord is found in Chapter 10 and Chapter 13.

TRAUMA

Trauma, such as fracture or luxation of the sacral or caudal lumbar vertebrae, is less likely in the absence of a known incident or acute onset, but should be considered in cases of sudden onset pain, paresis, or urinary/fecal incontinence. See Chapter 15 for more information on spinal trauma.

NEXT DIAGNOSTIC STEPS FOR THIS PATIENT

- Radiographs are an important first-line imaging modality in dogs with lumbosacral pain and deficits attributable to a lesion in the area. Radiographic signs of DLSS include narrowing of the L7–S1 intervertebral disc space, ventral spondylosis deformans, sclerosis of the vertebral endplates, and osteophyte formation at the articular processes (Figure 10.3.2). The diagnostic utility of radiography for detecting DLSS has been reported to range from 52% to 69%, with specificity often no better than chance unless advanced signs of bone remodeling or foraminal narrowing are present. Furthermore, radiographs cannot visualize the soft tissue structures critical to the pathogenesis of DLSS, such as the intervertebral disc itself, the ligamentum flavum, or the cauda equina. Radiographs can also help in searching for signs of discospondylitis (disc space narrowing or widening, lysis, or sclerosis of the vertebral endplates), but similar to DLSS, the diagnostic specificity is relatively low, and substantial bony changes are necessary before radiographic evidence is apparent. Similarly, neoplasia associated with vertebral lysis can be visualized on radiographs but requires extensive lysis to be radiographically apparent. Nonetheless, radiographs are an important first step in the diagnostic approach to these patients because they may be all that is required to diagnose discospondylitis or neoplasia.

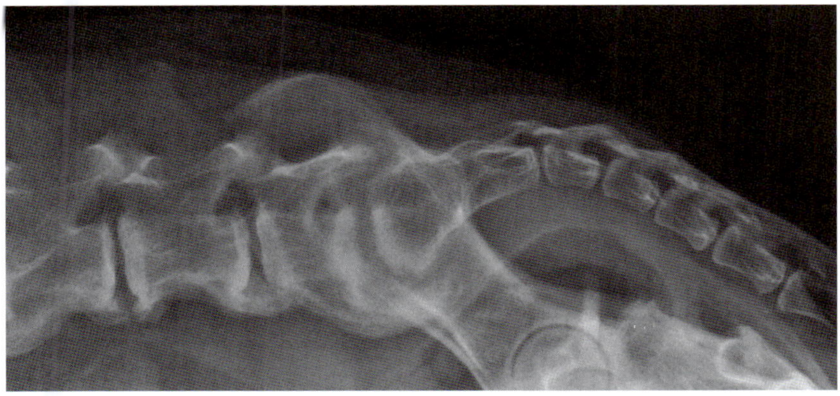

FIGURE 10.3.2 Lateral radiograph showing the typical findings that are supportive of a diagnosis of lumbosacral stenosis: sclerosis of the L7 and S1 vertebral endplates and spondylosis ventral to the vertebral bodies.

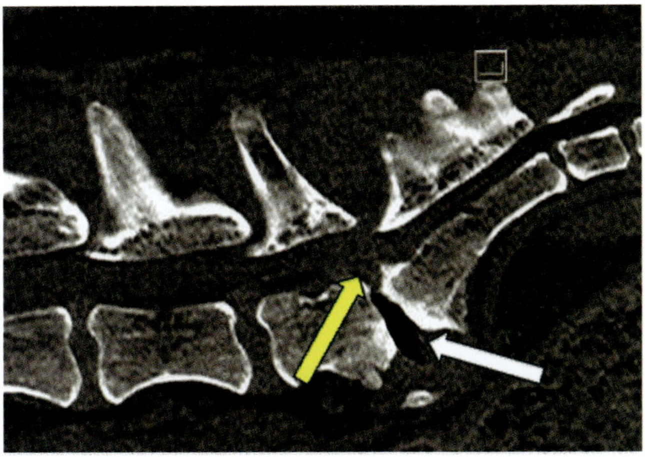

FIGURE 10.3.3 Computed tomography image of a dog with lumbosacral stenosis secondary to Hansen type II intervertebral disc protrusion of the L7–S1 intervertebral disc. The protruding material is subtly visible within the vertebral canal as hyperdense material (yellow arrow). Interestingly, this patient also exhibited a phenomenon called a "vacuum disc," in which gas is trapped within the space normally occupied by the intervertebral disc, leading to hypodensity in the region of the intervertebral disc (white arrow).

- Computed tomography (CT), particularly when performed with contrast myelography, offers markedly improved bony detail and allows more accurate visualization of the intervertebral foramina, articular processes and facets, intervertebral disc, and vertebral canal. CT can detect subtle changes in osseous alignment, mineralization of the disc, and encroachment into the vertebral canal by hypertrophied bone or soft tissue, as well as lysis associated with either infection or neoplasia. It is particularly valuable for identifying foraminal stenosis, one of the primary mechanisms of nerve root impingement in DLSS. However, CT still lacks the resolution to visualize the cauda equina and the dynamic nature of nerve root impingement during spinal extension. Although more sensitive than radiography, CT alone can miss lesions that involve soft tissue or epidural fibrosis. Its sensitivity and specificity in diagnosing DLSS have been reported to range between 70 and 85% depending on technique and interpretation, and are markedly improved with dynamic contrast studies or postural variation (Figure 10.3.3).
- Magnetic resonance imaging (MRI) is currently regarded as the most sensitive and specific modality for the diagnosis of DLSS, IVDD, discospondylitis, and neoplasia because of its unmatched ability to visualize both the neural elements and surrounding soft tissues. MRI allows direct assessment of the cauda equina nerve roots, the intervertebral disc, epidural fat, and supporting ligaments. It also permits evaluation of the foramina and subsequent neural compression (foraminal stenosis). 3D imaging techniques enable investigation of the entire radicular corridor. Sensitivity of MRI for detecting clinically significant DLSS has been reported in multiple studies to be over 90%, and specificity is similarly high when correlated with surgical or histopathologic confirmation (Figure 10.3.4). MRI and CT in combination likely provide the gold standard in comprehensive diagnostics.

TREATMENT AND PROGNOSIS

DLSS

The therapeutic approach to DLSS depends on the severity of clinical signs, degree of neurologic dysfunction, and imaging findings. While some dogs with mild signs can be managed conservatively, those with progressive or refractory pain, neurologic deficits, or cauda equina syndrome typically require surgical intervention.

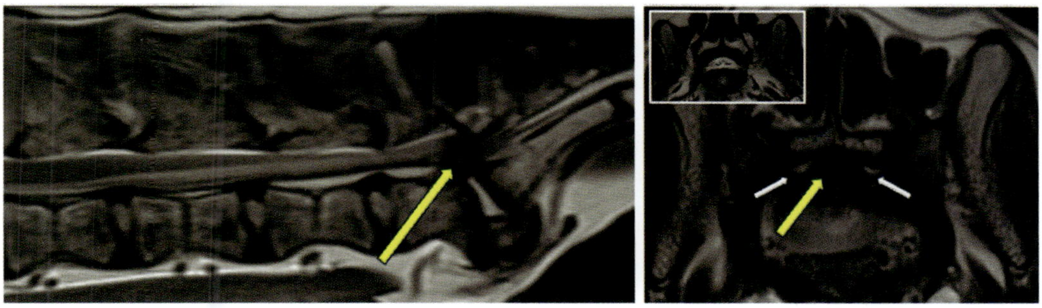

FIGURE 10.3.4 Magnetic resonance images of the same dog as in Figure 10.3.2. The compressive disc material is indicated by the yellow arrows on the sagittal (left) and transverse (right) images. Note that the disc material is occupying nearly the entire area of the vertebral canal at this transverse level. There remains only a small amount of epidural fat (white arrows) surrounding the emerging nerve roots, which are markedly compressed. For comparison, the insert shows a normal dog. Note the large amount of epidural fat (hyperintense material) surrounding nerve roots (hypointense, small circles) within the vertebral canal.

Medical management is often the first line of treatment in dogs with intermittent or mild signs of lumbosacral pain. This approach typically includes restricted activity, nonsteroidal anti-inflammatory drugs (NSAIDs) or glucocorticoids, gabapentin/pregabalin as a targeted analgesic, and physical rehabilitation. Strict exercise restriction is essential to prevent exacerbation of dynamic compression during lumbar extension. Adjunctive therapies, including laser therapy, acupuncture, or targeted strengthening exercises, may improve function and comfort. However, long-term success with conservative treatment is variable, and many patients relapse once activity resumes. It is estimated that 35–50% of medically managed dogs maintain sustained improvement over time, and recurrence is common.

A middle ground between conservative and surgical management involves epidural corticosteroid injections, which aim to reduce inflammation around the compressed nerve roots. Typically administered under sedation or light anesthesia, these injections deliver depot steroids such as methylprednisolone acetate into the lumbosacral epidural space, providing localized immunomodulation without systemic side effects. Clinical improvement in a modest majority of treated dogs has been observed. However, the benefits are often temporary – lasting weeks to months – and repeated injections may be necessary. Epidural injections are best considered as part of a multimodal plan or as a palliative option in nonsurgical candidates. More recently, the long-term value of this therapy has been questioned in the literature.

In patients with persistent pain, neurologic deficits, or imaging-confirmed nerve root compression, surgical intervention offers the most definitive treatment. The traditional approach to decompressing the cauda equina is a dorsal laminectomy, which involves removal of the dorsal lamina of L7 and the cranial sacrum to expose and relieve pressure on the nerve roots. This technique directly decompresses the vertebral canal and is effective in relieving central canal stenosis.

However, dorsal laminectomy alone may not sufficiently alleviate foraminal stenosis, particularly in cases with lateralized disc protrusion, articular process hypertrophy, or dynamic instability. To address this, distraction and stabilization procedures have been introduced, in which the L7 and sacrum are distracted to restore foraminal diameter and then stabilized with instrumentation, preventing further collapse. Modern surgical systems now employ polyaxial pedicle screws and contoured titanium rods to maintain alignment. The use of 3D-printed surgical guides, customized to the patient's anatomy, enhances screw placement accuracy and surgical efficiency, especially in complex or revision cases.

In some instances, intervertebral spacers – either titanium cages or cortical ring allografts – are placed into the disc space to maintain distraction and support fusion. These devices provide load sharing and preserve foraminal height while promoting osseous integration. When used in conjunction with rigid stabilization, they can restore biomechanics and improve long-term outcomes, particularly in working or athletic dogs.

Foraminotomy is another surgical technique used to directly widen the lateral recesses or foraminal corridors, particularly when nerve root impingement is localized. This technique allows targeted decompression of affected nerve roots, especially the L7 nerve exiting laterally. However, foraminotomy alone has limitations: it does not address central canal stenosis or instability and access to all nerve root corridors may not be feasible through a single window. For this reason, foraminotomy is often combined with dorsal decompression or stabilization in complex or recurrent cases.

Ultimately, the choice of surgical technique depends on the individual patient's pathology, surgeon expertise, and available equipment. While dorsal laminectomy remains effective in many cases, the addition of distraction, stabilization, and neural foramen management offers improved outcomes in cases with instability, foraminal collapse, or recurrence.

PATIENT OUTCOME

Radiographs of the lumbosacral region were unremarkable. The dog subsequently underwent an MRI, which showed that the L7–S1 intervertebral disc was protruding into the vertebral canal, causing cauda equina compression. The dog was started on an anti-inflammatory dose of prednisone (0.5 mg/kg/day), amantadine (4 mg/kg/day), and gabapentin (10 mg/kg every 8 hours). The dog responded well to therapy for 2 weeks. The prednisone dose was decreased, and the dog's discomfort returned. The dog subsequently underwent a dorsal laminectomy at L7–S1 without complication, which led to long-term resolution of his signs.

SUGGESTED READING

Dewey, C.W. and Da Costa, R.C. (2015). *Practical Guide to Canine and Feline Neurology*, 3e. Wiley.

De Lahunta, A., Glass, E., and Kent, M. (2020). *Veterinary Neuroanatomy and Clinical Neurology*, 5e. Saunders.

Platt, S., Olby, N. and Beltran, E. (2026). BSAVA Manual of Canine and Feline Neurology, 5e. British Small Animal Veterinary Association Publication.

Worth, A., Meij, B., and Jeffery, N. (2019). Canine degenerative lumbosacral stenosis: prevalence, impact and management strategies. *Vet. Med. (Auckl)* 10: 169–183. https://doi.org/10.2147/VMRR.S180448. Erratum in: Vet Med (Auckl). 2020 Feb 04;11:15. doi:10.2147/VMRR.S247481. PMID: 31819860; PMCID: PMC6875490.

Spinal Pain
Case 4—Lumbar Pain in a Cat

CHAPTER 10.4

Fred Wininger[1] and Susan A. Arnold[2]

[1] *The Animal Neurology Center, Saint Louis, MO, USA*
[2] *Department of Veterinary Clinical Sciences, University of Minnesota, St. Paul, MN, USA*

CASE HISTORY

A 9-year-old neutered male domestic shorthair cat was presented for evaluation of a 2–3-week history of progressive reluctance to jump, increasing sensitivity to touch over the lumbar spine, and episodes of self-mutilation. The owner reported that the cat frequently turned to look at or bite his lower back, often yowling or hissing, particularly when touched along the spine. These episodes appeared spontaneous at times and were occasionally triggered by petting or movement. In recent days, the owner observed the cat sitting in the litter box for extended periods – sometimes up to an hour – crying while attempting to defecate, without producing feces. The cat's tail appeared to hang lower than usual, with reduced movement and tone. Though the cat remained ambulatory and was eating, he had become increasingly reclusive and irritable. There was no known trauma, and the patient was a strictly indoor cat. The owner denied any recent changes in diet, medications, or household dynamics.

NEUROLOGIC AND PHYSICAL EXAMINATION (Video 10.4.1)

VIDEO 10.4.1 Cat with pelvic limb dysfunction and lumbar hyperesthesia.

On physical examination, the cat was bright and alert but highly reactive to handling, particularly when palpation of the thoracolumbar spine was attempted. Marked vocalization, growling, and attempts to bite were observed when pressure was applied over the L4–S1 region. The cat repeatedly turned to look at or bite toward the examiner's hand and intermittently licked and bit at his own lumbar area during the exam. Mild alopecia and several small, healing excoriations were noted over the lumbosacral region and base of the tail.

The tail was carried low, with diminished spontaneous movement and tone. During gait evaluation, the cat demonstrated a partially plantigrade stance in the pelvic limbs, walking with a crouched posture and pausing intermittently to vocalize or sit. A limited neurologic examination was possible due to fractious behavior; however, postural reactions were confirmed to be delayed in both pelvic limbs. Spinal reflexes were present but there was a subjectively diminished pelvic limb withdrawal reflex bilaterally. The thoracic limbs appeared normal during observation, and cranial nerve function was intact, with symmetrical menace, normal pupillary responses, and no abnormalities in facial tone or symmetry.

Key questions to consider

1. What is the likely lesion localization?
2. What are the most appropriate ranked differential diagnoses?
3. What are the best next diagnostic steps for this patient?

LESION LOCALIZATION

The clinical signs localize the lesion to the L6–S3 spinal cord segments and associated nerve roots, encompassing the cauda equina. The combination of lumbar spinal pain, low tail carriage, and self-mutilation focused on the lumbar and tail region suggests involvement of the dorsal cutaneous branches of the lumbar and sacral nerves, which carry sensory input from this region. The plantigrade posture, delayed pelvic limb proprioception, and diminished withdrawal reflexes support a neuroanatomical localization involving the sciatic nerve (L6–S1). The absence of incontinence or perineal reflex deficits suggests that the S2–S3 and pudendal nerves are currently spared.

DIFFERENTIAL DIAGNOSES

Feline Hyperesthesia Syndrome (FHS)

This condition is characterized by episodic, intense sensitivity over the dorsum, behavioral agitation, and self-directed mutilation. The cat's hyper-responsiveness to palpation, spontaneous tail-focused aggression, and prolonged, painful posturing in the litter box are all consistent with FHS. However, the plantigrade stance makes this differential less likely, as these patients rarely develop neurologic deficits. Feline Hyperesthesia Syndrome is a complex and incompletely understood condition characterized by paroxysmal episodes of skin twitching, vocalization, apparent spinal pain, and self-mutilation, most often directed at the lumbar area or tail. While the syndrome is most often diagnosed in young to middle-aged cats, it can affect older individuals as well. The etiology remains elusive, but several mechanisms have been proposed.

One prevailing hypothesis suggests that FHS represents a form of neuropathic pain, possibly due to irritation of the dorsal lumbar nerve roots or cutaneous sensory nerves. Electromyographic studies in affected cats have revealed spontaneous activity in epaxial muscles, consistent with denervation or myofascial pain. Others propose a behavioral component, citing the stereotypic nature of the episodes and their frequent association with stress or environmental change. In such cases, FHS may resemble obsessive-compulsive disorder (OCD) in humans, and some cats respond favorably to antidepressants.

Another hypothesis posits that FHS may be a focal seizure disorder, particularly affecting the temporal lobes. Although seizure activity is not observed in all patients, EEG abnormalities have been reported in a small subset. Lastly, myofascial pain syndrome, involving chronic trigger points in the lumbar musculature, has also been suggested, as some cats improve with laser therapy or physical rehabilitation.

Degenerative – Intervertebral Disc Disease (IVDD)

Intervertebral disc disease (IVDD) is also a possible consideration. Although less common in cats than in dogs, IVDD may cause pain, proprioceptive deficits, and tail or pelvic limb dysfunction when the lesion is located at the lumbosacral junction.

Neoplasia

Neoplasia, including lymphoma, nerve sheath tumors, or vertebral neoplasms, must also be considered in a cat of this age. Tumors can present with focal pain, tail dysfunction, or neuropathic signs. However, the episodic nature of this cat's signs makes neoplasia less likely, though not excluded.

Inflammatory – Discospondylitis

Discospondylitis, while uncommon in cats, remains a differential – particularly if the cat is immunosuppressed or feline leukemia virus or feline immunodeficiency virus-positive. Spinal pain and postural changes may arise from vertebral infection, although this typically produces systemic illness, fever, or radiographic abnormalities, none of which were evident.

NEXT DIAGNOSTIC STEPS FOR THIS PATIENT

- Performing a complete blood count, blood chemistry panel, and urinalysis is a good first diagnostic step. Rarely, feline lymphoma leads to changes in circulating lymphocytes, and various infectious diseases may lead to hematologic changes.
- Vertebral column radiographs could be performed to investigate signs of lysis that could suggest either discospondylitis or neoplasia. However, extensive lysis is necessary to be radiographically apparent, and many forms of neoplasia do not result in bony lysis.
- Magnetic resonance imaging (MRI) of the lumbar vertebral column is highly sensitive and specific for all the considered differential diagnoses for this patient.
- Cerebrospinal fluid (CSF) analysis can help evaluate for round cell tumors, especially lymphoma, as well as infectious etiologies.

TREATMENT AND PROGNOSIS

Feline Hyperesthesia Syndrome

Treatment for feline hyperesthesia syndrome is aimed at reducing episodes of discomfort. In severe cases, cats can mutilate their tails, requiring aggressive treatment to prevent substantial injury. Because the etiology of this condition remains poorly characterized and many possible inciting causes have been proposed, treatment approaches have also varied widely. Proposed therapies range from the use of fluoxetine to analgesics (typically gabapentin or pregabalin) to anticonvulsants to behavioral modifications. A recent study found that all cats treated with either fluoxetine alone or in combination with gabapentin achieved clinical remission within 1 year of the onset of signs. Overall, the prognosis for this condition is good, provided cats can be limited from causing self-trauma.

Intervertebral Disc Disease

Treatment of lumbosacral IVDD in cats may begin conservatively, especially in the absence of profound neurologic deficits. Medical management aims to reduce inflammation, alleviate pain, and prevent further disc extrusion through activity restriction. This typically includes strict confinement, analgesic support, and anti-inflammatory therapy.

Glucocorticoids such as prednisone exert their effect by inhibiting phospholipase A2, thereby decreasing the production of prostaglandins and leukotrienes. In IVDD, this reduces perineural edema and inflammation around the compressed nerve roots. While nonsteroidal anti-inflammatory drugs (NSAIDs) may be preferred in some cases due to their more favorable side effect profile, glucocorticoids are often chosen when pain is severe or nerve root inflammation is suspected.

Gabapentin is often selected as an adjunct analgesic due to its favorable safety profile in feline patients. Gabapentin binds to the α2δ subunit of voltage-gated calcium channels, decreasing the release of excitatory neurotransmitters such as glutamate and substance P. This leads to a dampening of nociceptive transmission, particularly in sensitized nerve roots. It is generally well-tolerated in cats, though sedation and ataxia may occur.

A related drug, pregabalin, shares a similar mechanism of action but has greater oral bioavailability, a longer half-life, and a higher binding affinity for the α2δ-1 subunit. These pharmacologic features make it potentially more effective for severe or refractory neuropathic pain, though its use in veterinary medicine is less established. Limited data suggest pregabalin may provide superior pain relief in cases where gabapentin is inadequate, though it comes at a higher cost and may be more sedating in cats.

Despite initial therapy, if the patient fails to show marked improvement within 2 weeks, or if pain worsens or neurologic deficits progress, surgical decompression is indicated.

Neoplasia

Treatment of neoplasia depends on the suspected cellular origin, location relative to the spinal cord, degree of invasiveness, and extent of disease. Some forms of neoplasia are amenable to surgical resection or minimally to debulking, whereas others respond to radiation therapy. For more details on the treatment of neoplasia of the vertebral column, see Chapter 12.

Discospondylitis

Treatment for discospondylitis consists of long-term antimicrobial therapy. For more details on the treatment of discospondylitis, see Chapter 10, Case 1.

PATIENT OUTCOME

MRI of the lumbosacral vertebral column was performed under general anesthesia. The MRI revealed a focal protrusion of the L6–L7 intervertebral disc. The protruded disc material was ventrally displacing the cauda equina nerve roots and reducing the volume of the vertebral canal at that level. No evidence of spinal cord signal change was noted, and there were no contrast-enhancing lesions suggestive of neoplasia or infectious disease. Mild reactive sclerosis was appreciated in the adjacent vertebral endplates, but there was no evidence of discospondylitis. The findings were confined to a single site and were most compatible with feline IVDD at the lumbosacral junction.

The cat was prescribed prednisolone, gabapentin for neuropathic pain control, and buprenorphine for short-term opioid analgesia. After 14 days of persistent lumbar pain and increasing postural changes, surgical intervention was elected. A dorsal hemilaminectomy was performed to decompress the L6–7 nerve roots. Intraoperative findings confirmed a chronic, broad-based disc protrusion with associated perineural fibrosis. No active disc extrusion or evidence of instability was present. Postoperative care included continued prednisolone tapering to minimize rebound inflammation, buprenorphine for short-term opioid analgesia, and maintenance dosing of gabapentin to support neuropathic comfort. The cat was confined for 4–6 weeks to allow healing of the surgical site and to limit dynamic stress on the recovering lumbosacral junction. Pain scores were assessed regularly, and gabapentin was gradually tapered over several weeks once functional improvement was evident.

SUGGESTED READING

Amengual Batle, P., Rusbridge, C., Nuttall, T. et al. (2019). Feline hyperaesthesia syndrome with self-trauma to the tail: retrospective study of seven cases and proposal for an integrated multidisciplinary diagnostic approach. *J. Feline Med. Surg.* 21 (2): 178–185. https://doi.org/10.1177/1098612X18764246. Epub 2018 Mar 29. PMID: 29595359; PMCID: PMC10814607.

Ebeling, R., Lorenz, N.D., Zablotski, Y. et al. (2025). EXPRESS: feline intervertebral disc disease - a systematic review and meta-analysis. *J. Feline Med. Surg.* 27 (12): 1098612X251385878. https://doi.org/10.1177/1098612X251385878. Epub ahead of print. PMID: 41006947.

Fowler, K.M., Pancotto, T.E., Werre, S.R. et al. (2022). Outcome of thoracolumbar surgical feline intervertebral disc disease. *J. Feline Med. Surg.* 24 (6): 473–483. https://doi.org/10.1177/1098612X211028031. Epub 2021 Jul 12. PMID: 34251296; PMCID: PMC11104248.

Gomes, S.A., Garosi, L.S., Behr, S. et al. (2022). Clinical features, treatment and outcome of discospondylitis in cats. *J. Feline Med. Surg.* 24 (4): 311–321. https://doi.org/10.1177/1098612X211020159. Epub 2021 Jun 8. PMID: 34100660; PMCID: PMC10812237.

Mayoral, V., Galvez, R., Ferrándiz, M. et al. (2025). Pregabalin vs. gabapentin in the treatment of neuropathic pain: a comprehensive systematic review and meta-analysis of effectiveness and safety. *Front. Pain Res. (Lausanne).* 5: 1513597. Published 2025 Jan 7. https://doi.org/10.3389/fpain.2024.1513597.

Pauciulo, C., Uccheddu, S., Corda, A. et al. (2025). Long-term clinical response to medical treatment, behavioral therapy, or their combination in cats with hyperesthesia syndrome. *J. Vet. Intern. Med.* 39 (4): e70174.

Rusbridge, C. (2024). Neuropathic pain in cats: mechanisms and multimodal management. *J. Feline Med. Surg.* 26: https://doi.org/10.1177/1098612X241246518. PMID: 38710218; PMCID: PMC11156241.

CHAPTER 11.1

Monoparesis

Case 1—Chronic Lameness in One Thoracic Limb in a Dog

Danielle Daw

MissionVet Specialty and Emergency, San Antonio, TX, USA

CASE HISTORY

A 9-year-old neutered male dachshund was presented for a chronic history of right thoracic limb lameness. The dog began with a mild, weight-bearing lameness of the right thoracic limb 4 months before presentation. This lameness gradually progressed over 4 months, to the point where the dog became non-weight-bearing. He was given a 7-day course of carprofen prior to presentation, but the lameness did not improve with this medication.

Before the onset of signs, the dog had no medical concerns. He had been routinely vaccinated and received monthly heartworm/flea/tick prevention.

NEUROLOGIC EXAMINATION

The dog was bright, alert, and responsive on presentation. The dog was ambulatory with a non-weight bearing, right thoracic limb lameness, carrying the limb flexed at the elbow. Postural reactions, including paw placement and hopping, were absent in the right thoracic limb. The dog had an absent withdrawal, marked muscle atrophy (Figures 11.1.1 and 11.1.2), and decreased tone in the right thoracic limb. There was no pain on paraspinal or axillary palpation, and there was normal cervical range of motion. An orthopedic examination did not show any other abnormalities.

1. **Where is the likely lesion localization?**
2. **What major disease processes should be considered?**
3. **What tests could you perform to help determine the diagnosis?**
4. **What is the expected outcome with each differential diagnosis?**

LESION LOCALIZATION

The patient's lameness alone would be concerning for either an orthopedic or a neurologic abnormality. In the absence of any obvious orthopedic abnormalities on exam, a neurologic cause is more highly considered. The patient's inability to support weight using the right thoracic limb is consistent with a lower motor neuron paresis, which is indicative of an abnormality in the right C6-T2 spinal cord segments and/or nerves. Further confirmation of the neuroanatomic lesion localization and differentiation from an orthopedic abnormality is based upon the absent withdrawal reflex and reduced tone. The significant muscle atrophy of the right limb in this case also

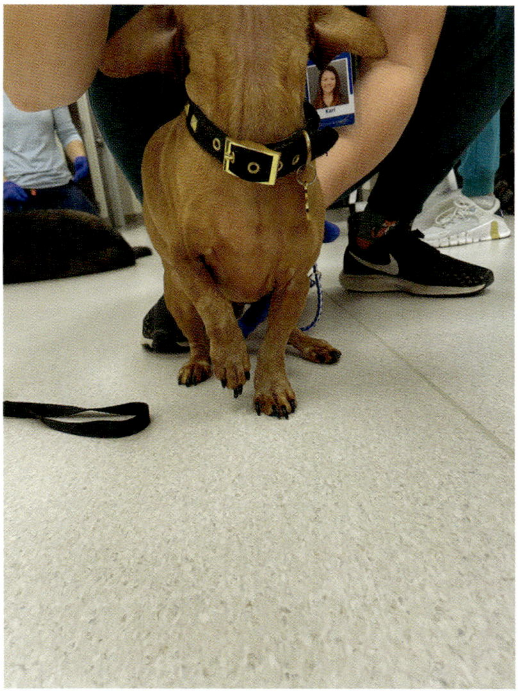

FIGURE 11.1.1 Dog with nerve root signature in the right thoracic limb.

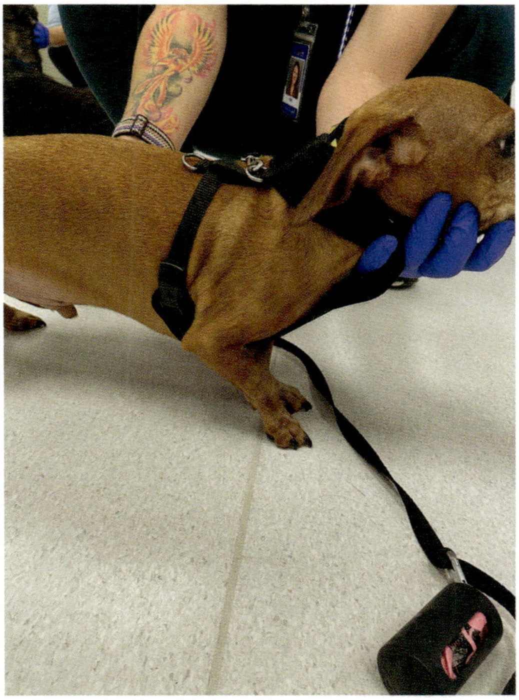

FIGURE 11.1.2 Side view of same patient as in Figure 11.1.1, showing the non-weight-bearing lameness and severe shoulder muscle atrophy.

supports the neuroanatomic lesion localization; however, this alone would not aid with differentiation in lesion localization as this may be secondary to disuse given the duration of signs.

WHAT MAJOR DISEASE PROCESSES SHOULD BE CONSIDERED? THE DIFFERENTIAL DIAGNOSIS

Neoplasia – Nerve Sheath Tumors

Nerve sheath tumors arise from either the Schwann cells or the associated connective tissue surrounding nerve fascicles or individual axons of the peripheral nervous system. Nerve sheath tumors are the most common nerve neoplasms in the dog, and they mostly affect the nerves or nerve roots associated with the brachial plexus. They typically affect dogs over the age of 7 years and signs are slowly progressive over an average of months. Early in the disease course, dogs typically display lameness, because these tumors cause compression of pain receptors associated with the affected nerves. Over time, other signs become apparent, including decreased spinal reflexes, decreased muscle tone, neurogenic atrophy, and lower motor neuron paresis or paralysis in advanced stages. For these reasons, this would be a highly likely differential for this case.

Nerve sheath tumors have a low rate of metastasis but are extensively locally aggressive and invasive. They spread slowly, both distally and proximally, affecting multiple nerves and nerve roots and eventually can invade the vertebral canal to cause spinal cord compression and resultant myelopathic clinical signs.

Inflammation – Chronic Neuritis

Chronic neuritis can be secondary to either immune-mediated or infectious processes. Hypertrophic neuritis and ganglioneuritis is a chronic demyelinating neuropathy that has presumed immune-mediated etiology. It most commonly affects the brachial plexus and can involve either one or both thoracic limbs. Hypertrophic (ganglio)neuritis causes signs that are very similar to nerve sheath tumors. As such, chronic neuritis is a strong alternative differential diagnosis for this patient. Infectious causes of neuritis include a protozoal infection, such as that with *Toxoplasma* or *Neospora*, or, less likely, with a fungal, viral, or bacterial organism. Overall, infectious causes of neuritis in adult dogs are rare.

Degenerative – Foraminal Stenosis

(i) Lateralized or foraminal intervertebral disc Nerve roots that emerge from and enter the spinal cord to travel to and from the limbs leave the vertebral canal through intervertebral foramina. These foramina are located dorsal to intervertebral disc spaces. A lateralized intervertebral disc protrusion or extrusion most commonly causes stenosis of the intervertebral foramina. A degenerative intervertebral disc that herniates laterally will compress the spinal ganglion and nerve within the vertebral canal (lateralized disc) or the foramen (foraminal disc), causing lameness and/or paresis, such as that seen in this case. The lameness arises because these nerve roots are innervated with pain receptors, such that compression elicits discomfort. Weight-bearing exacerbates the discomfort. The lameness that results from nerve root impingement is called a "nerve root signature." With enough compression, nerve dysfunction can lead to lower motor neuron dysfunction in the affected limb.

(ii) Far lateral or extraforaminal extrusions This type of disc extrusion occurs outside of the limits of the foramen; they can be combined with foraminal disc extrusions. These types of extrusions have been reported to affect the caudal lumbar intervertebral discs and occasionally the cervical intervertebral discs. Clinical signs associated with these types of extrusions are secondary to radicular and spinal nerve compression and could be misinterpreted as a primary orthopedic disorder. When affecting the cervical column, episodic or persistent signs of cervical pain, nerve root signature or abnormal cervical posture (cervical pseudodystonia) have been reported. Irritation or injury to spinal nerves can result in the clinical phenomenon of "peripheral nerve hyperexcitability", leading to electrical discharges in nerves and seemingly spontaneous muscle contractions termed "fasciculations". A far-lateral extruded disc will compress soft tissues adjacent to it, including spinal nerves and branches thereof as they course toward their intended targets. Fasciculations may be felt (palpated) or seen as flickers of muscle fibers contracting underneath the skin. Although these fasciculations are not voluntarily elicited (i.e. they are involuntary), they cannot be regarded as truly spontaneous since there is an identifiable cause for their occurrence in the case of nerve fiber compression. Alternatively, such muscle activity in the cervical region has been referred to as "cervical jerks" or myoclonus.

Neoplasia A cancerous mass within the intervertebral foramen is another, less likely, cause of stenosis and nerve compression of this region. Neoplasia that may behave in this manner include lymphoma or metastatic tumors. Vertebral body tumors may also cause narrowing of the intervertebral foramen to cause nerve root compression. For a more thorough review of these various neoplasms, please refer to Chapter 10, Case 4.

WHAT TESTS COULD YOU PERFORM TO HELP DETERMINE THE DIAGNOSIS?

A lower motor neuron monoparesis may be mistaken for an orthopedic lameness, especially in the absence of more supportive exam findings, such as spinal reflex deficits, significant muscle atrophy, or an obvious orthopedic abnormality. Orthopedic radiographs of the limb are helpful to exclude an underlying orthopedic condition. Electrodiagnostic testing, such as electromyography, may also be beneficial in differentiating an orthopedic from a neurologic abnormality, as this test would be expected to show evidence of denervation with the latter concern.

Nerve Sheath Tumors

Radiographs of the vertebral column and limbs are often normal in cases of nerve sheath tumors. However, enlargement of the affected intervertebral foramen may be observed on oblique views secondary to bone resorption caused by a thickened nerve root.

Magnetic resonance imaging (MRI) is the imaging modality of choice to identify a nerve sheath tumor. MRI features of this tumor typically consist of a circumscribed, T2 hyperintense, T1 iso- to hypointense, moderate to strong and heterogeneous contrast-enhancing mass (Figure 11.1.3). These tumors can occur at any location along the nerve, and those associated with the brachial plexus may show mild, tubular thickening of one or several branches. These tumors may also extend proximally, through the intervertebral foramen and into the vertebral canal to cause extradural spinal cord compression. However, if nerve roots are involved, the lesion may be intradural and extramedullary.

Muscle atrophy along the affected limb is often observed on MRI, and the atrophied muscles are often T2, STIR, and T1-hyperintense with minimal to no contrast enhancement.

Although less sensitive and specific, computed tomography (CT) can also be used to diagnose nerve sheath tumors.

While the above MRI characteristics are most indicative of a nerve sheath tumor, histopathology is required for definitive diagnosis. With a lesion that is affecting a nerve more distally, fine needle aspirate and cytology may also be performed, although this tumor type poorly exfoliates.

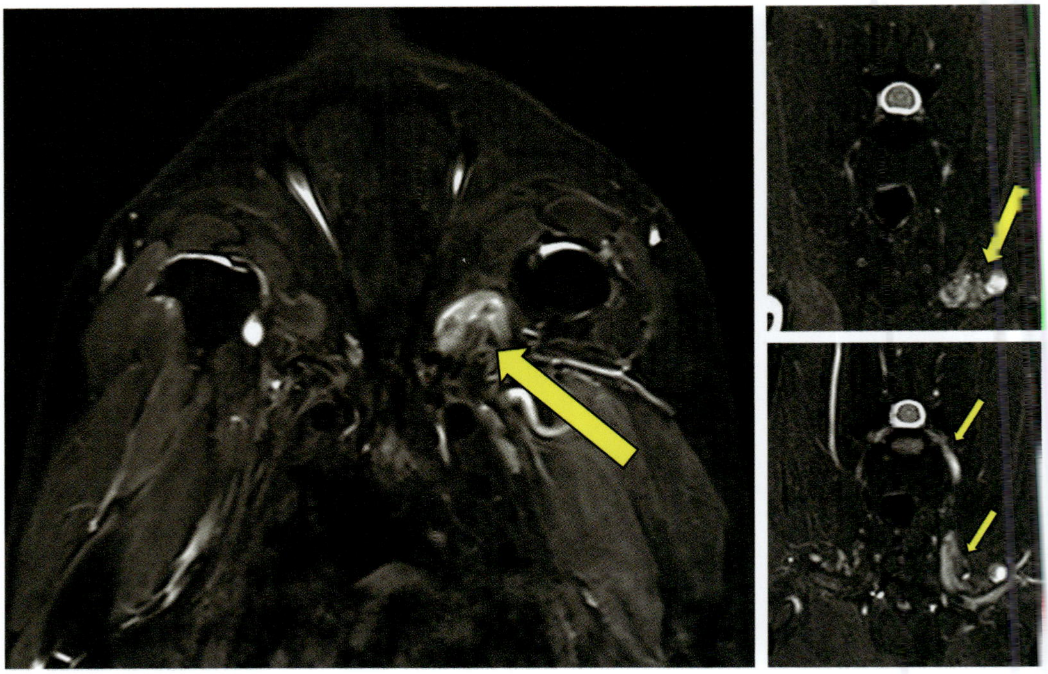

FIGURE 11.1.3 Magnetic resonance images of a 10-year-old spayed female Boston terrier with a nerve sheath tumor (yellow arrows). Left image: dorsal T2-weighted image showing a large, discrete, T2-weighted hyperintense mass in the region of the left brachial plexus. The right images are transverse images at different levels showing the mass at the level of the brachial plexus (top right image) and enlargement of the C8 nerve and nerve root (bottom right image).

Chronic Neuritis

Chronic neuritis, either due to infection or immune-mediated conditions, may have similar MRI characteristics to those of a nerve sheath tumor, showing T2-hyperintense, T1-hypointense, strong contrast-enhancing thickening of the affected nerve(s). If the observed abnormality extends to the vertebral canal and involves the subarachnoid space on MRI, cerebrospinal fluid (CSF) analysis may be helpful. Serology for specific infectious diseases based off suspicion/regionality may be considered. However, histopathology is often required for definitive diagnosis.

Foraminal Stenosis

Lateralized/foraminal intervertebral disc Vertebral radiographs may show signs suggestive of intervertebral foraminal stenosis due to a lateralized disc herniation, such as a calcified disc or soft tissue material within the intervertebral foramen, or enlargement of the affected intervertebral foramen. MRI is required for definitive diagnosis, with transverse images at the level of the affected intervertebral foramen being most helpful. The MRI will often show T2 hypointense material within the intervertebral foramen, causing a variable degree of spinal nerve compression.

Far lateral or extraforaminal extrusions As mineralized lesions and bone structures are well-evaluated from CT images, these lesions are readily apparent and easily diagnosed by parasagittal reconstructed CT or oblique radiographs. Mineralization may be more challenging to depict in

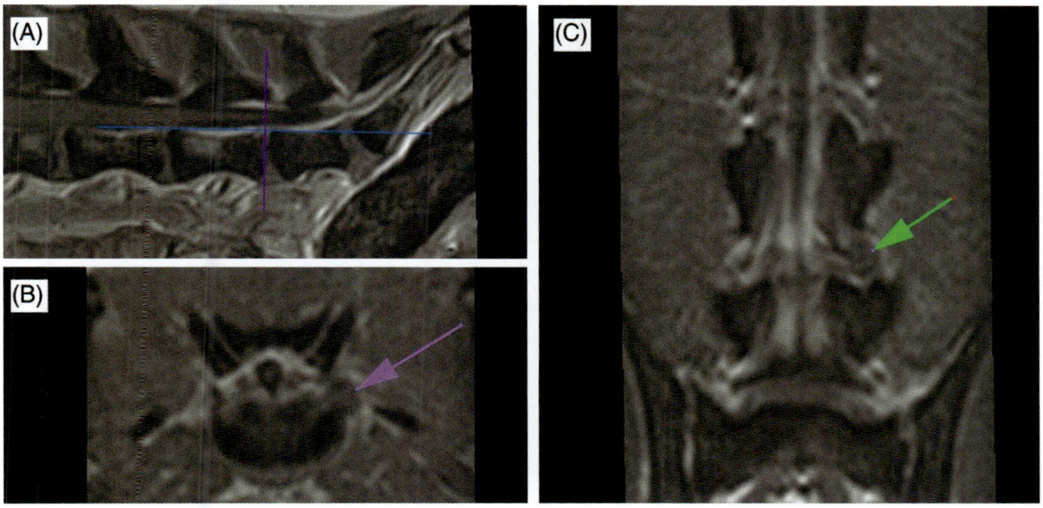

FIGURE 11.1.4 A T2W sagittal (A), transverse (B) and dorsal MRI (C) of a 7-year-old mixed-breed dog with a 1-week history of severe lumbar pain and left-sided monoparesis. There is a relatively well-defined, left-sided ovoid paravertebral lesion at L6-L7, lateral to the foramen (arrows), which was confirmed to be a far-lateral disc extrusion at surgery.

MRI studies; therefore, when suspecting a foraminal/far-distal disc extrusion, it is essential to include multiple sequences and planes (Figure 11.1.4). These can include (i) dorsal fat suppression sequences (such as STIR, Dixon), to assess any lateralized abnormal signal intensity in paravertebral and perineural tissues; and (ii) transverse T2W, T1W and T2* at the level of the suspected foramina/far-distal extrusion.

Neoplasia Radiographs of the vertebral column may show similar changes to those discussed with nerve sheath neoplasms. There may also be vertebral bone lysis present. However, even with neoplasms that cause osteolysis, radiographic changes are often not apparent unless there is substantial bone loss. Further, neoplasms that do not cause lysis are typically not radiographically apparent. Thus, neoplasm should not be ruled out based on unremarkable radiographs. Thoracic radiographs should also be performed to identify the presence of pulmonary metastasis, which can occur in a variety of primary and metastatic neoplasms.

CT is sensitive for diagnosing various neoplasms. The most sensitive and specific diagnostic imaging modality for assessing tumors is MRI. MRI appearance of neoplasms on various sequences varies by tumor type. Depending on the location of the mass, fluoroscopic-guided needle aspiration or surgical biopsy can be performed for definitive diagnosis.

WHAT IS THE EXPECTED OUTCOME WITH EACH DIFFERENTIAL DIAGNOSIS? TREATMENT AND PROGNOSIS

Nerve Sheath Tumors

Surgical resection is the treatment of choice for a nerve sheath tumor, although complete resection may be difficult due to the local invasiveness of the tumor into the vertebral canal. More distal neoplasms are more likely to be associated with curative resection, typically achieved with limb amputation. Local resection is also possible but is likely to result in substantial, permanent neurological deficits to the affected limb and is more likely to be associated with residual disease than amputation. For more proximal neoplasms, limb amputation combined with hemilaminectomy to achieve rhizotomies as close as possible to the spinal cord is necessary. In these cases, residual disease along the meninges is anticipated.

Nerve sheath tumors have a high rate of recurrence and long-term prognosis is considered poor. More proximally located tumors (nerve roots) respond more poorly to surgery with a median survival time of 1–5 months, whereas more distally located tumors (brachial plexus and peripheral nerves) have a median survival time of 7–9 months. However, if complete surgical resection with large margins is achieved in more distal neoplasms, then surgery can be curative.

Nerve sheath tumors can also be addressed with radiation therapy. This is a reasonable alternative treatment option for tumors that are not considered surgically resectable. However, there are limited data related to outcome with this treatment modality.

As an alternative to these definitive care options, palliative care for nerve sheath tumors consists of anti-inflammatory doses of corticosteroids and adjunctive analgesic medications, including gabapentin and amantadine.

Chronic Neuritis

Immune-mediated (ganglio)neuritis is treated with immunosuppressive doses of corticosteroids and has a poor to guarded prognosis. Infectious neuritis is typically treated with appropriate antimicrobial therapy and carries a guarded prognosis, although this may vary depending on the specific underlying infection identified.

Foraminal Stenosis

Lateralized/foraminal intervertebral disc Medical treatment with anti-inflammatory medications such as corticosteroids or non-steroidal anti-inflammatory drugs, pain medications, and activity restriction can alleviate signs of pain and paresis. However, the signs often recur following completion of medical management or do not respond to management.

Surgical removal of the extruded/protruded disc material within the intervertebral foramen is often recommended. The prognosis is good with appropriate decompression.

Far lateral or extraforaminal extrusions Regarding treatment options, both surgical and medical treatment are associated with good to excellent outcomes in 90% or more in dogs with thoracolumbar foraminal or far-lateral IVDEs. Most dogs with cervical foraminal IVDE are reported to recover completely with only medical therapy.

Neoplasia Neoplasia within the vertebral foramen to cause nerve root compression often carries a guarded to grave prognosis. Treatment is based on the tumor type and consists of either palliative care with pain management and corticosteroids or definitive therapy, such as radiation therapy, chemotherapy, and/or surgical decompression.

OUTCOME

The dog underwent an MRI, which confirmed a mass in the region of the right brachial plexus at the level of the shoulder joint. Based on the appearance, a nerve sheath tumor was prioritized as the top differential diagnosis. The dog underwent thoracic limb amputation, during which the mass was grossly visible. The nerves contributing to the brachial plexus were transected as proximally as possible. Histopathology confirmed a nerve sheath tumor with no tumor evident at the resection margins. The dog was lost to follow-up 6 months after surgery.

SUGGESTED READING

Cooper-Khan, R.S., Frankovich, A.N., Thompson, C.A. et al. (2024). Clinical findings and outcome in 30 dogs with presumptive or confirmed nerve sheath tumors. *Vet. Sci.* 11 (5).

de Lahunta, A. (2021). Chapter 5: lower motor neuron: spinal nerve, general somatic efferent system. In: *Veterinary Neuroanatomy and Clinical Neurology*, 5e, 106–162. Philadelphia, PA: Elsevier.

Lorenz, M.D., Coates, J.R., and Kent, M. (2012). Chapter 5: paresis of one limb. In: *Handbook of Veterinary Neurology*, 94–108. St. Louis, MO: Elsevier/Saunders.

Olby, N.J. and Flatt, S.R. (2014). Chapter 16: monoparesis. In: *BSAVA Manual of Canine and Feline Neurology*, 265–279. Gloucester, England: British Small Animal Veterinary Association.

Ródenas, S., Summers, B.A., Saveraid, T. et al. (2013). Chronic hypertrophic ganglioneuritis mimicking spinal nerve neoplasia: clinical, imaging, pathologic findings, and outcome after surgical treatment. *Vet. Surg.* 42 (1): 91–98. https://doi.org/10.1111/j.1532-950X.2012.01045.x.

Schachar, J., Bocage, A., Nelson, N.C. et al. (2024). Clinical and imaging findings in dogs with nerve root signature associated with cervical intervertebral disc herniation. *J. Vet. Intern. Med.* 38 (2): 1111–1119.

CHAPTER 11.2

Monoparesis

Case 2—Acute Onset of Unilateral Pelvic Limb Weakness in a Dog

Danielle Daw

MissionVet Specialty and Emergency, San Antonio, TX, USA

CASE HISTORY

A 4-year-old, intact female sheepadoodle was presented for an acute onset of dragging the left pelvic limb. The dog had been let outside unsupervised and was heard crying out once. When approached, the dog was found to be "dragging" the left pelvic limb and was immediately presented to an emergency clinic for evaluation. Before this incident, the dog was reportedly healthy with no concerns and on no medications other than monthly heartworm/flea/tick preventatives.

NEUROLOGIC EXAMINATION

The dog was bright, alert, and responsive on presentation. The dog was ambulatory with left pelvic limb monoparesis, where she would primarily knuckle and drag the left pelvic limb. Postural reactions, including paw placement and hopping, were absent in the left pelvic limb. The dog had a normal cutaneous trunci reflex cutoff bilaterally. The left pelvic limb had markedly decreased tone. The patellar reflex was normal to exaggerated in the left pelvic limb. The withdrawal reflex was reduced with incomplete flexion at the hip, stifle, and tarsus. The right pelvic limb was normal for all aspects of the neurological exam. The perineal reflex was normal, and there was strong anal tone. There was no evidence of pain or discomfort on paraspinal palpation.

1. **Where is the likely lesion localization?**
2. **What major disease processes should be considered?**
3. **What tests could you perform to help determine the diagnosis?**
4. **What is the expected outcome with each suspected disease process?**

LESION LOCALIZATION

The knuckling, abnormal spinal reflexes, and reduced muscle tone in the left pelvic limb are indicative of a lower motor neuron paresis. Given that the right pelvic limb is not showing any neurologic deficits, the gait abnormalities are consistent with a left-lateralized or unilateral lumbosacral myelopathy. An exaggerated patellar reflex may be seen in association with a loss of antagonistic (flexor) muscle function. Thus, the neurolocalization for this patient is a left-sided L6-S2 myelopathy.

DIFFERENTIAL DIAGNOSIS

Vascular – Ischemic Myelopathy

Ischemic myelopathies are a result of obstruction of the blood supply to the spinal cord. The most common reason for ischemic myelopathy in canine patients results from embolization of the spinal cord vasculature with fibrocartilaginous material, or a fibrocartilaginous embolic myelopathy (FCEM). There are various hypotheses to explain how the fibrocartilaginous material gains access to the spinal cord vasculature, with the prevailing hypothesis being that the material originates from a nearby intervertebral disc.

FCEMs occur most commonly in adult, large-breed dogs with a peracute onset during high physical activity. In addition to large-breed dogs, two types of small breed dogs also have a higher rate of FCEM occurrence: miniature schnauzers and Shetland sheepdogs. The reason for the higher rate of FCEM in these breeds is unknown. While the patient may show pain at the initial injury, the discomfort usually does not persist after a few hours, while the patient's neurologic deficits usually stabilize within 24 hours. There is often an asymmetry to the signs based on which vessel has become occluded.

With the patient's signalment, history, and lesion localization, an FCEM is a highly likely differential for this patient.

Vascular – Aortic Thrombus

Aortic thrombosis is the pathologic formation of a blood clot within the aorta, causing altered blood flow. This has been more commonly described in cats and less commonly described in dogs, but is suspected to have a higher prevalence than previously considered. In dogs, clinical signs are found to either be acute or chronic in onset and consist of mono/paraparesis or mono/paraplegia with diminished reflexes and tone, decreased/absent femoral pulses, cold and/or painful extremities, and cyanotic nail beds. Often, blood flow to the tail is maintained, such that on rectal palpation, the median sacral artery pulse quality will be observed to be normal. The clinical signs in dogs can otherwise be insidious and vague, with intermittent claudication being a common feature. Clinical signs can also wax and wane. This intermittency should prompt the clinician to consider this etiology, as few other diseases will cause such fluctuation in clinical signs. Few cases are reported to have single-limb involvement, and these cases are often found to have an acute onset of signs.

In dogs, an aortic thrombus can be associated with multiple underlying conditions, particularly those that promote a hypercoagulable state, including hyperadrenocorticism, neoplasia, infective endocarditis, diabetes mellitus, liver disease, or a protein-losing nephropathy or enteropathy.

Trauma

Nerve trauma that will result in pelvic limb monoparesis is typically a result of the sciatic nerve or its branches, primarily the common fibular nerve, being affected. Proximal sciatic nerve injuries can be a result of pelvic trauma, particularly those associated with fractures of the ilium, acetabulum, or sacroiliac joint. Injury to the sciatic nerve can also occur during surgical intervention of the pelvis or coxal joint or due to an intramuscular injection into the caudal thigh.

The common fibular branch of the sciatic nerve may be damaged, although uncommonly, as it courses along the lateral aspect of the stifle due to a lack of muscle coverage. This trauma can occur secondary to intramuscular injections, during stifle surgery, or from pressure associated with the placement of an orthopedic cast along the stifle.

Trauma to the femoral nerve is uncommon, as the hypaxial musculature provides sufficient protection of this nerve.

Given no evidence of trauma associated with the onset of this dog's signs, nerve trauma is considered unlikely for this patient.

NEXT DIAGNOSTIC STEPS FOR THIS PATIENT

Ischemic Myelopathy

Magnetic resonance imaging (MRI) will show an intramedullary lesion, a sharply demarcated lesion that extends over the vertebral body (Figure 11.2.1). The lesion is typically T2-weighted hyperintense relative to the surrounding normal spinal cord and does not contrast-enhance. The lesion often primarily affects the gray matter and is often lateralized, coinciding with the clinical signs. It is important to note that MRI can be normal in ischemic myelopathies. Therefore, a normal MRI seen in a patient with a typical history and exam is highly suggestive of an ischemic myelopathy.

Aortic Thrombus

There are several comparative tests that can be performed when an aortic thrombus is suspected. Comparing the systolic blood pressure in the affected limb versus the unaffected limbs may disclose a lower systolic blood pressure in the affected limb. Likewise, blood glucose concentration obtained from the affected limb may be lower than in unaffected limbs. Lactate obtained from the affected limb may be higher than in unaffected limbs. Finally, because of a lack of blood supply to the limb's musculature, ischemic necrosis develops. Creatine kinase leaks from myocytes, resulting in a frequently marked increase in serum creatine kinase concentration.

Abdominal ultrasound, performed by an experienced ultrasonographer, can be highly sensitive and specific for the identification of an aortic thrombus. On ultrasound, an aortic thrombus appears as a region of hyperechoic material within the aorta relative to the normally hypoechoic material (blood) expected to be within its lumen. Doppler flow ultrasound will further demonstrate decreased or absent flow past the thrombus in the aorta or external iliac artery.

CT is highly sensitive and specific for detecting aortic thrombi. MRI is also highly sensitive and specific for identifying the aortic thrombus. It is important to note that with MRI, an aortic thrombus can be overlooked if the study is focused exclusively on the spinal cord (in these cases, a "saturation band" may be placed over the aorta during MRI planning to reduce flow artifact, which can impact the interpretation of spinal cord changes). If such a saturation band is placed over the aorta, the thrombus may be missed.

Nerve Trauma

The diagnosis of a traumatic neuropathy is primarily based on history and clinical signs. Radiographs of the pelvis would determine the extent of orthopedic fractures and subluxations/luxations that may cause nerve damage. Computed tomography (CT) or MRI can be used to confirm a historical suspicion or to evaluate further comorbidities that may have occurred with trauma.

Electrodiagnostic testing, such as motor nerve conduction studies, can be performed to determine the integrity of the nerve.

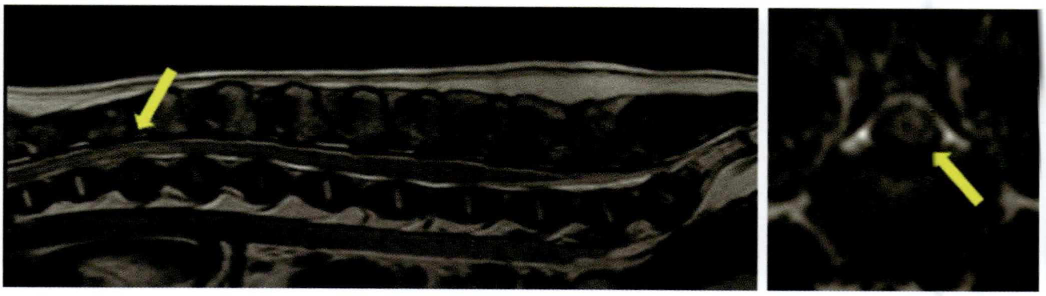

FIGURE 11.2.1 T2W MR images of fibrocartilaginous embolic myelopathy in a dog. Note the hyperintensity within the spinal cord (yellow arrows).

TREATMENT/PROGNOSIS

Ischemic Myelopathy

Treatment for an ischemic myelopathy is conservative and consists of nursing care and physical therapy. Most patients (80%) who retain motor function will recover over a 2–16-week period. Patients with loss of nociception and those with lower motor neuron involvement are shown to have a guarded prognosis.

Aortic Thrombus

Treatment for an aortic thrombus primarily consists of addressing the primary underlying cause, if found, along with thrombolytic drugs. Thrombectomy can also be performed. The prognosis for an aortic thrombus in dogs is guarded, and an acute presentation of signs was shown to have a shorter survival time compared to dogs who presented with chronic disease. See Chapter 12, Case 3 for information on the feline version of this disease.

Nerve Trauma

There is no specific treatment for a nerve trauma other than supportive care to protect the paw from injury and physical therapy. The prognosis for recovery is primarily based on the type of damage and the severity of the neurologic dysfunction. Nerves that have been compressed, stretched, or contused may regain function slowly, whereas nerves that are lacerated or avulsed rarely regain function.

Regarding neurologic status – if nociception is intact, prognosis for recovery is good. However, if nociception is absent, the prognosis is guarded.

OUTCOME

MRI confirmed FCEM in this dog. She was treated with supportive care and regained normal function of her limb 6 weeks after the onset of signs.

SUGGESTED READING

Cauzinille, L. (2000). Fibrocartilaginous embolism in dogs. *Vet. Clin. North Am. Small Anim. Pract.* 30 (1): 155–167. vii.

de Lahunta, A. (2021). Chapter 5: lower motor neuron: spinal nerve, general somatic efferent system. In: *Veterinary Neuroanatomy and Clinical Neurology*, 5e, 106–162. Philadelphia, PA: Elsevier.

Olby, N.J. and Platt, S.R. (2014). Chapter 16: monoparesis. In: *BSAVA Manual of Canine and Feline Neurology*, 265–279. Gloucester, England: British Small Animal Veterinary Association.

Williams, T.P., Shaw, S., Porter, A., and Berkwitt, L. (2017). Aortic thrombosis in dogs. *J. Vet. Emerg. Crit. Care (San Antonio)* 27 (1): 9–22.

CHAPTER 12.1

Pelvic Limb Ataxia, Paraparesis, and Paralysis

Case 1—Acute Paraparesis in a Chondrodystrophic Dog

Edward MacKillop

BluePearl Pet Hospital, Pittsburgh, PA, USA

CASE HISTORY

A 4-year-old neutered male miniature dachshund was presented for acute-onset difficulty walking with his pelvic limbs. Over the prior weekend, the dog seemed to be in pain and was not able to jump up onto elevated surfaces. He was evaluated by the primary care veterinarian and was prescribed prednisone for suspected intervertebral disc disease (IVDD). The dog remained ambulatory until that morning, at which point he was found to be suddenly unable to walk.

NEUROLOGICAL EXAMINATION (Video 12.1.1)

VIDEO 12.1.1 Neurological examination of a nonambulatory paraparetic dachshund.

The dog was friendly and interactive. He was nonambulatory due to the inability to use his pelvic limbs effectively. Both pelvic limbs exhibited strong voluntary motor function (non-ambulatory paraparesis), and the dog could propel himself forward with his pelvic limbs, taking exaggerated and stiff steps. If the dog was supported by a sling under his abdomen, he was able to walk, but pelvic limb movements were uncoordinated (displaying general proprioceptive ataxia), and he was prone to walking on the dorsum of the pes. Thoracic limb postural reactions were normal; pelvic limb postural reactions were absent. Cranial nerve exam did not disclose any deficits. Segmental spinal reflexes were brisk in both pelvic limbs, and limb tone was considered normal to slightly increased in both pelvic limbs. Spinal reflexes were normal in both thoracic limbs. The dog's cutaneous trunci reflex could be elicited in the caudal lumbar region bilaterally but was strengthened in the cranial lumbar region, at the level of the L1/L2 spinous processes. The dog did not generally seem painful, but a discrete pain response (vocalization) was noted with direct pressure on the thoracolumbar junction. The remainder of the physical and neurologic examination was unremarkable.

1. **Where is the likely lesion localization?**
2. **What major disease processes should be considered?**
3. **What tests could you perform to help determine the diagnosis?**
4. **What treatment options exist for the most common differential?**

LESION LOCALIZATION

The dog's neurologic deficits are restricted to the pelvic limbs only, and so the primary considerations for neuroanatomic diagnosis are either a thoracolumbar myelopathy (T3–L3) or a lumbosacral (L4–S3) myelopathy, radiculopathy, or neuropathy. The dog shows a combination of paraparesis (inability to walk unassisted) and proprioceptive ataxia, which are most commonly myelopathic in origin, rather than a radiculopathy or neuropathy. The pelvic limb reflexes are intact to slightly exaggerated (brisk), indicating normal lower motor neuron function. This, in combination with normal to increased limb tone, indicates an upper motor neuron paraparesis (T3–L3).

In domestic animals, the cutaneous trunci muscle is responsible for the movement of the skin in the dorsal thorax and lumbar region in response to a cutaneous stimulus (Figure 12.1.1). "Panniculus reflex" is a common misnomer for the cutaneous trunci reflex and should be avoided as the cutaneous trunci muscle is not in the panniculus layer of the skin. Stimulation of sensory afferents in the dermis initiates the reflex. Action potentials descend into the dorsal grey column and synapse on long spinal interneurons. The signal is conducted cranially through the thoracolumbar spinal cord in a deep white matter tract (fasciculus proprius) to the level of C8–T1. The impulse activates lower motor neurons whose axons exit the spinal cord to become the lateral thoracic nerve, which innervates the cutaneous trunci muscle. Stimulation of this reflex leads to a rippling movement of the skin dorsally along the thoracolumbar vertebral column. With severe thoracolumbar myelopathy, the transmission of impulses will be disrupted, and stimulation of the skin caudal to the lesion will not activate the reflex. A moderate lesion will cause a diminution of the reflex, whereas a transverse T3–L3 myelopathy (paraplegia with loss of nociception) will completely attenuate the reflex with a line of analgesia caudal to the region in which the reflex is observed. Dermal afferents for each segmental spinal nerve extend about two vertebrae caudally, and so the reflex will "cut off" about two segments caudal to the lesion. In this case, the cutaneous trunci reflex was weaker caudal to L1/L2, indicating a lesion around T12/T13. The dog also shows signs of discomfort (hyperesthesia) with direct palpation of this region. The sum of the dog's neurologic signs indicates a T3–L3 myelopathy with a more specific localization to the thoracolumbar junction.

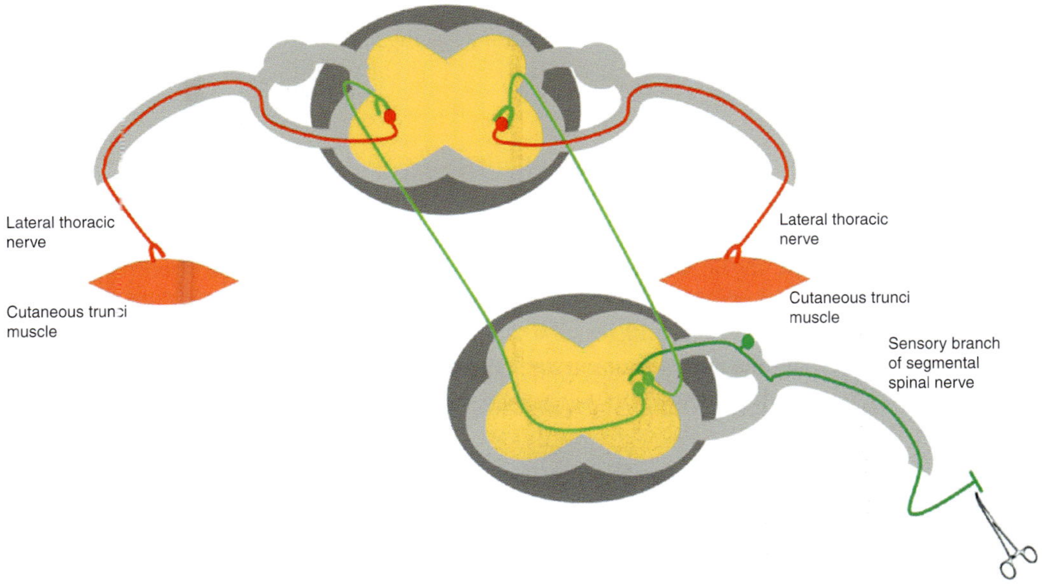

FIGURE 12.1.1 Illustration of the cutaneous trunci reflex.

WHAT MAJOR DISEASE PROCESSES SHOULD BE CONSIDERED?

Degenerative – Intervertebral Disc Herniation/Intervertebral Disc Extrusion

Intervertebral disc herniation is an umbrella term used to describe displacement of the intervertebral disc beyond its normal anatomic boundary. Chondrodystrophic dogs are prone to rupture of the annulus fibrosus with extrusion of degenerated nucleus pulposus (Hansen type I degeneration) into the epidural space. An acute intervertebral disc extrusion (IVDE) should be considered as the primary differential for any acutely myelopathic chondrodystrophic dog and is the top differential for this patient. Other differentials (see below) should be considered much lower on the differential diagnosis list.

Inflammatory – Meningomyelitis or Discospondylitis with Empyema

Infectious or primary inflammatory disease of the central nervous system may present with only myelopathic signs. Granulomatous meningomyelitis (part of the meningitis of unknown origin or etiology complex) is the most common inflammatory disorder of the central nervous system of dogs, and it is occasionally seen in dachshunds, but at a much lower frequency than IVDE. Discospondylitis will usually cause signs of pain, but myelopathy may develop in cases with secondary empyema (a collection of purulent material in the epidural space), or vertebral fracture, subluxation, or luxation, which lead to alterations in the vertebral canal trajectory and can cause spinal cord compression. Large-breed dogs and French bulldogs appear to be at a greater risk for discospondylitis. In French bulldogs, there is a predilection for discospondylitis to be associated with hemivertebrae. Overall, these considerations indicate a low likelihood of discospondylitis for this patient. For more information about discospondylitis, please refer to Chapter 10, Case 1.

Trauma – Traumatic Myelopathy

Fracture or subluxation should be considered in the differential, but there will typically be a known inciting cause (i.e. motor vehicle accident). Radiographs can be helpful in excluding traumatic myelopathy and will also help to screen for evidence of degenerative disc disease. Traumatic myelopathy may occur without vertebral fracture or subluxation and is termed spinal cord injury without radiographic abnormality (SCIWORA). For more information about traumatic myelopathy please refer to Chapter 15, Case 2.

Neoplasia

Spinal cord or vertebral neoplasia is occasionally seen in young animals. Lymphoma, osteosarcoma, and nephroblastoma are considerations, although they tend to be more common in large-breed dogs (See Chapter 13, Case 2 for more information).

Vascular – Hemorrhagic or Ischemic Myelopathy

Fibrocartilaginous embolic myelopathy (FCEM) is a rare occurrence in chondrodystrophic dogs. This dog's clinical history and examination are incompatible with FCEM; the dog had premonitory signs of pain, progressive myelopathy over the course of a week, and discomfort on palpation of the vertebral column, all of which are not seen with FCEM. More details about FCEM are found in Chapter 13, Case 1. Epidural hemorrhage, subarachnoid hemorrhage, and/or hematomyelia can cause progressive myelopathy and paraspinal hyperesthesia. Hemorrhage is usually secondary to trauma or disc extrusion but can occur spontaneously or secondary to coagulopathy (idiopathic thrombocytopenic purpura, Warfarin toxicity, von Willebrand's disease, or hemophilia).

WHAT TESTS COULD YOU PERFORM TO HELP DETERMINE THE DIAGNOSIS?

Radiographs

Orthogonal radiographs of the clinically affected area (i.e. region of neuroanatomic localization; in this case, including the thoracic and lumbar vertebral column regions) are the starting point for diagnosing disorders of the spinal cord and vertebral column. Radiographs are

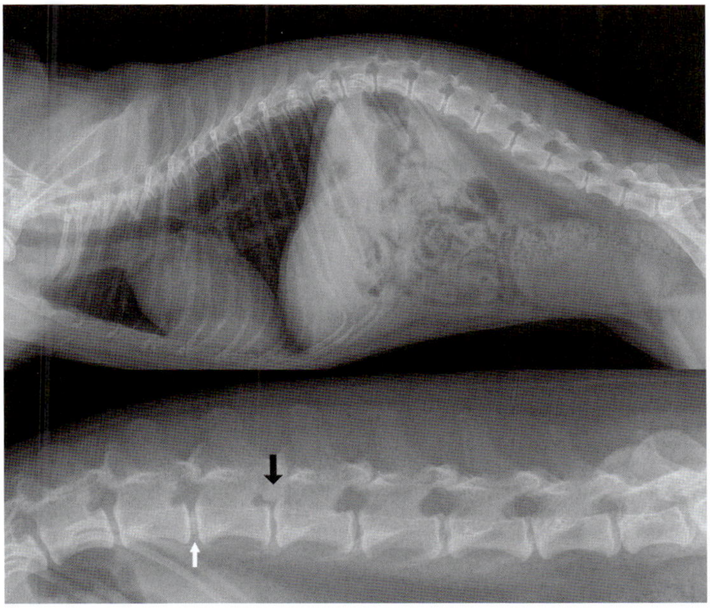

FIGURE 12.1.2 Upper: lateral whole-body radiograph of a bichon frise presented for paraparesis/ataxia. The radiograph is well-positioned but poorly collimated to the clinically affected area. Lower: cropping the image to focus on the thoracolumbar vertebral column clearly shows a mineral opacity within the foramen at L2–L3 (black arrow), suggesting a calcified disc extrusion. The L1–L2 intervertebral disc is mineralized in situ (white arrow), raising the possibility of a disc herniation at this level.

approximately 60% accurate for diagnosing the location of an intervertebral disc extrusion but should never be used as the exclusive modality when planning surgery. Appropriate positioning and collimation improve diagnostic accuracy but may require patient sedation. The radiographic (Roentgen) signs of a disc disease/herniation include calcification of the intervertebral disc *in situ*, collapse or wedging of the intervertebral disc space, the presence of mineral opacity in the intervertebral foramen, and a decrease in the size of the intervertebral foramen (Figure 12.1.2). Radiographs are also helpful in confirming a normal vertebral formula (13 thoracic vertebrae, 7 lumbar vertebrae) and the number/appearance of ribs, as transitional vertebrae are not uncommon and complicate localization at surgery if unidentified.

Myelography

With the advent of three-dimensional imaging (computed tomography/magnetic resonance [CT/MR]), myelography is less commonly used for the diagnosis of acute intervertebral disc extrusion but remains an option, especially if CT/MR is unavailable or provides equivocal results. Nonionic, iodinated contrast is injected into the subarachnoid space at L4–5 or L5–6 to create a silhouette of the spinal cord. Attenuation or deviation of the radiographic contrast columns identifies regions of significant spinal cord compression (Figure 12.1.3). The location of IVDE using myelography can be difficult in cases with significant cord swelling, and the lateralization (predominant side of compression) is not always clear. Myelography also carries some risk to the patient (e.g. neurologic deterioration, seizures), and so noninvasive imaging is typically preferred. If noncontrast CT of the vertebral column does not provide an accurate diagnosis (see below) and MR imaging is not available, then myelography or CT myelography can be pursued.

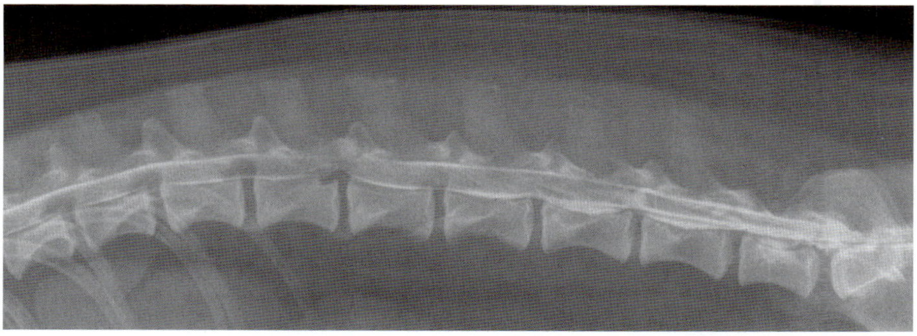

FIGURE 12.1.3 Lateral radiograph myelogram showing deviation of the ventral contrast column at the level of the L2–L3 intervertebral disc space, consistent with intervertebral disc extrusion at this level.

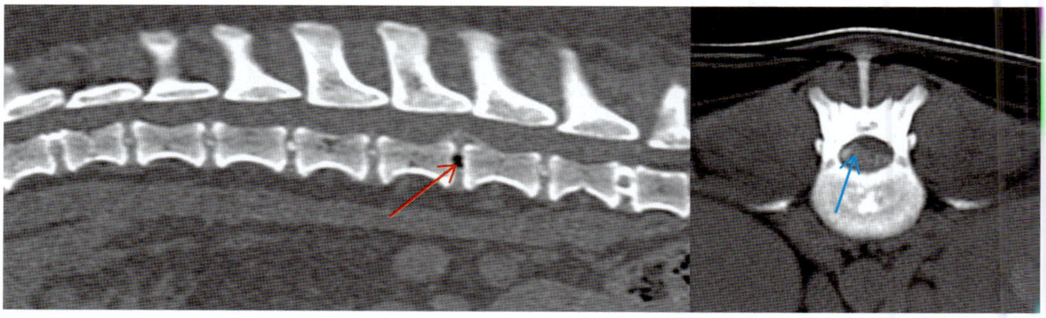

FIGURE 12.1.4 Sagittal reconstruction of a noncontrast CT of the lumbar vertebral column of a young chondrodystrophic dog. All visible intervertebral discs are calcified in situ. A significant extradural compression of the spinal cord can be seen at L4–L5 because of extruded hyperattenuating disc material. There is a focal region of hypoattenuation (black oval) representing nitrogen gas that has been drawn into the disc because of acute extrusion of nucleus pulposus (vacuum phenomenon - red arrow). Right: transverse noncontrast transverse CT image of an acute calcified disc extrusion (blue arrow). A large region of hyperattenuating material occupies about 75% of the vertebral canal.

Computed Tomography (CT)

Young chondrodystrophic dogs are prone to herniation of calcified nucleus pulposus, which can be easily detected by noncontrast CT of the vertebral column (Figure 12.1.4). Calcified nucleus pulposus in the epidural space is variably hyperattenuating depending on chronicity; acute herniations are moderately hyperattenuating (Hounsfield unit [HU] 100–400), whereas chronic herniations are more marked in attenuation (HU 400–1,000+). Acute intervertebral disc extrusions are often accompanied by epidural hemorrhage, which is also hyperattenuating (HU 40–100) relative to the spinal cord (HU 30 ± 10). Intervertebral disc extrusion in older chondrodystrophic patients is less consistently calcified, often comprised of fibrocartilaginous fragments of nucleus pulposus, and may not be visible on noncontrast CT, requiring subsequent myelography or CT myelography.

Magnetic Resonance Imaging

Magnetic resonance imaging (MRI) is the gold standard for diagnosing diseases of the spinal cord. Sagittal and transverse T2-weighted images are usually sufficient for the diagnosis of an acute intervertebral disc extrusion (Figure 12.1.5), but other sequences may be necessary and of prognostic value. A fat-saturated T2-weighted sequence, such as a short tau inversion-recovery (STIR), is helpful for identifying intraparenchymal spinal cord hyperintensity. In a study of 77 dogs with acute IVDE,

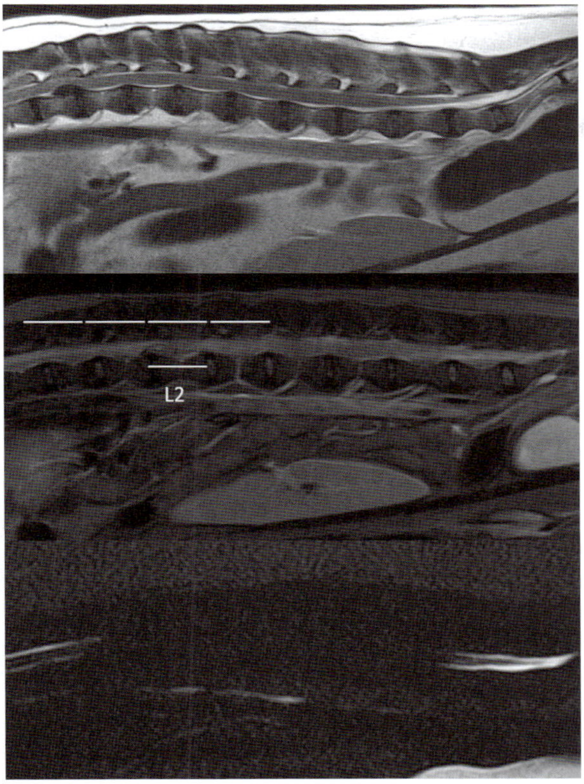

FIGURE 12.1.5 Upper: T2 sagittal MR image of a 3-year-old neutered male dachshund presenting for chronic ambulatory paraparesis/ataxia. A large region of hypointensity can be seen in the vertebral canal over the T12–T13 intervertebral disc, causing severe compression of the overlying spinal cord. MR changes are typical of a calcified disc herniation. Middle: sagittal STIR image of a severe disc extrusion at L1–L2 with marked spinal cord hyperintensity extending over at least four vertebral segments. Lower: sagittal HASTE image of the lumbar spinal cord showing a large region of CSF attenuation indicating extensive extradural compression or spinal cord swelling.

dogs with T2-weighted spinal cord hyperintensity greater than the length of the L2 vertebra had a significantly lower rate of functional neurological recovery after surgery. All dogs without segmental hyperintensity (n=44) recovered ambulation following surgery, whereas only 18/33 dogs (55%) with hyperintensity recovered ambulation. A heavily T2-weighted single-shot turbo spin echo sequence, such as HASTE (Half-Fourier Acquisition Single-shot Turbo spin Echo), clearly defines the subarachnoid space and can identify regions of spinal cord compression or cord swelling. A large region of cerebrospinal fluid (CSF) attenuation may carry a more guarded prognosis and is associated with progressive myelomalacia, although this condition can only be confirmed with postmortem histopathological evaluation. MR changes should be correlated with clinical signs, as signal changes may represent a reversible change, such as edema, rather than an irreversible process like myelomalacia.

TREATMENT OF INTERVERTEBRAL DISC EXTRUSIONS

Treatment is broadly divided into conservative management and surgical management:

- Conservative management consists of strict rest for 4 weeks. Ideally, dogs are confined to a kennel or small room to prevent them from actively extruding more disc material while the ruptured annulus fibrosus is undergoing fibrosis. Anti-inflammatory medications are the primary treatment for many medical conditions. Much debate has occurred regarding which option, steroidal or nonsteroidal, is superior. Ultimately, the author's opinion is that both are reasonable options (but not to be used together), provided the appropriate dose is used and the client is counseled regarding side effect profiles.

- For thoracolumbar intervertebral disc extrusions, surgical management typically consists of a hemilaminectomy or occasionally a pediculectomy or mini-hemilaminectomy, depending on the surgeon's preference.
- Supportive care consists of bladder emptying (either with manual expression or intermittent catheterization in some cases) in patients who cannot void on their own, sedatives to reduce anxiety associated with confinement, and additional analgesic support such as gabapentin, codeine, or amantadine.

Both treatment routes (conservative or surgical) are reasonable options, provided owners are counseled diligently regarding expectations for recovery. Dogs that have exclusively back pain or mild neurologic dysfunction often respond favorably to conservative management. Contrastingly, dogs that are paraplegic, with or without nociception, are less likely to recover with conservative management than they are with surgical management. Over 90% of dogs treated surgically, excepting those lacking nociception, achieve functional recovery with surgery. Between 50% and 60% of dogs lacking nociception achieve functional recovery with surgery (and fewer than 20% of these severely affected dogs achieve functional recovery with conservative management).

Alternative therapies, including acupuncture, holistic options, and chiropractic, have not been demonstrated to improve patient outcomes. Acupuncture has not been associated with adverse outcomes, but chiropractic manipulation is contraindicated in the presence of canine intervertebral disc extrusions. Adjustments predispose patients to the extrusion of additional disc material, which can lead to substantial pain and neurological deterioration.

Patients should be referred for surgery when:

- They fail to respond to conservative management after 2 weeks of therapy.
- Their pain or myelopathy worsens during conservative management.
- They are non-ambulatory, especially if paraplegic.
- They are paraplegic and lack nociception. In this circumstance, owners should be counseled that the likelihood of functional recovery even with surgery is lower than in dogs that maintain nociception.

Intervertebral disc extrusion can lead to a devastating, progressive, irreversible process of progressive myelomalacia. The greatest population at risk for this occurrence are dogs that are paraplegic and lack nociception, although a small subset of dogs that are paraplegic but retain nociception have also been described to develop the condition. Up to 15% of paraplegic, nociception-negative dogs experience progressive myelomalacia. This is ischemic necrosis of the spinal cord. It starts at the level of the disc extrusion and extends both cranially and caudally from this level. As the spinal cord cannot regenerate, this process leads to irreversible axonal loss and permanent paralysis. As it progresses to the lumbosacral intumescence, the pelvic limbs, tail, and external urethral and anal sphincters experience flaccid paralysis and areflexia. As it progresses cranially, the cutaneous trunci reflex cutoff progresses further cranially at each examination. If the process is allowed to continue, flaccid paralysis and areflexia of the thoracic limbs ensue. The diaphragm becomes denervated as the process reaches the C5–C7 region of the spinal cord, leading to hypoventilation and asphyxiation. Progressive myelomalacia occurs up to 2 weeks following intervertebral disc extrusion, but most often begins in the first 72 hours following the injury. If the cutaneous trunci cutoff reaches the cranial thorax, there is a high likelihood that it will reach the cervical spinal cord imminently, and prompt euthanasia is advised to prevent fatal respiratory distress.

OUTCOME

Given the dog's non-ambulatory paraparetic status, MRI was recommended to investigate the cause of his dysfunction. The MRI showed a disc extrusion at the level of the T12–T13 intervertebral disc, leading to marked compression of the spinal cord. A hemilaminectomy at this site was performed. A large amount of disc material was retrieved from the vertebral canal. Two days after surgery, the dog showed substantial improvement in neurological function. At his suture removal appointment 12 days later, he was ambulatory with mild paraparesis. He was crate rested for a total of 4 weeks, after which he was gradually reintroduced to activity. He was limited from engaging in high-impact activities for the rest of his life.

SUGGESTED READING

Aikawa, T., Fujita, H., Kanazono, S. et al. (2012). Long-term neurologic outcome of hemilaminectomy and disk fenestration for treatment of dogs with thoracolumbar intervertebral disk herniation: 831 cases (2000–2007). *J. Am. Vet. Med. Assoc.* 241 (12): 1617–1626.

Burkert, B.A., Kerwin, S.C., Hosgood, G.L. et al. (2005). Signalment and clinical features of diskospondylitis in dogs: 513 cases (1980–2001). *J. Am. Vet. Med. Assoc.* 227 (2): 268–275.

Gilmour, L.J., Jeffery, N.D., Miles, K., and Riedesel, E. (2017). Single-shot turbo spin echo pulse sequence findings in dogs with and without progressive myelomalacia. *Vet Radiol. Ultrasound* 58 (2): 197–205.

Grapes, N., Bertram, S., Gonçalves, R., and De Decker, S. (2024). Prevalence of discospondylitis and association with congenital vertebral body malformations in English and French bulldogs. *J. Vet. Intern. Med.* 38 (6): 3138–3143.

Ito, D., Matsunaga, S., Jeffery, N.D. et al. (2005). Prognostic value of magnetic resonance imaging in dogs with paraplegia caused by thoracolumbar intervertebral disk extrusion: 77 cases (2000–2003). *J. Am. Vet. Med. Assoc.* 227 (9): 1454–1460.

Jeffery, N.D., Levine, J.M., Olby, N.J., and Stein, V.M. (2013). Intervertebral disk degeneration in dogs: consequences, diagnosis, treatment, and future directions. *J. Vet. Intern. Med.* 27 (6): 1318–1333.

Moore, S.A., Tipold, A., Olby, N.J. et al. (2020). Current approaches to the management of acute thoracolumbar disc extrusion in dogs. *Front. Vet. Sci.* 7: 610.

Olby, N.J., Moore, S.A., Brisson, B. et al. (2022). ACVIM consensus statement on diagnosis and management of acute canine thoracolumbar intervertebral disc extrusion. J. Vet. Intern. Med. 36 (5): 1570–1596.

CHAPTER 12.2

Pelvic Limb Ataxia, Paraparesis, and Paralysis

Case 2—Chronic Progressive Paraparesis in a Large-Breed Dog

Edward MacKillop

BluePearl Pet Hospital, Pittsburgh, PA, USA

CASE HISTORY

An 8-year-old neutered male German shepherd dog was presented for chronic progressive paraparesis and pelvic limb ataxia. The owner had noticed problems with the dog's mobility for at least 6 months; he would often trip and fall with his pelvic limbs when running or turning. They had noticed that the dog would drag the left paw on the ground when walking and intermittently stand on the dorsum of the foot. The dog was purchased primarily for protection, and he undergoes Schutzhund training. When in his kennel, he will run around and jump to the top of the kennel. The owner feels he might have fallen and hurt himself. The dog is having difficulty posturing to defecate and urinate, but is still continent. He does not seem painful to the owner and still wants to do training exercises.

NEUROLOGICAL EXAMINATION

The animal's demeanor was normal: he was bright and interactive. He was strongly ambulatory with obvious spastic paraparesis and pelvic limb ataxia that was more apparent on the left side. When the right pelvic limb was placed with the dorsum on the ground (knuckling response or proprioceptive positioning), the speed of correction was slow, and the dog would not return the paw to the original location. If the dog's weight was displaced laterally to the right, the hopping response was slow in onset, but he would reposition. Left pelvic limb postural reactions were markedly decreased: the dog would rarely correct the paw position when knuckled and would almost fall over when hopped to the left. Thoracic limb postural reactions were normal, as was the cranial nerve exam. Spinal reflexes were considered normal, and the cutaneous trunci reflex could be clearly elicited in the caudal lumbar region. Limb tone was considered normal. The dog was not reactive to palpation of the vertebral column and did not show any posture suggesting pain (e.g. thoracolumbar kyphosis). Anal tone and perineal reflex were normal. Orthopedic examination did not identify any concurrent musculoskeletal abnormalities (i.e. stifle instability, joint pain, or effusion). The only notable abnormality on the physical exam was numerous cracked and broken teeth, likely from the dog chewing on its kennel door.

1. **What is the lesion localization for this case?**
2. **What are the three most likely differential diagnoses for this dog?**
3. **What changes on neurologic examination favor a focal versus diffuse thoracolumbar myelopathy?**

LESION LOCALIZATION

The dog's gait is typical of an upper motor neuron (UMN) spastic paraparesis with general proprioceptive (GP) ataxia, often abbreviated as a UMN/GP pelvic limb gait. Pelvic limb spasticity and extensor rigidity lead to a longer stride length, causing the pelvic limb to come close to or even touch the ipsilateral thoracic limb when walking. UMN dysfunction also causes the delayed onset of forward motion. GP ataxia results in crossing of the limbs toward or past the midline, or circumduction of the limbs. The net effect of UMN paresis and proprioceptive ataxia is stiff (spastic), uncoordinated movement, a longer-than-normal stride, and abnormal limb trajectory. This gait phenotype is distinctly different from a lower motor neuron paresis, which is characterized by a shorter stride length and/or flaccid movements of the limb. The dog's pelvic limb reflexes are normal, indicating appropriate lower motor function, and so the dog's localization is a focal or diffuse thoracolumbar (T3–L3) myelopathy, worse on the left side. The cutaneous trunci reflex extends to a normal level, which lowers the consideration of a focal myelopathy, as this would cause discrete disruption of the cutaneous trunci reflex approximately two segments caudal to the lesion. Focal myelopathy is still possible, as a dog with an isolated lesion at L2 or L3 would retain a cutaneous trunci reflex that extends to a normal level, given that the sensory axons that enter at L2–L3 originate in skin caudal to this spinal cord region, likely at the level at which the cutaneous trunci reflex is first appreciable.

WHAT ARE THE THREE MOST LIKELY DIFFERENTIAL DIAGNOSES FOR THIS DOG?

Neoplasia

A tumor of the spinal cord, vertebra, or adjacent tissue is a strong consideration for an older pet with progressive signs of myelopathy with or without concurrent hyperesthesia. Clinical signs are often insidious but may also progress acutely if there is a pathologic fracture or clinical decompensation. The presence of clinical signs for >6 months is less consistent with a tumor, as neurologic deterioration typically progresses more quickly.

Degenerative

(1) Chronic Intervertebral Disc Disease

This is an active and energetic working dog, and so there is a strong consideration for Hansen type II intervertebral disc degeneration and subsequent herniation. Dehydration of the intervertebral disc from age-associated loss of proteoglycans leads to fissures in the inner fibers of the annulus fibrosis. Subsequent weakening of the dorsal annulus leads to the disc protruding into the vertebral canal, compressing the spinal cord. German shepherd dogs are overrepresented for type II disc herniations. The thoracolumbar junction is the most common location, although herniations in the cranial thoracic vertebral column are also seen in this breed. Intervertebral disc protrusion may be on the midline and so hyperesthesia may not be seen if there is not significant nerve or nerve root compression. Disc protrusions may be isolated but are often multifocal, and signs may be the result of cumulative compression across multiple sites. Chronic degenerative disc herniation may also lead to a stepwise deterioration in function (i.e. episodes of acute worsening with subsequent stabilization of function or improvement), which was not seen in this dog.

Treatment for Hansen type II intervertebral disc protrusion consists broadly of conservative management or surgical management. Please refer to Chapter 12, Case 1, for a detailed description of conservative and surgical management of intervertebral disc disease. Note, however, that the prognostic guidance for Hansen type I intervertebral disc extrusions is different from the prognostic guidance for Hansen type II intervertebral disc protrusions. Given the chronic compression experienced with Hansen type II intervertebral disc protrusions, irreversible spinal cord degeneration can limit neurologic improvement following surgery. Thus, clients who pursue surgical management of Hansen type II intervertebral disc protrusion should be counseled that the goal of surgery is to prevent worsening of the myelopathy rather than reversal.

(2) Degenerative Myelopathy

A progressive disorder of axonal loss/demyelination in the thoracolumbar spinal cord of German shepherds was first described in 1973, referring to the disease as canine degenerative myelopathy. Histopathologic changes are first noted in the mid-to-caudal thoracic spinal cord, which explains the initial clinical signs of a thoracolumbar (T3–L3) myelopathy (Video 12.2.1). All funiculi of the spinal cord are involved, but changes are most evident in the dorsal portion of the lateral funiculus. Regions of axonopathy and myelin loss are often discontinuous early in the disease but eventually become confluent and progress to the cervical and lumbar spinal cord. Central axonopathy is accompanied by peripheral axonal degeneration and muscle atrophy. Diminution and eventual loss of the patellar reflex occurs later in the disease, often providing a clinical "clue," as this is not expected with a focal T3–L3 myelopathy. It should be noted that the patellar reflex can be reduced in strength in older dogs and can be hard to elicit if there is significant stifle disease (i.e. cruciate ligament disease, patellar luxation). Given sufficient time, all dogs with degenerative myelopathy will develop flaccid non-ambulatory paraparesis/paraplegia (Video 12.2.2) and eventually tetraparesis/tetraplegia (Video 12.2.3). Fecal and urinary continence are often retained until paraplegia develops. Bulbar (brainstem) signs and hypoventilation are seen in terminal cases.

VIDEO 12.2.1 Dog with early to mid-stage degenerative myelopathy. The dog is ambulatory with UMN paraparesis and general proprioceptive ataxia, localized as a T3–L3 myelopathy.

VIDEO 12.2.2 Dog with more advanced degenerative myelopathy than the dog featured in Video 12.2.1.

VIDEO 12.2.3 Dog with advanced degenerative myelopathy, now affecting all four limbs.

Histologically confirmed degenerative myelopathy has been reported in >20 breeds but is most often seen in German shepherd, Pembroke Welsh corgi (PWC), Bernese mountain dogs, and Boxer dogs. The age at onset of signs in large-breed dogs is 8–9 years of age, but later for PWC (mean age 11 years old). Progression of signs to non-ambulatory paraparesis is typically 6–9 months, although potentially longer in PWC. A homozygous mutation (E40K) in the superoxide dismutase 1 gene (SOD1a) has a strong association with the development of degenerative myelopathy. A second mutation (T18S or SOD1b mutation) has been exclusively found in Bernese Mountain dogs, and clinical disease has been reported in dogs that are homozygous for this mutation or are heterozygous for both mutations (compound heterozygote). Homozygous SOD1a/b mutation may be present in clinically normal dogs, indicating age-associated incomplete penetrance. The presence of a homozygous SOD1a/b mutation should be correlated with clinical history/neurologic examination, and magnetic resonance imaging and cerebrospinal fluid analysis are still considered the gold standard for excluding other potential causes of myelopathy.

Currently, there is no treatment for degenerative myelopathy. Rehabilitation can slow the progression of signs.

OUTCOME

Magnetic resonance imaging (MRI) in this case disclosed numerous chronic disc protrusions (Figure 12.2.1), most notable at T13-L1, but the degree of spinal cord compression was disproportionate to the dog's clinical signs, and nothing on MRI was lateralized to the left side. Based on the progression of clinical signs, age, breed, and lack of clear cause for the dog's signs on MRI, a presumptive diagnosis of degenerative myelopathy was made. Inflammatory etiologies were considered but thought to be improbable based on the progression of signs (chronic) and lack of abnormal contrast enhancement of the spinal cord or meninges on MRI. The dog was confirmed to be homozygous for the SOD1a mutation, confirming the clinical diagnosis of degenerative myelopathy. Over the subsequent 4 months, the dog deteriorated to a non-ambulatory status and was subsequently euthanized. The videos provided demonstrate the progression of degenerative myelopathy over the disease course.

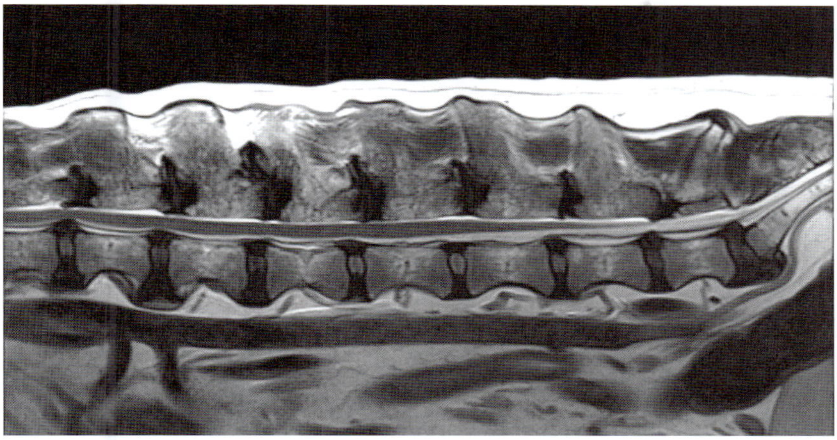

FIGURE 12.2.1 T2 sagittal MR image of an 8-year-old German shepherd. All intervertebral discs show a variable decrease in T2 signal, indicating degeneration/dehydration. Mild extradural compression can be seen at several levels, with the most notable compression at T13-L1. Proliferative osteophytosis of the lumbar articular processes can also be seen, although there is no associated compression of the spinal cord.

SUGGESTED READING

Awano, T., Johnson, G.S., Wade, C.M. et al. (2009). Genome-wide association analysis reveals a SOD1 mutation in canine degenerative myelopathy that resembles amyotrophic lateral sclerosis. *PNAS* 106 (8): 2794–2799.

Coates, J.R. and Wininger, F.A. (2010). Canine degenerative myelopathy. *Vet. Clin. North Am. Small Anim. Pract.* 40 (5): 929–950.

Gaitero, L., Nykamp, S., Daniel, R., and Monteith, G. (2013). Comparison between cranial thoracic intervertebral disc herniations in German Shepherd dogs and other large breed dogs. *Vet. Radiol. Ultrasound* 54 (2): 133–138.

Zeng, R., Coates, J.R., Johnson, G.C. et al. (2014). Breed distribution of SOD1 alleles previously associated with canine degenerative myelopathy. *J. Vet. Intern. Med.* 28 (2): 515–521.

CHAPTER 12.3

Pelvic Limb Ataxia, Paraparesis, and Paralysis

Case 3—Acute Paresis in a Cat

Anna Tauro

Access Specialty Animal Hospital, Pasadena, CA, USA

CASE HISTORY

A 7-year-old spayed female domestic long-haired cat was presented with a 48-hour history of acute progressive paraparesis and an inability to jump. The cat remained continent with respect to both urination and defecation throughout this period. The cat was up to date on vaccinations and preventive care. There was no history of trauma in association with the onset.

NEUROLOGICAL EXAMINATION (Video 12.3.1)

VIDEO 12.3.1 Neurological examination of a 7-year-old spayed female domestic long-haired cat, divided into "hands-off" and "hands-on" components. On hands-off assessment, the cat was bright and responsive, with ambulatory paraparesis, a long-strided gait, and pelvic limb general proprioceptive ataxia. On hands-on examination, postural reactions were severely reduced-to-absent in the pelvic limbs. Spinal reflexes were normal, although a crossed extensor reflex was present. Cranial nerve function was normal. Moderate discomfort was elicited on palpation of the mid-to-cranial thoracic vertebral column.

The neurological examination revealed a normal level of consciousness and behavior. The cat showed ambulatory paraparesis and pelvic limb general proprioceptive ataxia. The pelvic limb strides were long, and the cat tended to walk with a sloped back. Muscle mass was considered normal in all four limbs, with subjectively mildly increased extensor tone appreciated in the pelvic limbs. Postural reactions revealed severely reduced-to-absent paw placement and hopping responses in the pelvic limbs, more pronounced on the left side, while both tests were normal in the thoracic limbs. Spinal reflexes were present in all limbs, but a crossed-extensor reflex was noted in the pelvic limbs. The cutaneous trunci reflex was absent bilaterally. Tail movement and the perineal reflex were intact. Moderate discomfort was noted upon palpation of the mid-to-cranial thoracic vertebral column. Cranial nerve assessment was normal.

Note: Performing at least two postural reaction tests in an animal with spinal disease aids in assessing various components of the nervous system, including proprioceptive and motor pathways, and can help detect subtle deficits that might not be apparent with a single test.

1. **Where is the likely lesion localization?**
2. **What major disease processes should be considered?**
3. **What tests could you perform to help determine the diagnosis?**

LESION LOCALIZATION

Neuroanatomical localization was determined to be a T3–L3 spinal cord segment myelopathy. The normality of thoracic limb testing typically rules out an issue cranial to T3. This leaves three possible lesion localizations for a patient exhibiting solely pelvic limb dysfunction while retaining the perineal reflex: T3–L3 myelopathy, L4–S1 myelopathy, and a lesion affecting the nerve roots or the nerves emerging from the L4–S1 region of the spinal cord to provide innervation to the muscles of the pelvic limbs. Patients with L4–S1 myelopathies or radiculopathies/neuropathies exhibit lower motor neuron signs, including a short-strided gait, decreased muscle tone, and reduced or absent spinal reflexes. As these features were not observed in this cat, a lesion affecting L4–S1 or the nerves emerging from this region can be ruled out, supporting the remaining possibility of a T3–L3 myelopathy. A T3–L3 lesion localization is supported in this patient by the observation of long pelvic limb strides, which occur due to upper motor neuron dysfunction, the general proprioceptive ataxia, which occurs due to impedance of sensory projections coursing cranially through the spinal cord, the increased extensor tone, and intact pelvic limb reflexes. The sinking of the trunk in this cat suggests truncal weakness, further supporting a potential issue in the thoracic or lumbar spinal cord segments (T3–L3) or in their associated peripheral nerves, which innervate trunk-supporting muscles.

CAUTION: The cutaneous trunci reflex in cats can be unreliable when tested in a hospital setting, indicating the potential impact of stress. It should always be interpreted in the context of other neurological findings.

Note: The crossed extensor reflex is part of the normal supporting system of the animal when standing; if one limb is flexed, increased support is required of the opposite limb. This is considered an abnormal reflex if not standing. In the normal recumbent animal, the extensor response is inhibited, but if present, it indicates a lesion in ipsilateral descending pathways or upper motor neuron (UMN) disease, as these motor pathways arising in the brain normally descend in the spinal cord to regulate and predominantly inhibit lower motor neuron function. It is not a reliable indicator of severity.

WHAT MAJOR DISEASE PROCESSES SHOULD BE CONSIDERED?

Degenerative – Acute Disc Disease

Intervertebral Disc Extrusion (IVDE or Hansen Type I) Intervertebral disc extrusion (IVDE) is a potential differential diagnosis in this case. Intervertebral disc disease (IVDD), encompassing both Hansen type I and type II, has been sporadically reported in cats, with occurrences increasing with age and body weight. However, IVDE rather than intervertebral disc protrusion is typically the cause of presenting signs of myelopathy and is often associated with severe neurological signs in cats, which can be progressive.

Presumptive intramedullary IVDE has been reported in cats. This disc type is thought to share a similar pathophysiology with acute non-compressive nucleus pulposus extrusions (ANNPE; see below), where excessive force on intervertebral discs results in a high-velocity extrusion of a fragment of non-degenerate nucleus pulposus into the vertebral canal. The clinical signs are peracute or acute non-progressive and often lateralizing, which is similar to ANNPEs and ischemic myelopathies.

Acute Non-compressive Nucleus Pulposus Extrusion (ANNPE)

ANNPE is typically associated with an acute or peracute onset of non-progressive clinical signs, sometimes following a traumatic event, such as a road traffic accident or a fall from height. However, this condition is also observed in dogs and cats without a history of trauma. It is characterized by a poorly understood process in which a small tear in the annulus fibrosus develops, such that there is a small opening through which healthy, hydrated nucleus pulposus material can extrude through with high pressure and high velocity (think of water emerging from a garden hose in which the opening is partially occluded by one's thumb). This process leads to spinal cord contusion with minimal compression. Cats may or may not show signs of spinal hyperesthesia. The progressive nature of this cat's signs makes ANNPE a less likely differential diagnosis.

Trauma: Vertebral Fracture and/or Luxations

Although vertebral fractures and luxations often present acutely, the clinical history in this case does not suggest external trauma; however, it still cannot be completely ruled out. Animals involved in vehicle-related accidents are frequently assumed to have multiple traumatic injuries, so a thorough neurological examination should be approached cautiously to avoid exacerbating any vertebral instability. See Chapter 15 for more information on vertebral column trauma.

> **Note:** In animals struck by a vehicle, a lack of deep pain perception (nociception) often indicates a poor prognosis due to the high-impact trauma involved.

Vascular

Saddle Thrombus or Feline Aortic Thromboembolism (FATE)

Feline aortic thromboembolism (FATE) is the most common cause of acute paraparesis, paraplegia, and severe pain in cats. It can occur at any age, with over 70% of affected cats being male. The condition can result from cardiogenic causes (such as hypertrophic cardiomyopathy), non-cardiogenic causes (such as coagulopathies or metastatic disease), or unknown factors. In FATE, a thromboembolus becomes lodged in the aortic bifurcation, which is located in the caudal lumbar region. This leads to a lack of blood supply to the pelvic limbs, causing an ischemic neuromyopathy. Skin sensation is reduced to absent due to the ischemia, which affects not only the musculature (in particular, the distal muscles such as the cranial tibial muscle) but also the peripheral nerve fibers. Affected muscles might appear firm and cold on palpation, which the animal perceives as painful. Spinal reflexes are reduced to absent. The femoral pulses are diminished to absent, and the nailbeds and/or footpads are cyanotic. Because of the common cardiac origin in cats, dyspnea, heart murmur, gallop sound, or arrhythmias may be present.

This condition is an unlikely differential diagnosis for this cat, given the cat's lesion localization is a T3–L3 myelopathy. Cats with FATE display pelvic limb dysfunction that resembles L4–S1 myelopathies.

Ischemic Myelopathy (IM)

Ischemic myelopathy is a consequence of spinal cord vasculature occlusion and resultant infarction of the territory supplied. IM has characteristic clinical and magnetic resonance imaging (MRI) features, yet histopathology is required for a definitive diagnosis. Fibrocartilaginous embolic myelopathy (FCEM) is the most common cause of IM, although other causes include embolization of thrombi, parasitic or septic emboli, vasculopathy, and hypercoagulable state. In cats, potential risk factors predisposing to thrombosis or embolization include hyaline arteriopathy, chronic kidney disease (CKD), hypertension, cardiomyopathy, and hyperthyroidism.

Feline IM could be considered in this case, as it occurs in older cats and has a peracute-to-acute onset. However, this condition is a non-progressive, non-painful myelopathy with a predilection for the cervical spinal cord segments. A feline-specific condition called hyaline arteriopathy leads to hyaline deposition in the cervical spinal cord arterial walls, which leads to luminal narrowing/occlusion of the basilar or ventral spinal artery.

- **Fibrocartilaginous embolic myelopathy (FCEM)**
  FCEM, as a cause of IM, is a condition in which a piece of fibrocartilage, presumably from a regional intervertebral disc, becomes dislodged and embolizes into a nearby blood vessel supplying a region of the spinal cord. This process leads to peracute, nonprogressive, and often lateralized signs of a myelopathy. Although animals may display evidence of pain or discomfort at the time of the embolic event, FCEM is not associated with subsequent signs of pain. The progressive component of this cat's myelopathy makes FCEM less likely.

Inflammatory Spinal Cord Disease

Inflammatory diseases of the meninges and central nervous system (CNS), whether sterile or infectious in origin, can cause an acute-onset myelopathy, with clinical signs being progressive and dependent on the location of the inflammatory process. Examples of infectious diseases include bacterial spinal epidural empyema, feline infectious peritonitis (FIP), and protozoal, rickettsial, algal, and fungal diseases.

- **Protozoal myelitis**
  Toxoplasma gondii infection can cause a focal or disseminated myelopathy in cats. Although a subacute or chronic clinical cause is often seen, disseminated or progressive multifocal neurological signs of protozoal infection can also present acutely. In cats, *T. gondii* infection can result in an acute onset of paresis or proprioceptive ataxia, depending on the location of the spinal cord lesion, which may be focal or diffuse and can be restricted to the spinal cord only in some cats.
- **Feline infectious peritonitis virus myelitis**
  Most cats with FIP are under 3 years old, though cats of any age can contract the disease. Clinical signs vary depending on lesion distribution and may include vague signs indicating multiple organ involvement, such as fever, weight loss, dullness, and loss of appetite. Neurological signs often develop slowly but can also appear suddenly, presenting as focal, diffuse, or multifocal issues and sometimes occurring without systemic symptoms. Signs of spinal cord involvement related to FIP may include paresis, proprioceptive ataxia, and paraspinal hyperesthesia. Cats often show signs of intracranial disease like central vestibular dysfunction and obtundation, reflecting brain involvement in most neurological cases.

  FIP is a common feline viral disease caused by a mutated form of the widespread feline enteric coronavirus (FeCoV). It is an immune complex disease involving the virus, antibodies, and complement. FIP can present in two forms: non-effusive (dry) and effusive (wet). CNS involvement, including the spinal cord, is most frequent with the dry, pyogranulomatous form, although it can occur with the wet form. Histological findings in the CNS include granulomatous inflammation of the meninges, periventricular ependymal cells, and choroid plexus of the brain. Spinal cord pathology may include hydromyelia and myelitis.

Neoplasia

Neoplasia affecting the vertebrae, encroaching into the vertebral canal, or emerging from the spinal cord itself can all cause myelopathy with variable degrees of associated pain or discomfort. Although neoplasia can have a more chronic and insidious onset, acute signs are also possible. For example, feline lymphoma is often referred to as the "great pretender" due to its potential to present with acute clinical signs. This characteristic makes lymphoma a key differential diagnosis in cases with an acute onset of signs. In cats, lymphoma of the nervous system accounts for 13% of all lymphomas, most commonly as a secondary event in a multicentric neoplastic disease. It represents the most common tumor affecting the spinal cord (38.8%), followed by vertebral osteosarcoma (16.5%).

Feline lymphoma can occur at any age and is commonly associated with spinal hyperesthesia and progressive neurological deficits. A recent study of 27 cats with spinal lymphoma found that the most frequent neurological signs were rapidly progressive paraparesis (62 9%) or paraplegia (22.2%), with pain being present in 1/3 of cases. A bimodal age distribution was found with 40.7% of cats aged ≤2.5 years (63.6% of them FeLV positive), and 44.4% of cats aged ≥8 years (16.7% of them FeLV positive).

WHAT TESTS COULD YOU PERFORM TO HELP DETERMINE THE DIAGNOSIS?

Acute Disc Disease

Intervertebral Disc Extrusion (IVDE or Hansen Type I)

Radiographic studies can reveal narrowed intervertebral disc (IVD) spaces and mineralized IVDs; however, radiographs alone are insufficient for diagnosing IVDE. Myelography, which consists of the administration of non-ionic contrast media into the subarachnoid space, typically administered between L4–L5 or L5–L6, provides additional detail by aiding in the detection of extradural spinal cord compression and can confirm the side to which material has extruded. With the advent of computed tomography (CT) and MRI, myelography is now rarely performed. CT and CT myelography are generally sensitive for the diagnosis of IVDE, but are less sensitive in small-sized animals. Thus, CT and CT myelography would be inferior to MRI for diagnosing IVDE in this cat while MRI is considered a more sensitive and safer diagnostic method. Due to the often-severe nature of the signs in feline patients, surgical decompression via hemilaminectomy is frequently necessary, typically leading to a good to excellent recovery. The precise identification of the location of compressive extradural material is vital to the success of surgical therapy (Figure 12.3.1C and D). Furthermore, MRI can confirm an intramedullary extrusion, which is less amenable to surgical treatment (Figure 12.3.1E and F).

Acute Non-compressive Nucleus Pulposus Extrusion (ANNPE)

MRI is the preferred diagnostic tool for identifying ANNPE. Typical MRI findings include a focal intramedullary hyperintensity on T2W images (T2WI) observed over the IVD space, associated with a small amount of material in the epidural space and minimal or absent spinal cord compression. The nucleus pulposus shows reduced volume compared with adjacent discs, yet remains hyperintense on T2WI, supporting its hydrated state. In cases of ANNPE, an ill-defined hyperintensity on T2WI in the epaxial muscles, likely due to contusion, edema, or hemorrhage, may also be observed if related to trauma or due to muscular inflammation and degeneration secondary to disc disease. Since ANNPE is a nonsurgical condition, most cases respond well to supportive treatment, resulting in favorable outcomes.

Trauma: Vertebral Fracture and/or Luxation

The thoracolumbar junction (T10–L2) is a common site for vertebral column fractures, but imaging the entire vertebral column, as well as the chest and abdomen, is crucial for a comprehensive assessment of injury extent. CT is often preferred for its detailed visualization of spinal structures and reduced need for patient manipulation. MRI is preferred to rule out extradural and intramedullary pathology in relation to the vertebral column lesions. Prognosis varies, with a poorer outcome for cats lacking pain sensation in the affected limbs, indicating severe spinal cord injury. See Chapter 15 for more information on spinal trauma.

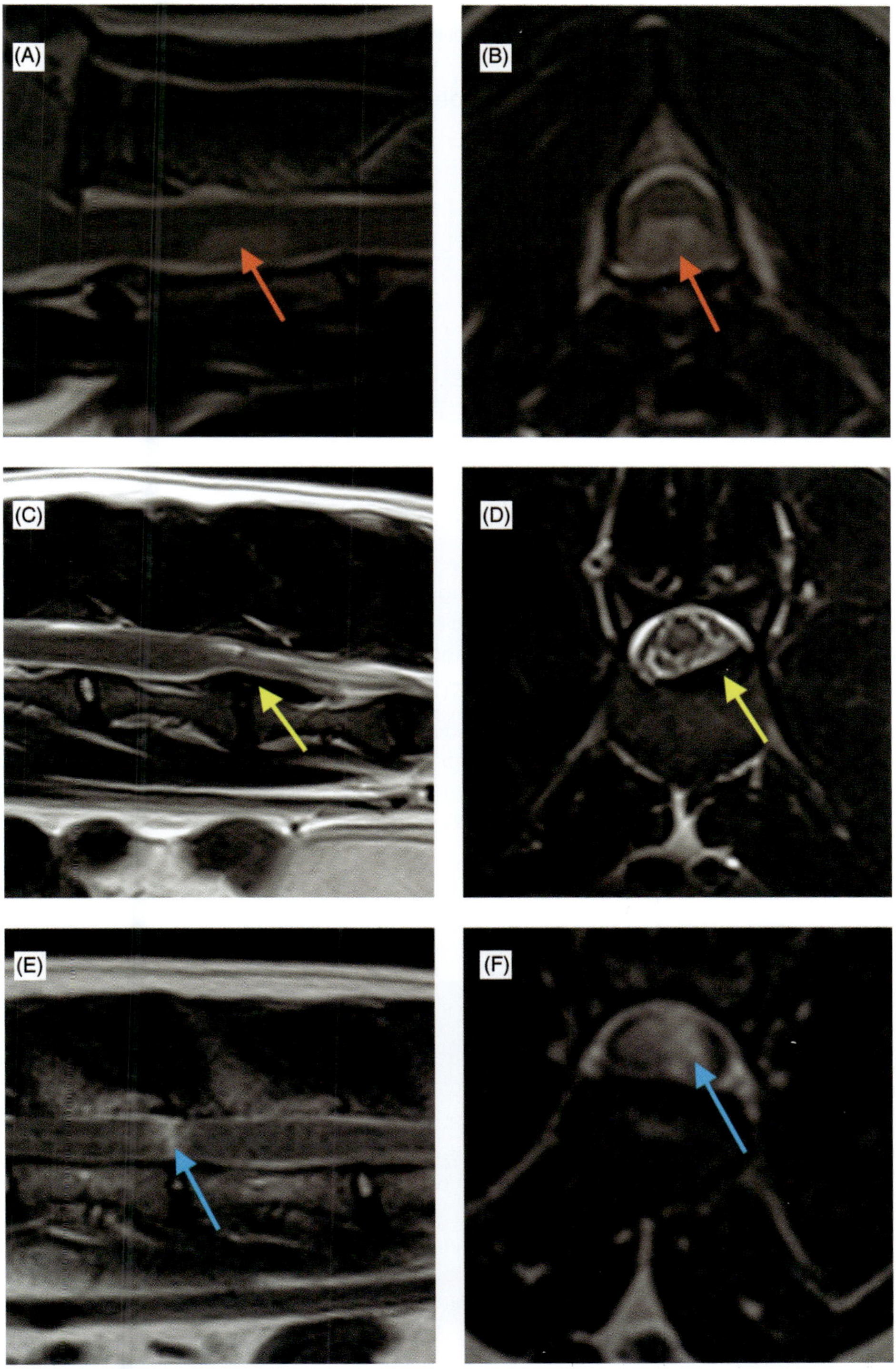

FIGURE 12.3.1 MR images of acute onset feline spinal cord diseases. (A) Sagittal and (B) transverse T2W images at the level of the cranial cervical spinal cord of a 16-year-old domestic short-haired cat with tetraplegia. A ventral midline hyperintense intramedullary lesion (red arrows) is noted over the C2 vertebral body. This lesion is compatible with ischemic myelopathy secondary to ventral spinal artery disease (hyaline arteriopathy). (C) Sagittal and (D) transverse T2W images at the level of the caudal lumbar vertebral column of an 8-year-old domestic short-haired cat with ambulatory painful paraparesis. A ventral hypointense extradural lesion (yellow arrows) is noted over the narrowed L4–L5 disc space on the left ventrolateral aspect of the spinal cord. The lesion is compatible with an intervertebral disc extrusion. (E) Sagittal and (F) transverse T2W images at the level of the caudal lumbar vertebral column of a 7-year-old domestic short-haired cat with paraplegia. A linear hyperintense intramedullary lesion (blue arrows) is noted above the disc space of L4–L5, which itself exhibits a reduced nucleus pulposus size. The lesion is compatible with an intramedullary intervertebral disc extrusion.

Saddle Thrombus or Feline Aortic Thromboembolism (FATE)

The "5P rule" can aid in the diagnosis of FATE on physical examination:

1. Pallor (e.g. cyanotic or pale toes),
2. Polar/poikilothermy (e.g. cold extremities),
3. Pulselessness,
4. Paralysis/paresis, and
5. Pain.

Other diagnostic aids include the absence of Doppler flow in the affected limb, direct visualization of a thrombus on ultrasound (Figure 12.3.2), infrared thermal imaging, or angiography. Additionally, low glucose or high lactate levels in the affected limb(s) compared with the normal limbs can be indicative of the condition. Medical management of the acute phase of ischemic neuromyopathy comprises the following:

- Anticoagulants (e.g. unfractionated or low-molecular weight heparins, warfarin, rivaroxaban, and apixaban). Rivaroxaban and apixaban are two of the newest groups of anticoagulant medications, which include direct factor Xa inhibitors and direct thrombin inhibitors known as direct small molecule inhibitors.
- Antithrombotics (e.g. clopidogrel, aspirin). Clopidogrel (2–4 mg/kg every 24 hours) is recommended over aspirin due to evidence of superior platelet inhibition compared to aspirin. Clopidogrel administration has also been associated with a significantly reduced likelihood of recurrent arterial thromboembolism compared to aspirin, with a longer median time to recurrence.

The prognosis for cats is typically poor, with 26–66% of cats euthanized in the acute phase, a reported rate of survival to discharge of 0–50% and a 6-month recurrence rate of 45–75%. Only 2%

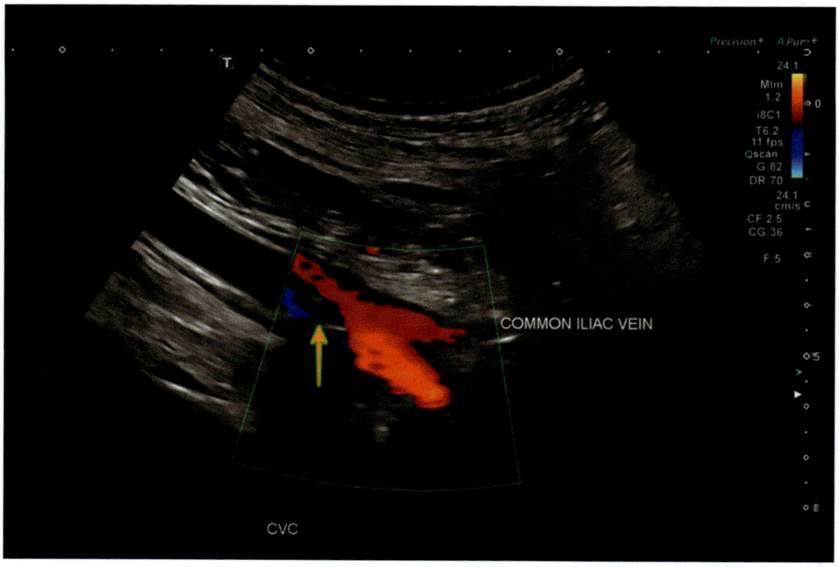

FIGURE 12.3.2 An Ultrasound image depicting an internal iliac arterial thrombus in a cat (yellow arrow), characterized by hyperechoic material obstructing blood flow within the vessel lumen.

of 250 cats in one study survived over a year. Low rectal temperature, bradycardia, and multiple limb involvement have all been associated with decreased survival rate in cats. Surgical aortic thrombectomy may be considered as a treatment option for cats with FATE, particularly when timely presentation allows for early intervention. Cats undergoing surgical aortic thrombectomy for FATE showed a 53.8% survival rate to discharge, with 71.4% of survivors achieving full recovery of limb motor function.

Ischemic Myelopathy (IM) and Fibrocartilaginous Embolic Myelopathy (FCEM)

IM is typically associated with exercise, trauma, or concurrent disorders, including renal disease, hyperthyroidism, hypertension, and hypertrophic cardiomyopathy. The diagnosis of IM is based on a combination of clinical signs, intramedullary T2-w hyperintensity on MRI (Figure 12.3.1A and B), and a normal to neutrophilic cerebrospinal fluid analysis.

While FCEM is a recognized cause of acute spinal cord infarction in both feline and canine patients, other potential causes of vascular occlusion should be considered in cats, including bacterial, parasitic, neoplastic, vasculopathies, or hypercoagulable states. Therefore, it is recommended to investigate feline patients thoroughly and address any underlying disorders.

The long-term prognosis is favorable in most cases. However, in feline patients, the extent and severity of the lesion or concurrent systemic disorders may lead to poor recovery, recurrence of clinical signs, and ultimately euthanasia.

Inflammatory Spinal Cord Disease

- **Protozoal Myelitis**
  MRI findings include multifocal lesions within the spinal cord and other regions of the CNS, while CSF analysis typically shows a mixed cell or mononuclear pleocytosis with an elevated protein concentration. While serology for *T. gondii* antibodies is often positive, it is essential to consider that this may indicate recent exposure rather than active infection. Marked antibody elevations, particularly of immunoglobulin (Ig)M in the case of *T. gondii*, alongside consistent clinical signs and exclusion of common differentials, can be used to make a presumptive antemortem diagnosis. Polymerase chain reaction (PCR) of the CSF, in combination with diagnostic imaging, CSF analysis, and serology, can be used to confirm the diagnosis.

  Early treatment for at least 4 weeks with combinations of trimethoprim-sulfadiazine or ormetoprim-sulfadimethoxine and clindamycin may improve clinical signs. Pyrimethamine may be added to the regimen, but it can cause bone marrow suppression in young animals. Early antibiotic treatment may improve clinical signs, but recovery is often incomplete.

- **Feline infectious peritonitis virus myelitis**
  Confirmation of FIP antemortem is very difficult. Hematological findings are not specific but can include leukocytosis with lymphopenia and neutrophilia, accompanied by mild to moderate anemia. Hyperglobulinemia is reported in up to 90% of cats with FIP. Many cats with FIP (up to 63%) also have hyperbilirubinemia. FCoV-specific tests include antibody testing and FCoV detection by reverse transcriptase PCR assay (RT-PCR). Serum tests for anti-coronavirus antibodies are often positive but have low specificity. In addition, a negative serum titer (i.e. a complete absence of antibody) does not exclude the possibility of FIP-associated neurological disease because soluble antibodies can form immune complexes and escape detection by standard tests. Detecting high levels of FCoV RNA in blood, effusion, tissue, and/or aqueous humor by RT-PCR can be highly supportive of a diagnosis of FIP FCoV. CSF analysis can also contribute to the diagnosis; however, the risk of CSF collection

must be weighed against the potential benefits, especially if there is a suggestion of increased intracranial pressure based on clinical signs and/or imaging findings. Results of CSF analysis are variable. The characteristic finding is a marked neutrophilic to pyogranulomatous pleocytosis, with cell counts often in the hundreds, and an associated increase in protein concentration to >200 mg/dL. However, the CSF can be normal, show a mild mononuclear pleocytosis, or have a normal cell count with an elevated protein concentration. Positive CSF titers can be a useful antemortem indicator of neurological disease, but must be interpreted with respect to the integrity of the blood–brain barrier. More recently, RT-PCR assays for feline coronavirus RNA and immunostaining of FCoV antigen in CSF samples have proven useful in supporting a diagnosis of neurological FIP.

MRI evidence of ventriculomegaly and ependymal and meningeal contrast enhancement of the brain can be used to support a diagnosis of FIP in cats that present with clinical signs of a myelopathy. Biopsy confirmation of FIP viral antigen in infected tissue is the only method to diagnose FIP definitively, which is usually not feasible with spinal cord parenchymal lesions.

The aims of treatment should focus on modifying the cat's immune response and inhibiting the viral replication. The use of corticosteroids can provide some palliative treatment; however, the disease will continue to progress, and some cats with FIP may only survive for days to months from the time of diagnosis without further treatment. Recent developments in antiviral therapy have changed the fatal outcome of FIP to a more favorable prognosis if the cats survive the first 48 hours after presentation.

- *The antiviral compound GS-441524*, a nucleoside analog and active metabolite of remdesivir (GS-5734), has been most widely studied in cats with FIP and has shown promising results for treating and controlling the disease. Survival rates range from 55% to 100%, but are on the lower side in cats with neurological involvement. A 42-day treatment course appears to be as effective as the commonly recommended treatment duration of 84 days.
- *Remdesivir* is the prodrug of GS-441524, which is painful on subcutaneous injection and cost-prohibitive for many cat owners. Therefore, a compounded oral version is often used, which has a good bioavailability in cats compared to other species; 80–90% of cats survive more than 6 months with this treatment. An intravenous formulation is also available with documented clinical success.
- *Unlicensed antiviral molnupiravir (EIDD-2801)* is an antiviral prodrug that is orally bioavailable and appears to be another effective treatment for cats with FIP, either as a first-line therapy or as a rescue therapy when the patient fails treatment with remdesivir. Survival with this drug has been documented to be 80–90% for effusive FIP.

Neoplasia Affecting the Vertebral Column, Canal, or Spinal Cord

Vertebral column radiographs and CT imaging can detect vertebral lysis, fractures, and bone destruction from tumors, but MRI remains superior for evaluating spinal cord tumors. Feline spinal lymphoma shows variable, nonspecific MRI findings, typically as ill-defined, enhancing masses with meningeal and nerve root involvement (Figure 12.3.3). Lesions commonly affect the thoracic and lumbosacral regions, involving extradural, intradural, or intramedullary spaces. They may extend to extraneural tissues with paravertebral masses extending into the vertebral canal or with vertebral involvement that spares the cortical bone.

CSF analysis may reveal an elevated cell count and detect tumor cells, especially in cases with lymphoma. Diagnosis usually requires tissue sampling via CT- or fluoroscopy-guided aspiration or biopsy, with molecular diagnostics or immunohistochemistry aiding differentiation from other spinal tumors.

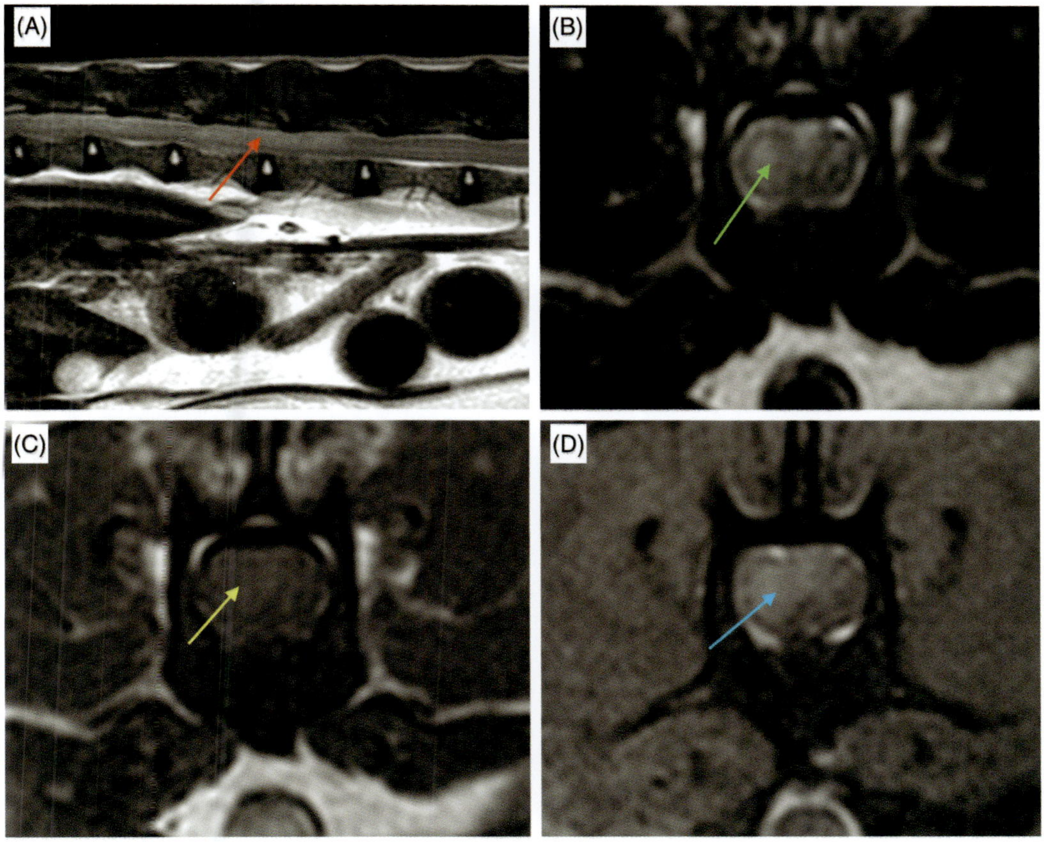

FIGURE 12.3.3 A sagittal T2W (A), transverse T2W (B), T1W (C), and T1W post-contrast (D) with fat saturation MRI of the thoracolumbar vertebral column of a 14-year-old cat with chronic progressive paraparesis. There is an extensive, ill-defined, and irregular intramedullary hyperintensity over several vertebral bodies (red arrow), which is predominantly right-sided (green arrow) and is mildly T1W hyperintense (yellow arrow) to normal cord, with diffuse moderate contrast enhancement (blue arrow). Pathology confirmed lymphoma.

Feline nervous system lymphoma is typically treated with surgical decompression (for histopathological confirmation), chemotherapy, and/or radiation therapy. Outcomes depend on the disease stage and treatment response, with early intervention improving quality of life; however, prognosis is poor in advanced cases with one study documenting a mean 4.5-month survival.

OUTCOME

The cat described in this case underwent an MRI of the thoracolumbar vertebral column, which identified an intradural-intramedullary lesion over the cranial thoracic vertebrae. Lumbar CSF revealed an elevated cell count, with 100% lymphocytes that were morphologically abnormal and the cat was diagnosed with lymphoma. The cat progressed rapidly despite chemotherapy.

SUGGESTED READING

Chow, K., Beatty, J.A., Voss, K., and Barrs, V.R. (2012). Probable lumbar acute non-compressive nucleus pulposus extrusion in a cat with acute onset paraparesis. *J. Feline Med. Surg.* 14 (10): 764–767.

Coggins, S.J., Govendir, M., Norris, J.M. et al. (2025). Pharmacokinetics of GS-441524 following intravenous remdesivir in six cats and results of therapeutic drug monitoring during treatment of feline infectious peritonitis: 22 cases (2021-2024). *J. Small Anim. Pract.* 66 (7): 495–506.

Cosaro, E., Pires, J., Castillo, D. et al. (2023). Efficacy of oral remdesivir compared to GS-441524 for treatment of cats with naturally occurring effusive feline infectious peritonitis: a blinded, non-inferiority study. *Viruses* 15 (8): 1680.

De Decker, S., Warner, A.-S., and Volk, H.A. (2017). Prevalence and breed predisposition for thoracolumbar intervertebral disc disease in cats. *J. Feline Med. Surg.* 19 (4): 419–423.

Durand, A., Keenihan, E., Schweizer, D. et al. (2022). Clinical and magnetic resonance imaging features of lymphoma involving the nervous system in cats. *J. Vet. Intern. Med.* 36 (2): 679–693.

Eberlé, O., Pouzot-Nevoret, C., Thomas-Cancian, A. et al. (2022). Ultrasonographic findings of feline aortic thromboembolism. *J. Feline Med. Surg.* 24 (12): e588–e594.

Felten, S. and Hartmann, K. (2019). Diagnosis of feline infectious peritonitis: a review of the current literature. *Viruses* 11 (11): 1068.

Gokalsing, E., Ferrolho, J., Gibson, M.S. et al. (2025). Efficacy of GS-441524 for feline infectious peritonitis: a systematic review (2018-2024). *Pathogens* 14 (7): 717.

Guillaumin, J. (2024). Feline aortic thromboembolism: recent advances and future prospects. *J. Feline Med. Surg.* 26 (6): 1098612X241257878.

Guillaumin, J., DeFrancesco, T.C., Scansen, B.A. et al. (2022). Bilateral lysis of aortic saddle thrombus with early tissue plasminogen activator (BLASTT): a prospective, randomized, placebo-controlled study in feline acute aortic thromboembolism. *J. Feline Med. Surg.* 24 (12): e535–e545.

Heaselgrave, T., De Risio, L., Domínguez, E. et al. (2025). Presumptive intramedullary intervertebral disc extrusion in 12 cats: clinical presentation, MRI findings, treatment and outcome. *J. Feline Med. Surg.* 27 (7): 1098612X251349712.

Jeffery, N.D. (2010). Vertebral fracture and luxation in small animals. *Vet. Clin. North Am. Small Anim. Pract.* 40 (5): 809–828.

Kennedy, M.A. (2020). Feline infectious peritonitis: update on pathogenesis, diagnostics, and treatment. *Vet. Clin. North Am. Small Anim. Pract.* 50 (5): 1001–1011.

Klainbart, S., Kelmer, E., Vidmayer, B. et al. (2014). Peripheral and central venous blood glucose concentrations in dogs and cats with acute arterial thromboembolism. *J. Vet. Intern. Med.* 28 (5): 1513–1519.

Knipe, M.F., Vernau, K.M., Hornof, W.J., and LeCouteur, R.A. (2001). Intervertebral disc extrusion in six cats. *J. Feline Med. Surg.* 3 (3): 161–168.

Li, J., Zhou, Y., Liu, Y. et al. (2025). Surgical treatment and outcomes in feline aortic thromboembolism: a retrospective study of 13 cats. *Front. Vet. Sci.* 12: 1618435.

Lorenzo, V., Ribeiro, J., Bernardini, M. et al. (2022). Clinical and magnetic resonance imaging features, and pathological findings of spinal lymphoma in 27 cats. *Front. Vet. Sci.* 9: 980414.

MacKay, A.D., Rusbridge, C., Sparkes, A.H., and Platt, S.R. (2005). MRI characteristics of suspected acute spinal cord infarction in two cats, and a review of the literature. *J. Feline Med. Surg.* 7 (2): 101–107.

Mella, S.L., Cardy, T.J., Volk, H.A., and De Decker, S. (2020). Clinical reasoning in feline spinal disease: which combination of clinical information is useful? *J. Feline Med. Surg.* 22 (6): 521–530.

Mikszewski, J.S., Van Winkle, T.J., and Troxel, M.T. (2006). Fibrocartilaginous embolic myelopathy in five cats. *J. Am. Anim. Hosp. Assoc.* 42 (3): 226–233

Paushter, A.M., Hague, D.W., Foss, K.D., and Sander, W.E. (2020). Assessment of the cutaneous trunci muscle reflex in neurologically abnormal cats. *J. Feline Med. Surg.* 22 (12): 1200–1205.

Pouzot-Nevoret, C., Barthélemy, A., Goy-Thollot, I. et al. (2018). Infrared thermography: a rapid and accurate technique to detect feline aortic thromboembolism. *J. Feline Med. Surg.* 20 (8): 780–785.

Reagan, K.L., Brostoff, T., Pires, J. et al. (2024). Open label clinical trial of orally administered molnupiravir as a first-line treatment for naturally occurring effusive feline infectious peritonitis. *J. Vet. Intern. Med.* 38 (6): 3087–3094.

Renner, K.A., Cattin, R., Kimble, B. et al. (2025). Efficacy of oral remdesivir in treating feline infectious peritonitis: a prospective observational study of 29 cats. *J. Feline Med. Surg.* 27 (5): 1098612X251335189.

Rossi, G., Stachel, A., Lynch, A.M., and Olby, N.J. (2020). Intervertebral disc disease and aortic thromboembolism are the most common causes of acute paralysis in dogs and cats presenting to an emergency clinic. *Vet. Rec.* 187 (10): e81.

Rylander, H., Eminaga, S., Palus, V. et al. (2014). Feline ischemic myelopathy and encephalopathy secondary to hyaline arteriopathy in five cats. *J. Feline Med. Surg.* 16 (10): 832–839.

Soteras, M.P., Dominguez, E., Suñol, A. et al. (2024). Spinal magnetic resonance imaging in cats: differences in clinical significance of intervertebral disk extrusion, intervertebral disk protrusion, and degenerative lumbosacral stenosis. *J. Am. Vet. Med. Assoc.* 262 (9): 1193–1200.

Tasker, S. (2018). Diagnosis of feline infectious peritonitis: Update on evidence supporting available tests. *J. Feline Med. Surg.* 20 (3): 228–243.

Taylor-Brown, F.E. and De Decker, S. (2017). Presumptive acute non-compressive nucleus pulposus extrusion in 11 cats: clinical features, diagnostic imaging findings, treatment and outcome. *J. Feline Med. Surg.* 19 (1): 21–26.

Theobald, A., Volk, H.A., Dennis, R. et al. (2013). Clinical outcome in 19 cats with clinical and magnetic resonance imaging diagnosis of ischaemic myelopathy (2000-2011). *J. Feline Med. Surg.* 15 (2): 132–141.

Tsai, C.-Y. and Chang, Y.-P. (2022). Assessment of the cutaneous trunci muscle reflex in healthy cats: comparison of results acquired by clinicians and cat owners. *J. Feline Med. Surg.* 24 (8): e163–e167.

Zuzzi-Krebitz, A.M., Buchta, K., Bergmann, M. et al. (2024). Short treatment of 42 days with oral GS-441524 results in equal efficacy as the recommended 84-day treatment in cats suffering from feline infectious peritonitis with effusion-a prospective randomized controlled study. *Viruses* 16 (7): 1144.

CHAPTER 12.4

Pelvic Limb Ataxia, Paraparesis, and Paralysis

Case 4—Acute Paraparesis in a Non-Chondrodystrophic Dog

Anna Tauro

Access Specialty Animal Hospital, Pasadena, CA, USA

CASE HISTORY

An 8-year-old spayed female golden retriever was presented with an acute onset of non-ambulatory paraparesis, more pronounced on the right side. The condition developed after the dog played with another dog in the household. Prior to the play event, the dog was reportedly normal. The dog whimpered when she was lifted into the car. The dog was up to date with vaccinations and preventive care.

NEUROLOGICAL EXAMINATION

A neurological examination, conducted within 3 hours of the onset, revealed a normal level of consciousness and behavior. The dog was non-ambulatory owing to pelvic limb dysfunction but able to take 10 consecutive steps unassisted using three limbs (both thoracic limbs and the left pelvic limb). She was unable to rise without assistance and showed a tendency to fall when turning. The dog exhibited paresis in the left pelvic limb and plegia in the right pelvic limb. Pelvic limb postural reactions revealed absent paw placement bilaterally, with hopping delayed in the left pelvic limb and absent in the right pelvic limb. The patellar reflex was present bilaterally. The flexor withdrawal reflex was slightly reduced in the left pelvic limb and absent in the right pelvic limb. Thoracic limb function and cranial nerve reflexes were normal. The cutaneous trunci reflex was absent caudal to the L4 vertebra, bilaterally. Tail movement and perineal reflex were intact. No discomfort was noted upon vertebral column palpation. Given lack of motor function in the right pelvic limb, nociception was evaluated in that limb and was confirmed to be intact. (Video 12.4.1)

VIDEO 12.4.1 Neurological examination of an 8-year-old spayed female golden retriever, divided into "hands-off" and "hands-on" components. On hands-off assessment, the dog was bright and responsive, with paresis in the left pelvic limb and plegia in the right pelvic limb. On hands-on examination, pelvic limb postural reactions showed absent paw placement bilaterally, with hopping delayed on the left and absent on the right. Patellar reflexes were present bilaterally. The flexor withdrawal reflex was slightly reduced in the left pelvic limb and absent in the right, with preservation of the remaining spinal reflexes. Cranial nerve function was normal, and no discomfort was elicited on spinal palpation.

> **Note:** Ambulatory status is defined as the ability to rise and take at least 10 consecutive weight-bearing steps using all limbs unassisted without falling.

1. **Where is the likely lesion localization?**
2. **What major disease processes should be considered?**
3. **What tests could you perform to help determine the diagnosis?**

LESION LOCALIZATION

Since only the pelvic limbs are affected, the lesion must be somewhere caudal to T3. The dog's reduced pelvic limb withdrawal reflexes may initially point to a focal lesion in the spinal cord (L6-S1) or the bilateral sciatic nerves. However, such a focal lesion in the spinal cord to cause only these signs without affecting adjacent regions to impact the patellar and perianal reflexes is uncommon. A more likely localization is a T3-L3 myelopathy with spinal shock.

Following spinal shock, the anal sphincter reflex usually recovers within 15 minutes of spinal cord injury in dogs, and the patellar reflex returns hours after injury, whereas the withdrawal reflex can take days to weeks to return.

Note: Acute spinal cord injuries in dogs can be associated with spinal shock, a reversible phenomenon characterized by the temporary loss of spinal reflexes and muscle tone in the pelvic limbs. Although spinal shock typically occurs with acute onset and severe lesions between T3 and L3, its presentation may resemble that of an L4–S3 lesion, complicating the neurolocalization.

CAUTION: To distinguish T3–L3 myelopathy with spinal shock from L4–S3 myelopathy, clinicians should:

1. **Monitor spinal reflexes over time** to identify transient loss, which is typical of spinal shock and gradually recovers as the spinal cord stabilizes.
2. **Evaluate the patellar and perianal reflexes**, as they return rapidly after spinal shock and the patellar reflex is more resilient to synaptic pathway disruptions.
3. **Assess the cutaneous trunci reflex**, which helps localize the lesion, typically located two vertebrae cranial to the site of the absent reflex.

Note: Ataxia is a neurological sign characterized by a lack of voluntary coordination of muscle movements. It can be appreciated in ambulatory dogs; however, in the case described, it was difficult to assess, as the dog was walking on three limbs. When present, ataxia signifies a lesion affecting the spinal cord due to involvement of ascending sensory projections carrying information about limb location and movement (kinesthesia) to the cerebral cortex.

WHAT MAJOR DISEASE PROCESSES SHOULD BE CONSIDERED?

Degenerative – Intervertebral Disc Disease (IVDD)

Acute Non-compressive Nucleus Pulposus Extrusion (ANNPE) There has been considerable variation in the terminology used historically to describe this condition, including: traumatic intervertebral disc (IVD) extrusion, IVD explosion, traumatic IVD prolapse, missile disks, high-velocity low-volume disc extrusion, and (Hansen) Type III IVDD. The term ANNPE has become widely accepted in the veterinary literature as the most descriptive terminology for this condition and is therefore used here.

Given the asymmetric signs, the acute onset, and the short-lasting pain, ANNPE is a strong differential diagnosis to consider. It can coincide with an external trauma, such as a road traffic accident or a fall from a height; however, reports have shown that at the onset, most dogs are exercising vigorously.

Neurological deficits in ANNPE cases typically do not progress beyond 24–48 hours from the initial presentation. In ANNPE, a small tear in the annulus fibrosus develops, allowing the hydrated nucleus pulposus material to extrude through this small opening with high pressure and high velocity. It impacts the spinal cord, effectively causing a "contusion." ANNPE can occur at any age, predominantly affecting non-chondrodystrophic dogs, and most often occurs between the T3 and L3 spinal cord segments, but any IVD can be affected. Dogs with ANNPE may exhibit transient, mild, or absent pain on palpation of the vertebral column.

Hansen Type I Intervertebral Disc Disease (IVDD) The acute onset of signs suggests IVD extrusion as a likely differential, though the extrusion would need to be quite lateralized in this case to cause the difference in severity between sides. Disc extrusions generally do not cause this degree of difference. Hansen Type I IVDD commonly affects young to middle-aged chondrodystrophic breeds like dachshunds, beagles, and poodles, but can occur, albeit less frequently, in non-chondrodystrophic breeds. This condition involves chondroid degeneration of the nucleus pulposus, leading to extrusion of material that compresses the spinal cord (see Case 1 in this chapter). Clinical signs include spinal pain often evidenced by an arched back posture (i.e. antalgic posture) and acute neurological deficits, which can range from paresis (partial loss of voluntary motor function) to paralysis (complete loss of voluntary motor function) of the limbs.

Acute thoracolumbar IVD extrusions can lead to multilevel epidural hemorrhage caused by laceration of the internal vertebral venous plexus. Sometimes, this hemorrhage can be substantial, resulting in multilevel spinal cord compression and forming a hematoma. The term disc extrusion with extensive epidural hemorrhage (DEEH) describes this specific phenomenon. Usually, affected dogs develop sudden paraparesis that quickly progresses to paraplegia, often accompanied by severe spinal pain. Most commonly, medium to large breeds, such as Pit Bull Terriers, American Staffordshire terriers, Labradors, German shepherds, and Rottweilers, are affected; however, small and giant breeds can also be susceptible.

Intradural/Intramedullary Intervertebral Disc Extrusion (IIVDE) While extruded nucleus pulposus material typically stays in the extradural space during IVD extrusion and ANNPE, there have been reports of nuclear material penetrating the dura mater. In such cases, the extruded material may remain extramedullary but within the intradural space or enter the spinal cord tissue itself, becoming intramedullary. The term "Intradural/Intramedullary Disc Extrusion" (IIVDE) describes these instances. IIVDE is a rare diagnosis. Most reported cases occur around the thoracolumbar junction, similar to ANNPE and Hansen Type I IVD extrusion. However, IIVDE has also been found in the cervical spinal cord region of dogs.

Hydrated Nucleus Pulposus Extrusion (HNPE) HNPE is a subtype of acute herniation involving a partially or nondegenerate nucleus pulposus, leading to varying degrees of extradural spinal cord compression. In dogs, reports of acute compressive HNPE usually describe well-hydrated extradural material over the IVD, indicating a connection with the annulus fibrosus and accompanying spinal cord compression. The exact cause of this herniation remains unclear, but it may be similar to ANNPE, where a small tear in the annulus fibrosus occurs after sudden increases in intradiscal pressure.

Most cases of canine HNPE documented in veterinary studies involve the cervical spinal cord region, suggesting a regional anatomical vulnerability that matches the typical clinical signs

Nonetheless, thoracolumbar HNPE has been observed in dogs, particularly in older, non-chondrodystrophic breeds. These cases often present with a nonprogressive, sudden onset, usually linked to trauma during exercise, and may show a lateralized clinical presentation, although bilateral dysfunction is more common.

Trauma: Vertebral Fracture and/or Luxations

Vertebral fractures and luxations typically present acutely, though this case lacks a history of trauma. In dogs with possible vehicle-related injuries, proceed cautiously with neurological exams to avoid worsening any instability. See Chapter 15 for more details on vertebral trauma.

Vascular: Fibrocartilaginous Embolic Myelopathy (FCEM)

This phenomenon likely arises from the embolization of fibrocartilaginous material originating from IVDs into arterial and/or venous structures within the spinal cord, leading to focal ischemic myelopathy. It can occur at any age but is most common in large non-chondrodystrophic breed dogs and can affect any region of the spinal cord.

The signs of FCEM are peracute, lateralized, and nonprogressive, resembling ANNPE. FCEM is a non-painful condition, although animals can exhibit signs of pain or discomfort at the time of embolization.

Neoplasia

Neoplasia affecting the vertebral column, canal, or spinal cord is more common in dogs over 5 years of age. Given the younger age and acute onset of neurological signs in this case, neoplasia is less likely but remains a differential diagnosis to consider, as neoplasia can cause acute pain and myelopathy. Tumors can be extradural, intradural-extramedullary, and intramedullary (Figure 12.4.1).

- Extradural tumors, generally affecting the vertebrae, are the most common location for neoplasia. Possible tumor types include osteosarcoma, chondrosarcoma, fibrosarcoma, and undifferentiated sarcoma. Hematopoietic tumors such as plasma cell tumors, lymphoma, and hemangiosarcoma can also lead to extradural tumors.

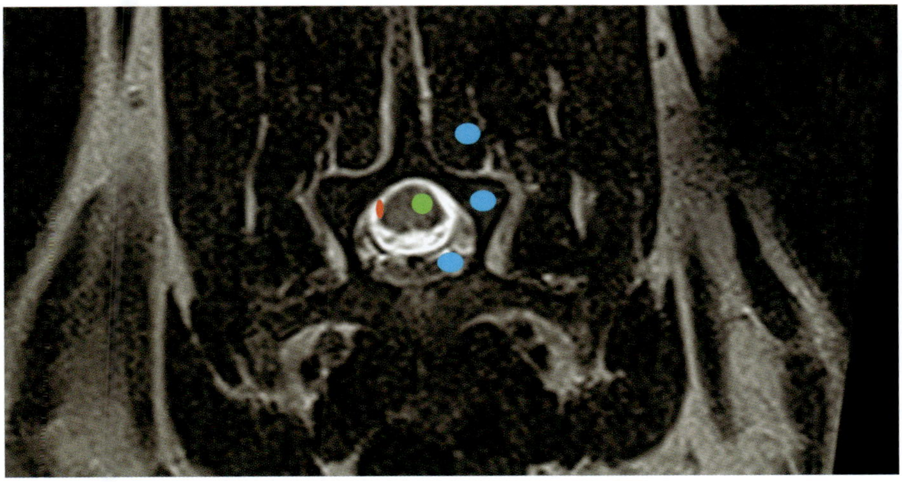

FIGURE 12.4.1 A transverse T2W MRI of a cervical vertebral body and associated spinal cord, illustrating the descriptive locations of neoplasia. Blue ovals = extradural (vertebral canal, vertebral bone, and paravertebral tissues); red oval = intradural-extramedullary; green oval = intramedullary.

- Intradural-extramedullary tumors arise from the meninges or nerve sheaths (meningiomas and nerve sheath tumors, respectively). Other tumors affecting this space include nephroblastomas in young dogs and round cell tumors such as lymphoma.
- Least commonly, intramedullary tumors within the spinal cord itself include gliomas, ependymomas, and round cell neoplasms.

Depending on the tumor location, affected animals may or may not exhibit pain. Extradural neoplasms that cause bony lysis generally lead to observable pain and can result in pathologic fractures that lead to acute neurological decline.

WHAT TESTS COULD YOU PERFORM TO HELP DETERMINE THE DIAGNOSIS?

Intervertebral Disc Disease (IVDD)

Acute Non-compressive Nucleus Pulposus Extrusion (ANNPE) ANNPE is best diagnosed with magnetic resonance imaging (MRI), showing a focal, asymmetric T2-weighted hyperintensity within the spinal cord near an IVD space and a small extradural lesion with minimal or no spinal cord compression. Additional findings include decreased T2-weighted signal of the nucleus pulposus and possible narrowing of the affected disc space (Figure 12.4.2). Gradient echo imaging may reveal an intramedullary hypointensity, indicating potential hemorrhage due to the traumatic disc extrusion. ANNPE is managed nonsurgically with rest, nursing care and medications for pain and inflammation. Intensive physical rehabilitation therapy should be considered early in the recovery process. The prognosis is generally favorable, particularly when nociception remains intact. One study reported that 75% of dogs without nociception eventually recovered nociception, although the presence of spinal shock at presentation is a poor prognostic indicator.

Hansen Type I Intervertebral Disc Disease (IVDD) Vertebral column radiographs and computed tomography (CT) are valuable tools for identifying mineralized discs within the vertebral canal and narrowing of IVD spaces caused by disc degeneration. Mineralized discs appear radiopaque

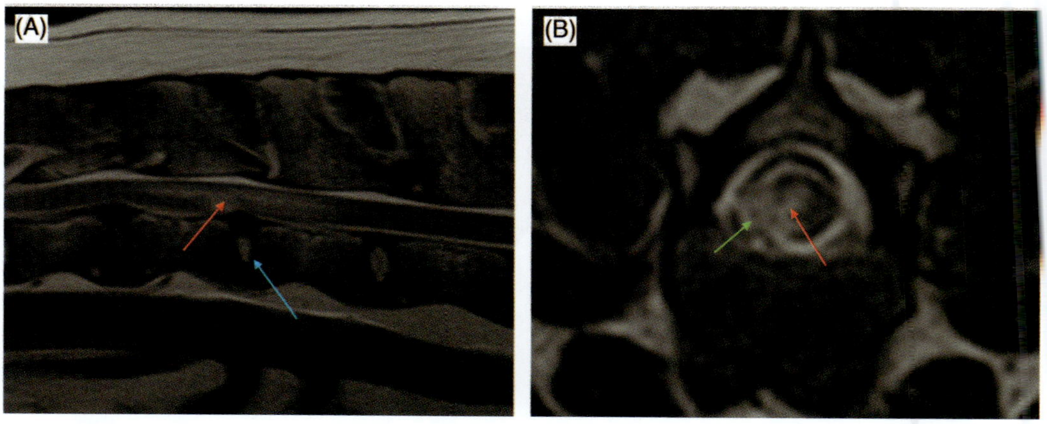

FIGURE 12.4.2 T2-weighted sagittal (A) and transverse (B) MR images of the thoracolumbar vertebral column in the dog in this case study with a T13–L1 acute non-compressive nucleus pulposus extrusion (ANNPE). The images demonstrate a focal, asymmetric T2 hyperintensity within the spinal cord (red arrows) at the level of the intervertebral disc, and a small extradural lesion with minimal to no spinal cord compression (green arrow). Notable features include decreased T2 signal intensity of the nucleus pulposus (blue arrow) and narrowing of the affected disc space, consistent with disc extrusion.

on radiographs and hyperattenuated on CT. Additional findings associated with IVDD include endplate sclerosis and spondylosis deformans.

> **Note**: Radiographs do not provide visualization of the contents of the vertebral canal; thus, the degree of spinal cord compression cannot be evaluated, nor can they be used to determine the side of extruded material. As a result, radiographic findings can suggest the possibility of IVD extrusion but are not diagnostic.

While myelography remains an option when MRI or CT is unavailable, its use has declined due to risks of associated neurological deterioration, as well as its inferior sensitivity and specificity compared to cross-sectional imaging. MRI is the most sensitive and specific modality for confirming compressive lesions, particularly in diagnosing noncalcified disc extrusions, distinguishing extrusions from protrusions, and assessing intramedullary changes that can impact prognosis. Greater T2-weighted intramedullary hyperintensity and HASTE subarachnoid signal loss are linked to worse outcomes.

Recovery is favorable, with the return of deep pain perception; however, fecal and urinary continence may not fully resolve in one-third of cases in which continence has been lost. Progressive myelomalacia (PMM) is a fatal complication that occurs in 10–17.5% of paraplegic dogs without pain perception, typically developing within 14 days of IVD extrusion. PMM is characterized by ischemic and hemorrhagic necrosis of the spinal cord, which progresses cranially and caudally from the initial site of extrusion. As the necrosis courses cranially, the cutaneous trunci reflex will be lost progressively further cranially over time. Eventually, when the necrosis reaches the cervicothoracic intumescence, lower motor neuron paralysis develops in the thoracic limbs, and respiratory paralysis follows shortly thereafter. On MRI, spinal cord swelling and intramedullary T2-weighted hyperintensity are concerning for the development of myelomalacia (Figure 12.4.3), but are not consistently predictive of the condition. Diagnosis of PMM is only possible post-mortem, but imaging and clinical findings guide early recognition, often necessitating euthanasia to prevent suffering.

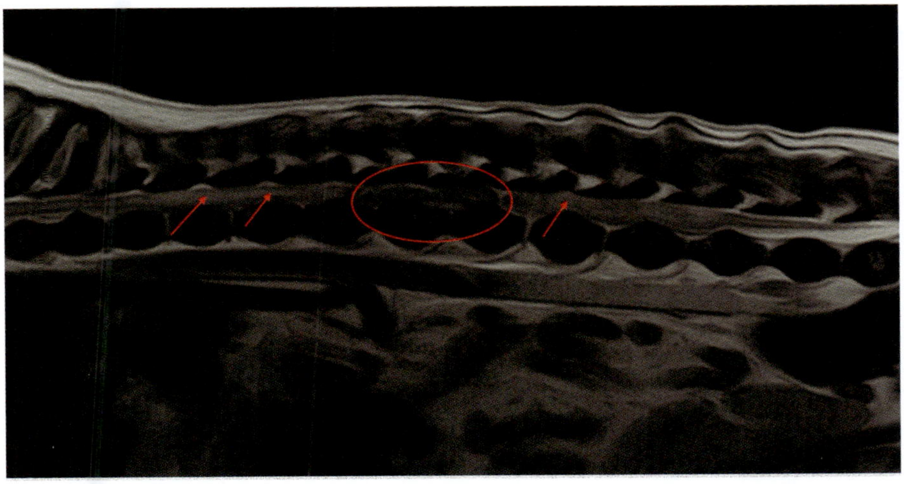

FIGURE 12.4.3 A T2W sagittal MR image of the thoracolumbar vertebral column of a 4-year-old male Dachshund with an acute onset of paraplegia with loss of nociception. There is extensive extradural compression of the cord associated with an intervertebral disc extrusion (oval) over L1–L3. Cranial and caudal to this lesion, there is diffuse intramedullary hyperintensity (red arrows), which was confirmed to be myelomalacia.

Intradural/Intramedullary Intervertebral Disc Extrusion (IIVDE) Due to the similar clinical presentations of dogs with intramedullary IVD extrusion (IIVDE), Hansen Type I IVD extrusion, or acute non-compressive nucleus pulposus extrusion (ANNPE; traumatic IVD extrusion), antemortem diagnosis relies heavily on precise interpretation of diagnostic imaging or surgical confirmation of intradural or intramedullary disc material. Early reports on IIVDE indicated that myelography could reveal intramedullary contrast, a "golf-tee" sign suggesting intradural-extramedullary material, or contrast leakage indicating a dural tear at the suspected extrusion site. More recent studies suggest that specific high-field MRI characteristics – such as intramedullary hypointensity on T2-weighted, T1-weighted, and gradient echo (T2*) images above a disc with decreased nucleus pulposus volume, as well as a linear tract extending from the IVD to the spinal cord (Figure 12.4.4) – may support an IIVDE diagnosis. Recently, a case series reported that CT-myelography was more effective than low-field MRI in diagnosing IIVDE due to its ability to accurately identify focal filling defects within the subarachnoid space from intradural-extramedullary disc material.

Further research is needed to assess outcomes of surgical and nonsurgical management in these rare cases. Accurate classification of degenerative versus nondegenerative IVD material may help determine whether subclassifying IIVDE types has clinical utility.

Hydrated Nucleus Pulposus Extrusion (HNPE) While the clinical presentation can strongly suggest a diagnosis of HNPE, differential diagnoses typically include IVDE, IIVDE, ANNPE, and fibrocartilaginous embolic myelopathy (FCEM). MRI, is the preferred modality for confirming HNPE. Reported MRI features characteristic of HNPE (Figure 12.4.5) include:

- Ventral, midline extradural material (T2 hyperintense, T1 hypointense) over the affected disc space
- Spinal cord compression, with or without intramedullary T2 hyperintensity
- A bilobed, "seagull"-shaped appearance of the extradural material
- Reduced volume of the T2 hyperintense nucleus pulposus signal in the affected disc

Although these MRI features are most commonly used to diagnose canine HNPE, a recent study indicates that contrast-enhanced CT can also effectively diagnose HNPE, with a sensitivity of 91% and a specificity of 100%.

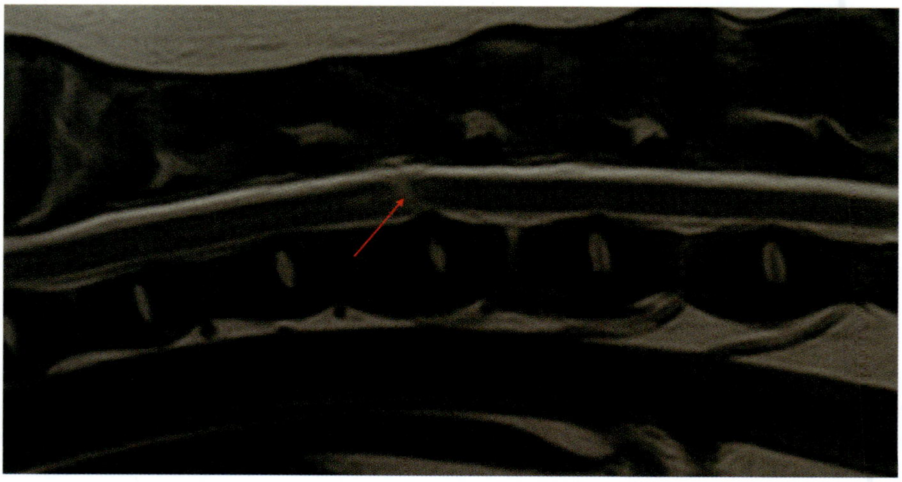

FIGURE 12.4.4 A T2W sagittal MR image of the thoracolumbar vertebral column of a 7-year-old Cocker spaniel with a linear intramedullary T2W hyperintensity (arrow) over the T12-T13 intervertebral disc space. This lesion was confirmed to be an intramedullary intervertebral disc extrusion.

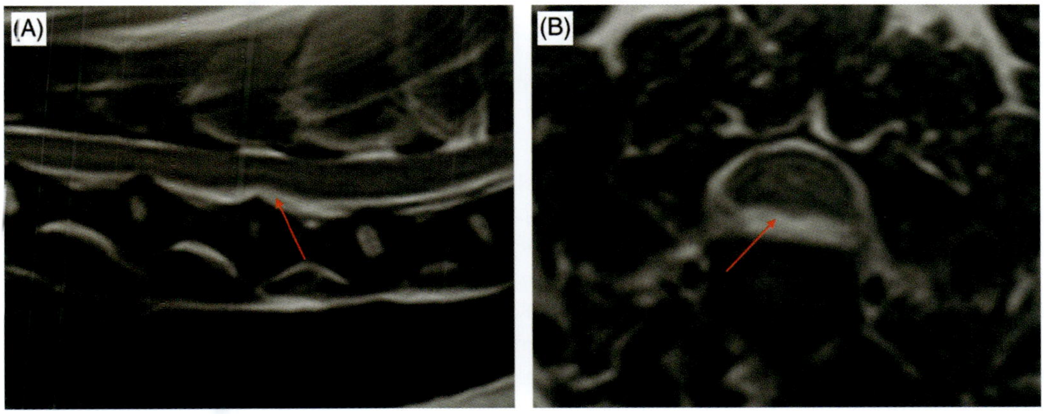

FIGURE 12.4.5 A T2W sagittal (A) and transverse (B) MR image of the cervical vertebral column of a 5-year-old mixed-breed dog with a hydrated nucleus pulposus extrusion. The lesion can be challenging to differentiate from ventral epidural fat signal on sagittal images, but on transverse images, a distinct ventral extradural bilobed "seagull" sign is often noted (arrow).

Trauma: Vertebral Fracture and/or Luxations

Radiographs are a valuable diagnostic tool for examining patients for vertebral fractures, luxations, and subluxations. All myelopathic patients with a history of trauma should receive vertebral column radiographs. Importantly, injuries affecting one region of the spinal cord, such as the L4–S1 region of the spinal cord, can mask the ability to appreciate other lesions cranial to the apparent one, such as injuries affecting the T3–L3 region of the spinal cord. Therefore, entire vertebral column radiographs are recommended in all cases of trauma. Although radiographs are sensitive and specific for such traumatic injuries, not all lesions are readily visible with this modality, especially in patients with lesions in the region of clinically silent vertebral anomalies such as hemivertebrae. Additionally, radiographs may not provide sufficient information for surgical planning, if necessary. Therefore, a CT or MRI (or ideally both) should be performed in all patients in whom trauma is suspected and for whom there is consideration for surgical management. Complete imaging of the vertebral column, thorax, and abdomen is necessary to assess the full extent of the injury. Therefore, CT is often preferred for its detailed imaging and minimal patient handling. Depending on the extent of injury and degree of instability, vertebral column trauma may be managed surgically or with conservative management consisting of strict rest for at least 6–8 weeks, anti-inflammatory medications, other analgesics, and sedatives to facilitate rest. The prognosis for recovery is generally good, except in cases of absent nociception, where recovery is unlikely. Further information on spinal trauma can be found in Chapter 15.

Note: Nociception is the only reliable neurological feature that influences the prognosis in plegic dogs.

Fibrocartilaginous Embolic Myelopathy (FCEM)

FCEM is best diagnosed with MRI, which reveals a sharply defined, asymmetric T2W hyperintensity within the spinal cord, predominantly affecting the gray matter due to edema and myelomalacia around the embolic event. This feature is often centered over the vertebral body rather than the disc space and extends along the length of the spinal cord, helping to distinguish FCEM from ANNPE. Additionally, there is no sign of extradural material. CSF analysis can be normal in about half of cases, while the rest show variable, nonspecific changes. It is important to note that fibrocartilage within blood vessels can only be identified after death, so imaging suggests ischemic myelopathy. Histopathology indicates that FCEM is the most common cause of ischemic myelopathy in dogs. Like ANNPE, FCEM is a nonsurgical condition and is treated with supportive care, including physical therapy, hydrotherapy, and nursing care. The prognosis is generally good, but the absence of pain perception indicates a severe spinal cord injury and poor prognosis, with one study documenting that only 8% of nociception-negative dogs recovered independent ambulation.

Neoplasia

Neoplasms involving the vertebral column, vertebral canal, or spinal cord can be identified using radiographs or CT scans, which reveal vertebral lysis and pathological fractures. However, MRI offers better specificity for detecting tumors affecting the spinal cord (Figures 12.4.6 and 12.4.7). While some features may overlap, specific imaging characteristics can help narrow down differential diagnoses for extradural neoplasia. Features suggesting round cell neoplasia include maintained vertebral shape, uniform contrast enhancement, and lesions centered on the bone. Conversely, mesenchymal neoplasia is indicated by altered vertebral shape, mixed contrast enhancement, and lesions centered in the surrounding soft tissues. Both epithelial and mesenchymal neoplasms are more likely to cause cortical lysis, have cavitary soft tissue components, and present medium to large soft tissue masses.

CSF analysis may reveal tumor cells, particularly in the presence of lymphoma or histiocytic sarcoma, but a biopsy is typically required for a definitive diagnosis. Treatment options include palliative care, surgery, radiation therapy, or their combination. Prognosis varies based on tumor type, location, and neurological severity, with metastatic and intramedullary tumors often carrying a poorer outcome due to invasiveness and limited surgical options.

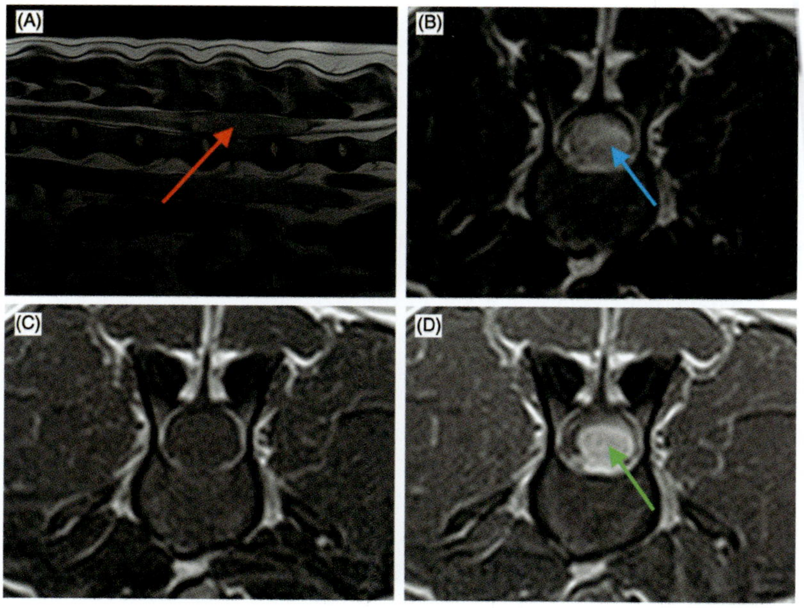

FIGURE 12.4.6 T2W sagittal (A), T2W transverse (B), T1W transverse (C), and a T1W transverse post-contrast (D) MR images of the lumbar vertebral column of a 7-year-old Labrador that was presented with left-sided chronic progressive paraparesis and sudden-onset recumbency. There is a well-defined, elongated, and ovoid intradural and extramedullary mass extending over the L4–L5 and L5–L6 disc spaces (red arrow). The lesion is located on the left ventrolateral aspect of the cord, markedly compressing it, and appears T2W hyperintense (blue arrow) and homogeneously contrast-enhancing (green arrow). The lesion was confirmed to be a histiocytic sarcoma. T2W sagittal (E), T2W transverse (F), T1W transverse (G), and T1W transverse post-contrast MR images of the lumbar column of a 10-year-old mixed-breed dog with a chronic, painful ambulatory paraparesis due to an extradural vertebral body neoplasia. There is T2W heterogeneous hypointensity of the L5 vertebral body along with dorsal and ventral soft tissue paravertebral extension (yellow arrows). The dorsal aspect is extradural and compressing the cord. There is an ill-defined and irregular extradural vertebral canal lesion on the right ventrolateral aspect of the cord, moderately compressing it (indicated by orange arrows). The lesion is isointense to the cord on T1W and mildly hyperintense on T2W with peripheral contrast enhancement. The paravertebral lesion peripherally enhances (purple arrow). The lesion was confirmed to be an undifferentiated sarcoma (H).

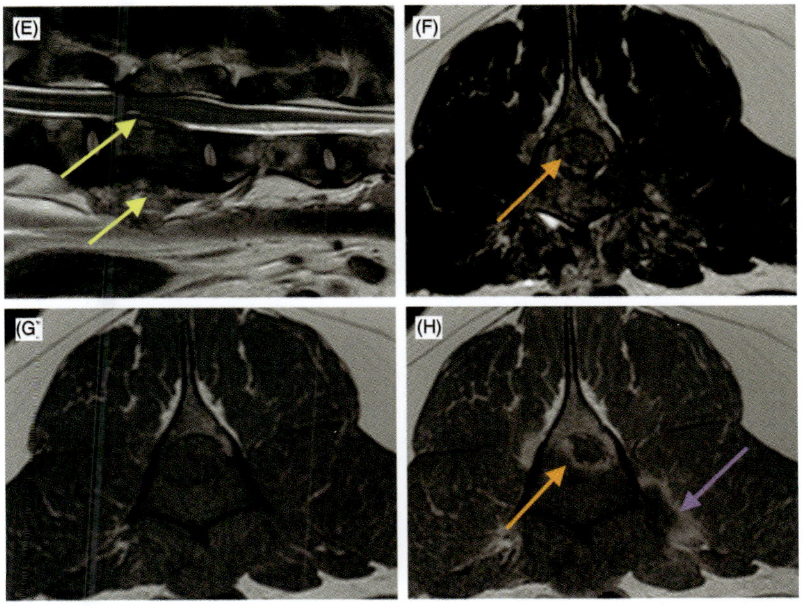

FIGURE 12.4.6 (Continued)

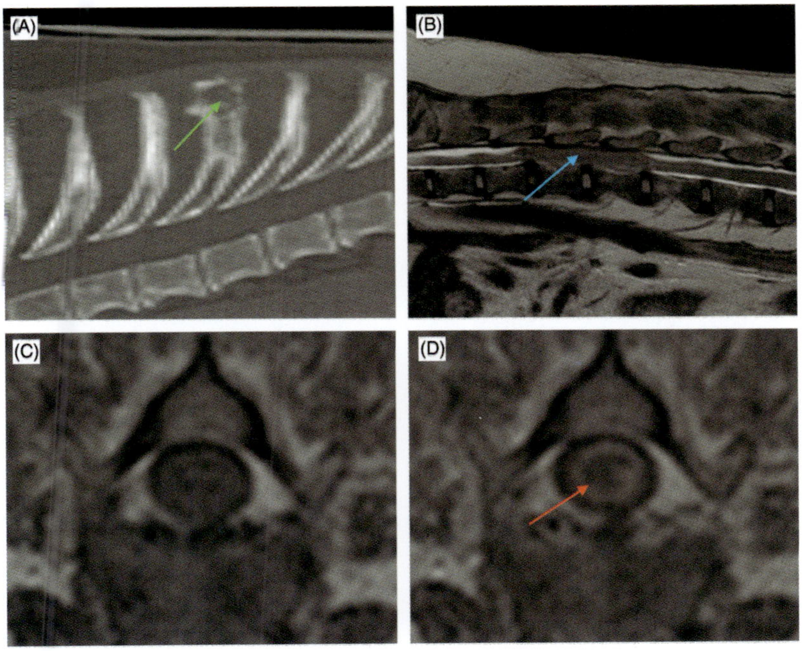

FIGURE 12.4.7 A 3D reconstructed sagittal CT image of the cranial thoracic vertebral column of an 8-year-old poodle with chronic back pain (A). There is an ill-defined and irregular expansile lesion centered on the spinous process of T4 (green arrow). There is lysis and periosteal proliferation. There are no spinal cord lesions noted in association, but this cannot be confirmed on the CT images in this case. The lesion was one of several carcinomatous metastases. Sagittal T2W (B), T1W transverse (C), and T1W transverse post-contrast (D) MR images of the thoracolumbar vertebral column of a 9-year-old boxer dog with rapidly progressive paraparesis. There is an ill-defined and irregular elongated vertebral canal lesion noted overlying several vertebral bodies (blue arrow). The lesion is confirmed to be intramedullary on transverse images with ring-like enhancement (red arrow). Post-mortem confirmed a high-grade glioma.

OUTCOME

Based on the lack of pain detected on examination of the dog shortly after the acute onset of the neurological signs, initially described as painful by the owner, consideration was given to the possibilities of ANNPE and FCEM. An MRI strongly supported ANNPE as the diagnosis. With supportive and rehabilitative care, the dog was ambulatory within 4 weeks and was considered normal by the owners within 12 weeks.

SUGGESTED READING

Alcoverro, E., Schofield, I., Spinillo, S. et al. (2024). Thoracolumbar hydrated nucleus pulposus extrusion and intervertebral disc extrusion in dogs: comparison of clinical presentation and magnetic resonance imaging findings. *Vet. J.* 306: 106178.

Alvarez Sanchez, A., Mullins, R.A., Hoey, S., and Kirby, B.M. (2008). What is your diagnosis? Discal cysts associated with the intervertebral disc: magnetic resonance imaging observations in seven dogs. *Vet. Surg.* 37 (1): 94–101.

Bresciani, L., Trevail, R., Clarke, S. et al. (2021). Lumbosacral intervertebral disk extrusions in 13 dogs. *Vet. Surg.* 50 (4): 823–832.

Bridges, J., Windsor, R., Stewart, S.D. et al. (2022). Prevalence and clinical features of thoracolumbar intervertebral disc-associated epidural hemorrhage in dogs. *J. Vet. Intern. Med.* 36 (4): 1365–1372.

Castel, A., Olby, N.J., Mariani, C.L. et al. (2017). Clinical characteristics of dogs with progressive myelomalacia following acute intervertebral disc extrusion. *J. Vet. Intern. Med.* 31 (6): 1782–1789.

Cudia, S.P. and Duval, J.M. (1997). Thoracolumbar intervertebral disk disease in large, nonchondrodystrophic dogs: a retrospective study. *J. Am. Anim. Hosp. Assoc.* 33 (5): 456–460.

Da Costa, R.C., De Decker, S., Lewis, M.J. et al. (2020). Diagnostic imaging in intervertebral disc disease. *Front. Vet. Sci.* 7: 588338.

De Risio, L. (2015). A review of fibrocartilaginous embolic myelopathy and different types of peracute non-compressive intervertebral disk extrusions in dogs and cats. *Front. Vet. Sci.* 2: 24.

Falzone, C. (2017). Canine acute cervical myelopathy: Hydrated nucleus pulposus extrusion or intraspinal discal cysts? *Vet. Surg.* 46 (3): 379–385.

Fenn, J. and Olby, N. (2020). Classification of intervertebral disc disease. *Front. Vet. Sci.* 7: 579025.

Gomes, S.A., Volk, H.A., Packer, R.M. et al. (2016). Clinical and magnetic resonance imaging characteristics of thoracolumbar intervertebral disk extrusions and protrusions in large breed dogs. *Vet. Radiol. Ultrasound* 57 (4): 417–426.

Gouveia, D., Cardoso, A., Carvalho, C. et al. (2022). Influence of spinal shock on the neurorehabilitation of ANNPE dogs. *Animals (Basel)* 12 (12): 1557.

Gouveia, D., Carvalho, C., Vong, N. et al. (2023). Spinal shock in severe SCI dogs and early implementation of intensive neurorehabilitation programs. *Res. Vet Sci.* 164: 105018.

Henke, D., Gorgas, D., Flegel, T. et al. (2013). Magnetic resonance imaging findings in dogs with traumatic intervertebral disk extrusion with or without spinal cord compression: 31 cases (2006-2010). *J. Am. Vet. Med. Assoc.* 242 (2): 217–222.

Kang, B.J., Jung, Y., Park, S., and Lee, K. (2015). Discal cysts of the cervical spine in two dogs. *J. Vet. Sci.* 16 (4): 543–545.

Lewis, M.J., Jeffery, N.D., Olby, N.J., and Canine Spinal Cord Injury Consortium (CANSORT-SCI) (2020). Ambulation in dogs with absent pain perception after acute thoracolumbar spinal cord injury. *Front. Vet. Sci.* 7: 560. Published 2020 Aug 26.

Mari, L., Behr, S., Shea, A. et al. (2017). Outcome comparison in dogs with a presumptive diagnosis of thoracolumbar fibrocartilaginous embolic myelopathy and acute non-compressive nucleus pulposus extrusion. *Vet. Rec.* 181 (11): 293.

Mari, L., Behr, S., Shea, A. et al. (2019). Predictors of urinary or fecal incontinence in dogs with thoracolumbar acute non-compressive nucleus pulposus extrusion. *J. Vet. Intern. Med.* 33 (6): 2693–2700.

McBride, R., Parker, E., Garabed, R.B. et al. (2022). Developing a predictive model for spinal shock in dogs with spinal cord injury. *J. Vet. Intern. Med.* 36 (2): 663–671.

Müller, M.K., Ludewig, E., Oechtering, G. et al. (2013). The vacuum phenomenon in intervertebral disc disease of dogs based on computed tomography images. *J. Small Anim. Pract.* 54 (5): 253–257.

Olby, N.J., Moore, S.A., Brisson, B. et al. (2022). ACVIM consensus statement on diagnosis and management of acute canine thoracolumbar intervertebral disc extrusion. *J. Vet. Intern. Med.* 36 (5): 1570–1596.

Tartarelli, C.L., Baroni, M., and Borghi, M. (2005). Thoracolumbar disc extrusion associated with extensive epidural haemorrhage: a retrospective study of 23 dogs. *J. Small Anim. Pract.* 46 (10): 485–490.

Togawa, G., Lewis, M.J., and Devathasan, D. (2024). Outcome in paraplegic dogs with or without pain perception due to thoracolumbar fibrocartilaginous embolic myelopathy or acute non-compressive nucleus pulposus extrusion. *Front. Vet. Sci.* 11: 1406843.

Weber, W.J., Berry, C.R., and Kramer, R.W. (1995). Vacuum phenomenon in twelve dogs. *Vet. Radiol. Ultrasound* 36 (6): 493–498.

CHAPTER 13.1

Tetraparesis and Hemiparesis

Case 1—Acute Tetraparesis with Thoracic Limbs Worse Than Pelvic Limbs

Amanda R. Taylor

Southeast Veterinary Neurology, Miami, FL, USA

CASE HISTORY

A 5-year-old spayed female German shepherd was presented for a peracute onset of a gait abnormality affecting all four limbs. The morning of her presentation, she was running in the backyard playing with her ball when she cried out and suddenly became unable to walk. Before the incident the dog had no known health concerns, had been routinely vaccinated since she was a puppy, and was not receiving any medications other than heartworm and flea/tick preventatives. The dog had been unable to lift her head or move her limbs since becoming affected, according to the clients.

NEUROLOGICAL EXAMINATION

The dog was bright, alert, and responsive on presentation. She was non-ambulatory with minimal to no motor present in her thoracic limbs and mild motor present in her pelvic limbs. Muscle tone was subjectively decreased in both thoracic limbs and normal in both pelvic limbs. Superficial nociception was tested in the thoracic limbs and found to be normal. Postural reactions were absent in all limbs based on proprioceptive positioning. Withdrawal reflexes were lacking in the thoracic limbs and normal in the pelvic limbs. Patellar reflexes were normal in both pelvic limbs. Cutaneous trunci and perineal reflexes were normal. The cranial nerve exam was considered normal. There was no evidence of overt pain or discomfort on palpation of the head, neck, or back; however, when the patient's neck was manipulated in range of motion, there was resistance to movement.

1. **Where is the likely lesion localization?**
2. **What major disease processes should be considered?**
3. **What diagnostics should you perform to help determine the diagnosis?**

LESION LOCALIZATION

Non-ambulatory tetraparesis with reduced reflexes in the thoracic limbs is typically consistent with a C6–T2 myelopathy. In cases where the thoracic limbs are more affected than the pelvic limbs, a lesion is considered likely to be more centrally located within the spinal cord (referred to as "central cord syndrome"). This is because the tracts of the thoracic limbs are more internally located in the spinal cord than the tracts of the pelvic limbs. Because withdrawal reflexes can also be reduced in patients with C1–C5 myelopathy, it would also be appropriate to assign a broader localization to this patient of C1–T2 myelopathy. The acute onset of severe spinal cord injury can also cause a condition known as "spinal shock," where descending motor tracts are inhibited, and lower motor neuron signs occur in the affected limbs, in this case, the thoracic limbs, although the intumescence is not directly affected.

WHAT MAJOR DISEASE PROCESSES SHOULD BE CONSIDERED?

Degenerative - Intervertebral Disc Extrusion (Hansen Type I Intervertebral Disc Disease)

This is the most common cause of myelopathy in dogs, and given the acute onset of her signs, her localization, and her signalment, it is considered highly likely.

In contrast to cervical Hansen type II IVDD (see Chapter 13, Case 2), with Hansen Type I IVDD, the nucleus pulposus degenerates and loses its water content, resulting in a structure that cannot withstand the normal forces and physics applied to the vertebral column during motion. Hansen Type I IVDD occurs most commonly in young to middle-aged chondrodystrophic breeds such as the French bulldog and dachshund, but any breed may be affected. Type I IVDD occurs most commonly in the thoracolumbar region, followed by the cervical region of the vertebral column. Dogs typically have an acute or peracute onset of signs. The most common presentation is an ambulatory patient with difficulty walking (paresis) and proprioceptive ataxia in affected limbs. However, the signs of disease can be much more severe in cases with more significant spinal cord injury, and loss of motor function or sensation is possible. This degree of injury is more common with thoracolumbar cases than cervical cases. While this disease can be identified and diagnosed via computed tomography (CT), a magnetic resonance imaging (MRI) study is the most accurate test available.

Vascular – Fibrocartilaginous Embolism (FCE)

Fibrocartilaginous embolism is sometimes referred to as a spinal cord stroke and consists of blockage of spinal vasculature secondary to an embolus of cartilage from the intervertebral disc. There are multiple hypotheses as to how the cartilage is embolized into the blood vessels that have not been confirmed. FCE causes a peracute or acute onset of signs of spinal cord dysfunction. In many cases, it is reported to occur during exercise, with a dog vocalizing and then becoming unable to walk. This condition can affect the spinal cord in the cervical, thoracic, lumbar, or sacral regions. Affected dogs typically do not progress in the severity of clinical signs after the initial few hours. These dogs are nonpainful and are often more affected on one side of their body in the severity of their signs. FCE can only be distinguished from Type I IVDD or hydrated nucleus pulposus extrusion (HNPE) based on the results of an MRI study.

Traumatic – Hydrated Nucleus Pulposus Extrusion (HNPE)

HNPE, previously referred to as intraspinal or discal cyst, is a clinical condition where a large portion of the hydrated nucleus pulposus of the intervertebral disc herniates or ruptures through the annulus fibrosus, resulting in spinal cord compression. HNPE most commonly occurs in the cervical region but has also been reported to affect the thoracolumbar region of the vertebral column. Another version of disc extrusion, called an acute, non-compressive nucleus pulposus extrusion (ANNPE), is a similar process to HNPE, except that the amount of extruded nucleus pulposus material with ANNPE is smaller, is even more hydrated than HNPE material, and does not result in spinal cord compression but rather "contusive" injury to the spinal cord. The clinical signs associated with this condition cannot be distinguished from Type I IVDD, FCE, or ANNPE, other than the fact that, unlike cases of Type I IVDD, HNPE, FCE, and ANNPE, cases may not display signs of discomfort on physical examination. HNPE can only be distinguished from Type I IVDD, FCE, or ANNPE based on the results of an MRI study.

Inflammatory – Meningomyelitis of Unknown Origin and Bilateral Brachial Plexus Neuritis

Meningomyelitis of unknown origin (MUO) is an immune-mediated disease associated with inflammatory infiltration of the spinal cord. As a sole entity (rather than in conjunction with meningoencephalitis of unknown origin), it is uncommon, but has a higher prevalence in large-breed compared to small-breed dogs. This is the spinal cord correlate of meningoencephalitis of unknown etiology, which is reviewed extensively in Chapter 3, Case 1. Bilateral brachial plexus neuritis has rarely been reported in dogs. This disease has been proposed as an idiopathic inflammatory condition comparable to a chronic inflammatory disease in humans, known as hypertrophic neuritis. The onset of signs can be subacute to acute, progressive, and affect both thoracic limbs. The pelvic limbs are not involved, which rules out this condition in this tetraparetic patient. The primary sign in the thoracic limbs is weakness with decreased reflexes. There should be no evidence of neck pain.

Trauma – Fracture / Luxation

Trauma causing fracture or luxation is not considered a likely differential for a dog that is not known to have had a traumatic event, such as a vehicular trauma, running into something such as a wall, being kicked by a horse, etc. This differential category is reviewed elsewhere within this text (Chapter 15).

Neoplasia

Neoplasia is not considered a likely differential in a younger dog with an acute onset of signs of spinal cord dysfunction. This differential category is well reviewed in Chapter 13, Case 2.

WHAT DIAGNOSTICS SHOULD YOU PERFORM TO HELP DETERMINE THE DIAGNOSIS?

Type I Disc Disease

Common radiographic abnormalities associated with Hansen type I IVDD include narrowing of the intervertebral disc space, minimization of the intervertebral foramen, increased overlap of the vertebral articular processes, and mineralization of the intervertebral disc in situ or mineralized disc material present within the vertebral canal. Hansen type I IVDD can be diagnosed by myelography, computed tomography (CT), and MRI. Due to the invasive nature of myelography and higher sensitivity for diagnosis compared to CT, MRI is considered the imaging modality of choice for dogs with Hansen type I IVDD.

Specific MRI characteristics have been identified to aid in predicting Type I IVDD:

- Lateralized intervertebral disc herniation is predictive of a diagnosis of Type I IVDD.
- The intervertebral discs in the MRI study will have signs of complete degeneration, resulting in dehydration of the intervertebral discs (T2-weighted hypointense intervertebral discs).

- The presence of a single intervertebral disc herniation is predictive of a diagnosis of Type I IVDD.
- Herniated material dispersed beyond the boundaries of the intervertebral disc space is predictive of a diagnosis of Type I IVDD.
- Herniated material is typically T2-weighted hypointense or of mixed intensity when associated with hemorrhage.

Fibrocartilaginous Embolism (FCE)

Fibrocartilaginous embolism cannot be diagnosed via radiographs, myelogram, CT, or CT myelogram. A suspected diagnosis of FCE can only be made via MRI or confirmed in post-mortem histopathologic evaluation. Typical MRI findings include T2-weighted hyperintensity within the spinal cord (intramedullary), often affecting the gray matter more than the white matter, and worse on one side of the spinal cord. This area may extend over several vertebral bodies and is often indistinctly marginated.

Hydrated Nucleus Pulposus Extrusion

HNPE cannot be diagnosed via radiographs, myelogram, CT, or CT myelogram. MRI should identify a T2-hyperintense extradural spinal cord compression centered over an intervertebral disc space. The disc that has herniated will have decreased volume and T2-weighted signal intensity on MRI. The remaining intervertebral discs are often normal in comparison.

MUO and Bilateral Brachial Plexus Neuritis

MUO is diagnosed based on MRI and cerebrospinal fluid analysis findings. Refer to Chapter 3, Case 1 for more details. Brachial plexus neuritis cannot be diagnosed via radiographs, myelogram, CT, or CT myelogram. MRI could be normal or identify enlargement of nerve roots associated with the brachial plexus with concurrent contrast enhancement. Should the patient be affected for a week or longer, there could be changes identified on electrodiagnostic testing, such as a reduced thoracic limb motor nerve conduction velocity and spontaneous abnormal discharges on electromyogram.

OUTCOME

The dog underwent an MRI of the cervical spinal cord. The C2–C3 intervertebral disc was confirmed to have extruded, causing substantial compression of the spinal cord (Figures 13.1.1 and 13.1.2). The dog underwent a ventral slot to remove the compressive disc material. The dog made steady improvement and was ambulatory 10 days postoperatively (Videos 13.1.1–13.1.3).

VIDEO 13.1.1 Patient 4 days after ventral slot at C2–C3.

VIDEO 13.1.2 Patient 7 days after ventral slot at C2–C3.

VIDEO 13.1.3 Patient 10 days after ventral slot at C2–C3.

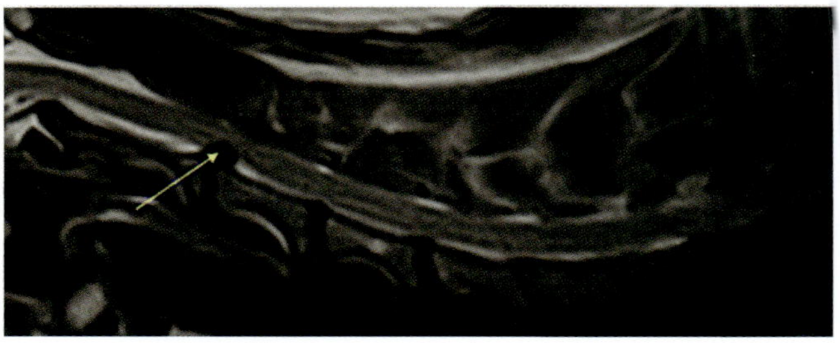

FIGURE 13.1.1 Sagittal T2W MRI of intervertebral disc extrusion at C2–C3.

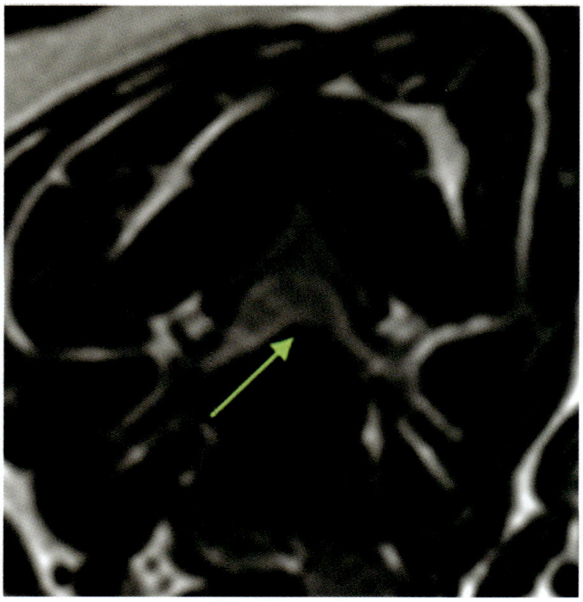

FIGURE 13.1.2 Transverse T2W MRI of intervertebral disc extrusion at C2–C3.

SUGGESTED READING

Dewey, C.W. and Da Costa, R.C. (ed.) (2015). *Practical Guide to Canine and Feline Neurology*. John Wiley & Sons.

Platt, S. and Garosi, L. (2012). *Small Animal Neurological Emergencies*. CRC Press.

Tetraparesis and Hemiparesis
Case 2—Chronic Tetraparesis in a Large-Breed Dog

CHAPTER 13.2

Jill Niederhuth

BluePearl, Des Moines, IA, USA

CASE HISTORY

A 9-year-old neutered male standard poodle was presented for a chronic onset of a gait abnormality affecting all four limbs. The dog began with an abnormality of the pelvic limb gait approximately 3 months earlier, which slowly progressed in severity to involve the thoracic limbs over the last month. Before the onset of signs, this dog had no known health concerns, had been routinely vaccinated since puppyhood, and was not receiving any medications other than heartworm and flea/tick preventatives. The dog was continent and not evidently in pain, but the owners had noted a reluctance to lower his neck to the food bowl.

NEUROLOGICAL EXAMINATION

The dog was bright, alert, and responsive on presentation. He was ambulatory with a short-strided gait in the thoracic limbs and a long-strided gait in the pelvic limbs, which also displayed ataxia (Video 13.2.1). Postural reactions were abnormal, as indicated by the hopping evaluation in the thoracic limbs and proprioceptive positioning in the pelvic limbs; the responses were slightly worse on the left side. Spinal reflexes were normal in the pelvic limbs, but there was a bilateral reduced withdrawal reflex in the thoracic limbs. The thoracic limbs also demonstrated reduced tone and proximal atrophy. The cranial nerve exam was considered normal. There was no evidence of pain or discomfort on thoracolumbar or cervical palpation; however, there was resistance to cervical range of motion. Extension of the neck resulted in the dog becoming recumbent in the pelvic limbs.

VIDEO 13.2.1 Neurological examination of a 9-year-old neutered male standard poodle with tetraparesis.

1. **Where is the likely lesion localization?**
2. **What major disease processes should be considered?**
3. **What tests could you perform to help determine the diagnosis?**

LESION LOCALIZATION

A wide-based general proprioceptive ataxia and upper motor neuron paresis of the pelvic limbs, in combination with a short and stilted gait in the thoracic limbs, is referred to as a "two-engine" or "disconnected" gait and can be considered suggestive of a lesion affecting the C6–T2 region of the spinal cord. In dogs with a chronic cervical spinal cord compression, it can be

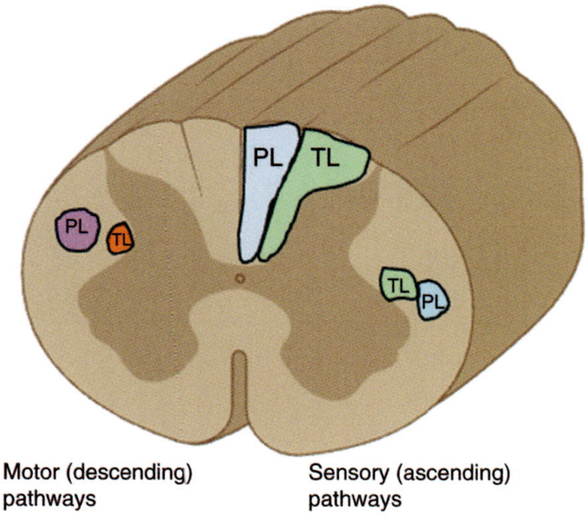

FIGURE 13.2.1 Schematic showing the distribution of white matter tracts within the spinal cord. Note that most of the pelvic limb tracts are lateral to the thoracic limb tracts.

particularly difficult to localize the lesion to the cervical spinal cord segments. Affected dogs can demonstrate obvious general proprioceptive ataxia and paresis in the pelvic limbs with only mild to no appreciable gait abnormalities in the thoracic limbs, especially in large-breed dogs. Lack of thoracic limb abnormalities in these cases is due to the specific anatomical organization of the neuronal tracts in the cervical spinal cord. Tracts involved with pelvic limb function are located laterally, while the tracts involving the thoracic limbs are located more medially in the cervical spinal cord white matter (Figure 13.2.1). A progressive extradural cervical spinal cord compression will therefore initially compress the tracts involving the pelvic limbs prior to those involving the thoracic limbs, making it challenging to differentiate a cervical from a thoracolumbar chronic myelopathy. Confirmation of the C6–T2 localization is based on the reduced thoracic limb spinal reflexes as well as the loss of tone in these limbs, in the presence of intact reflexes in the pelvic limbs.

CAUTION: Although spinal hyperesthesia is often noted in the early stages of a chronic compressive disease, it may not be present once the animal develops apparent gait abnormalities. This is due to an adaptation of the nociceptors.

DIFFERENTIAL DIAGNOSIS

Degenerative – Hansen Type II Intervertebral Disc Disease (IVDD)

This is a highly likely differential diagnosis for this patient, based on his signalment, the lesion localization, and the speed of onset of clinical signs.

In contrast to cervical Hansen type I IVDD (see Chapter 13, Case 1), Hansen type II IVDD involves fibrous metaplasia of the intervertebral disc. This is a more gradual process than the chondroid metaplasia of Hansen type I IVDD, leading to disc bulging (protrusion) rather than rupture of the annulus fibrosus and disc extrusion (Figure 13.2.2). Although Hansen type II IVDD occurs most commonly in older, large non-chondrodystrophic dog breeds, it has become apparent that similar degenerative changes are seen in the intervertebral discs of chondrodystrophic dog breeds. Most affected dogs are approximately 9 years old, and the German shepherd, English Staffordshire terrier,

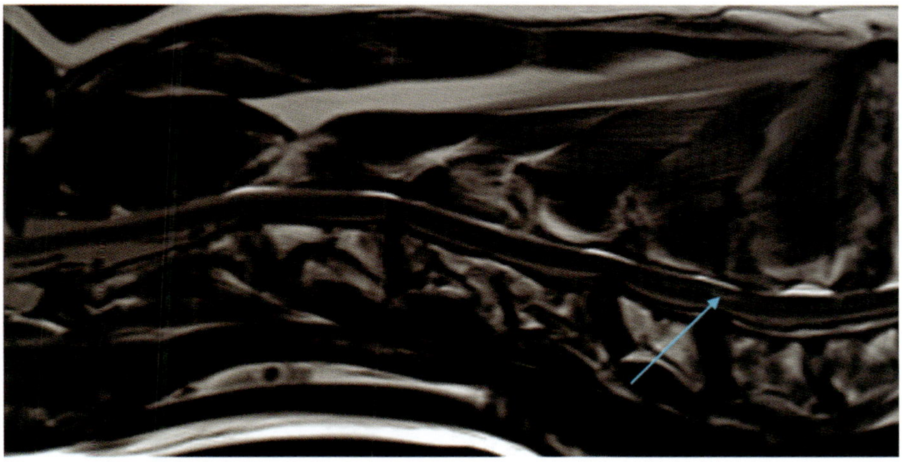

FIGURE 13.2.2 Sagittal T2-weighted MRI of the cervical vertebral column of a dog with disc protrusion. Several of the intervertebral discs are protruding, leading to mild compression of the spinal cord. At the level of the C6–C7 intervertebral disc, there is intramedullary hyperintensity in the spinal cord (arrow), which likely represents gliosis secondary to chronic compression from the protruding C6–C7 intervertebral disc.

Labrador retriever, and basset hound are the most commonly affected breeds. Type II IVDD occurs most often in the caudal cervical, thoracolumbar, and lumbosacral regions. The nature of clinical signs is reflected by the location of the lesion along the vertebral column. The signs are typically characterized by an insidious onset and are slowly progressive. Ambulatory paresis with proprioceptive ataxia is the most common clinical presentation. Clinical signs can, however, vary from spinal hyperesthesia to non-ambulatory paraparesis and can occur or exacerbate more acutely.

Degenerative – Cervical Spondylomyelopathy ("Wobbler Syndrome")

Cervical spondylomyelopathy (CSM) is a multifactorial neurological syndrome also referred to as cervical vertebral malformation-malarticulation syndrome, caudal cervical spondylomyelopathy, wobbler syndrome, cervical stenotic myelopathy, and cervical vertebral instability. Focal vertebral canal stenosis can be caused by a combination of bone and soft-tissue structures and the involvement of several static and dynamic factors.

The two forms of CSM are disc-associated (DA-CSM) and osseous-associated cervical spondylomyelopathy (OA-CSM), which are associated with differences in signalment, different pathological abnormalities, imaging findings, and different surgical techniques.

- **Disc-associated cervical spondylomyelopathy**
  DA-CSM is most commonly seen in older (>7 years of age) large-breed dogs. The Doberman pinscher appears to be predisposed, but many breeds, such as the Dalmatian, Weimaraner, and Rottweiler, can be affected. Spinal cord compression is predominantly caused by one or more Hansen Type II intervertebral disc herniations. The caudal cervical intervertebral disc spaces are most often affected, and multiple sites of spinal cord compression are seen in up to half of cases. Additionally, one or more of the following abnormalities are present: dorsal spinal cord compression caused by ligamentum flavum hypertrophy, abnormalities in the shape and position of the vertebral body and the dorsal lamina, the latter often resulting in a funnel-shaped vertebral canal, and foraminal stenosis. Alongside these static factors, dynamic factors result in changes in the dimensions of the cervical vertebral canal when the animal makes physiologic movements of the neck.

- **Osseous-associated cervical spondylomyelopathy**
  This type of CSM is seen most often in younger (between 6 and 48 months old) giant breed dogs, such as the Great Dane, Dogue de Bordeaux, and bullmastiff. Spinal cord compression and foraminal stenosis are predominantly caused by hypertrophy of articular processes, resulting in lateral and dorsolateral spinal cord compression. Other abnormalities that can be observed include ligamentum flavum hypertrophy and vertebral arch malformations, which can result in additional dorsal spinal cord compression. Multiple sites of spinal cord compression are seen in up to 85% of affected cases.

Neoplasia

Tumors affecting the spinal cord are categorized as extradural, intradural-extramedullary, and intramedullary based on their location (see Chapter 12, Case 4, Figure 1). Tumors involving the vertebral body can cause secondary spinal cord compression.

- Extradural tumors include primary bone tumors, metastatic tumors, and hematopoietic tumors (e.g. lymphomas and plasma cell tumors). Extradural tumors are estimated to represent around 50% of spinal tumors in dogs.
- Intradural–extramedullary tumors include meningiomas, neuroepitheliomas, nerve sheath tumors, and histiocytic sarcoma. Intradural-extramedullary tumors are estimated to represent around 35% of spinal tumors in dogs.
- Intramedullary tumors represent around 15% of canine spinal tumors, with 66% being primary tumors. Primary tumors include gliomas (e.g. oligodendrogliomas, astrocytomas, and undefined gliomas). Although this type of tumor can occur over the entire length of the vertebral column, they occur commonly in the cervical region of younger dogs (mean age, 5.9 years) and the caudal cervical region of cats (median, 8 years). Secondary tumors represent metastatic tumors. Metastases of transitional cell carcinoma and hemangiosarcoma are the most common secondary intramedullary spinal tumors in dogs.

Spinal meningiomas

Spinal meningiomas are the most common primary spinal cord tumor in cats >8 years of age. The mean age of onset of spinal meningiomas in dogs is 9 years; they occur most commonly in the cranial cervical region, and boxers and golden retrievers are most commonly affected. Meningiomas of the spinal cord in dogs and cats cause progressive ataxia and paresis, often accompanied by spinal hyperesthesia. The clinical signs indicate the region of the spinal cord involved.

Vertebral body tumors

Vertebral body tumors are primary or metastatic tumors and are most frequently reported in large- and giant-breed dogs. Commonly described tumors in dogs include osteosarcomas, fibrosarcomas, chondrosarcomas, hemangiosarcomas, undifferentiated sarcomas, plasma cell tumors, metastatic carcinomas, lymphomas, and liposarcomas. Small-breed dogs have a higher rate of vertebral metastasis than large-breed dogs. In cats, the most commonly described vertebral body tumor is osteosarcoma.

Clinical signs may be focal or multifocal depending upon the extension of the tumor. Clinical signs include spinal hyperesthesia, ataxia, paresis, and plegia. Although clinical signs are usually chronic, pathological vertebral fractures can result in an acute onset or exacerbation of clinical signs.

INVESTIGATION

Type II Disc Disease

Common radiographic abnormalities associated with Hansen type II IVDD include sclerosis of the vertebral endplates, spondylosis deformans, and narrowing of the intervertebral disc space. Hansen type II IVDD can be diagnosed by myelography, computed tomography myelography (CTM), and magnetic resonance imaging (MRI). Because of the invasive nature of myelography and CTM, MRI is considered the imaging modality of choice. MRI studies of dogs with Hansen type II IVDD often reveal multiple sites of intervertebral disc herniation and associated spinal cord compression. This complicates clinical decision-making, and differentiating between clinically relevant and irrelevant spinal cord compressions is challenging.

Specific MRI characteristics have been identified to aid in predicting the type of IVDD:

- Midline instead of lateralized intervertebral disc herniation is predictive of a diagnosis of type II IVDD.
- Partial instead of complete dehydration of the nucleus pulposus is predictive of a diagnosis of type II IVDD.
- The presence of a single intervertebral disc herniation instead of multiple intervertebral disc herniations is predictive of a diagnosis of type I IVDD.
- Herniated material dispersed beyond the boundaries of the intervertebral disc space is predictive of a diagnosis of type I IVDD.

Cervical Spondylomyelopathy

Although radiographic abnormalities can be suggestive, a diagnosis of DA-CSM cannot be confirmed by survey radiographs. A diagnosis of DA-CSM can be confirmed by myelography, CTM, or MRI. Each of these techniques is associated with specific advantages and limitations for diagnosing DA-CSM. In myelography, the lateral view can reveal abnormalities in both the ventral and dorsal contrast columns. One or more ventral extradural disc-associated compressions are the most common finding. Dorsal extradural compression related to ligamentum flavum hypertrophy can also be seen. The use of dynamic studies, and traction studies in particular, has been discussed in dogs with DA-CSM. Different methods have been described to apply linear traction to the head. A lesion is termed "dynamic" or "traction responsive" when the degree of spinal cord compression decreases with traction. In contrast, a lesion is termed "static" when the degree of spinal cord compression remains unchanged after applying traction. It has traditionally been suggested that traction-responsive lesions benefit from distraction-stabilization surgical techniques, while static lesions benefit from direct decompressive surgical techniques.

Spinal cord compression, intervertebral disc degeneration, intervertebral disc herniation, vertebral abnormalities, and intraparenchymal intensity changes are abnormalities commonly observed on MRI studies of dogs with DA-CSM (Figure 13.2.2). The occurrence of a T2-weighted hyperintense intraparenchymal signal intensity change is considered the most reliable morphologic variable to differentiate between dogs with and without clinical signs of DA-CSM. Traction-responsive studies have also been routinely performed by MRI.

Spinal Tumors

MRI and CT-myelography reveal an extradural or an intradural-extramedullary compressive lesion or occasionally a swollen cord compatible with an intramedullary lesion (Figure 13.2.3). Survey radiographs can reveal lysis and pathological fractures secondary to tumor destruction of the bone. CT provides a 3D assessment of bone involvement, important for osseous tumors. Cerebrospinal fluid (CSF) evaluation is rarely specifically helpful for the diagnosis except for in neoplasms associated with exfoliation, such as lymphoma, which occasionally are diagnosed based on CSF results. Fluoroscopic-guided needle aspiration or surgical biopsy can be used to obtain a definitive diagnosis.

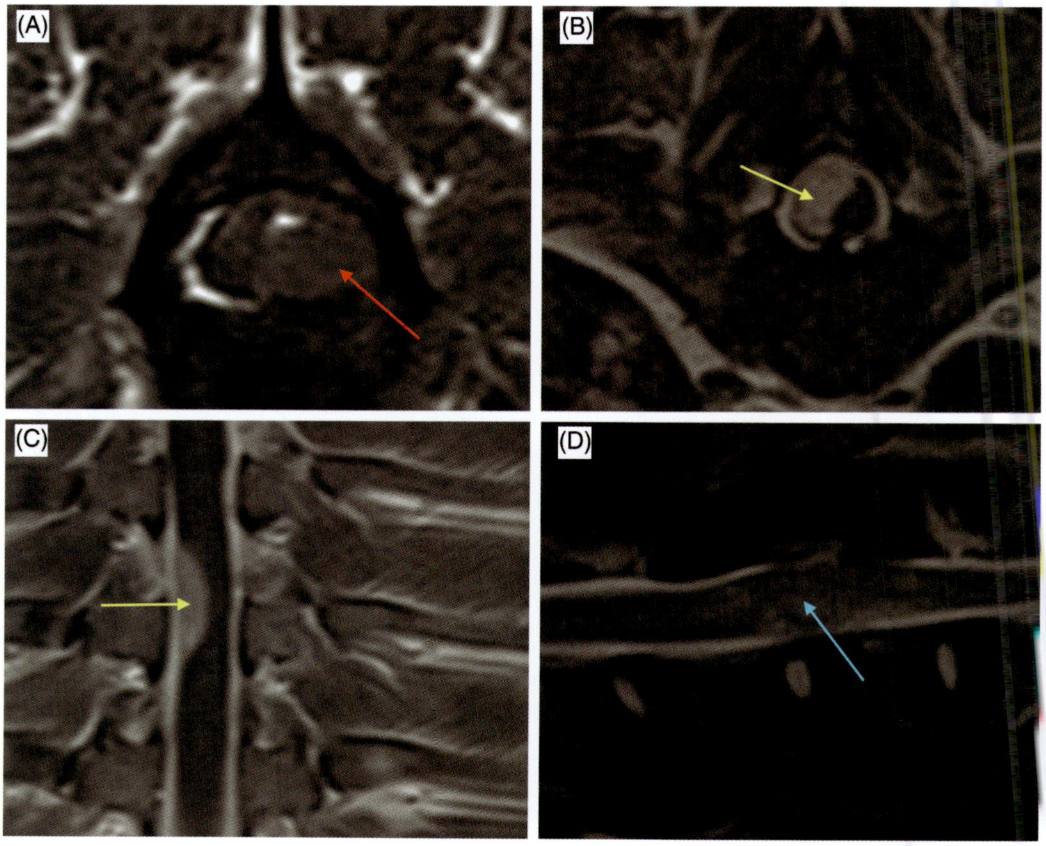

FIGURE 13.2.3 (A) A T1W post-contrast transverse MR image at the level of L5 showing a left-sided extradural lesion within the vertebral canal. The lesion had extended from the vertebral body and was confirmed to be an undifferentiated sarcoma. (B) T1W post-contrast transverse and (C) dorsal MR images at the level of T10 showing a right-sided intradural-extramedullary neoplastic mass, which was confirmed to be lymphoma. (D) A T2W sagittal MR image at the level of C6–C7 showing an intramedullary neoplasia with regional cord swelling. The lesion was confirmed as an undifferentiated glioma.

OUTCOME

MR imaging of the cervical vertebral column of the standard poodle described in this case revealed a moderate cord compression secondary to a type II intervertebral disc. Four weeks of crate rest with anti-inflammatory medications was associated with mild improvement. Subsequently, a decompressive surgery was performed with a ventral slot at C6–C7. The dog made an excellent recovery and was considered nearly normal by 2 weeks after the surgery.

SUGGESTED READING

Platt, S.R., Olby, N., and Beltran, E. *BSAVA Manual of Canine and Feline Neurology*, 5th ed. (2026) British Small Animal Veterinary Association Publishing.

de Lahunta, A., Glass, E.N., and Kent, M. *Veterinary Neuroanatomy and Clinical Neurology*, 5th edition. Elsevier Enhanced Digital Version ISBN: 9780323696111.

Tetraparesis and Hemiparesis

Case 3—Acute Tetraparesis in a Small Dog

CHAPTER 13.3

Amanda R. Taylor

Southeast Veterinary Neurology, Miami, FL, USA

CASE HISTORY

A 2-year-old spayed female miniature dachshund was presented for an acute onset of a gait abnormality affecting all four limbs, worse on the right side. Two days prior to the presentation, she had fallen down several stairs and, since that time, had been unable to ambulate normally. Before the incident, the dog had no known health concerns, had been routinely vaccinated since she was a puppy, and was not receiving any medications other than heartworm and flea/tick preventatives. Since the incident occurred, the clients have noted that the dog regularly cries out when moving her head and is unwilling to walk on her leash.

NEUROLOGICAL EXAMINATION

The dog was bright, alert, and responsive on presentation. She was ambulatory with hemiparesis of her right side, and she would spontaneously knuckle her right thoracic limb (Video 13.3.1). Subjectively, she had increased tone in her right limbs compared to her left limbs. Postural reactions were absent on the right side but relatively normal on the left side based on proprioceptive positioning (Video 13.3.2). Withdrawal reflexes were normal in all limbs. Patellar reflexes were normal in both pelvic limbs. Cutaneous trunci and perineal reflexes were normal. The cranial nerve exam was normal. There was marked discomfort in her neck, particularly when lifting her head upward.

VIDEO 13.3.1 A 2-year-old miniature Dachshund with tetraparesis; gait assessment.

VIDEO 13.3.2 A 2-year-old miniature Dachshund with tetraparesis; proprioceptive positioning testing

1. **Where is the likely lesion localization?**
2. **What major disease processes should be considered?**
3. **What diagnostics should you perform to help determine the diagnosis?**

LESION LOCALIZATION

Ambulatory right-sided hemiparesis with cervical discomfort and normal reflexes in the thoracic limbs is consistent with a C1–C5 myelopathy, worse on the right side.

WHAT MAJOR DISEASE PROCESSES SHOULD BE CONSIDERED?

Degenerative – Intervertebral Disc Extrusion (Hansen Type I Intervertebral Disc Disease)

This is the most common cause of difficulty walking in the dog, and given the acute onset of her signs, her localization, and her signalment, it is considered highly likely. This disease was previously reviewed in this chapter (see Chapter 13, Case 1).

Anomalous – Atlantoaxial Subluxation

Atlantoaxial subluxation typically affects young, small, or toy breed dogs such as Yorkshire terriers or Chihuahuas. There may be a congenital abnormality associated with this condition, where the dog has a malformed or absent dens process on the cranial aspect of the second cervical vertebra (the axis). The dog may also lack critical ligamentous connections between the first cervical vertebra (atlas) and the second cervical vertebra (axis). Some dogs have normal anatomy of these two vertebrae and solely have abnormalities of the ligamentous connections. Atlantoaxial subluxation may occur spontaneously in dogs with malformations or secondary to trauma in dogs with normal anatomy. When the connection between the atlas and axis is disrupted, the axis slides craniodorsally, resulting in compression of the spinal cord. Atlantoaxial subluxation causes a peracute or acute onset of signs of spinal cord dysfunction in most cases, but in congenital atlantoaxial subluxation that goes undetected, animals may exhibit waxing and waning signs of neck pain and myelopathy over several months to years. This condition can affect the spinal cord in the cervical region, and in some cases, there are signs of brainstem dysfunction. These dogs often experience pain in the cervical region

Inflammatory – Meningoencephalomyelitis of Unknown Origin (MUO)

Meningoencephalomyelitis of Unknown Origin or Etiology (MUO and MUE are considered equivalent) is a clinical condition with a proposed immune-mediated cause. Clinical signs result from inflammation and edema within the nervous system. This condition may be granulomatous or necrotizing in nature, although cases where the spinal cord is affected are typically granulomatous. MUO most commonly affects multiple areas of the nervous system at once. Of note, this disease category is also common in small or toy breed dogs, similar to atlantoaxial subluxation. In dogs with myelopathy signs only, this condition cannot be distinguished from other differentials based on examination. MUO can only be distinguished from other diseases based on the results of a magnetic resonance imaging (MRI) study and cerebrospinal fluid analysis. This disease is reviewed elsewhere within this text (see Chapter 3, Case 1). Infectious causes of CNS inflammation and discospondylitis should also be considered.

Trauma

Trauma is considered a differential for this case due to the history of a fall down several stairs. This differential category is reviewed elsewhere within this text (Chapter 15).

Neoplasia

Neoplasia is not considered a likely differential in a younger dog with an acute onset of myelopathy. This differential category is well reviewed in Chapter 13, Case 2.

INVESTIGATION

Type I Disc Disease

Diagnostic investigation of Type I IVDD is reviewed in Chapter 13, Case 1.

Atlantoaxial Subluxation

Craniodorsal displacement of the axis relative to the atlas can be observed in radiographs. There can be increased space identified between the first two cervical vertebrae (Figure 13.3.1). In

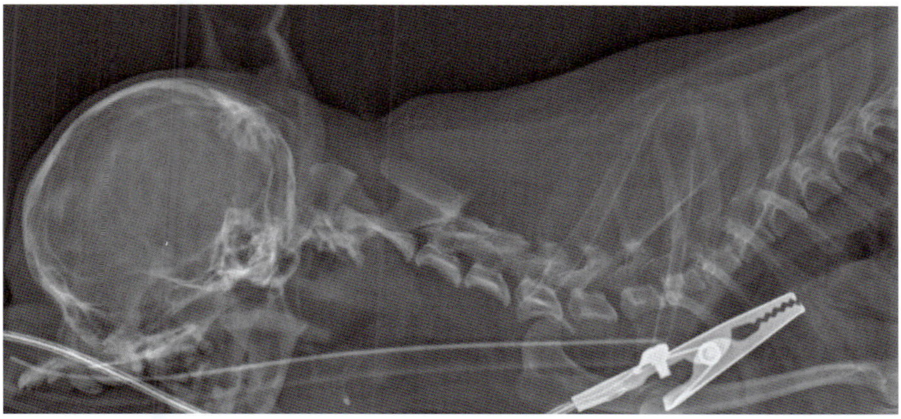

FIGURE 13.3.1 Lateral radiograph of a dog with an absent dens process and atlantoaxial subluxation.

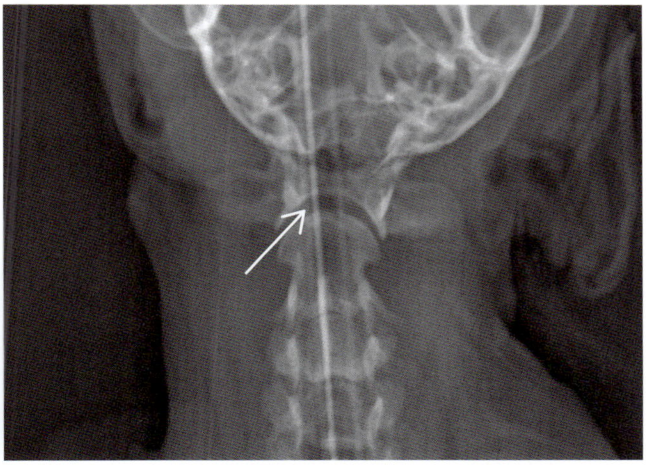

FIGURE 13.3.2 Ventrodorsal view of the same patient as in Figure 13.3.1. Note the widening of the atlantoaxial joint space and the absence of a dens (arrow).

patients with congenital abnormalities, the dens may be absent (Figure 13.3.2). Cases with a history of trauma may have concurrent fractures noted on radiographs. In cases where a neutral radiograph does not identify the luxation, a gently flexed view may allow the change to be identified. Computed tomography (CT) scans will identify the luxation and can determine with further clarity whether other fractures or luxations are present (Figure 13.3.3). CT is also typically utilized in surgical planning. MRI is performed to determine whether there are changes within the spinal cord parenchyma consistent with contusion or edema secondary to the luxation, to determine whether other congenital changes are present, and to rule out other diseases such as meningoencephalomyelitis or Type I IVDD (Figure 13.3.4). Both of these imaging modalities will identify craniodorsal displacement of the axis relative to the atlas and compression of the spinal cord. The prognosis for this disease is guarded to good depending on chronicity, changes within the spinal cord parenchyma, and treatment route (coaptive bandage alone versus surgical correction).

Meningoencephalomyelitis of Unknown Origin (MUO)

MUO is diagnosed with MRI and concurrent cerebrospinal fluid analysis in most cases once infectious causes have been ruled out. Diagnostics for this disease are reviewed in Chapter 3.

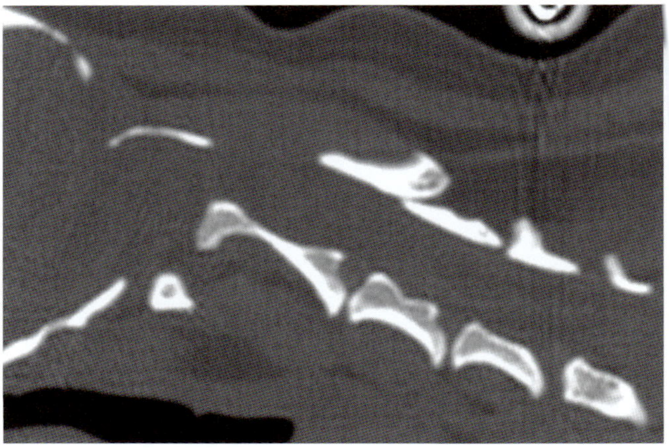

FIGURE 13.3.3 Sagittal CT view of a dog with an absent dens process and atlantoaxial subluxation.

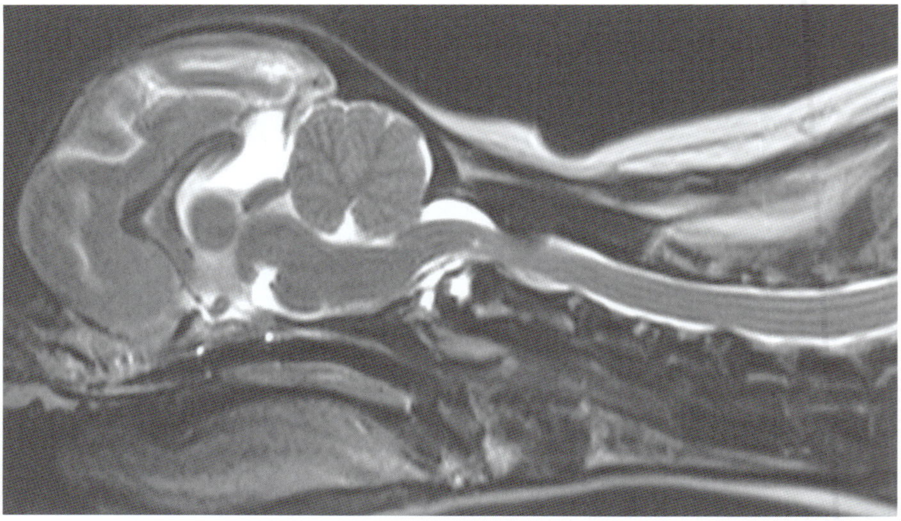

FIGURE 13.3.4 Sagittal MRI view of a dog with an absent dens process and atlantoaxial subluxation. Note that less bone detail is evident using this modality, but the associated spinal cord parenchyma can be evaluated.

OUTCOME

Radiographs and MRI confirmed the absence of a dens process in the dog, as well as atlantoaxial subluxation. The dog underwent surgical stabilization in which transarticular pins were inserted across the C1–C2 joint space, and cortical screws were inserted into the ventral aspect of C1 and C2. The pins and screws were subsequently embedded in polymethylmethacrylate. Postoperative radiographs confirmed the reduction of the subluxation. The dog recovered well following surgery (Video 13.3.3).

VIDEO 13.3.3 A 2-year-old miniature dachshund with atlantoaxial subluxation, 1 week after surgical stabilization.

SUGGESTED READING

Dewey, C.W. and Da Costa, R.C. (ed.) (2015). *Practical Guide to Canine and Feline Neurology*. John Wiley & Sons.

Platt, S. and Garosi, L. (2012). *Small Animal Neurological Emergencies*. CRC Press.

CHAPTER 14.1

Urinary and Fecal Dysfunction

Case 1—Urinary and Fecal Incontinence in a Cat

Sergio A. Gomes

Dovecote Veterinary Referrals, Derby, UK

CASE HISTORY

A 4-year-old spayed female cat was presented with a loss of tail function that occurred 3 days prior to presentation, in conjunction with a road traffic accident. The cat had been dragging her tail since the accident and was having both urinary and fecal accidents in the house. Her owners were unsure of how often she voided in the household litter boxes, as there were multiple cats in the house. Before referral to the present clinic, she had been hospitalized for 24 hours with her primary veterinarian. At that time, bladder expression was deemed difficult to perform.

NEUROLOGICAL EXAMINATION (Video 14.1.1)

VIDEO 14.1.1 Video examination of a 4-year-old spayed female cat was presented with a loss of tail function that occurred 3 days prior to presentation, in conjunction with a road traffic accident.

On neurological examination, the cat was bright, alert, and responsive. She had a normal gait and normal posture. Hopping of the left pelvic limb was subjectively slightly delayed compared to the right pelvic limb. Spinal reflexes were normal in all four limbs, as was the cutaneous trunci reflex bilaterally. Cranial nerve function was normal. The cat's tail hung behind her. No overt voluntary tail movement was observed. When palpated, no tail tone was appreciated. The perineal reflex was absent. The anus was subjectively dilated and did not contract when the perianal skin was pinched anywhere encircling the anus. When the tail was pinched with hemostats, the cat showed no conscious response to the painful stimulus. A response to this painful stimulus was not observed along the entire length of the tail, or with pinching the perianal region. Upon abdominal palpation, the bladder was soft, and with moderate manual pressure on the abdomen, urine dribbled out of the urethra.

1. **Where is the likely lesion localization?**
2. **What major disease processes should be considered?**
3. **What tests could you perform to help determine the diagnosis?**

LESION LOCALIZATION

Flaccid paralysis of the tail, dilated anus, and easily expressible bladder are consistent with lower motor neuron dysfunction affecting the tail, the anal sphincter, and the external urethral sphincter, respectively. The lower motor neurons that innervate the tail are located in the caudal spinal cord segments, which were previously referred to as coccygeal segments. The lower motor neurons that innervate the anal and external urethral sphincters are located in the S1–S3 spinal cord segments. A lesion affecting these spinal cord segments, or the nerves that emerge from them as the cauda equina, results in the signs observed in this cat.

A NOTE REGARDING URINARY AND FECAL INCONTINENCE

There are broadly two forms of incontinence: upper motor neuron incontinence and lower motor neuron incontinence (Figure 14.1.1).

Upper motor neuron incontinence results from a lesion cranial to the S1–S3 spinal cord segments and is characterized by spastic paresis or paralysis of the external urethral sphincter. This results in urinary retention until the hydrostatic pressure within the bladder exceeds the sphincter's capacity. At this point, urine exits the bladder through the urethra until equilibrium of pressure is reached. This is often referred to as "overflow incontinence." Although the anal sphincter similarly experiences upper motor neuron paresis or paralysis with a spinal cord lesion cranial to the S1–S3 spinal cord segments, constipation or fecal retention is uncommon; there can, however, be a lack of sensory awareness of a full rectum in these cases, and feces can "drop out" without a voluntary effort being witnessed.

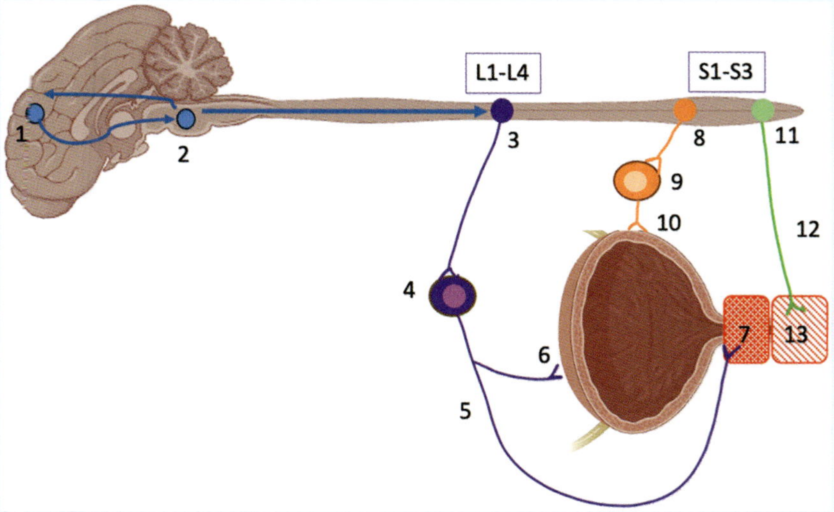

FIGURE 14.1.1 Schematic illustration of the innervation of the lower urinary tract (Created with www.biorender.com). (1) Cortical neurons for conscious awareness of bladder filling and voluntary control of sphincters and micturition. (2) Pontine micturition center. (3) Sympathetic pre-ganglionic cell bodies. (4) Caudal mesenteric ganglion. (5) Hypogastric nerve. (6) Beta-receptors cause the detrusor muscle to relax. (7) Alpha-receptors innervate the smooth muscle of the urethral internal smooth-muscle sphincter, causing contraction. (8) Parasympathetic pre-ganglionic cell bodies. (9) Pelvic nerve and ganglia. (10) Cholinergic receptors cause the detrusor muscle to contract. (11) Cell bodies of the pudendal nerve. (12) Pudendal nerve with sensory and motor fibers. (13) External skeletal urethral sphincter with nicotinic receptors for acetylcholine. During the storage phase of micturition, the detrusor muscle is innervated by the sympathetic nervous system (3, 4, 5, 6, and 7), which facilitates urine storage by relaxing the bladder wall and contracting the internal sphincter. This is supported by the pudendal nerve causing external sphincter contraction (11, 12, and 13). During the voiding phase of micturition, the detrusor muscle is innervated by the parasympathetic nervous system (8, 9, and 10), causing contraction of the detrusor muscle. This occurs in response to bladder wall stretching, which stimulates the pons and cerebral cortex (1 and 2) responsible for coordinating urethral sphincter relaxation through inhibition of the hypogastric and pudendal nerves.

Lower motor neuron incontinence results from a lesion affecting the S1–S3 region of the spinal cord. It is characterized by flaccid paresis or paralysis of the external urethral sphincter and the anal sphincter. This results in dilated sphincters through which urine and feces can pass freely, leading to constant emission of urine and feces or constipation/obstipation.

WHAT MAJOR DISEASE PROCESSES SHOULD BE CONSIDERED?

Trauma to the Sacral and Caudal Spinal Cord Segments or Cauda Equina

This is a highly likely differential diagnosis for this patient, based on clinical history. Traction injury to the tail (also called "tail pull injury") results in stretching or severing (avulsion) of the nerve roots of the cauda equina. Sacrocaudal luxation or fractures can contribute to damage to the sacral and caudal spinal cord segments and the cauda equina, not only by causing stretching or severing but also by compressing these regions. Commonly implicated causes of tail pull injuries in cats include vehicular accidents, getting their tails stuck in crevices or under doors, or having their tails pulled by children. In cases of vehicular trauma, other fractures and luxations are often observed. Neurological manifestations of a lesion in this region include flaccid tail paresis or paralysis, decreased to absent anal tone, a dilated anus, decreased to absent perianal reflex, and lower motor neuron urinary and fecal incontinence. In the most severe cases, animals that lack motor function in the tail may also lack sensation. Caudal nerve lesions are responsible for tail paralysis, while damage to either the pelvic or pudendal nerves can result in urinary and fecal dysfunction.

A clinical grading system has been proposed, as follows:

Grade 1: Tail paresis without additional signs;

Grade 2: Tail paralysis with sensitivity at the base of the tail;

Grade 3: Tail paralysis without sensitivity at the base of the tail, but presence of anal tone and perineal reflex;

Grade 4: Tail paralysis without sensitivity at the base of the tail, absence of anal tone and perineal reflex, and urinary incontinence with increased bladder tone;

Grade 5: Tail paralysis without sensitivity at the base of the tail, absence of anal tone and perineal reflex, and urinary incontinence with decreased bladder tone or a flaccid bladder.

A higher neurological grade decreases the chances and lengthens the recovery time for voluntary urination. Typically, cats with lower motor neuron urinary and fecal incontinence who retain sensation at the base of the tail are more likely to regain continence. In cases where sensation at the tail base is absent, about 60% will recover continence. Around 50% of cats with a neurological grade 5 recover the ability to urinate. Nearly 90% of those who recover will do so within the first 30 days. Additionally, half of the cats with lost defecatory function regain voluntary defecation.

Early tail amputation is advised to alleviate ongoing nerve tension caused by continuous movement at the fracture site and the weight of the paralyzed, atonic tail. However, tail movement may take several months to recover, so it is recommended to wait 4–6 weeks before reassessing tail function.

Alongside cauda equina injury, the most frequently concomitantly observed injuries include fractures of the pelvic floor, followed by sacroiliac luxations, ilial body fractures, and, least commonly, sacral wing fractures. Although these comorbidities do not directly contribute to tail and sphincter dysfunction, they are important to identify, as surgical repair may be necessary, particularly if weight-bearing capacity or pelvic canal size is affected.

Degenerative – Intervertebral Disc Disease

Intervertebral disc disease (IVDD) in cats is less prevalent than in dogs, but it is a consideration in this case. Clinical signs include vertebral column pain and myelopathic signs, which include paresis or paralysis and general proprioceptive ataxia. Urinary and fecal incontinence are possible with injury anywhere along the spinal cord, with lesions cranial to the S1 spinal cord segment resulting in urinary retention (upper motor neuron incontinence) and lesions affecting the S1–S3 spinal cord segments resulting in constant urinary and fecal voiding (lower motor neuron incontinence). Typically, the severity of motor dysfunction observed in the pelvic limbs approximates the severity of paresis of the external urethral and anal sphincters. Animals that are paraplegic are therefore "bladder plegic," and are unable to void normally. Similar to dogs, a distinction should be made between an intervertebral disc extrusion (IVDE) and an intervertebral disc protrusion (IVDP). IVDE occurs more frequently in older cats (ages of ~8–9 years), and males appear to be overrepresented.

Therapeutic interventions for IVDE in cats are similar to those in dogs, encompassing both conservative and surgical management strategies. Conservative management typically involves strict confinement to restrict movement and minimize further disc extrusion and spinal cord compression. Analgesia, with nonsteroidal anti-inflammatory drugs (NSAIDs), gabapentin, or pregabalin, is provided. Adjunctive therapies such as physiotherapy, hydrotherapy, and acupuncture may be implemented to aid in neurological recovery. Bladder management, including manual expression or catheterization, may be necessary in cases of urinary dysfunction. Surgical decompression of extruded disc material is typically considered in nonambulatory cases, persistent pain despite medication, or lack of improvement with conservative management. Interestingly, the prognosis appears to be favorable in the majority of cats, even those with paraplegia and no pain perception. Additionally, similar successful outcomes and survival times were reported for cats managed conservatively and surgically, even though surgically treated cats presented with a more severe neurological status. This suggests that conservative management may be a viable option for many cats with IVDE.

Acute Non-compressive Nucleus Pulposus Extrusion

This is a possible differential for this acutely affected cat, although most cases of this condition occur in regions of the spinal cord that would also result in paraparesis or paraplegia. Acute non-compressive nucleus pulposus extrusion (ANNPE) was previously referred to as traumatic intervertebral disc extrusion (TIVDE), type III intervertebral disc extrusion, or a high-velocity low-volume disc extrusion. ANNPE, similarly to IVDE, describes a peracute extrusion of nucleus pulposus through an annular tear. ANNPE, however, differs in the type of material extruded (hydrated), and in its more frequent occurrence during vigorous activity or trauma. The spinal cord injury arises from the impact (contusion) with minimal or no spinal cord compression. See Chapter 12, Cases 3 and 4. The prognosis for cats diagnosed with ANNPE is generally favorable, with approximately 90% of cats regaining ambulatory status and restoring urinary and fecal continence. Residual neurologic deficits are possible in any case.

Vascular – Fibrocartilaginous Embolic Myelopathy

Similarly to ANNPE, this condition is also possible but considered less likely as a differential diagnosis for this cat, given the lack of pelvic limb dysfunction.

Clinically, fibrocartilaginous embolic myelopathy (FCEM) is indistinguishable from ANNPE. See Chapter 12, Cases 3 and 4. In cats, the domestic shorthair is the most represented breed, with an age at diagnosis ranging from 6 months to 17 years (median, 10 years). Management of FCEM in cats is similar to that of ANNPE, being conservative, without indication of surgery. Standard treatment protocols include supportive care, physiotherapy, and analgesia as needed.

INVESTIGATION

Sacrocaudal Luxation and Cauda Equina Injury

Sacrocaudal luxation and cauda equina syndrome often occur due to traction injuries to the tail and frequently occur in conjunction with pelvic fracture or luxation. Alongside tail fractures (Figure 14.1.2) or dislocation, the most frequently concomitant observed injuries include fractures of the pelvic floor, followed by sacroiliac luxations, ilial body fractures, and, least commonly, sacral wing fractures. An in-depth review of pelvic fracture management is outside the scope of this book. Although not strictly neurological, it is important to always check if the bladder is intact and has not been ruptured.

Intervertebral Disc Disease

Imaging features of IVDD in cats are similar to that in dogs. Magnetic resonance imaging (MRI) is considered the most detailed modality for visualizing the spinal cord and surrounding soft tissues, allowing for the identification of disc extrusion (IVDE), disc protrusion (IVDP), ANNPE and the rare intradural-intramedullary intervertebral disc extrusion (IIVDE). Computed tomography (CT) with or without contrast may be utilized, although both the spinal cord and disc material visualization are inferior to MRI. Myelography, while historically used, is less common with the increased availability of advanced cross-sectional imaging. The specific type of IVD herniation, such as IVDE versus IVDP, may be suggested by the imaging characteristics, although overlap, such as IVDE-on-P, can occur.

For more details, refer to Chapter 12.

Acute Non-compressive Nucleus Pulposus Extrusion

MRI is the modality of choice for the diagnosis of ANNPE, as it relies heavily on intraparenchymal or intradiscal changes that CT would not be able to reveal. CT could nonetheless often reveal a vacuum artifact within the affected intervertebral disc compatible with an acute herniation. Characteristic MRI features include: (1) focal intramedullary hyperintensity on T2-weighted sequences directly overlying or in proximity to an intervertebral disc, (2) evidence of loss of nucleus pulposus signal intensity or focal annular disruption, and (3) lack of evidence of an extradural compression (Figure 14.1.3). These imaging features, in conjunction with the clinical presentation,

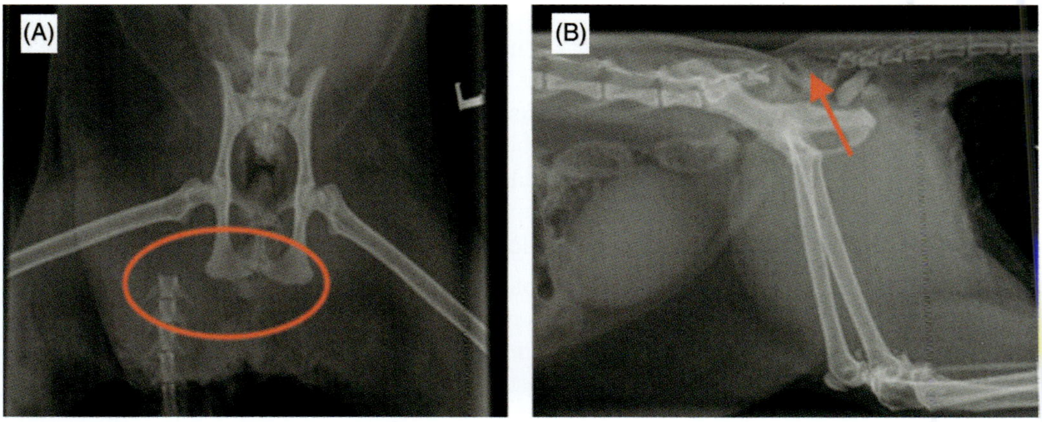

FIGURE 14.1.2 Ventrodorsal (A) and lateral (B) radiographs of the pelvic region of a cat, revealing a complete tail avulsion with sacrocaudal fracture.

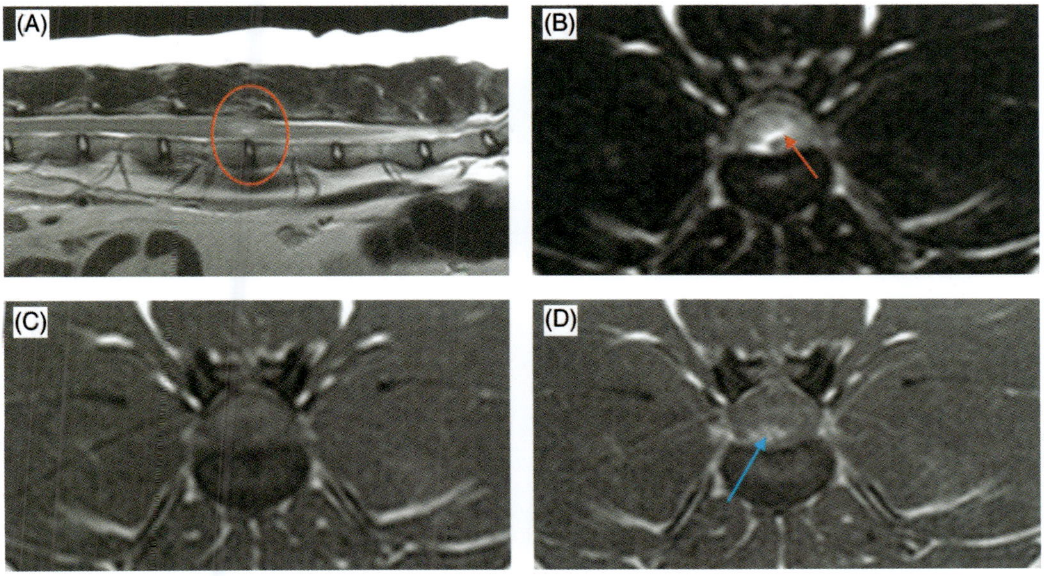

FIGURE 14.1.3 Sagittal T2W (A), transverse T2W (B), transverse T1W pre-contrast (C), and post-contrast (D) magnetic resonance images of an ANNPE in a cat. There is a loss of size and intensity of the nucleus pulposus at the L4–L5 disc space above which there is an ill-defined, irregular, heterogeneous intramedullary hyperintensity affecting the cord (red oval). The transverse images show an ill-defined and irregular heterogeneous hyperintense T2W lesion (red arrow) as well as an ill-defined ventral extradural lesion, which is mildly contrast-enhancing (blue arrow) and minimally compressive.

allow for a presumptive diagnosis. Although a definitive diagnosis of ANNPE can only be achieved through histopathological evaluation, imaging features alongside clinical presentation are often enough, considering that prognosis is positive in the vast majority of cases.

FCEM

MRI is the modality of choice for the diagnosis of FCEM. MRI features suggestive of FCEM include: (1) focal, relatively sharply demarcated intramedullary, and often lateralized lesion (edematous infarcted tissue), (2) predominantly involving the gray matter that is hyperintense to normal gray matter on T2-weighted images and iso- or hypointense to normal gray matter on T1-weighted images, (3) the intramedullary hyperintensity lesion length on T2-weighted images is generally longer than one vertebral body (see Chapter 12). When an MRI is performed within the first 24–72 hours after the onset of neurological signs, a lesion might not be identified. FCEM cannot be directly visualized with CT, with only a mild indication of spinal cord swelling possible.

OUTCOME

A luxation of the tail at the level of the second caudal vertebra was documented on radiographs in this case. The owner declined surgery but agreed to medical supportive care with manual bladder expression as well as pharmacological support (see Case 3 in this chapter). The cat regained voluntary urination within 3 weeks, with no return of normal tail movement. Intermittent fecal incontinence was noted until 3 months after the injury, when the cat was lost to follow-up.

SUGGESTED READING

Amey, J.A., Liatis, T., Cherubini, G.B. et al. (2024). Outcomes of surgically and conservatively managed thoracolumbar and lumbosacral intervertebral disc herniations in cats. *J. Vet. Intern. Med.* 38 (1): 247–257.

Bibbiani, L., Gelendi, S., Bernardini, M. et al. (2022). Prevalence, clinical presentation and MRI of intervertebral disc herniations in cats. *J. Feline Med. Surg.* 24 (12): e443–e452.

Couper, E. and De Decker, S. (2020). Evaluation of prognostic factors for return of urinary and defecatory function in cats with sacrocaudal luxation. *J. Feline Med. Surg.* 22 (10): 928–934.

De Risio, L. (2015). A review of fibrocartilaginous embolic myelopathy and different types of peracute non-compressive intervertebral disk extrusions in dogs and cats. *Front. Vet. Sci.* 2: 24.

Meeson, R. and Corr, S. (2011). Management of pelvic trauma: neurological damage, urinary tract disruption and pelvic fractures. *J. Feline Med. Surg.* 13 (5): 347–361.

Meeson RL, Geddes AT. Management and long-term outcome of pelvic fractures: a retrospective study of 43 cats. J. Feline Med. Surg. 2017; 19(1): 36–41.
Pisco V, Gomes SA. Feline neurological disease in a veterinary referral hospital in the UK: clinical diagnosis, neuroanatomical localisation and VITAMIN D-based aetiological distribution. J. Feline Med. Surg. 2026, 28.1: 1098612X251394770.

Simpson, K.M., De Risio, L., Theobald, A. et al. (2014). Feline ischaemic myelopathy with a predilection for the cranial cervical spinal cord in older cats. *J. Feline Med. Surg.* 16 (12): 1001–1006.

Taylor-Brown, F.E. and De Decker, S. (2017). Presumptive acute non-compressive nucleus pulposus extrusion in 11 cats: clinical features, diagnostic imaging findings, treatment and outcome. *J. Feline Med. Surg.* 19 (1): 21–26.

Theobald, A., Volk, H.A., Dennis, R. et al. (2013). Clinical outcome in 19 cats with clinical and magnetic resonance imaging diagnosis of ischaemic myelopathy (2000–2011). *J. Feline Med. Surg.* 15 (2): 132–141.

Urinary and Fecal Dysfunction

Case 2—Fecal Incontinence in a Pug

CHAPTER 14.2

Sergio A. Gomes

Dovecote Veterinary Referrals, Derby, UK

CASE HISTORY

An 8-year-old intact male pug was presented for investigation of a chronic (6 months) progressive history of non-painful pelvic limb ataxia and paraparesis, stumbling over the back feet, and dragging both legs. The dog also started urinating and defecating in the house over the same time period. Many times, the dog would urinate while he walked, apparently unaware of voiding (Video 14.2.1). The dog also occasionally stumbled and fell on both pelvic limbs, struggled to go up the stairs, and bunny-hopped. No medication trials had been attempted prior to referral.

VIDEO 14.2.1 An 8-year-old pug is seen to keep walking while urinating. Gait analysis revealed that the dog was ambulatory with paraparesis and general proprioceptive ataxia.

NEUROLOGICAL EXAMINATION

The dog was bright, alert, and responsive on presentation. Gait analysis revealed ambulatory paraparesis, characterized by hyperextension, lack of flexion, and spastic movements with general proprioceptive ataxia. When stationary, the dog frequently stood with the left pelvic limb knuckled. His tail carriage was no longer that typically observed in pugs (upright, curled over the back) and was instead hanging behind him. Postural reactions were abnormal based on severely delayed or absent placing and hopping tests in both pelvic limbs; the responses were slightly worse on the left side. Spinal reflexes were normal in all four limbs. The perineal reflex was normal. The cutaneous trunci reflex cutoff was at the level of the thoracolumbar junction bilaterally. The mentation and cranial nerve assessment were considered normal. There was no evidence of pain or discomfort on palpation of the whole vertebral column.

1. **Where is the likely lesion localization?**
2. **What major disease processes should be considered?**
3. **What tests could you perform to help determine the diagnosis?**
4. **What treatment options exist for the common differentials?**

LESION LOCALIZATION

All neurological deficits in this dog are restricted to the pelvic limbs and the presence of urinary and fecal incontinence.

With normal thoracic limbs, pelvic limb dysfunction localizes to three broad areas: the T3–L3 region of the spinal cord, the L4-caudal region of the spinal cord, and the nerves that emerge from the lumbosacral intumescence to innervate the pelvic limbs, external urethral sphincter, and anal sphincters. The paraparesis observed in this dog is consistent with upper motor neuron dysfunction, localizing to the T3–L3 region of the spinal cord. Typically, general proprioceptive ataxia of the pelvic limbs, as observed in this dog, is more apparent with T3–L3 lesions than lesions affecting L4-caudal region and the peripheral nervous system. This further strengthens a localization of a T3–L3 myelopathy for this dog. Spinal reflexes can help distinguish T3–L3 lesions from L4-caudal lesions or peripheral neuropathies. Both patellar and withdrawal reflexes can be reduced or incomplete with L4-caudal lesions or with lesions affecting the nerves that emerge from this region, whereas these reflexes will be normal or exaggerated with a T3–L3 lesion. The abnormally cranial cutaneous trunci cutoff in this patient further validates the localization of T3–L3. A final important consideration is that this dog is reported to be both urinary and fecally incontinent.

Incontinence can also occur due to lower motor neuron dysfunction or upper motor neuron dysfunction, with these two localizations leading to different forms of incontinence. Lower motor neuron incontinence occurs due to a lesion affecting the S1–S3 region of the spinal cord or the nerves that emerge from this region to innervate the external urethral sphincter and anal sphincter. Animals with lesions affecting one of these two regions will have decreased or absent perineal reflexes, perianal hypalgesia or analgesia, a dilated anus, will drop feces frequently and urinate with minimal pressure applied to the abdomen. Conversely, animals with lesions affecting the T3–L3 region will exhibit normal perineal reflexes, normal anal sphincter tone, and will only occasionally drop feces due to colonic overloading while experiencing overflow urination. This dog's perineal reflex and anal tone were normal, and the fecal and urinary incontinence had an intermittent, rather than near-constant, characterization. It is hypothesized that urinary and fecal incontinence secondary to T3–L3 myelopathies occur when the lesion is predominantly dorsal or dorsolateral within the spinal cord. These regions convey sensory input cranially to the somatosensory cortex, providing information about 'fullness' or distension in the colon and urinary bladder. With impaired sensory information, animals with T3–L3 myelopathies are unaware of the need to urinate and defecate.

WHAT MAJOR DISEASE PROCESSES SHOULD BE CONSIDERED?

Anomalous –

(1) Subarachnoid Diverticulum

Subarachnoid diverticulum (SAD) refers to a localized abnormal dilation of the subarachnoid space accompanied by fluid buildup. This consequently leads to compressive myelopathy and disruption of cerebrospinal fluid (CSF) flow, leading to neurological dysfunction. Historically, this pathology has been identified by several terms, including spinal meningeal cyst, meningeal cyst, arachnoid cavitation, arachnoid pseudocysts, spinal intradural arachnoid cysts, and arachnoid or subarachnoid cysts. The origins of SAD are unclear, with both congenital and acquired types noted. Potential causes include congenital anomalies, effects from biomechanical stresses, trauma, or bleeding, or arising in association with other spinal conditions like intervertebral disc extrusion or inflammatory disorders. Most SAD lesions have dorsal or dorsolateral locations relative to the spinal cord. Commonly affected breeds include the pug, French bulldog, Rottweiler, and French mastiff.

Clinical signs are consistent with a non-painful, progressive myelopathy. The thoracolumbar region is most commonly affected, but lesions can also develop in the cervical spinal cord region, especially in Rottweilers and French mastiffs. Urinary and fecal incontinence are common with thoracolumbar lesions.

(2) Constrictive Myelopathy

Constrictive myelopathy (CM), also known as meningeal fibrosis, bears resemblances to SAD. CM is characterized as an acquired, circumferential narrowing of the spinal cord, thought to arise due to fibrosis and adhesion between the pia-arachnoid membranes. Similarly to SAD, this process obstructs CSF flow, causing spinal cord compression and resultant neurological dysfunction.

Clinical signs are indistinguishable from SAD, including a non-painful progressive thoracolumbar myelopathy. Like SAD, fecal and urinary incontinence are common complaints. Commonly affected breeds include the pug and the French bulldog. Despite similarities with SAD, particularly at the clinical presentation level, CM is recognized as a separate condition with distinctive diagnostic imaging features. CM is also believed to have a poorer long-term prognosis and a higher likelihood of recurrence compared to SAD. The compression of the spinal cord, although not necessarily restricted to the dorsal portions, also compromises the pathways relating to urinary and fecal control.

Pugs, French bulldogs, and English bulldogs have a high prevalence of a congenital anomaly called vertebral facet hypoplasia or aplasia. Technically, the actual anatomic components involved are the thoracolumbar caudal articular processes. These articular processes arise from the caudal aspect of a vertebra to form a joint with the cranial articular process of the vertebra immediately caudal. These processes overlap with each other like 'stacked plates'. This joint surface is the facet. Caudal articular process hypoplasia is found in many dogs that are neurologically normal. However, it has also been associated with constrictive myelopathy in pugs.

Degenerative - Intervertebral Disc Disease: Intervertebral Disc Protrusion or Hansen Type II

Intervertebral disc protrusion (IVDP), also referred to as Hansen type II intervertebral disc herniation, is characterized by chondroid metaplasia of the nucleus pulposus. This is a slow process that leads to the gradual expansion of the nucleus pulposus and an overall bulging of an intact intervertebral disc. The disc causes focal compression of the spinal cord. IVDP typically occurs most often in large, older, nonchondrodystrophic dogs. Typically, progressive signs develop gradually over several months. Thoracolumbar lesion localizations are most common. Evidence of pain or discomfort with vertebral column palpation is variable. Given the ventral location of intervertebral discs relative to the spinal cord, the ventral and ventrolateral regions of the spinal cord experience the most compression with IVDP Urinary and fecal incontinence can still occur, but may be less likely than with conditions affecting the dorsal region of the spinal cord. Refer to Chapter 12, Case 2, for additional details about IVDP.

Neoplasia

Tumors affecting the spinal cord are categorized as extradural, intradural-extramedullary, and intramedullary based on their location relative to the spinal cord. Tumors are also classified as primary tumors arising *in situ* or as metastatic tumors that have spread from elsewhere in the body. The rate of clinical sign progression depends on the tumor type and location. All tumor types can cause slowly progressive myelopathic signs and urinary and fecal incontinence. Please refer to Chapter 10, for more details about neoplasia affecting the vertebral column and spinal cord.

WHAT TESTS COULD YOU PERFORM TO HELP DETERMINE THE DIAGNOSIS?

Subarachnoid Diverticulum

Plain radiographs and non-contrasted computed tomography (CT) have poor sensitivity for SAD. Myelogram and CT myelogram can reveal a collection of contrast medium in the subarachnoid space at the affected area, typically characterized by a tear-drop shape. Focal compression of the spinal cord at the same level is evident. Ultimately, magnetic resonance imaging (MRI) is the most sensitive and specific imaging modality to distinguish between SAD and alternative differential diagnoses (Figure 14.2.1). MRI features of SAD include enlargement or dilation of the subarachnoid space, T2-weighted hyperintensity, and T1-weighted hypointensity compatible with a CSF-filled dilation, causing a compressive myelopathy. Two additional MRI sequences that are valuable for the visualization of SAD are the half-Fourier acquisition single-shot turbo spin-echo pulse sequence (HASTE) and the 3D constructive interference in steady state (3D-CISS). These sequences are sometimes referred to as

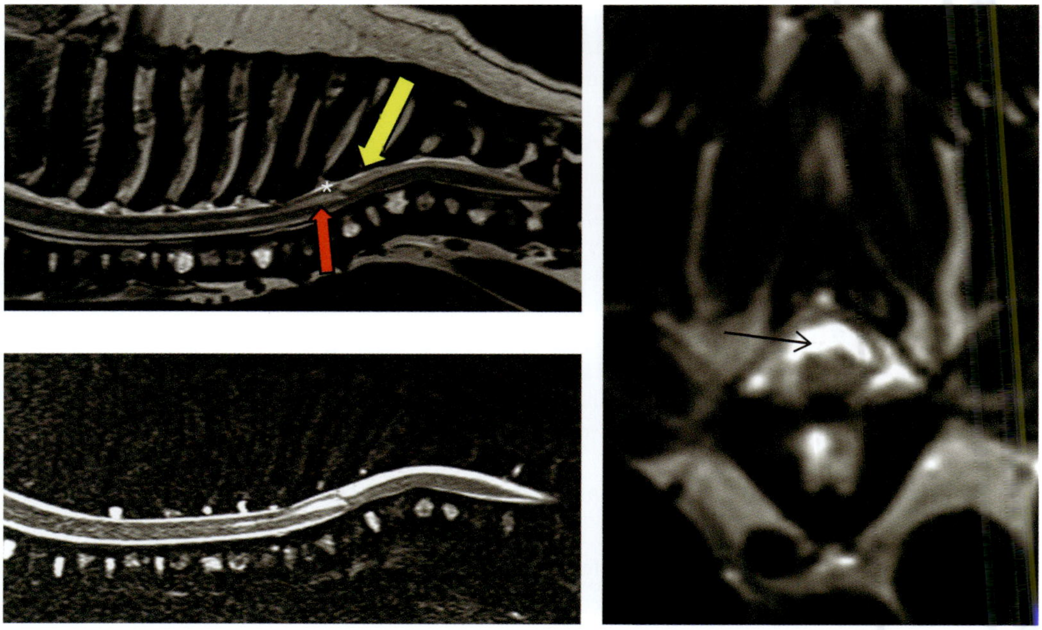

FIGURE 14.2.1 Magnetic resonance images of the thoracic spinal cord of a dog with a SAD. On the T2-W sagittal image (top left), there is dilation of the dorsal subarachnoid space (yellow arrow) that ends abruptly due to the presence of a fibrous tag (white arrowhead). Cranial to this fibrous tag, there is fluid accumulation within and surrounding the central canal (red arrow). The fibrous tag obstructs the flow of cerebrospinal fluid, causing the accumulations observed here. The HASTE sequence (bottom left), confirms the accumulation of pure fluid in these dilations, consistent with cerebrospinal fluid. The T2-W transverse image (right) shows a large amount of accumulated cerebrospinal fluid dorsal to the spinal cord (arrow).

"myelogram" sequences because they increase the signal intensity of CSF and diminish the signal intensity of fat. This makes the SAD much more visibly apparent. SAD can have a cranial or caudal direction, and syringomyelia (fluid accumulation within the spinal cord) can be found concurrently.

Constrictive Myelopathy

MRI is the diagnostic test of choice for diagnosing constrictive myelopathy (Figure 14.2.2). MRI features of constrictive myelopathy include intramedullary hyperintensity on T2-weighted and STIR sequences; reduced spinal cord diameter; and a linear meningeal contrast-enhancement pattern [4]. Unlike SAD, constrictive myelopathy may lead to visibly thickened meninges in the absence of focal CSF accumulation (hypointense on T1-weighted images) relating to pia-arachnoid adhesions. Reduced spinal cord diameter, a stellate appearance of the spinal cord in the transverse plane, with multiple hypo-intense bands crossing the arachnoid space, can also be identified. As with SAD, syringomyelia (fluid accumulation within the spinal cord) can be found concurrently.

Intervertebral Disc Protrusion (IVDP)

Although IVDP can be diagnosed in myelography, currently, cross-sectional imaging is mostly used in its diagnosis, including both CT and MRI. CT features are less well-described but are typically characterized by a ventral extradural spinal cord compression with soft tissue attenuating characteristics, overlying and not exceeding the intervertebral disc space. On MRI, IVDP appears as an extradural, compressive lesion ventral to the spinal cord. The nucleus pulposus of the affected intervertebral disc

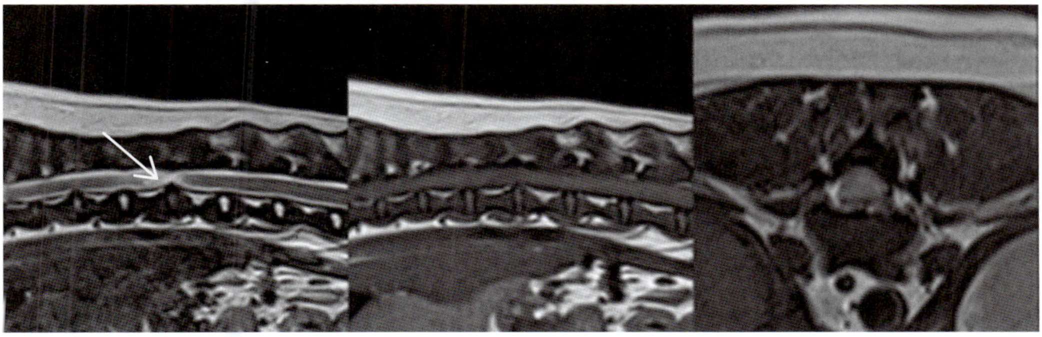

FIGURE 14.2.2 Magnetic resonance images of the thoracolumbar spinal cord of a pug with constrictive myelopathy. The T2-weighted sagittal image (left) shows focal hyperintensity within the spinal cord (arrow). At this level, the spinal cord appears to be being "cinched" dorsally and ventrally due to circumferential adhesions that are creating compression. The T1-weighted sagittal image (middle) reveals that this hyperintensity is caused by fluid accumulation. The T2-weighted transverse image (right) shows that there is intramedullary hyperintensity within the spinal cord at the level of the constrictive adhesions.

is often hypointense relative to adjacent intervertebral discs. Additionally, IVDP is more often linked to multiple intervertebral disc herniations being present in imaging rather than a single one.

Neoplasia

MRI would be the modality of choice in most cases where a neoplasia causing myelopathy is suspected. Please refer to Chapter 10 for more details.

WHAT TREATMENT OPTIONS EXIST FOR THE COMMON DIFFERENTIALS?

Subarachnoid Diverticulum

Broadly, subarachnoid diverticula can be managed conservatively or surgically. Conservative management involves the use of corticosteroids to reduce cerebrospinal fluid production and inflammation, along with activity modification. Mild cases are amenable to conservative management. More severe or progressive cases may benefit from surgical management. A variety of techniques have been described to address the diverticulum, including durotomy/durectomy with transection of the fibrous adhesions, marsupialization of the dura mater, and using a catheter to create a shunt within the subarachnoid space. Surgery is typically associated with stabilization of the current neurologic status or improvement.

Constrictive Myelopathy

As opposed to arachnoid diverticula, constrictive myelopathy has a worse prognosis and might not respond to surgical management. Although pugs may experience temporary neurological improvement post-operatively, most show progression of their myelopathy. Studies investigating stabilization of caudal articular hypoplasia and secondary constrictive myelopathy found similarly that stabilization temporarily improved outcomes, but this improvement was short-lived.

IVDP

The reader is encouraged to review Chapter 12, Case 2, for details regarding the treatment of IVDP.

Neoplasia

The reader is encouraged to review Chapter 10, for details regarding the treatment of neoplasia.

OUTCOME

The dog underwent a thoracolumbar MRI, which revealed T2-weighted hyperintensity and circumferential compression of the spinal cord at the T12 and T13 vertebral levels, deemed compatible with a constrictive myelopathy diagnosis. A short course of prednisone did not improve the clinical signs. The dog continued to have a slow progression of its T3–L3 myelopathy and incontinence for several more years, until it died from an unrelated disease.

SUGGESTED READING

Ban, J., Park, J., Kim, H. et al. (2023). Investigation of canine caudal articular process dysplasia of thoracic vertebrae using computed tomography: prevalence and characteristics. *Front. Vet. Sci.* 10: 1066420.

Bertram, S., Ter Haar, G., and De Decker, S. (2018). Caudal articular process dysplasia of thoracic vertebrae in neurologically normal French bulldogs, English bulldogs, and pugs: prevalence and characteristics. *Vet. Radiol. Ultrasound* 59 (4): 396–404.

De Frias, J.M., De Decker, S., De Stefani, A., and Llabres-Diaz, F. (2024). Description and clinical relevance of the variable conformation of canine spinal arachnoid diverticula. *Vet. Radiol. Ultrasound* 65 (4): 344–351.

Driver, C.J., Rose, J., Tauro, A. et al. (2019). Magnetic resonance image findings in pug dogs with thoracolumbar myelopathy and concurrent caudal articular process dysplasia. *BMC Vet. Res.* 15: 182.

Fenn, J., Olby, N.J., The Canine Spinal Cord Injury Consortium (CANSORT-SCI) et al. (2020 [cited 2025 Nov 4]). Classification of intervertebral disc disease. *Front. Vet. Sci.* 7: 579025. Available from: https://www.frontiersin.org/journals/veterinary-science/articles/10.3389/fvets.2020.579025/full.

Fisher, S.C., Shores, A., and Simpson, S.T. (2013). Constrictive myelopathy secondary to hypoplasia or aplasia of the thoracolumbar caudal articular processes in Pugs: 11 cases (1993-2009). *J. Am. Vet. Med. Assoc.* 242 (2): 223–229.

Gomes, S.A., Volk, H.A., Packer, R.M. et al. (2016). Clinical and magnetic resonance imaging characteristics of thoracolumbar intervertebral disk extrusions and protrusions in large breed dogs. *Vet. Radiol. Ultrasound* 57 (4): 417–426.

Gomes, S.A., Targett, M., Mignan, T. et al. (2025). Postsurgical outcome and recurrence rates in thoracolumbar arachnoid diverticula undergoing durotomy alone or alongside a modified technique of subdural shunt-placement in dogs. *Vet. Surg.* 54 (5): 972–982.

Jones, B., Behr, S., Shaw, T. et al. (2022). Surgical techniques used in the management of intra-arachnoid diverticula in dogs across four referral centres and their immediate outcome. *J. Small Anim. Pract.* 63 (7): 520–525.

Lourinho, F., Holdsworth, A., McConnell, J.F. et al. (2020). Clinical features and MRI characteristics of presumptive constrictive myelopathy in 27 pugs. *Vet. Radiol. Ultrasound* 61 (5): 545–554.

Mauler, D.A., De Decker, S., De Risio, L. et al. (2014). Signalment, clinical presentation, and diagnostic findings in 122 dogs with spinal arachnoid diverticula. *J. Vet. Intern. Med.* 28 (1): 175–181.

Seiler, G.S., Robertson, I.D., Mai, W. et al. (2012). Usefulness of a half-fourier acquisition single-shot turbo spin-echo pulse sequence in identifying arachnoid diverticula in dogs. *Vet. Radiol. Ultrasound* 53 (2): 157–161.

Smith, C.J. and Guevar, J. (2020). Spinal subarachnoid diverticula in dogs: a review. *Can. Vet. J.* 61 (11): 1162–1169.

Tauro, A., Kurihara, M., Macri, J. et al. (2025 [cited 2025 Nov 4]). Case report: 3D-CISS and PC-MRI in the diagnosis and surgical planning of hydrocephalus secondary to presumptive lateral aperture obstruction in a dog. *Front. Vet. Sci.* 12: 1646137. Available from: https://www.frontiersin.org/journals/veterinary-science/articles/10.3389/fvets.2025.1646137/full.

Tauro, A., Driver, C.J., Rose, J. et al. (2025 [cited 2025 Nov 4]). Case report: long-term surgical outcomes in pug dogs with articular facet dysplasia-associated thoracolumbar myelopathies. *Front. Vet. Sci.* 12: 1648444. Available from: https://www.frontiersin.org/journals/veterinary-science/articles/10.3389/fvets.2025.1648444/full.

Urinary and Fecal Dysfunction

Case 3—Urinary and Fecal Incontinence in a Large-Breed Dog

CHAPTER 14.3

Sergio A. Gomes

Dovecote Veterinary Referrals, Derby, UK

CASE HISTORY

A 10-year-old intact male Staffordshire bull terrier was presented for evaluation due to a chronic, progressive condition that had been ongoing for over 6 months. The owner reported a gradual worsening of signs, including frequent spontaneous yelping episodes, particularly when the dog attempted to stand up from rest. Over time, he also developed a marked reluctance or complete inability to jump onto elevated surfaces or climb stairs (Video 14.3.1). These difficulties were notably aggravated following periods of physical activity. As the dysfunction progressed, pelvic limb dysfunction and urinary and fecal incontinence developed. Initial medical management included treatment with carprofen and gabapentin, which provided only partial relief, as the clinical signs persisted and were not fully controlled with this therapeutic approach.

VIDEO 14.3.1 A dog showing difficulty climbing the stairs due to lower motor neuron (LMN) dysfunction of the pelvic limbs.

NEUROLOGICAL EXAMINATION

General clinical examination was largely unremarkable, with no pertinent findings besides consistent pain on bilateral extension of the hips. Neurological examination revealed dysfunction limited to the pelvic limbs, tail, and anal sphincter. Both when the dog was stationary and when ambulating, a bilateral plantigrade stance was present. The dog was ambulatory with moderate paraparesis. During the swing phase of the gait, minimal flexion at the stifle and tibiotarsal joint bilaterally was appreciated. Instead, the dog appeared to flip the tarsi forward to prevent landing on the dorsal aspect of the pes. Mild general proprioceptive ataxia was observed in both pelvic limbs. Palpation of the pelvic limbs revealed moderate, generalized muscle atrophy and decreased tone bilaterally. The tail was held low and had similarly decreased tone as well. Postural reactions were mildly delayed in both pelvic limbs. The patellar reflex was present bilaterally and seemed exaggerated. The withdrawal reflex was abnormal in both pelvic limbs: flexion was present at the hip joints bilaterally, reduced at the stifle joints bilaterally, and absent at the tibiotarsal joints bilaterally. Rectal examination revealed decreased anal tone and an absent perineal reflex. On caudal lumbar palpation, the dog demonstrated evidence of discomfort.

1. **Where is the likely lesion localization?**
2. **How should this dog's urinary incontinence be managed?**

LESION LOCALIZATION

Given that the thoracic limbs are normal, there are two possible lesion localizations leading to pelvic limb dysfunction and urinary and fecal incontinence. This patient is displaying signs of LMN dysfunction pertaining to the pelvic limbs. Specifically, the plantigrade stance, "tarsal flip" during ambulation, and the reduced pelvic limb withdrawal reflexes bilaterally point to dysfunction of the sciatic nerve, the L7–S1 nerve roots, or the L7–S1 spinal cord segments. The absent perineal reflex and decreased anal tone similarly reflect LMN dysfunction, specifically pertaining to the S1–S3 spinal cord segments, the S1–S3 nerve roots, or the pudendal nerve. Finally, the decreased tail movement and tone indicate LMN dysfunction of the tail as a result of a lesion in the caudal spinal cord, caudal nerve roots, or caudal nerves. The combination of signs observed in this patient is consistent with a lesion affecting the cauda equina, which is the terminal region of the spinal cord.

Cauda equina syndrome is a multifactorial condition centered on compression or infiltration of the nerves emerging from the caudal aspect of the spinal cord, referred to as the "cauda equina," or horse's tail. In dogs, the cauda equina includes the L7, S1–S3, and caudal nerve roots. As such, impingement or irritation of these nerve roots leads to:

- Pelvic limb dysfunction from L7 and S1 compression, characterized by LMN paraparesis, a plantigrade stance, decreased tone, and reduced withdrawal reflexes, particularly at the tibiotarsal joint.
- LMN urinary and fecal incontinence from S1–S3 nerve root compression, characterized by inability to retain urine and feces, and decreased anal tone
- Low tail carriage and decreased tail tone from caudal nerve root compression

For more details regarding the differential diagnoses for this lesion localization, please refer to Chapter 10. The reader should also be aware that urinary incontinence can rarely occur secondary to a condition called dysautonomia. While this is not a differential diagnosis for the case presented herein, it is nonetheless an important disease with which practitioners should be familiar.

Dysautonomia is a neurodegenerative disorder that affects the autonomic nervous system through degeneration of autonomic ganglia. Primary dysautonomia has been observed in dogs cats, horses, and rabbits. In cats in the United Kingdom, the disease is often referred to as "Key-Gaskell syndrome." Canine dysautonomia was subsequently reported, mostly in the United States. The underlying etiology remains elusive, but there is strong suspicion for an environmental cause. In the United States, most dogs that develop dysautonomia live in the Midwest or western United States. A pathogen in soil has been suspected but never definitively identified. Typically, dogs that develop this disease are young and spend substantial time outdoors in rural areas, often in close proximity to cattle and wildlife [1].

Clinical signs of dysautonomia are consistent with both sympathetic and parasympathetic dysfunction. The most commonly reported clinical signs include dysuria and urinary retention, bilateral mydriasis with absent pupillary light reflexes, raised third eyelids, decreased anal tone, vomiting and regurgitation, and decreased saliva and tear production [2]. Thoracic radiographs may reveal megaesophagus. Abdominal radiographs may disclose ileus and gastric distension. The typical disease course is 14 days. The prognosis is grave.

Although definitive diagnosis requires postmortem evaluation of the autonomic ganglia, pharmacologic testing in addition to the observation of the above-listed clinical signs can provide support for a presumptive antemortem diagnosis:

- Pilocarpine diluted to 0.05–0.1% will result in miosis within 45 minutes in patients with dysautonomia. Pilocarpine is a parasympathomimetic drug. In dysautonomia, the autonomic ganglion denervation deprives effector cells of neurotransmitters. This makes these receptor cells supersensitive to low doses of parasympathomimetic drugs. In healthy dogs, this low concentration of pilocarpine would not lead to miosis within this time period.

- In healthy dogs, an intradermal injection of histamine results in both a wheal and flare. Dogs with dysautonomia develop a wheal, which is dependent on the direct action of histamine on local blood vessels, but they do not develop flare. Flare is mediated by sympathetic neurons [1].
- There are additional tests that can be performed, but they are associated with higher risk profiles and are therefore not typically performed.

Currently, as the definitive cause of dysautonomia is unknown, there is no definitive therapy for this devastating condition. Relative to this chapter, dogs with dysautonomia have urinary retention. One aspect of their supportive care is assisting with elimination.

MANAGING URINARY INCONTINENCE

Incontinence is defined as the inability to voluntarily void normally. There are broadly two forms of urinary and fecal incontinence: upper motor neuron (UMN) incontinence and LMN incontinence. These are described in Chapter 14, Case 1.

Both forms of incontinence result in urinary retention, which predisposes animals to urinary tract infections and can also cause detrusor atony in UMN bladders. Thus, the cornerstone of incontinence management is assisting with voiding. There are several techniques, each with benefits and drawbacks:

- *Manual expression:* This is the most common and generally the easiest technique to perform (Video 14.3.2). Expression can be performed in lateral recumbency or with the patient supported in a modified standing position, based on operator preference and patient compliance. The hands are placed on either side of the abdomen, and gentle, steady pressure is applied to initiate voiding. This steady pressure is continued until the urine stream stops.

VIDEO 14.3.2 Video demonstrating and narrating technique for bladder expression in lateral recumbency.

  - Expressing a LMN bladder typically requires little exertion, given that the external urethral sphincter is experiencing flaccid paralysis with a lesion that causes LMN dysfunction.
  - Expressing an UMN bladder typically requires a substantial amount of steady pressure, given that the external urethral sphincter is experiencing spastic paralysis with a lesion that causes UMN dysfunction.

> Note: Use caution when expressing the urinary bladders of cats with UMN incontinence. If too much pressure is placed on the bladder, it may rupture.

- **Catheterization:**
  - Indwelling catheters are generally used temporarily, in-hospital, in patients who are not amenable to bladder expression, either due to patient temperament or because they are large and expression is difficult to perform. Indwelling catheters should only remain in place for up to several days, and ideally should be cultured following removal, since they can be a source of urinary tract infections.
  - Intermittent catheterization is generally used in male dogs that are not amenable to bladder expression. Clients can be instructed on how to perform catheterization and how to sterilize them for repeated use.

- *Decompressive cystocentesis:* This procedure, in which a sterile needle is inserted into the bladder lumen, is typically only performed as single events when expression or catheterization is either contraindicated or not possible. Decompressive cystocentesis should therefore not be used as a routine voiding assistance technique.

There are a variety of medications that can aid with bladder expression. Typically, pharmacologic intervention is not necessary when assisting a patient with an LMN bladder, as expression is typically relatively easy against a flaccid external urethral sphincter. Contrastingly, UMN bladders may become easier to express with urinary sphincter relaxants.

- Diazepam is a skeletal muscle relaxant that works at the level of the external urethral sphincter. A dose of 0.5–1 mg/kg PO can be given to dogs about 30 minutes prior to bladder expression. Cats can develop idiosyncratic fulminant hepatic necrosis with repeated use of oral benzodiazepines, so their use should be avoided in cats. The most common side effect of diazepam is sedation. The author has used dantrolene, another muscle relaxant, successfully in several cats to aid in bladder expression.
- Prazosin and phenoxybenzamine are alpha-adrenergic antagonists that work at the level of the internal urethral sphincter. For phenoxybenzamine, a dose of 0.25–0.5 mg/kg PO every 12 hours can be used. For prazosin, a dose of 1 mg per 15 kg of body weight PO every 8–12 hours can be used. Both are safe in cats. The most common side effects are hypotension and weakness.
- Bethanechol is generally not used in patients with UMN incontinence and is instead used in the treatment of patients with detrusor atony. It is a muscarinic receptor agonist, leading to increased detrusor muscle contraction. For dogs, 2.5–25 mg as the total dose PO every 8 hours can be used. For cats, 1.25–7.5 mg as the total dose PO every 8 hours can be used. The most common side effects are salivation, lacrimation, urination, and defecation. Do not use bethanechol without using medications to relax the urethral sphincters, as bladder rupture has been documented to occur in these cases.

Preventing urinary tract infections: Dogs and cats with urinary and fecal incontinence should have the regions cleaned anytime following elimination to avoid the development of urinary tract infections. Non-scented baby wipes are a good option.

Treating urinary tract infections: Urinary tract infections are a source of discomfort in patients who have retained sensation in their bladders. Bladder infections can also progress to ascending urinary tract infections. Clients should be instructed to monitor for signs of a urinary tract infection, including hematuria and malodorous urine. Dogs and cats that have some urinary control may display pollakiuria if they are experiencing a urinary tract infection.

In patients with chronic myelopathies, repeated treatment of urinary tract infections can lead to antibiotic-resistant urinary tract infections. Therefore, treatment with antibiotics should be reserved for patients who show discomfort associated with a urinary tract infection or patients who show signs consistent with an ascending infection (fever, malaise, anorexia, vomiting, azotemia, and isosthenuria).

MANAGING FECAL INCONTINENCE

If urinary incontinence is present, fecal incontinence is typically also present. The colon and rectum are efficient smooth muscle organs that continue to experience peristalsis in cases of myelopathies. Myelopathic dogs and cats with UMN lesions may defecate less often due to decreased colonic stimulation from limb movements. Feces will be evacuated whenever the rectum fills sufficiently with decreased conscious control in cases with UMN lesions. Should a more regular schedule be desired, pet owners can be instructed to insert a lubricated thermometer into the rectum, which can sometimes stimulate defecation.

LMN fecal incontinence is associated with a dilated external anal sphincter, out of which feces will constantly drip. There is no direct treatment for LMN fecal incontinence. Animals living indoors may need to wear diapers to prevent house soiling. LMN fecal incontinence predisposes dogs, especially female dogs, to urinary tract infections, since animals with LMN fecal incontinence typically also have LMN urinary incontinence, and bacteria from feces can easily traverse the dilated external urethral sphincter.

SUGGESTED READING

Caines, D., Pinard, C.L., Kruth, S. et al. (2011). Autonomic dysfunction in a Jack Russell terrier. *Can. Vet. J.* 52 (3): 297–299.

Dewey, C.W. and Da Costa, R.C. (2015). *Practical Guide to Canine and Feline Neurology*, 3e. Wiley.

Granger, N., Olby, N.J., and Nout-Lomas, Y.S. (2020). Canine Spinal Cord Injury Consortium (CANSORT-SCI). Bladder and bowel management in dogs with spinal cord injury. *Front. Vet. Sci.* 7: 583342.

Harkin, K.R., Andrews, G.A., and Nietfeld, J.C. (2002, [cited 2025 Nov 4]). Dysautonomia in dogs: 65 cases (1993–2000). *J. Am. Vet. Med. Assoc.* 220 (5): 633–639. Available from: https://avma.ournals.avma.org/view/journals/javma.220/5/javma.2002.220.633.xml.

CHAPTER 15.1

Neurological Trauma

Case 1—Head Trauma

Juliet Armstrong

Blue Pearl Pet Hospital, Richmond, VA, USA

CASE HISTORY

A 12-year-old spayed female Pomeranian was presented on emergency following a dog bite to the head. Immediately after being bitten on the head, she collapsed and began convulsing. Initial evaluation was performed by her primary care veterinarian, at which time an intravenous (IV) catheter was placed, and a single dose of intravenous midazolam (0.5 mg/kg) was administered before transfer to a multispecialty center. Prior medical history included a grade III/VI systolic heart murmur for which she was managed on enalapril (0.3 mg/kg by mouth every 12 hours) and a compound antebrachial fracture, which had been surgically repaired years prior. She was up to date on vaccines and received regular monthly preventatives.

TRIAGE EXAMINATION AND POINT-OF-CARE ASSESSMENT

At presentation, she was severely obtunded. She was non-ambulatory tetraparetic with a tendency to turn to the left, and a generalized seizure event was observed upon arrival. Cardiothoracic auscultation identified a grade IV/VI left apical systolic murmur. She was tachycardic (pulse rate of 140 beats/minute) with no evidence of pulse deficits, and femoral pulses were of good quality. Oral mucous membranes were light pink and moist with a capillary refill time of 2 seconds. Her eyes, ears, and nares were free of any discharge or debris, although she was noted to be anisocoric with a miotic left pupil. She had a mild increase in respiratory rate (40 breaths/minute) and effort, but no crackles or wheezes were auscultated. Abdominal palpation was tense with no obvious evidence of organomegaly or fluid waves. Palpable peripheral lymph nodes were of normal size and symmetry. A rectal examination was not performed.

She was normothermic (rectal temperature of 98 °F), and her blood pressure, measured at presentation (Doppler, systolic on a thoracic limb), was 80 mmHg. Pulse oximetry without supplemental oxygenation was 95%, and a brief electrocardiogram identified a sinus tachycardia. Point-of-care bloodwork revealed a packed cell volume of 47%, total solids of 6.4 g/dL, and blood glucose of 120 mg/dL. Abdominal focused assessment and sonography for trauma (AFAST) identified no free fluid and an intact bladder. Thoracic focused assessment and sonography for trauma (TFAST) identified occasional left-sided B-lines and no evidence of pleural or pericardial effusion.

1. **What systemic factors should be closely evaluated/monitored?**
2. **What diagnostics should be urgently performed to assess the extent of trauma?**

SYSTEMIC EVALUATION

Irrespective of the type of trauma sustained, assessment and management of life-threatening injuries should be prioritized (Figure 15.1.1). In cases of head trauma, aside from an initial

1. Oxygenation
   - Provide flow by oxygen taking care not to struggle with a face mask or nasal prongs if the patient will not tolerate
   - Intubate and ventilate based on assessment of $PaCO_2$, and respiratory rate/effort
2. Continuous ECG
   - It is common to encounter tachycardia, premature complexes, and ventricular tachycardia secondary to trauma and hemodynamic instability
3. Intravenous catheter and bloodwork
   - PCV/TS/BG/Lactate
   - Point-of-care bloodwork: blood gas, i-STAT, epoc®, etc.
4. Blood pressure (decisions for intervention dependent upon patient comorbidities)
   - If hypotensive/tachycardic or other signs of hemodynamic instability are noted, consider crystalloid bolus (10ml/kg IV over 15–20 minutes)
   - May need administration of hyperosmolar agent or additional crystalloid boluses based on reassessment
5. Brief assessment of other body cavities
   - Abdominal focused assessment with sonography for trauma (AFAST)
   - Thoracic focused assessment with sonography for trauma (TFAST)
6. Perform brief neurologic assessment
   - Assign modified Glasgow Coma Scale score
   - Administration of anticonvulsants for observed seizure activity
7. Elevate head/neck
   - Do not compress/obstruct jugular veins as that will risk increasing intracranial pressure
8. Hyperosmolar therapy
   - 2–5 mL/kg of 7.2% hypertonic saline IV over 15 minutes
   - 0.5–1.5 g/kg mannitol IV over 15 minutes administered via a filter
   - It is important to reassess both blood pressure and neurologic status following treatment
9. Administration of analgesia
   - Titrate dose carefully while monitoring/assessing mentation and neurologic status
10. Administration of GI medications

FIGURE 15.1.1 Stepwise approach to initial patient assessment and stabilization for patients presenting for head trauma. Initial assessment and triage focus on systemic factors with neurologic assessment and intervention occurring secondarily. BG= blood glucose; ECG = electrocardiography; PCV = packed cell volume; TS = total solids.

evaluation focusing on the triage parameters of heart rate, respiratory rate, mucous membrane color, capillary refill time, pulse quality, level of consciousness, and oxygen saturation, interventions to address hypotension, hypovolemia, and ventilation are critical. As hypoxemia and hypovolemia are strongly correlated with increased intracranial pressure (ICP) for these patients, medical interventions to stabilize these parameters may affect patient prognosis.

INITIAL DIAGNOSTIC APPROACH (Table 15.1.1)

Initial point-of-care and patient-side diagnostic testing should include measurements of blood pressure (with serial reassessments), packed cell volume, total protein, blood glucose, lactate, electrolytes, and coagulation parameters. Abdominal and thoracic focused assessments and sonography

Table 15.1.1 Suggested staged diagnostic approach for traumatic brain injury/head trauma patients.

Diagnostic test	Patient selection	Additional considerations
Point of care/initial diagnostics		
Blood Pressure	All patients	
Complete Blood Count	All patients	
Chemistry Profile with electrolytes (emphasis on blood glucose, lactate)	All patients	
PCV/TS	All patients	
Coagulation Testing (PT/PTT)		
ECG	All patients	
AFAST/TFAST	All patients	
Modified Glasgow Coma Scale Assessment	All patients	Take care in moving the patient; serial examination is the key component for prognostication
Once a patient has been stabilized		
Radiographs	All patients when stable/able to be safely moved	Consider thoracic AND abdominal/pelvic radiographs to screen for concurrent trauma
As guided by neurologic status and response to therapies; completed with consultation from specialists		
Computed Tomography	Those with moderate to severe trauma or who seem refractory to supportive care measures	To be performed when the patient can be safely moved; administer contrast only if hemodynamically stable
Magnetic Resonance Imaging	Those with moderate to severe trauma or who seem refractory to supportive care measures	Consider anesthetic risk or adjustments to protocols based on patient's hemodynamic stability

Items included are grouped by initial/emergent diagnostics, those diagnostics that should be considered once a patient is stabilized, and those for which consultation with specialists is advised.

for trauma (AFAST/TFAST) are also recommended to evaluate for the presence of concurrent injuries such as pneumothorax, pleural effusion, pulmonary contusions, and abdominal effusion and to evaluate for the presence of an intact bladder.

The animal trauma triage (ATT) score is a veterinary illness severity score that numerically classifies the degree of trauma in an attempt to quantify mortality risk probability. The ATT score is based on a 0–3 scale (0 indicating slight or no injury, 3 indicating severe injury), with assessment of six independent components (perfusion, cardiac, respiratory, eye/muscle/integument, skeletal, and neurologic) that contribute equally to the overall predictive score (Table 15.1.2). Dogs with an ATT score of 9 have approximately a 50% probability of survival with the score having an overall linear relationship with mortality and suggested to be a better predictor than the MGCS.

Once life-threatening abnormalities have been addressed and the patient is hemodynamically stabilized, additional diagnostics including a complete blood count, chemistry profile, and thoracic and abdominal radiographs, should be obtained. Thoracic screening for trauma patients is recommended, as neurogenic/noncardiogenic pulmonary edema can develop rapidly as peripheral vasoconstriction causes an increase in sympathetic activity. This vasoconstriction can lead to systemic and pulmonary capillary hypertension and therefore pulmonary edema. As edema develops, dyspnea, hypoxemia, hypercapnia, and potentially increased ICP may occur. Although

Table 15.1.2 Animal trauma triage (ATT) score.

Perfusion	
MMs pink/moist, CRT 2 seconds, T ≥ 100 °F strong or bounding femoral pulse quality	0
MMs hyperemic or pale pink, MMs tacky, CRT 0–2 seconds, T ≥ 100 °F, fair femoral pulses	1
MMs very pale pink and tacky, CRT 2–3 seconds, T < 100 °F, detectable but poor pulses	2
MMs grey/blue/white, CRT >3 seconds, T < 100 °F, nonpalpable femoral pulses	3
Cardiac	
HR canine: 60–140 bpm; feline: 120–200 bpm, normal sinus rhythm	0
HR canine: 140–180 bpm; feline: 200–260 bpm, NSR or VPC < 20/minute	1
HR canine: >180 bpm; feline: >260 bpm, consistent arrhythmia	2
HR canine: <60 bpm; feline: ≤120 bpm, erratic arrhythmia	3
Respiratory	
Regular respiratory rate with no stridor, no abdominal component to respiration	0
Mildly increased respiratory rate and effort ± abdominal component, mild upper airway sounds	1
Moderately increased respiratory rate and effort, some abdominal component, elbow abduction, moderately increased upper airway sounds	2
Marked respiratory effort or gasping/agonal respiration, little/no air passage	3
Eye/muscle/integument	
Abrasion/laceration – none or partial thickness. Eye – no fluorescein uptake	0
Abrasion/laceration – full thickness, no deep tissue involved. Eye – corneal laceration, not perforation	1
Abrasion/laceration – full thickness, deep tissue involved, artery/nerve/muscle intact. Eye: corneal perforation, punctured globe, or proptosis	2
Penetration of abdomen/thorax. Abrasion/laceration, full thickness, deep tissue involvement, artery/nerve/muscle compromised	3
Skeletal	
Weight bearing three or four limbs. No palpable fracture/joint laxity	0
Closed limb fracture/rib fracture or any mandibular fracture. Single joint laxity/luxation (including sacroiliac). Pelvic fracture with unilateral intact sacroiliac – ilium – acetabulum. Single limb open/closed fracture at or below carpus/tarsus	1
Multiple grade 1 conditions, single long bone open fracture above carpus/tarsus with cortical bone preserved. Nonmandibular skull fracture	2
Vertebral body fracture/luxation except coccygeal, multiple long bone open fractures above tarsus/carpus, single long bone open fracture above tarsus/carpus with loss of cortical bone	3
Neurological	
Central: alert to slightly dull. Peripheral: normal spinal reflexes; purposeful movement and nociception in all limbs	0
Central: dull/depressed/withdrawn. Peripheral: abnormal spinal reflexes with purposeful movement and nociception intact in all limbs	1
Central: unconscious, responds to noxious stimuli. Peripheral: absent purposeful movement with intact nociception in two or more limbs or nociception absent in one limb, decreased anal or tail tone	2
Central: nonresponsive to all stimuli ± refractory seizures. Peripheral: absent nociception in two or more limbs, absent tail or perianal nociception	3

bpm, beats per minute; CRT, capillary refill time; HR, heart rate; MMs, mucous membranes.

edema formation is typically self-limiting, it can also be exacerbated by continued seizure activity in head trauma patients.

Depending on patient stability and technical availability, whole-body trauma computed tomography (CT) could also be considered. CT may help to screen for concurrent limb, vertebral column, thoracic, and abdominal trauma and better evaluate the severity of the sustained head trauma.

NEUROLOGICAL EXAMINATION AT PRESENTATION

At presentation, the patient was severely obtunded and experienced a generalized seizure. She was non-ambulatory tetraparetic with a tendency to turn to the left. She had an absent menace bilaterally with a noted anisocoria (left pupil miosis) and sluggish pupillary light reflexes (PLRs). She had normal tone and reflexes in all limbs but no appreciable paraspinal pain.

1. **What is the patient's modified Glasgow Coma Scale score?**
2. **What additional diagnostics could be considered for neurologic assessment?**
3. **What medical and/or surgical interventions should be considered?**

ASSIGNING A MODIFIED GLASGOW COMA SCALE SCORE

The modified Glasgow Coma Scale should be performed and serially re-evaluated in patients who have sustained a traumatic brain injury. This scale (Figure 15.1.2) aims to objectively measure the level of consciousness, motor activity, and brainstem reflexes, providing a 48-hour prognostication. Each category of assessment receives a score of 1–6 with a total potential score of 18, such that the lower the score, the poorer the prognosis. Serial measurements using this scoring system enable clinicians to monitor improvements and deterioration over the course of hospitalization.

For this patient, her severely obtunded mentation (score: 3), non-ambulatory tetraparesis (motor activity score: 5), and brainstem reflexes (score: 5) yielded a total score of 13, suggesting a poor to guarded 48-hour prognosis.

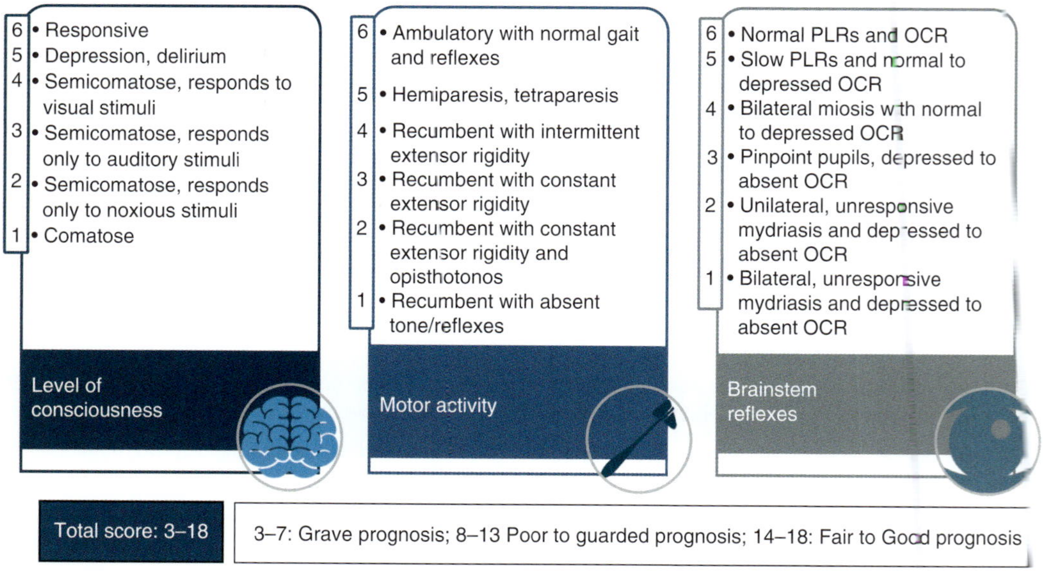

FIGURE 15.1.2 Modified Glasgow Coma scale; PLRs: pupillary light reflexes; OCR: oculocephalic reflex.

ADDITIONAL DIAGNOSTICS TO CONSIDER FOR NEUROLOGIC ASSESSMENT

In the absence of the availability of CT or magnetic resonance imaging (MRI), skull radiographs may be considered. Skull radiographs may reveal evidence of depressed skull fractures, but generally are considered unlikely to alter the course of therapeutic decision-making.

CT, when technically available and performed once patients are hemodynamically stabilized, is the modality of choice for cases of moderate and severe acute head trauma (Figure 15.1.3). The speed and accuracy of CT allow for the detection of abnormalities that may alter clinical case management, including compressive fractures, intracranial hemorrhage, edema, and herniation. Additionally, if a skull CT is being considered, added imaging of the thorax, limbs, abdomen, and pelvis may better screen for concurrent injuries without much added time for image acquisition.

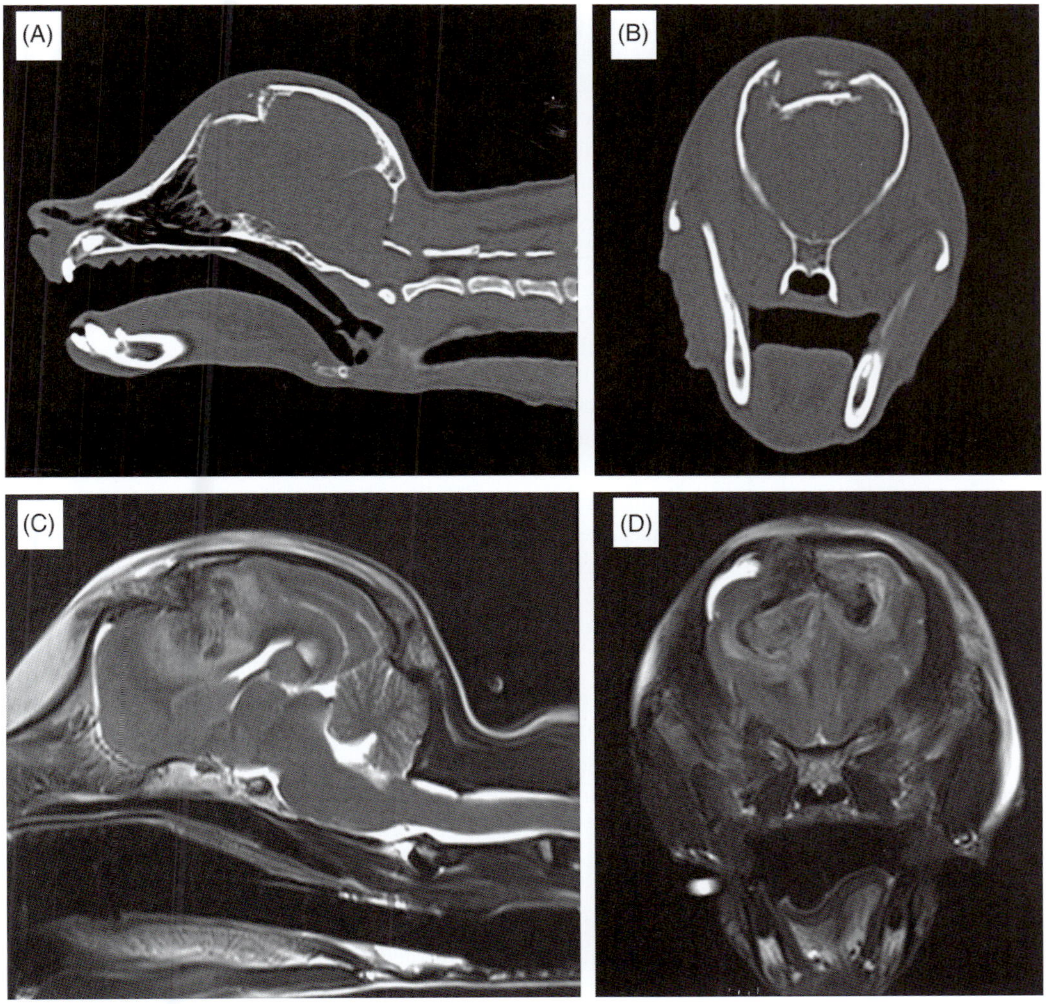

FIGURE 15.1.3 Sagittal (A) and Transverse (B) images from skull CT in a bone window demonstrating a comminuted, compression fracture of the dorsal aspect of the frontal bone, predominantly right of midline. Sagittal T2-weighted (C) and transverse T2-weighted (D) MRI images from the same patient demonstrating a large bony fragment originating from the frontal bone compressing the underlying frontal lobe of the brain with associated hemorrhage and edema.

MRI is indicated when CT fails to explain the neurologic signs associated with head trauma and is preferred in cases of subacute or chronic traumatic brain injuries. Within MRI sequencing, proton density, T2-weighted and fluid-attenuated inversion recovery (FLAIR) sequences provide the most diagnostic information, allowing for improved detection of contusions, axonal injury, subarachnoid hemorrhage, and extracranial soft tissue trauma (Figure 15.1.3).

MEDICAL AND SURGICAL INTERVENTIONS TO CONSIDER

Therapies for head trauma patients are directed at minimizing the effects of secondary brain injury: the delayed injury that can include cerebral swelling (related to vasogenic and cytotoxic edema), post-traumatic ischemia and infarction, brain herniation, and infection related to penetrating injuries to the skull. These changes occur within minutes to weeks after the primary injury and are exacerbated by perfusion compromises and alterations in mean arterial blood pressure.

Medical therapies include the management of ICP and maintenance of cerebral perfusion through intravenous fluid therapy and the use of hyperosmolar agents (e.g. mannitol or hypertonic saline), as well as oxygenation and ventilatory support, pain management, and seizure prophylaxis. Intensive nursing care is also critical to limit the potential for complications to arise, such as coagulopathies, aspiration pneumonia, electrolyte derangements, and sepsis.

Supplemental oxygen should be administered initially via flow by, as oxygen cages are usually ineffective because constant monitoring of the patient does not allow for a closed system. Nasal oxygen catheters or transtracheal catheters can be used to supply at 40% inspired oxygen concentration with flow rates of 100 mL/kg/min or 50 mL/kg/min, respectively. Mechanical ventilation is recommended for animals with impaired consciousness (e.g. MGCS < 8), progressive hypercapnia ($PaCO_2$ > 60 mmHg), refractory hypoxemia despite oxygen supplementation, or when spontaneous respiratory effort is insufficient.

Initial resuscitation usually involves intravenous administration of hypertonic saline and/or synthetic colloids. Use of these solutions allows rapid restoration of blood volume and pressure while limiting the volume of fluid administered.

Hypertonic saline, typically administered as 3-7.2% solutions, is preferred for its ability to rapidly draw water from the cerebral interstitium into the vascular compartment, thereby reducing brain swelling and ICP. It also enhances mean arterial pressure and microvascular perfusion with minimal fluid volume, making it particularly useful in hypovolemic patients. Recommended dosing ranges from 2 to 5 mL/kg intravenously over 15 minutes.

Mannitol should be administered as a bolus over a 15-minute period (rather than as an infusion) to obtain the plasma-expanding effect. Its effect on brain edema takes approximately 15–30 minutes to establish and lasts between 2 and 8 hours. Doses of 0.5–1.5 g/kg appear to be equally effective in lowering ICP, but the duration of effect is shorter with lower doses.

Surgical intervention for head trauma patients should be considered in cases of depressed or open skull fractures and to remove contaminated bone fragments or foreign material lodged within the brain parenchyma. Surgical intervention by way of a decompressive craniotomy should also be considered in cases that deteriorate neurologically despite appropriate aggressive medical therapy (Figure 15.1.4).

The duration of hospitalization for a given patient is dependent upon the severity of the traumatic brain injury, concurrent injuries, and response to medical or surgical interventions. The suggested discharge criteria include maintenance of an adequate neurologic status while on oral medications, hemodynamic and respiratory stability, an ability to prehend and swallow food and water independently or with minimal assistance, and seizure control. It is important to note that severe head trauma cases are still likely to be abnormal at the time of discharge and may have altered vision, gait changes, and require additional supportive care at home. Seizures may also occur at the time of trauma or develop months to years later.

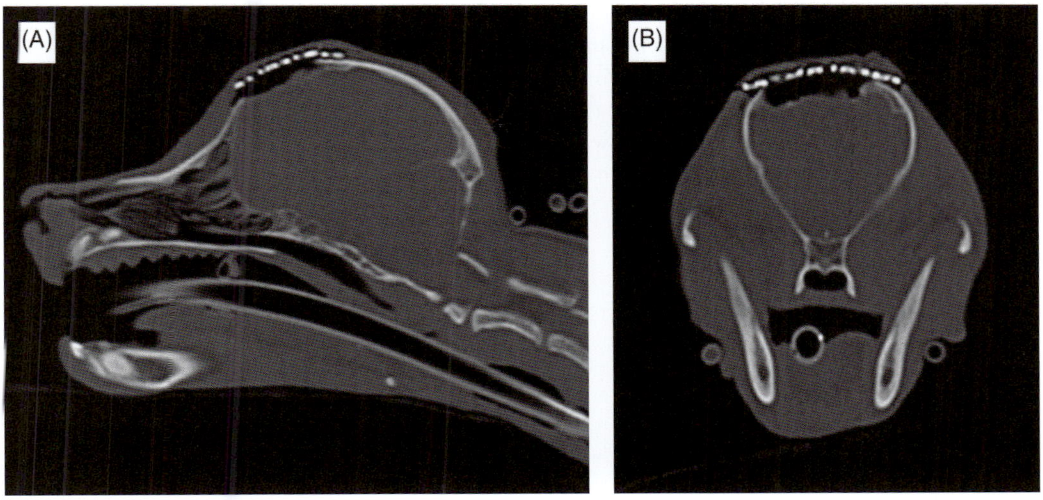

FIGURE 15.1.4 Sagittal (A) and Transverse (B) postoperative skull CT images from the same patient as Figure 15.1.3. Images obtained following a decompressive craniotomy and titanium mesh placement.

OUTCOME

The dog was initially stabilized with hypertonic saline and oxygenation via flow-by. The MGCS following this systemic stabilization was 13. Intravenous fluids were administered, temperature and pain were controlled, and seizure activity was treated at the time of occurrence. Antibiotics were also started intravenously given the bite wound. The dog underwent an MRI and CT and subsequent surgical decompression of its skull fracture. The neurological examination mildly improved over the next 4 days, but the patient continued to have a decreased appetite and due to the concern that her caloric intake was not being met, a nasogastric tube was placed. Despite making continued neurologic improvements, on day 19 of her hospitalization, the patient experienced an acute respiratory decompensation requiring oxygen support. Despite aggressive treatment for possible congestive heart failure and suspected aspiration pneumonia, the patient suffered cardiopulmonary arrest and succumbed to her comorbidities.

SUGGESTED READING

Ash, K., Hayes, G.M., Goggs, R., and Sumner, J.P. (2019). Performance evaluation and validation of the animal trauma triage (ATT) score and modified Glasgow coma scale (mGCS) with suggested category adjustment in dogs – a VetCOT registry study. *J. Vet. Emerg. Crit. Care (San Antonio)* 28 (3): 192–200.

Cameron, S., Weltman, J.G., and Fletcher, D.J. (2022). The prognostic value of admission point-of-care testing and modified Glasgow Coma Scale score in dogs and cats with traumatic brain injuries (2007–2010): 212 cases. *J. Vet. Emerg. Crit. Care* 32: 75–82.

Chesnut, R.M. (1997). The management of severe traumatic brain injury. *Emerg. Med. Clin. North Am.* 15 (3): 581–604.

Danel, A. and Shores, A. (2023). Head trauma management in small animals. *Today Vet. Pract.* March/April: 104–114.

Dewey, C.W. (2000). Emergency management of the head trauma patient. Principles and practice. *Vet. Clin. North Am. Small Anim. Pract.* 30 (1): 207–225. vii–viii.

DiFazio, J. and Fletcher, D.F. (2013). Updates in the management of the small animal patient with neurologic trauma. *Vet. Clin. Small Anim.* 43: 915–940.

Platt, S.R., Radaelli, S.T., and McDonnell, J.J. (2001). The prognostic value of the modified Glasgow coma scale in head trauma in dogs. *J. Vet. Intern. Med.* 15 (6): 581–584.

Sande, A. and West, C. (2010). Traumatic brain injury: a review of pathophysiology and management. *J. Vet. Emerg. Crit. Care* 20 (2): 177–190.

Wart, M., Edwards, T.H., Rizzo, J.A. et al. (2024) Traumatic brain injury in companion animals: pathophysiology and treatment. *Top. Companion Anim. Med.* 63: 100927.

Neurological Trauma

Case 2—Traumatic Vertebral Fractures and Luxations

CHAPTER 15.2

Juliet Armstrong

Blue Pearl Pet Hospital, Richmond, VA, USA

CASE HISTORY

A 5-year-old intact female German shepherd dog was presented on emergency after being hit by a tractor on a family farm. Before the accident, she was up to date on vaccines, had no past pertinent medical history, and was receiving no routine medications aside from monthly preventatives. Once freed from underneath the tractor, she was noted to walk away from the accident but seemed generally weak and had labored breathing.

TRIAGE EXAMINATION AND POINT-OF-CARE ASSESSMENT

At presentation, she was normothermic (rectal temperature of 98 °F), tachycardic (160 beats/minute palpable pulse rate with a normal electrocardiogram), tachypneic (50 breaths/minute) with increased respiratory effort, and moderately hypotensive (Doppler systolic blood pressure of 70 mmHg). Her oral mucous membranes were pale pink with a capillary refill time of 2 seconds. Cardiothoracic auscultation revealed muffled heart sounds and suspected borborygmus. An intact bladder without evidence of peritoneal free fluid was identified on abdominal focused assessment and sonography for trauma (AFAST), and thoracic focused assessment and sonography for trauma (TFAST) identified scant pleural effusion and hepatized tissue in the thoracic cavity. Gait analysis was not performed, but the patient was noted to move her tail voluntarily.

1. **What systemic factors should be closely evaluated/monitored?**
2. **What diagnostics should be urgently performed to assess the extent of trauma?**

INITIAL EVALUATION AND STABILIZATION

The initial evaluation and stabilization should aim to maintain adequate blood flow, blood pressure, and oxygenation, which can be achieved by providing appropriate intravenous fluid therapy and oxygen supplementation (Figure 15.2.1). It is crucial to identify and address systemic abnormalities and life-threatening injuries that have occurred because of the trauma in an effort to prevent secondary spinal cord injury.

During this initial evaluation, to prevent iatrogenic spinal cord damage and progressive neurologic dysfunction, limited manipulation and/or immobilization is recommended. Analgesic or anxiolytic medications should be administered once a brief neurologic assessment has been made.

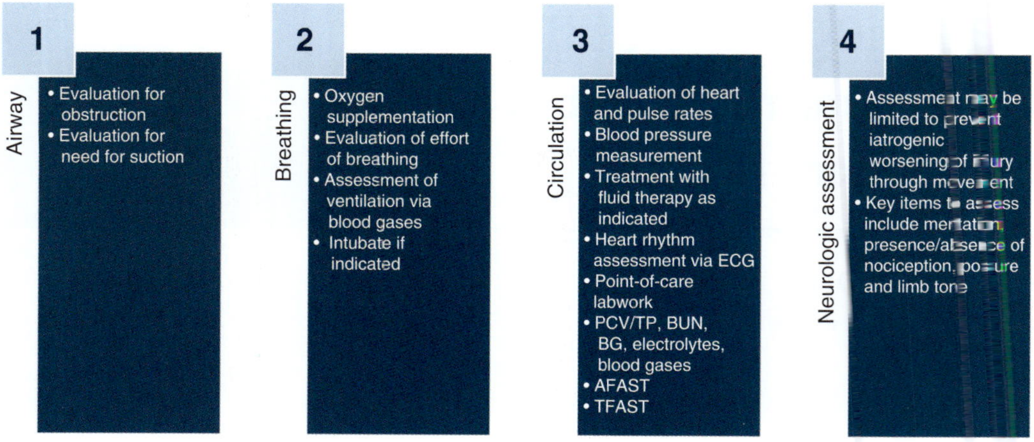

FIGURE 15.2.1 Stepwise approach to assessment for polytrauma patients with suspected spinal cord injuries. Life-threatening injuries and cardiovascular stability should be addressed as a priority.

It is essential to titrate these medication doses to effect in consideration of mentation monitoring, as well as to provide pain relief without an accompanying over-relaxation of epaxial muscles, which may result in destabilization of a vertebral fracture or luxation.

INITIAL DIAGNOSTIC APPROACH

Point-of-care/patient-side diagnostic testing for polytrauma patients with concerns for spinal injury should include measurements of blood pressure (with serial reassessment), pulse oximetry, and brief blood work (packed cell volume, blood glucose, lactate, total solids, and coagulation parameters). Additional point-of-care diagnostics, including AFAST/TFAST, are also recommended. Once life-threatening abnormalities have been addressed and the patient stabilized, additional diagnostics may be pursued.

Survey radiographs for polytrauma patients serve as a rapid way to evaluate for evidence of vertebral column trauma. As multiple injuries may occur, obtaining radiographs of the entire vertebral column from the base of the skull to the coccygeal vertebra is recommended. Similarly, thoracic and abdominal radiographs should be obtained to screen for concurrent trauma.

Concurrent thoracic trauma, reported to occur in 15–35% of patients who sustain vertebral column injuries, may include the presence of a pneumothorax, rib fractures, pulmonary contusions, and traumatic diaphragmatic hernia. Concurrent abdominal trauma, such as hemoabdomen, uroabdomen, and gastrointestinal or hepatobiliary injuries, has been reported in 6–15% of spinal trauma patients. Additionally, in 14–48% of cases with documented traumatic vertebral column fractures or luxation, concurrent pelvic and appendicular fractures have been reported. Some of these concurrent injuries, most notably pulmonary contusions, may worsen in the first one to two days following the initial trauma and, with progression, can become of significant concern for anesthesia, pursuit of diagnostic and therapeutic interventions, and prognosis.

For this dog, initial systemic evaluation identified tachypnea, tachycardia, mild hypotension, and muffled heart sounds. Following placement of an intravenous catheter, fluid resuscitation, and provision of analgesia, complete bloodwork and thoracic radiographs were obtained. Bloodwork was largely unremarkable, and thoracic radiographs (Figure 15.2.2) identified a traumatic diaphragmatic hernia. Given her clinical status, the patient underwent emergency surgical correction of her traumatic diaphragmatic hernia.

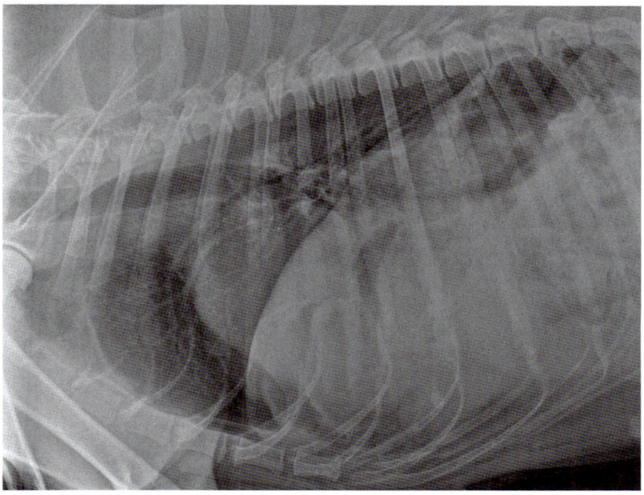

FIGURE 15.2.2 Lateral radiograph of the thorax demonstrating evidence of a traumatic diaphragmatic hernia.

NEUROLOGICAL EXAMINATION

On initial presentation, the patient had an appropriate mentation with a normal cranial nerve assessment. Tone and reflexes in her thoracic limbs, pelvic limbs, and tail were normal. She had a normal perineal reflex and anal tone. A cutaneous trunci reflex was not assessed at the time of presentation, and a gait assessment was not completed prior to the pursuit of surgery to address her traumatic diaphragmatic hernia – although it was noted during the triage examination that she was able to wag her tail and was initially observed to walk away from the accident.

The morning after her diaphragmatic surgery repair, the patient was noted to be non-ambulatory, severely paraparetic with normal tone and reflexes in her thoracic limbs and pelvic limbs. She had retained normal sensation in her pelvic limbs and tail. She had normal tail tone, anal tone, and a normal perineal reflex. A thoracolumbar junction cutoff to her cutaneous trunci reflex was identified. She was slightly sedated from the analgesics administered postoperatively and had no noted cranial nerve abnormalities.

1. **Where is the likely lesion localization?**
2. **What additional diagnostics should be performed?**

LESION LOCALIZATION

As part of a polytrauma evaluation, a neurologic assessment is warranted so that prognostication and the extent of sustained injuries can be addressed appropriately. In some cases of suspected spinal trauma, the neurologic examination may be initially limited to avoid iatrogenic damage to the spinal cord with patient manipulation. This is especially important to consider, as some injuries to the vertebral column may result in instability and be dynamic. Initial neurologic examination in this patient was determined to be normal following her triage and systemic evaluation immediately post-trauma. However, gait analysis and assessment of motor function (aside from notation of tail movement) were not initially performed in favor of addressing her life-threatening diaphragmatic hernia.

When this patient was noted to be non-ambulatory the morning after her diaphragmatic hernia repair, a more complete neurologic assessment was performed. Given her normal cranial

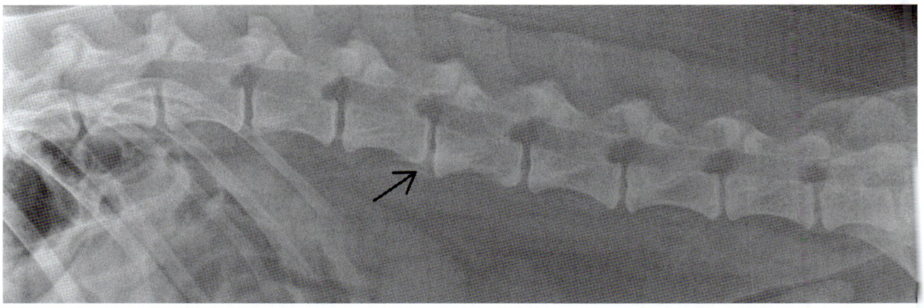

FIGURE 15.2.3 Single lateral radiograph of the thoracolumbar vertebral column (patient has eight lumbar vertebrae) demonstrating a mild subluxation, widening, and step defect centered at the L3–L4 intervertebral disc space (arrow).

nerves, mentation, and normal thoracic limbs, the patient was determined to have a thoracolumbar myelopathy. More specifically, with the normal pelvic limb tone and reflexes, as well as normal tail and anal tone, the patient was localized to a T3–L3 myelopathy.

DIAGNOSTICS

Radiography may be used as a screening for traumatic vertebral column injuries (Figure 15.2.3). However, it has only moderate sensitivity for identifying fractures (around 70%) and subluxations (around 75%) and cannot be used to reliably identify unstable or subtle lesions.

Further evaluation, with cross-sectional imaging such as computed tomography (CT) (Figure 15.2.4) or magnetic resonance imaging, should be considered under the guidance of specialists and to aid in surgical planning. Of these modalities, CT is the most sensitive and specific for diagnosing vertebral fractures and luxation.

1. **What is the patient's prognosis for recovery?**
2. **What treatment options could be considered both medically and surgically?**

PROGNOSTICATION

Initial grading of the severity of neurologic injury at the time of presentation, more specifically the presence or absence of nociception, is the most important clinical feature affecting prognosis (Table 15.2.1). For patients who present following a traumatic vertebral fracture or luxation that also lack nociception, the prognosis for recovery of voluntary motor function is grave,

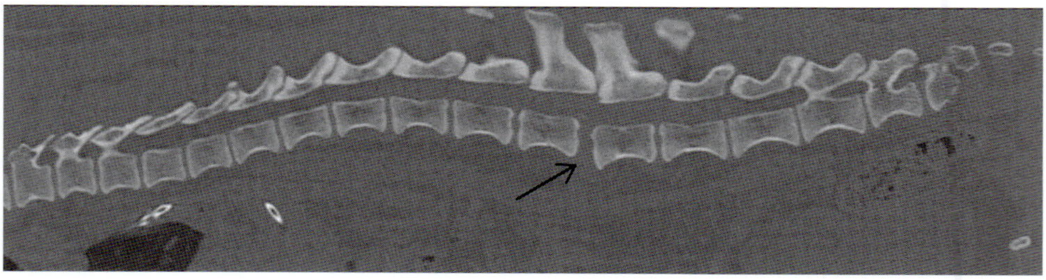

FIGURE 15.2.4 Sagittal computed tomography of the thoracolumbar vertebral column (patient has eight lumbar vertebrae) demonstrating a mild subluxation, marked widening, and a mild step defect centered at the L3–L4 intervertebral disc space (arrow).

Table 15.2.1 Negative prognostic indicators for patients with traumatic spinal fracture and luxation.

• Lack of nociception (especially for longer than 48 hours)
• Spinal cord intumescences are affected (C6–T2 and L4–S3)
• More than two vertebrae are affected
• Older or large/giant breeds
• Concurrent historical disease or injury

reported as anywhere between 0% and 10% of cases. Of note, within some of those recovered cases, patients did not return to normal neurologic function and instead regained coordinated reflex walking patterns known as spinal walking.

Other prognostic indicators, extrapolated from causes of spinal cord injury such as intervertebral disc herniation and fibrocartilaginous embolism due to the limited literature discussing exact outcomes for vertebral fractures and luxation, include the duration of the injury, neurolocalization, lesion extent, and concurrent diseases.

For this patient, her non-ambulatory paraparetic status in the face of an acute injury with a T3–L3 localization predicts a fair to good prognosis for return to function.

MEDICAL AND SURGICAL TREATMENT OPTIONS

Determining if conservative (medical) management or surgical intervention should be pursued for a traumatic vertebral fracture or luxation is dependent upon the degree of suspected spinal cord compression and vertebral column instability.

For patients with minimal neurologic deficits, pain that responds to medical management, and little instability, conservative therapy is appropriate. This consists of strict confinement for 4–6 weeks with provision of adequate analgesia and anxiolytics as needed. Should a patient deteriorate or have refractory pain, reassessment should be regularly performed throughout this management; surgical intervention may need to be reconsidered.

Decompression and stabilization of vertebral column trauma is recommended for unstable and compressive injuries (i.e. those associated with hematoma formation, traumatic disc herniations, or displaced bone fragments). These factors may be best evaluated with the pursuit of a CT to also allow for concurrent surgical implant planning. In cervical, thoracolumbar, and lumbosacral injuries, fixation with a combination of a laminectomy and placement of monocortical or bicortical screws within antibiotic-impregnated polymethylmethacrylate (PMMA) is most common (Figure 15.2.5). Other techniques, such as external skeletal fixation, plates, or 3D-printed patient-specific implants, are also used. Prompt decompression improves outcomes and is associated with improved survival rates; however, it is essential to remember that surgery should be pursued once a patient has been hemodynamically stabilized, so that the reduction in blood pressure often associated with anesthesia does not increase the risk of worsening neural injury. Aside from risks of anesthesia, the primary complications associated with pursuit of surgical fixation for spinal fractures and luxations include iatrogenic injury to neural tissue and vascular supply, implant-related complications (such as implant loosening or failure), and infection.

Regardless of the treatment pursued, adequate nursing and supportive care are essential and can be intensive. Recumbency care and cautious patient manipulation, skin monitoring, and provision of appropriate padding to prevent the development of decubital ulcers, urinary bladder management, and nutritional support are all essential facets of this nursing care.

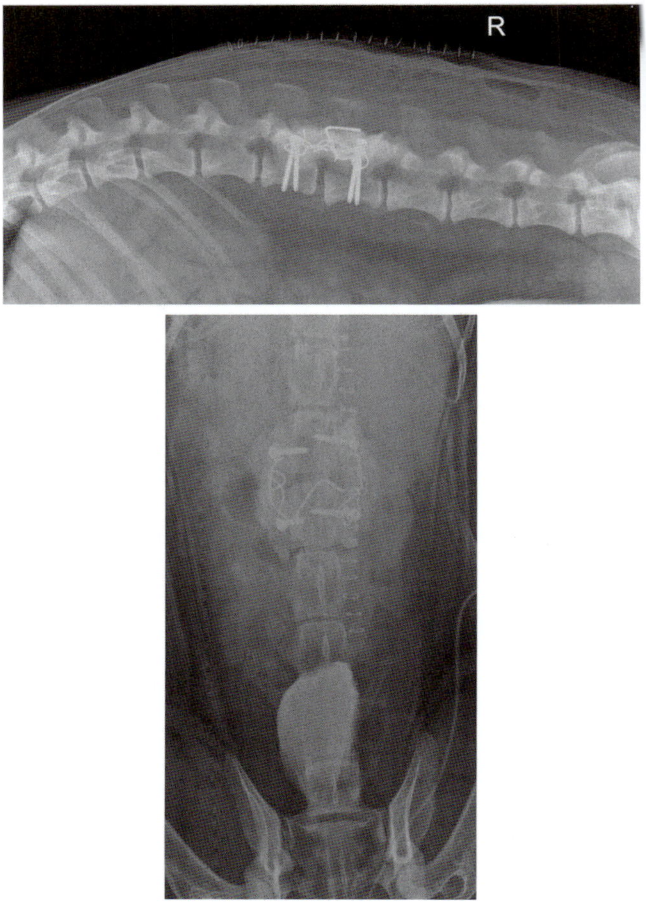

FIGURE 15.2.5 Immediate postoperative lateral and ventrodorsal radiograph of the thoracolumbar vertebral column (patient has eight lumbar vertebrae) demonstrating stabilization of the L3–L4 subluxation.

OUTCOME

Following surgical repair of the L3–L4 subluxation (Figure 15.2.5), the patient was strictly rested but began an immediate escalating regimen of rehabilitative therapy. Under two weeks into her recovery, she was acutely paraplegic and had retained sensation in both pelvic limbs and tail. She was re-evaluated and it was identified that her implants had failed. Her L3-4 subluxation repair was explanted and surgically revised. Following her second surgery, she again began an escalating regimen of rehabilitative therapy and within 4 weeks was ambulatory paraparetic and at an 8 week postoperative recheck was ambulatory with a mild paraparesis and proprioceptive ataxia. At that time, a gradual return to normal activity was resumed.

SUGGESTED READING

Bruce, C.W., Brisson, B.A., and Gyselinck, K. (2008). Spinal fracture and luxation in dogs and cats: a retrospective evaluation of 95 cases. *Vet. Comp. Orthop. Traumatol.* 21 (3): 280–284.

DiFazio, J. and Fletcher, D.F. (2013). Updates in the management of the small animal patient with neurologic trauma. *Vet. Clin. Small Anim.* 43: 915–940.

Ganie, F.A., Lone, H., Lone, G.N. et al. (2013). Lung contusion: a clinic-pathological entity with unpredictable outcome. *Bull. Emerg. Trauma* 1 (1): 7–16.

Grasmuek, S. and Steffen, F. (2004). Survival rates and outcomes in cats with thoracic and lumbar spinal cord injuries due to external trauma. *J. Small Anim. Pract.* 45 (6): 284–288.

Jeffery, N.D. (2010). Vertebral fracture and luxation in small animals. *Vet. Clin. North Am. Small Anim. Pract.* 40 (5): 809–828.

Orgonikova, I., Brocal, J., Bruto Cherubini, G., and Palus, V. (2021). Vertebral fractures and luxations in dogs and cats, part II: treatment and surgery options. *Companion Anim.* 26 (3): 15–19.

Orgonikova, I., Brocal, J., Bruto Cherubini, G., and Palus, V. (2021). Vertebral fractures and luxations in dogs and cats, part 1: evaluation of diagnosis and prognosis. *Companion Anim.* 26 (2): 1–10.

Penderis, J. (2008). Spinal cord injury in the dog; features of the neurological examination affecting prognosis. Presented at 33rd congress of world small animal veterinary association proceedings, Dublin, Ireland (20–24 August 2008).

Shores, A. (1992). Fractures and luxations of the vertebral column. *Vet. Clin. North Am. Small Anim. Pract.* 22 (1): 171–180.

Turner, W.D. (1987). Fractures and fracture-luxations of the lumbar spine: a retrospective study in the dog. *J. Am. Anim. Hosp. Assoc.* 23: 459–464.

Index

A

B

C

D

E

F

G

O

P

W

X

Z